POINT MUTATION

Edited by **Colin Logie**

Point Mutation
Edited by Colin Logie

Published by InTech
Janeza Trdine 9, 51000 Rijeka, Croatia

Publishing Process Manager Sandra Bakic

Technical Editor Teodora Smiljanic

Cover Designer InTech Design Team

Additional hard copies can be obtained from orders@intechopen.com

Point Mutation, Edited by Colin Logie
p. cm.
ISBN 978-953-51-0331-8

For EU product safety concerns:
IN TECH d.o.o., Prolaz Marije Krucifikse Kozulić 3, 51000 Rijeka, Croatia,
info@intechopen.com or visit our website at intechopen.com.

Meet the editor

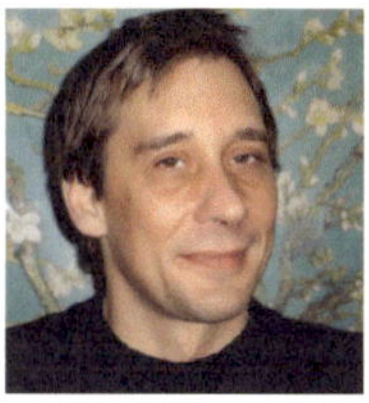

Dr. Colin Logie developed steroid-regulated site-specific DNA recombination for his PhD (1995) at EMBL, Heidelberg, Netherlands. Later on, he went on to engineer nucleosome remodeling assays at UMASS in Worcester in the late nineties and has since then been a group leader at the Nijmegen Centre for Molecular Life Sciences in the Netherlands, studying chromatin.

Contents

Preface

Point mutation is a vast subject that could not be captured in a set of fifteen vignettes. This book therefore reflects the interest of its authors, who are, for the most part, medically oriented scientists from all over the world, from Latin America to Russia and from Africa to Asia. A diverse array of research fields are broached, with an effort to bring the reader up to date with the knowledge amassed since the year 2000. After an introductory chapter on point mutation, current theory is expounded in two chapters on human point mutation. This is followed by five chapters on point mutation in viral genomes, going from adaptation of HIV to current therapies to antiviral vaccination and point mutation. Next, current trends in our knowledge of bacterial adaptation to quinolone antibiotics is described. This is followed by point mutagenesis in eukaryotic genomes, going from drug resistance in malaria to the nefarious effects of cigarette smoking. Finally, two contemporary synthetic point mutagenesis methodologies are described.

Colin Logie
Nijmegen Centre of Molecular Life Sciences,
Nijmegen,
The Netherlands

Part 1

Current Views on Point Mutation Theory

1

Point Mutations, Their Transition Rates and Involvements in Human and Animal Disorders

Viliam Šnábel
Parasitological Institute, Slovak Academy of Sciences, Košice, Slovakia

1. Introduction

Point mutation or single base substitution is the replacement of a single base nucleotide with another nucleotide of the genetic material. Point mutations can be divided into transitions, changes between the purines A and G, or changes between the pyrimidines C and T, and transversions, changes between purines and pyrimidines. A fundamental aspect of DNA point mutation is the observation that transitional nucleotide changes commonly occur with greater frequency than transversional changes. This bias is primarily due to the biochemical structure of the nucleotide bases and the similar chemical properties of complementary base pairing (Topal & Fresco, 1976). Estimates of the bias are important for understanding the mechanisms of nucleotide substitution, assessing mode and strength of natural selection, and the relative abundance of transitional and/or transversional mutations has important consequences in epidemiological research as each class is associated with different diseases (Wakeley, 1996; Martínez-Arias et al., 2001). This review addresses the issue to which extent transition bias is ubiquitous among living organisms and whether this is similar in different species, along with the screening of point mutations associated with diseases and disorders.

2. Point mutations and transitional bias

Within coding sequences, transitional changes are often synonymous whereas transversional changes are not. When both types of changes lead to a change in protein sequence, the transitional change is often less severe with respect to the chemical properties of the original and mutant amino acids (Zhang, 2000). In mammalian nuclear DNA, transition mutations appear to be approximately twice as frequent as transversions as is evident from the substitution patterns of mammalian pseudogenes (Gojobori et al., 1982), in synonymous and non-coding SNPs in humans (Cargill et al., 1999), and in SNPs in mice (Lindblad-Toh et al., 2000). On the other hand, transitions are about as common as transversions in synonymous and intron SNPs in *Drosophila* DNA (Moriyama and Powell, 1996). In contrast to the modest transition bias observed in mammalian nuclear DNA, transitions appear to be about 15 times as frequent as transversions in human mitochondrial (mt) DNA (Tamura & Nei, 1993). In a detailed analysis of mtDNA Belle et al. (2005)

investigated the transition bias by assessing polymorphism in the cytochrome *b* gene (*cyt-b*) in 70 species distributed amongst mammals, birds, reptiles, amphibians, and fish, considering a total of 1823 mutations. The authors found that the bias towards transitions is widespread and the ts / tv ratio was always greater or equal to 1, and it varied from an average ratio of 2.4 in amphibians to 7.8 in birds. This is in sharp contrast with plant mtDNA where a transversion bias has been recorded (Wolfe et al., 1987), suggesting that the mitochondrial genomes of plants and animals follow very different patterns of evolution. Data of Belle et al. (2005) indicated little evidence for variation within orders or genera and between closely related species such as the great apes. For these primates, an advantage was that complete mtDNA sequences for humans, chimpanzees, gorillas and orangutans are available. Though humans displayed the greatest ts / tv ratio among these species (humans 13.75, chimpanzees 11.00, orangutans 6.87, gorillas 5.67), there was no evidence of significant variation ($\chi^2 = 5.8$, $df = 3$, $p = 0.12$) between species, suggesting that the parameter has not changed much during the evolution of the great apes. Generally, the majority of the variation appeared to be at higher phylogenetic levels, between orders and classes. No evidence that the metabolic rate affects the ts / tv ratio was found in surveyed species.

Rosenberg et al. (2003) conducted a similarly designed analysis of 4,347 mammalian protein-coding genes from seven species (human, mouse, rat, cow, sheep, pig, macaque) as well as from the introns and multiple intergenic regions from human, chimpanzee and baboon primates. Estimates showed that genes and regions with widely varying base composition exhibit uniformity of transition mutation rate both within and among mammalian lineages, with no relationship to intrachromosomal or interchromosomal effects. This points to similarity in point mutation processes in genomic regions with substantially different GC-content biases. Knowledge of the mutational transition/transversion rate bias also allows a prediction of time to saturation of substitutions at fourfold-degenerate sites. From mutation parameters the above authors derived that transversions become more common than transition after 250 Myr, i.e. the time about which transitions become saturated (at ~25% of sites). Transversions become saturated much more slowly, beginning to reach 50% after about 750 Myr. In addition, the observed number of transitional substitutions accumulates approximately linearly for about 100 Myr, whereas the transversional substitutions accumulate linearly for about 250 Myr.

The accumulation of base substitutions not subject to natural selection is the neutral mutation rate. Most CpGs (regions of DNA where a cytosine nucleotide occurs next to a guanine nucleotide, separated by one phosphate) in mammals are uniquely hypermutable (e.g., Hwang & Green, 2004). The Cs of most CpGs are methylated (Ehrlich & Wang, 1981; Miranda & Jones, 2007), which enhances the deamination of C that produce in this case a T:G mismatch. The net result is that methyl-CpGs mutate at 10–50 times the rate of C in any other context (Sved & Bird, 1990), or of any other base (Hwang & Green 2004). Consequently, CpGs not under selection are replaced over time by TpG/CpAs. Mammals thus exhibit two dramatically different neutral mutation rates: the CpG mutation rate and the non-CpG rate. Walser et al. (2011) determined the neutral non-CpG mutation rate as a function of CpG content by comparing sequence divergence of thousands of pairs of neutrally evolving chimpanzee and human orthologs that differ primarily in CpG content. Both the mutation rate and the mutational spectrum (transition/transversion ratio) of non-CpG residues changed in parallel as sigmoidal function of CpG content. As different mechanisms generate transitions and transversions, these results indicate that both mutation rate and mutational processes are contingent on the local CpG content. Authors assessed that a threshold CpG content of ~0.53% must be attained before the non-CpG mutation rate is markedly affected, and the CpG effect reaches saturation at levels above ~0.63% CpG. Methyl-CpG may mediate the recruitment of various DNA- or histone-binding proteins and other factors (Cedar & Bergman, 2009), which could conceivably affect the susceptibility of the DNA to mutation. In this case the correlation between non-CpG mutations and CpG content would mean that chromatin states promoted by CpG methylation, or that result in it, render DNA more susceptible to mutation than DNA not in such states. There is some evidence that the mutation rate of compact heterochromatin (closed, inactive formation of chromosome) is higher than euchromatin (opened, transcribed chromosome portion) (Prendergast et al., 2007).

In attempting to quantify the context dependence of nucleotide substitution rates, Zhang et al. (2007) generated sequence data in baboon, chimpanzee and human by the NISC Comparative Sequencing Program. The study confirmed that C→T substitutions are enhanced at CpG sites compared with other transitions, and are relatively independent of the identity of the preceding nucleotide. While, as expected, transitions in general occurred more frequently than transversions, the most frequent transversions involved the C at CpG sites, with their rate comparable to the rate of transitions at non-CpG sites. A four-class model of the rates of context-dependent evolution in primate DNA sequences, CpG transitions > non-CpG transitions ≈ CpG transversions > non-CpG transversions, was consequently inferred from the observed mutation spectrum.

To relate establishment of mitochondrial mutations to environmental stress, Khrapko et al. (1997) investigated whether point mutations accumulated during a human lifetime were different from those that arise in human cell cultures in the absence of added xenobiotic chemicals. They found that human organs such as colon, lung, muscle and their derived tumors share nearly all mitochondrial hotspot point mutations that indicate that they are primarily spontaneous in nature and arise either from DNA replication error or reactions of DNA with endogenous metabolites. The hypothesis that environmental mutagens are important contributors to mitochondrial point mutagenesis thus no longer seems tenable. Assessments of the types of point mutations observed as polymorphisms have shown that both G→A and A→G transitions occur more frequently than transversions that was consistent with previous observations in human mtDNA (Aquadro & Greenberg, 1983; Horai & Hayasaka, 1990). In TK6 cells (human lymphoblast cells with normal P53 function) and in human tissues the mitochondrial point mutation rate appeared to be more than two orders of magnitude higher than the nuclear point mutation rate.

2.1 Mitochondrial and nuclear DNA mutations related to disorders

Although much smaller than the nuclear genome, mitochondrial DNA is equally important as it has been hypothesized to play a crucial role in ageing and carcinogenesis. This is mainly due to the fact that mitochondria represent the major site for the generation of cellular oxidative stress and play a key role in mediating programmed cell death (Birch-Machin, 2006). The first primary pathological mutations in mtDNA were discovered over 20 years ago (Holt et al., 1988; Wallace et al., 1988), and since then more than 100 mutations of mtDNA have been linked to human disease. The vast majority of these mutations fall into two classes: point mutations and large-scale rearrangements. The latter can be partial deletions (D) or duplications involving 1–10 kb of DNA (Holt et al., 2010). Nevertheless, the rearranged mtDNA invariably coexists with wild type molecules, a situation termed heteroplasmy, which is also frequently (Saada et al., 2001), but not universally (Van Goethem et al., 2001) found among pathological point mutations of mtDNA. Cellular dysfunction usually occurs when the ratio of mutated to wild-type mtDNA exceeds a threshold level (Birch-Machin, 2000). Mitochondrial DNA is wholly dependent on the nucleus for its maintenance and replication, and so mutations in nuclear DNA can also produce defects in mtDNA, or mtDNA loss (Zeviani et al., 1989; Moraes et al., 1991).

Incomplete oxygen reduction within the mitochondrial respiratory chain can lead to the formation of the superoxide radical, the first molecule in the pathway responsible for the production of reactive oxygen species (ROS), often inducing DNA strand breaks (Kang & Hamasaki, 2003). Growing evidence suggests that cancer cells exhibit increased intrinsic ROS stress, due in part to oncogenic stimulation, increased metabolic activity and mitochondrial malfunction (e.g., Pelicano et al., 2004; Sedelnikova et al., 2010). As the mitochondrial respiratory chain is a major source of ROS generation and the exposed mtDNA molecule is in close proximity to the source of ROS, the vulnerability of the mtDNA to ROS-mediated damage appears to be a mechanism to amplify ROS-stressing cancer cells. Coupled with this phenomenon is free-radical theory of Harman (2001) who attributed ageing in a wide range of species by postulating that the production of intracellular ROS is the major determinant of life span. Intracellular ROS are primarily generated by the mitochondrial respiratory chain and thus constitute a prime target for oxidative damage. According to this theory, mtDNA mutations caused by ROS accumulate within the cell, leading to impaired respiratory chain proteins, thereby generating more ROS, which in turn causes higher mtDNA mutation rates. Although there are data supporting a direct functional role of mtDNA in ageing and photoageing (Trifunovic et al., 2004; Birch-Machin & Swalwell, 2010), there is still considerable debate about the type of mtDNA associated with ageing. For example, the most frequently reported DNA region under assumption presents 4977-bp common deletion, but its significance is under debate (Thayer et al., 2003; Meissner et al., 2010). In addition, there are single somatic mtDNA control region mutations associated with ageing in tissues including skin, but their functional significance is still unclear (Liu et al., 1998; Wallace, 2005). This process of chronological ageing can be accelerated in skin by chronic exposure to ultraviolet radiation, which has been shown to be associated with a further increase in mtDNA damage. Mitochondria have further been implicated in the carcinogenic process because of their role in apoptosis and other aspects of tumour biology, alongside ROS generation (Jakupciak et al., 2005). In many types of human malignancy such as colorectal, liver, breast, pancreatic, lung, prostate, bladder and skin cancer somatic mtDNA mutations have been detected (Durham et al., 2003; Dasgupta et al., 2008; Fry et al., 2008; Yin et al., 2010; Choi et al., 2011; Namslauer et al., 2011; Potenza et al., 2011). Furthermore, sequence variations of mtDNA have been observed in preneoplastic lesions, which suggest generation of mutations early in tumour progression (Parr et al., 2006).

Human cells lacking mtDNA, so-called ρ^0 (rho zero) cells, can be repopulated with mitochondria derived from healthy subjects or patients with suspected mtDNA defects, to produce cytoplasmic hybrids, or cybrids. If the respiratory capacity of the cybrid cell is impaired then the deficiency can be ascribed to the mitochondrial, as opposed to the nuclear, genome (Chomyn et al., 1991). The cybrid cell culture system has enabled the discovery of the biased segregation of human mtDNA variants (Hayashi et al., 1991). Zastawny et al. (1998) compared oxidative base damage levels in mitochondrial and nuclear DNA of endogenous pig liver cells using gas chromatography. Higher levels (4.4 to 42.4 times) of five measured bases were found in mtDNA in relation to nuclear DNA. The higher rate of oxidatively modified bases may be due to the large amount of ROS produced in mitochondria, the absence of bound histones in mtDNA, and deficiency of DNA repair enzymes in some restoring routes.

Defects in oxidative phosphorylation (OXPHOS) are genetically unique because the key components involved in this process, respiratory chain enzyme complexes I, III, IV, V, are encoded by both nuclear and mitochondrial genes. Therefore, Rubio-Gozalbo et al. (2000) examined whether there are clinical differences in patients suffering from OXPHOS defects caused by nuclear or mtDNA mutations. 16 families with >=2 two siblings bearing a genetically established OXPHOS deficiency were studied, in four families due to a nuclear gene mutation and twelve due to a mtDNA mutation. Differences in age at onset, severity of clinical course, outcome, and intrafamilial variability in patients affected by an OXPHOS defect due to nuclear or mtDNA mutations were observed. Patients with nuclear mutations became symptomatic at a young age, and had a severe clinical course. Patients with mtDNA mutations showed a wider clinical spectrum of age at onset and severity. Reported differences are of importance regarding the choice of type of genome in further studies of affected patients.

2.2 Point mutations in pathogens

The challenge to identify point mutations accounting for resistance against antiparasitic drugs has been often addressed in veterinary pharmacology. For drug resistance in *Plasmodium*, causative organisms of malaria, a multitude of tests have been available and used for detecting parasites resistant to multiple drugs over the past 15 years (Hunt, 2011). Although the mechanisms by which malaria parasites develop resistance to drugs are unclear, current knowledge suggests that a main mechanism of resistance is the alteration of target enzymes by point mutation. Mutations in dihydrofolate reductase (dhfr) and dihydropteorate synthatase (dhps) cause anti-folate resistance in human malaria parasites against drugs sulphadoxine and pyrimethamin with synergystic anti-malarial effect (Prajapati et al., 2011). A constant monitoring is necessary to keep information about newly emerging drug resistance in *Plasmodium*, e.g. due to *ATP6* gene variants implicated in artemisin resistance (Menegon et al., 2008), and to detect new gene variants associated with resistance to older drugs, e.g. *cyt-B* gene variants in atovoquone resistance (Sutherland et al., 2008).

The principal mechanism of resistance to benzimidazoles is likely to involve changes in the primary structure of beta-tubulins, the building blocks of microtubules (Lacey, 1988). Specifically, point mutations in the beta-tubulin isotype 1 gene leading to amino acid substitutions in codons 167, 198, and 200 are widely thought to be associated with resistance in nematodes and DNA-based assays have been developed to monitor single nucleotide polymorphisms (SNP) (Silvester & Humbert, 2000; Von Samson-Himmelstjerna et al., 2009). These SNPs offer a means to detect the presence of resistance within populations and to monitor the development of resistance. As research progresses, however; it has become clear that other genes may be implicated in benzimidazole resistance and further aspects of anthelmintic resistance/susceptibility (Blackhall et al., 2008). Pan et al. (2011) identified heat-shock protein 60 (HSP 60) as one of the most frequently expressed biomolecules after albendazole treatment of patients that could be connected with beta-tubulin gene isoform 2 which exhibits a conserved point mutation indicative of benzimidazole resistance in tapeworm *Echinococcus granulosus*.

Detection of point mutations has been beneficial in allowing consistent differentiation of closely related parasitic organisms. By examining the ITS1 region Zhu et al. (1999) established six fixed nucleotide differences between sibling species of *Ascaris suum* (pig nematode) and *A. lumbricoides* (human nematode) that are impossible to distinguish by mitochondrial genes due to existence of different lineages before host affiliations (Levkut et al., 1999; Dubinský et al., 2000; Criscione et al., 2007). The *rrnS* mitochondrial gene was found to be a useful genetic marker for related genotypes G1 (sheep strain) and G3 (buffalo strain) of *Echinococcus granulosus* complex, revealing a total nucleotide uniformity within genotypes and two point mutations (166T→G, 205A→G) between these variants (Busi et al., 2007; Šnábel et al., 2009).

3. Conclusion

DNA base substitutions (mutations) are the most frequent class of genetic variants. Determining the factors that affect the base mutation rate remains a major concern of geneticists and molecular evolutionists. In mammalian nuclear DNA, transition mutations appear to be approximately twice as frequent as transversions. In human mitochondrial (mt) DNA transitions appear to be as much as about 15 times more frequent than transversions. In evaluating 70 species of mammals, birds, reptiles, amphibians, and fish, the ts / tv ratio varied from average of 2.4 in amphibians to 7.8 in birds in mtDNA. This contrasts with plant mtDNA with recorded transversion bias, suggesting that the mitochondrial genomes of plants and animals follow very different patterns of evolution. In mammalian protein-coding genes, it was estimated that transversions become more common than transition after 250 Myr, i.e. the time about which transitions become saturated (at ~25% of sites). Transversions become saturated much more slowly, beginning to reach 50% after about 750 Myr. The observed number of transitional substitutions accumulates approximately linearly for about 100 Myr, whereas the transversional substitutions accumulate linearly for about 250 Myr. Most CpG sites, particularly those in transposable elements, are preferred sites of C methylation. Therefore, the correlation between CpG content and non-CpG mutations could be due to an effect of methyl-CpG per se, to its spontaneous deamination to produce a T:G mismatch and subsequent recruitment of error-prone DNA repair mechanisms, or both. According to the present knowledge, more than 100 mutations of mtDNA have been proved to be linked to human disease. The majority of these mutations are point mutations and large-scale rearrangements (partial deletions or duplications involving 1–10 Kb of DNA). Mitochondria are implicated in the carcinogenic process because of their role in apoptosis and other aspects of tumour biology, and because of generating ROS (reactive oxygen species), presented as major determinant of life span. Intracellular ROS are primarily generated by the mitochondrial respiratory chain and thus constitute a prime target for oxidative damage. Many types of human malignancy such as colorectal, liver, breast, pancreatic, lung, prostate, bladder and skin cancer harbor somatic mtDNA mutations. Mitochondrial DNA is wholly dependent on the nucleus for its maintenance and replication, and so mutations in nuclear DNA can also produce defects in mtDNA, or mtDNA loss.

4. Acknowledgement

The study was supported by the Slovak Grant Agency VEGA (contract No. 2/0213/10).

5. References

Aquadro, C. F. & Greenberg, B. D. Human mitochondrial DNA variation and evolution: analysis of nucleotide sequences from seven individuals. Genetics, Vol. 103, No. 2, (Feb 1983), pp. 287-312, ISSN 0016-6731

Belle, E. M. S.; Piganeau, G.; Gardner, M. & Eyre-Walker, A. An investigation of the variation in the transition bias among various animal mitochondrial DNA. Gene, Vol. 355, (Aug 2005), pp. 58-66, ISSN 0378-1119

Birch-Machin, M. A. Mitochondria and skin disease Clinical and Experimnental Dermatology, Vol. 25, No. 2, (Mar 2000), pp. 141-146, ISSN 0307-6938

Birch-Machin, M. A. The role of mitochondria in ageing and carcinogenesis. Clinical and Experimental Dermatology, Vol. 31, No. 4, (Jul 2006), pp. 548-552, ISSN 0307-6938

Birch-Machin, M. A. & Swalwell, H. How mitochondria record the effects of UV exposure and oxidative stress using human skin as a model tissue. Mutagenesis, Vol. 25, (Mar 2010), No. 2, pp. 101-107, ISSN 0267-8357

Blackhall, W. J.; Prichard, R. K. & Beech, R. N. P-glycoprotein selection in strains of *Haemonchus contortus* resistant to benzimidazoles. Veterinary Parasitology, Vol. 152, No. 1-2 (Mar 2008), pp. 101–107, ISSN 0304-4017

Busi, M.; Šnábel, V.; Varcasia, A.; Garippa, G.; Perrone, V.; De Liberato, C. & D´Amelio, S. Genetic variation within and between G1 and G3 genotypes of *Echinococcus granulosus* in Italy revealed by multilocus DNA sequencing. *Veterinary Parasitology*, Vol. 150, No. 1-2, (Nov 2007), pp. 75-83, ISSN 0304-4017

Cargill, M.; Altshuler, D.; Ireland, J.; Sklar, P.; Ardlie, K.; Patil, N.; Shaw, N.; Lane, C. R.; Lim, E. P.; Kalyanaraman, N.; Nemesh, J.; Ziaugra, L.; Friedland, L.; Rolfe, A.; Warrington, J.; Lipshutz, R.; Daley, G. Q. & Lander, E. S. Characterization of single-nucleotide polymorphisms in coding regions of human genes. Nature Genetics, Vol. 23, No. 3, (Nov 1999), pp. 373-373, ISSN 1061-4036

Cedar, H. & Bergman, Y. Linking DNA methylation and histone modification: patterns and paradigms. Nature Review Genetics, Vol. 10, No. 5, (May 2009), pp. 295-304, ISSN 1471-0056

Choi, S. J.; Kim, S. H.; Kang, H. Y.; Lee, J.; Bhak, J. H.; Sohn, I.; Jung, S. H.; Choi, Y. S.; Kim, H. K.; Han, J.; Huh, N.; Lee, G.; Kim, B. C. & Kim, J. Mutational hotspots in the mitochondrial genome of lung cancer. Biochemical and Biophysical Research Communications, Vol. 407, No. 1, (Apr 2011), pp. 23-27, ISSN 0007-0920

Chomyn, A.; Meola, G; Bresolin, N.; Lai, S. T.; Scaralato, G. & Attardi, G. 0270-7306

Criscione, C. D.; Anderson J. D.; Sudimack, D.; Peng, W.; Jha, B.; Williams-Blangero, S. & Anderson, T. J. C. Disentangling hybridization and host colonization in parasitic roundworms of humans and pigs. Proceedings of the Royal Society B, Vol. 274, No. 1626, (Nov 2007), pp. 2669-2677.

Dasgupta, S.; Hoque, M. O.; Upadhyay, S. & Sidransky, D. Mitochondrial Cytochrome B gene mutation promotes tumor growth in bladder cancer. Cancer Research, Vol. 68, No. 3, (Feb 2008), pp. 700-706, ISSN 0008-5472

DiFrancesco, J. C.; Cooper, J. M.; Lam, A.; Hart, P. E.; Tremolizzo, L.; Ferrarese, C. & Schapira, A. H. MELAS mitochondrial DNA mutation A3243G reduces glutamate transport in cybrids cell lines. Experimental Neurology, Vol. 212, No. 1, (Jun 2008), pp. 152-156, ISSN 0014-4886 | View Record in Scopus | | Full Text via CrossRef

Dubinský, P.; Švický, E.; Kováč, G.; Lenhardt, L.; Krupicer, I.; Vasilková, Z.; Dvorožňáková, E.; Levkut, M.; Papajová, I. & Moncol, D. J. Pathogenesis of *Ascaris suum* in repeated infection of lambs. Acta Veterinaria Brno, Vol. 69, No. 3 (Sep 2000), pp. 201-207, ISSN 0001-7213

Durham, S. E.; Krishnan, K. J.; Betts, J. & Birch-Machin, M. A. Mitochondrial DNA damage in non-melanoma skin cancer. British Journal of Cancer, Vol. 88, No. 1, (Jan 2003), pp. 90-95, ISSN 0007-0920

Ehrlich, M. & Wang R. Y. 5-Methylcytosine in eukaryotic DNA. Science 212, No. 4501, (Jun 1981), pp. 1350–1357, ISSN 0036-8075

Fry, L. C.; Monkemuller, K. & Malfertheiner, P. Molecular markers of pancreatic cancer: development and clinical relevance. Langenbecks Archives of Surgery, Vol. 393, No. 6, (Nov 2008), pp. 883-890, ISSN 1435-2443

Gojobori, T.; Li, W. H. & Graur, D. Patterns of nucleotide substitution in pseudogenes and functional genes. Journal of Molecular Evolution, Vol. 18, No. 5 (Mar 1982), pp. 360–369, ISSN 0022-2844

Harman, D. Aging: overview. Annals of the New York Academy of Sciences, Vol. 928 (Mar 2001), pp. 1–21, ISBN 1-57331-285-1

Hayashi, J. I.; Ohta, S.; Kikuchi, A.; Takemitsu, M.; Goto, Y. & Nonaka, I. Introduction of disease-related mitochondrial DNA deletions into HeLa cells lacking mitochondrial DNA results in mitochondrial dysfunction. Proceedings of the National Academy of Sciences of the United States of America, Vol. 88, No. 23 (Dec 1991), pp. 10614-10618, ISSN 0027-8424

Holt, I. J. Zen and the art of mitochondrial DNA maintenance. Trends in Genetics, Vol. 26, No. 3, (Mar 2010), pp. 103-109, ISSN 0168-9525

Holt, I. J.; Harding, A. E. & Morganhughes, J. A. Deletions of muscle mitochondrial DNA in patients with mitochondrial myopathies. Nature, Vol. 331, No. 6158, (Feb 1988), pp. 717–719, ISSN 0028-0836

Horai, S. & Hayasaka, K. Intraspecific nucleotide-sequence differences in the major noncoding region of human mitochondrial-DNA. American Journal of Human Genetics, Vol. 46, No. 4, (Apr 1990), pp. 828-842, ISSN 0002-9297

Hunt, P. W. Molecular diagnosis of infections and resistance in veterinary and human parasites. Veterinary Parasitology, Vol. 180, No. 1-2, Special Issue SI, (Aug 2011), pp. 12-46, ISSN 0304-4017

Hwang, D. G. & Green, P. Bayesian Markov chain Monte Carlo sequence analysis reveals varying neutral substitution patterns in mammalian evolution. Proceedings of the National Academy of Sciences of the United States of America, Vol. 101, No. 39, (Sep 2004), pp. 13994-14001, ISSN 0027-8424

Jakupciak, J. P.; Wang, W.; Markowitz, M. E.; Ally, D.; Coble; M.; Srivastava, S.; Maitra, A.; Barker, P. E.; Sidransky, D. & O'Connell, C. D. Mitochondrial DNA as a cancer biomarker. Journal of Molecular Diagnostics, Vol. 7, No. 2, (May 2005), pp. 258-267, ISSN 1525-1578

Kang, D. & Hamasaki, N. Mitochondrial oxidative stress and mitochondrial DNA. Clinical Chemistry and Laboratory Medicine, vol. 4, no. 10, (Mar 2003), pp. 1281-1288, ISSN 1434-6621

Khrapko, K.; Coller, H. A.; Andre, P. C.; Li, X. C.; Hanekamp, J. S. & Thilly, W. G. Mitochondrial mutational spectra in human cells and tissues. Proceedings of the National Academy of Sciences of the United States of America, Vol. 94, No. 25, (Dec 1997), pp. 13798-13803, ISSN 0027-8424

Lacey, E. The role of the cytoskeletal protein, tubulin, in the mode of action and mechanism of drug resistance to benzimidazoles. International Journal for Parasitology, Vol. 18, No. 7 (Nov 1988), pp. 885–936, ISSN 0020-7519

Levkut, M.; Revajová, V.; Dvorožňáková, E.; Reiterová, K.; Dubinský, P.; Krupicer, I. & Moncol, D. J. Effect of *Ascaris suum* reinfection on immunoreactivity in lambs. Helminthologia, Vol. 36, No. 2, (Jun 1999), pp. 69-74, ISSN 0440-6605

Lindblad-Toh, K.; Winchester, E.; Daly, M. J.; Wang, D. G.; Hirschhorn, J. N.; Laviolette, J. P.; Ardlie, K.; Reich, D. E.; Robinson, E.; Sklar, P.; Shah, N.; Thomas, D.; Fan, J. B.; Gingeras, T.; Warrington, J.; Patil, N.; Hudson, T. J. & Lander, E. S. Large-scale discovery and genotyping of single-nucleotide polymorphisms in the mouse. . Nature Genetics, Vol 24, No. 4, (Apr 2000), pp 381-386, ISSN 1061-4036

Liu, V. W. S.; Zhang, C. F.; Pang, C. Y.; Lee, H. C.; Lu, C. Y.; Wei, Y. H. & Nagley, P. Independent occurrence of somatic mutations in mitochondrial DNA of human skin from subjects of various ages. Human Mutation, Vol. 11, No. 3, (Mar 1998), pp. 191-196, ISSN 1059-7794

Martínez-Arias, R.; Mateu, E.; Bertranpetit, J. & Calafell, F. Profiles of accepted mutation: From neutrality in a pseudogene to disease-causing mutation on its homologous gene. Human Genetics, Vol 109, No. 1, (Jul. 2001), pp. 7-10, ISSN 0340-6717

Meissner, C. & Ritz-Timme, S. Molecular pathology and age estimation. Forensic Science International Vol. 203, No. 1-3, (Dec 2010), pp. 34-43, ISSN 0379-0738

Menegon, M.; Sannella, A. R.; Majori, G. & Severini, C. Detection of novel point mutations in the *Plasmodium falciparum* ATPase6 candidate gene for resistance to artemisinins. Parasitology International, Vol. 57, No. 2, (Jun 2008), pp. 233-235, ISSN 1383-5769

Miranda, T. B. & Jones, P. A. DNA methylation: The nuts and bolts of repression. Journal of Cellular Physiology Vol. 213, No. 2, (Nov 2007), pp. 384-390, ISSN 0021-9541

Moraes, C. T.; Shanske, S.; Tritschler, H. J.; Aprille, J. R.; Andreetta, F.; Bonilla, E.; Schon, E. A. & DiMauro, S. mtDNA depletion with variable tissue expression: a novel genetic abnormality in mitochondrial diseases. American Journal of Human Genetics, Vol. 48, No. 3 (Mar 1991), pp. 492–501, ISSN 0002-9297

Moriyama, E. N. & Powell, J. R. Intraspecific nuclear DNA variation in *Drosophila*. Molecular Biology and Evolutoion, Vol. 13, No. 1, (Jan 1996), pp. 261–277, ISSN 0737-4038

Namslauer, I.; Dietz, M. S. & Brzezinski, P. Functional effects of mutations in cytochrome *c* oxidase related to prostate cancer. Biochimica et Biophysica Acta-Bioenergetics, Vol. 1807, No. 10, Special Issue SI, (Oct 2011), pp. 1336-1341, ISSN 0005-2728

Pan, D.; Das, S.; Bera, A. K.; Bandyopadhyay, S.; Bandyopadhyay, S.; De, S.; Rana, T.; Das, S. K.; Suryanaryana, V. V.; Deb, J. & Bhattacharya, D. Molecular and biochemical mining of heat-shock and 14-3-3 proteins in drug-induced protoscolices of *Echinococcus granulosus* and the detection of a candidate gene for anthelmintic resistance. Journal of Helminthology, Vol. 85, No. 2, (Jun 2011), pp. 196-203, ISSN 0022-149X

Parr, R. L.; Dakubo, G. D.; Thayer, R. E.; McKenney, K. & Birch-Machin, M. A. Mitochondrial DNA as a potential tool for early cancer detection. Human Genomics, Vol. 2, No. 4, (Jan 2006), pp. 252-257, ISSN 1479-7364

Pelicano, H.; Carney, D. & Huang, P. ROS stress in cancer cells and therapeutic implications. Drug Resistance Updates, Vol. 2004, No. 7, (Apr 2004), pp. 97–110, ISSN 1368-7646

Potenza, L.; Calcabrini, C.; De Bellis, R.; Guescini, M.; Mancini, U.; Cucchiarini, L.; Nappo, G.; Alloni, R.; Coppola, R.; Dugo, L. & Dacha, M. Effects of reactive oxygen species on mitochondrial content and integrity of human anastomotic colorectal dehiscence: A preliminary DNA study. Canadian Jouirnal of Gastroenterology, Vol. 25, No. 8, (Aug 2011), pp. 433-439, ISSN 0835-7900

Prajapati, S. K.; Joshi, H.; Dev, V. & Dua, V. K. Molecular epidemiology of *Plasmodium vivax* anti-folate resistance in India. Malaraia Journal, Vol. 10, (Apr 2011), pp. 102-102, ISSN 1475-2875

Prendergast, J. G. D.; Campbell, H.; Gilbert, N.; Dunlop, M. G.; Bickmore, W. A. & Semple, C. A. M. Chromatin structure and evolution in the human genome. BMC Evolutionary Biology, Vol. 7, (May 2007), pp. 72-72, ISSN 1471-2148

Rubio-Gozalbo, M. E.; Dijkman, K. P.; van den Heuvel, L. P.; Sengers, R. C.; Wendel, U. & Smeitink, J. A. Clinical differences in patients with mitochondriocytopathies due to nuclear versus mitochondrial DNA mutations. Human Mutation, Vol. 15, No. 6, (Apr 2000), pp. 522-32, ISSN 1059-7794

Rosenberg, M. S.; Subramanian, S. & Kumar, S. Patterns of transitional mutation biases within and among mammalian genomes. Mol. Biol. Evol., Vol. 20, No. 6, (Jun 2003), pp. 988–993, ISSN 0737-4038

Saada, A.; Shaag, A.; Mandel, H.; Nevo, Y.; Eriksson, S. & Elpeleg, O. Mutant mitochondrial thymidine kinase in mitochondrial DNA depletion myopathy. Nature Genetics, Vol. 29, No. 3, (Nov 2001), pp. 342-344, ISSN 1061-4036

Sedelnikova, O. A.; Redon, C. E.; Dickey, J. S.; Nakamura, A. J.; Georgakilas, A. G. & Bonner, W. M. Role of oxidatively induced DNA lesions in human pathogenesis. Mutation Research-Reviews in Mutation Research, Vol. 704, No. 1-3, Special Issue: SI, (Apr-Jun 2010), pp. 152-159, ISSN 1383-5742

Silvestre, A. & Humbert, H. F. A molecular tool for species identification and benzimidazole resistance diagnosis in larval communities of small ruminant parasites. Experimental Parasitology, Vol. 95, No. 4, (Aug 2000), pp. 271–276, ISSN 0014-4894

Šnábel, V.; Altintas, N.; D'Amelio, S.; Nakao, M.; Romig, T.; Yolasigmaz, A.; Gunes, K.; Turk, M.; Busi, M.; Hüttner, M.; Ševcová, D.; Ito, A.; Altintas, N. & Dubinský, P. Cystic echinococcosis in Turkey: genetic variability and first record of the pig strain (G7) in the country. In Parasitology Research, vol. 105, no. 1, (Jul 2009), pp. 145-154, ISSN 0932-0113

Sutherland, C. J.; Laundy, M.; Price, N.; Burke, M.; Fivelman, Q. L.; Pasvol, G.; Klein, J. L. & Chiodini, P. L. Mutations in the *Plasmodium falciparum* cytochrome b gene are associated with delayed parasite recrudescence in malaria patients treated with atovaquone-proguanil. Malaria Journal, Vol. 7, Article Number 240, (Nov 2008), ISSN 1475-2875

Sved, J. & Bird A. The expected equilibrium of the CpG dinucleotide in vertebrate genomes under a mutation model. Proceedings of the National Academy of Sciences of the United States of Americ, Vol. 87, No. 12, (Jun 1990) pp. 4692-4696, ISSN 0027-8424

Tamura, K. & Nei, M, Estimation of the number of nucleotide substitutions in the control region of mitochondrial DNA in humans and chimpanzees. Molecular Biology and Evolution, No. 10, (May 1993), pp. 512–526, ISSN 0737-4038

Topal, M. D. & Fresco, J. R. Base pairing and fidelity of in codon-anticodon interaction. Nature, Vol. 263, No. 5575, (May 1976), pp. 289-293, ISSN 0028-0836

Trifunovic, A.; Wredenberg, A.; Falkenberg, M.; Spelbrink, J. N.; Rovio, A. T.; Bruder, C. E.; Bohlooly-Y, M.; Gidlof, S.; Oldfors, A.; Wibom, R.; Tornell, J.; Jacobs, H. T. & Larsson, N. G. Premature ageing in mice expressing defective mitochondrial DNA polymerase. Nature, Vol. 429, No. 6990, (May 2004), pp. 417-423, ISSN 0028-0836

Thayer, R.; Wittock, R.; Parr, R.; Zullo, S. & Birch-Machin, M. A. A maternal line study investigating the 4977-bp mitochondrial DNA deletion. Experimental Gerontology, Vol. 38, No. 5, (May 2003), pp. 567-571, ISSN 0531-5565

Van Goethem, G.; Dermaut, B.; Lofgren, A.; Martin, J. J. & Van Broeckhoven, C. Mutation of POLG is associated with progressive external ophthalmoplegia characterized by mtDNA deletions. Nature Genetics, Vol. 28, No. 3, (Jul 2001), pp. 211-212, ISSN 1061-4036

Von Samson-Himmelstjerna, G.; Walsh, T. K.; Donnan, A. A.; Carriere, S.; Jackson, F.; Skuce, P. J.; Rohn, K. & Wolstenholme, A. J. Molecular detection of benzimidazole resistance in *Haemonchus contortus* using real-time PCR and pyrosequencing. Parasitology, Vol. 136, No. 3, (Mar. 2009), pp. 349–58, ISSN 0031-1820

Wakeley, J. The excess of transitions among nucleotide substitutions: new methods of estimating transition bias underscore its significance. Trends in Ecology & Evolution 11 (Apr 1996), pp. 158-163, ISSN 0169-5347

Wallace, D. C.; Singh, G.; Lott, M. T.; Hodge, J. A.; Schurr, T. G.; Lezza, A. M. S.; Elsas, L. J. & Ninkoskelainen, E. K. Mitochondrial DNA mutation associated with Leber's hereditary optic neuropathy. Science, Vol. 242, No. 4884, (Dec 1988), pp. 1427-1430, ISSN 0036-8075

Wallace, D. C. A mitochondrial paradigm of metabolic and degenerative diseases, aging, and cancer: a dawn for evolutionary medicine. Annual Review of Genetics, Vol. 39, (May 2005), pp. 359–407, ISSN 0066-4197

Walser, J. C.; Furano, A. V. The mutational spectrum of non-CpG DNA varies with CpG content. Genome Research, Vol. 20, No. 7, (Jul 2010), pp. 875-882, ISSN 1088-9051

Wolfe, K. H.; Li, W. H. & Sharp, P. M. Rates of nucleotide substitution vary greatly among plant mitochondrial, chloroplast, and nuclear DNAs. Proceedings of the National Academy of Sciences of the United States of America, Vol. 84, No. 24, (Dec 1987), pp. 9054–9058, ISSN 0027-8424

Yin, P. H.; Wu, C. C.; Lin, J. C.; Chi, C. W.; Wei, Y. H. & Lee, H. C. Somatic mutations of mitochondrial genome in hepatocellular carcinoma. Mitochondrion, Vol. 10, No. 2, (Mar 2010), pp. 174-182, ISSN 1567-7249

Zastawny, T. H.; Dabrowska, M.; Jaskolski, T.; Klimarczyk, M.; Kulinski, L.; Koszela, A.; Szczesniewicz, M.; Sliwinska, M.; Witkowski, P. & Olinski, R. Comparison of oxidative base damage in mitochondrial and nuclear DNA. Free Radical Biology and Medicine, Vol. 24, No. 5, (Mar 1998), pp. 722-725, ISSN 0891-5849

Zeviani, M.; Servidei, S.; Gellera, C.; Bertini, E.; DiMauro, S. & Didonato, S. An autosomal dominant disorder with multiple deletions of mitochondrial DNA starting at the D-loop region. Nature, Vol. 339, No. 6222, (May 1989), pp. 309–311, ISSN 0028-0836

Zhang, J. Rates of conservative and radical nonsynonymous nucleotide substitutions in mammalian nuclear genes. Journal of Molecular Evolution, Vol. 50, No. 1, (Jan 2000), pp. 56-68, ISSN 0022-2844

Zhang, W.; Bouffard, G. G.; Wallace, S. S. & Bond, J. P. Estimation of DNA sequence context-dependent mutation rates using primate genomic sequences. Journal of Molecular Evolution, Vol. 65, No. 3, (Sep 2007), pp. 207-214, ISSN 0022-2844

Zhu, X.; Chilton, N. B.; Jacobs, D. E.; Boes, J. & Gasser, R. B. Characterisation of *Ascaris* from human and pig hosts by nuclear ribosomal DNA sequences. International Journal for Parasitology, Vol. 29, No. 3, (Mar 1999), pp. 469-478, ISSN 0020-7519

2

Bioinformatical Analysis of Point Mutations in Human Genome

Branko Borštnik and Danilo Pumpernik
National Institute of Chemistry Ljubljana, Slovenia

1. Introduction

1.1 The bioinformatical resources

The carrier of biological information is a DNA molecule that is packed in the cell nucleus. In the case of human species the genome consists of roughly three billion of base pairs that are packed into the chromosomes 1 through 22, and two sex chromosomes *x* and *y*. The genomic data acquisition witnessed a strong push in recent years. Ever more versatile sequencing technologies enable the sequencing laboratories to maintain a high throughput regime of work. Genomic data are freely available at several locations such as the National Center for Biotechnology Information (http://www.ncbi.nlm.nih.gov) and European Molecular Biology Laboratory

(http://www.ebi.ac.uk/embl/) web sites. Also the aligned genomic sequences are available (Kuhn et al. 2009). The first draft of human genome was published in 2001 (Lander et al. 2001). A few years later Mikkelsen et al. (2005) produced the chimpanzee genome. Soon followed the rhesus genome (Gibbs et al. 2007) and also a great part of genomic sequences of orangutan and gorilla are available today.

The processes on the molecular level that are responsible for passing the genetic information between subsequent generations are prone to errors, causing the temporal modification of the genetic 'text'. In the primate branch of the phylogeny the error rate is approximately one point mutation per generation (Kumar and Subramanian 2002). Some changes eventually spread among a large part of the population, and the others die out. This happens within the period of approximately one million years (Myr) that is called the coalescence time. The differences between the human individuals that exist due to the mutations that did not yet reach their final destiny (i.e. extinction or spread over the entire population) represent the genetic polymorphism of a species. The richest amount of polymorphic data is available in the case of human species. We shall be only concerned with the so called single nucleotide polymorphism (*snp*). The word "single" in the *snp* phrase is to some extent misleading because the *snp* databases also contain entries with variations in the genetic text in the form of several consecutive variations of the nucleotide sequence of an individual with respect to the master sequence. The *snp* databases encompass more than 10 million entries (http://www.ncbi.nlm.nih.gov/snp). The problem is in validation of the *snp* data. Various levels of validation are possible, but only a limited number of *snps* fulfill the most stringent validation criteria.

The split times of the human species with chimpanzee, orangutan, gorilla and rhesus macaque are in the range of 6 to 25 Myrs. Multiple sequence alignments reveal an order of magnitude of tens of millions of point mutations. This represents a decent basis for statistical evaluation of the evolutionary models. The human - chimpanzee sequence comparison (Mikkelsen et al. 2005) provides the most important set of data because their common ancestor lived 5 to 7 Myrs ago. Each nucleotide difference that is detected when comparing these two species is in the greatest extent the result of a single event. However, the double alignment does not uncover the directionality of the mutations (Jiang and Zhao 2006). In order to assess more complete information about the mutational processes one needs to align at least three genomic sequences. This means that one needs to go deeper in the evolutionary history by adding to the human - chimpanzee pair additional primate species, as mentioned above. Going deeper in the evolutionary history cannot be at no cost. The differences that are inferred from the multiple alignments do not need to represent the genuine replacements but a result of a combination of the events that might have taken place at the same DNA site. This is likely to occur at the hypermutable sites such as CpG dinucleotides (Fryxell and Moon 2005, Fryxell and Zuckerkandl 2000, Jabbari and Bernardi 2004, Ollila et al. 1996).

1.2 Nucleotide replacements

The single nucleotide replacement events can be categorized in several ways. There are 12 possible replacements - two pairs of transitions (A<=>G, C<=>T) and four pairs of transversions (A<=>C, A<=>T, G<=>C, G<=>T). The replacements are context dependent. On a coarse grained scale the contextual categories can be identified in terms of the DNA functionalities: transcribed and non-transcribed regions, regulatory regions and the remaining sequences. The regions are subjected to variable functional constraints and the mutational spectra would differ for various regions. One can also define the context on micro scale in terms of the flanking nucleotides (Siepel and Haussler 2004; Fryxell and Moon 2005; Zhao and Zhang 2006). One can choose only one nucleotide as the context defining element: the left or the right neighbor of the mutated site. In such a case the mutated site plus the nucleotide defining the context is a dinucleotide entity (Gentles and Karlin 2001). There are 16 distinct dinucleotides and the replacement counts and the replacement probabilities can be represented by 16x16 matrices. Two kinds of matrices will be the subject of our interest. The **A** matrices will represent the replacement counts and the **W** matrices will represent the replacement probabilities. The other possibility is that the context is defined in terms of right and left neighbor. In this case the above mentioned matrices are of rank 64. However, one does not need to deal with all 64x64=4096 matrix elements. If the 12 above mentioned transitions and transversions are inserted within 16 possible left/right nucleotides defining the context one obtains altogether 192 replacement types that need to be examined in terms of their frequencies of appearance and their probabilities.

The counts can be extracted from the genomic alignments and single nucleotide polymorphism data. In order to unravel the evidence regarding the compositional changes one should gain access to the directionality of the replacements, meaning that when two different nucleotides are found in two genomes at a certain site one should be able to tell, which is the ancestral and which is the newly replaced nucleotide. The identity of the ancestral sequence elements can be determined by the analyses of multiple sequence alignments. The majority principle is usually applied. This means that the nucleotide that is found most frequently at a certain site is supposed to be the ancestral one. In the case of multiple events taking place at a single site the majority principle does not lead to proper results, which can be corrected by computer simulation.

We shall adhere to the convention that the A_{ij} element represents the number of j to i replacements. On the basis of the **A** matrix one can define the replacement probability matrix **W** following the simple philosophy that the number of replacement events is equal to the number of the sites multiplied by the replacement probability

$$A_{ij} = W_{ij} N f_j . \tag{1}$$

$N=\Sigma_i \Sigma_j A_{ij}$ denotes the total number of dinucleotides and f_j are the elements of the dinucleotide composition vector ($f_j = \Sigma_i A_{ij} / N$). The **W** matrix has the property that each column sums to unity:

$\Sigma_i W_{ij} = 1$.

1.3 Mutations produced by the replication slippage

A rather potent mechanism of DNA modification is the modification of the length of short tandem repeats or microsatellites (Cox and Mirkin 1997, Borštnik and Pumpernik 2002, 2005, Borštnik et al. 2008). The human genome contains approximately 2% of sequences having the form of short tandem repeats of nucleotides, dinucleotides, trinucleotides and so forth. In the DNA replication process the repetitive parts of DNA sequences are likely to be incorrectly reproduced. The repeats can become elongated or shortened. This is because the two complementary DNA strands retain the complementarity also in the case when one or the other strand slips forward or backward for an integer number of repeat units. In a series of subsequent cell divisions a tandem repeat can thus lead to a substantial elongation or, in the other extreme, may even lead to the disappearance of the repeat. The high mutability of repeats makes them usable in genotyping purposes. Microsatellite markers exhibit mutation rates that exceed the average mutation rates by two orders of magnitude. In this work we shall put under scrutiny whether the nucleotide replacement process and the replication slippage mechanism produce comparable densities of mutational changes.

1.4 The distribution of mutations along the chromosomes

Since stochasticity is an essential component of the mutational processes one can expect that the locations of the mutated sites will be randomly distributed along the DNA sequence. According to our opinion it is worth to study in detail the spatial distribution of the mutated sites. We shall be concerned with three types of point mutations: nucleotide replacements produced by the genomic and *snp* mutations and replication slippage events. There are several possible realizations of mutation density studies. One can look for the differences between genomic and *snp* nucleotide replacements and replication slippage mutations. Further, one can compare the mutation densities occurring in the human genome to those occurring within the genomes of other primate species. This can be done if one can trace the directionality of the mutations. By aligning several primate species one can first determine the ancestral state of the sequence and then one can identify the species that was subjected to the mutation.

1.5 The neutrality hypothesis

It is not easy to explain the Darwinian principle of the survival of the fittest in terms of the changes taking place at the DNA level. The idea that the mutations can be divided into two classes – the ones giving a positive contribution to fitness, and the others reducing the fitness of the organisms is an oversimplification. Kimura (1968) has shown that the majority of changes at the molecular level are neutral and do not affect fitness. Stochasticity is the main characteristic of molecular evolution. The changes are generated at random times and random positions along the chromosomes. The driving force of the mutations is the non-ideality of the DNA replication apparatus. If the selective coefficient belonging to the change that the mutation produces is small enough, the mutated variants would eventually spread among the population since there is no impact upon the functioning of the organisms. Studies of the patterns of neutral mutations can offer an insight into the cellular machinery that is responsible for DNA replication.

1.6 Scope of the work

In what follows we present new results on the mutational propensities in the human lineage. In the next section the results obtained by a simple four parameter model of nucleotide replacements will show that the mutational changes are amenable to statistical predictions. In the next section the model is expanded to a multi-parameter form and it is shown that the agreement between the model and the results of the alignment of natural sequences become very close. The mutational analyses are then expanded in two respects. The comparison between the processes leading to the diversity and divergence is performed on the ground of the nucleotide replacements. Further, two competing mutational mechanisms are compared: the nucleotide replacements and the replication slippage mechanism. The question is also addressed how to search the genetic basis of human phenotypical characteristics.

2. Results

2.1 Nucleotide replacements

Let us first present the results obtained by a simple four parameter model of nucleotide replacements. The model is defined as follows. A nucleotide sequence with the 60:40 A+T:C+G composition is subjected to a process of one-nucleotide replacement at random positions in such a way that transitions are four times more probable than transversions. The CpG dinucleotides are taken to be five times less frequent and two times more mutable than the average dinucleotides. A computer simulation procedure was set up. An artificial sequence was randomly subjected to the nucleotide replacements. After enough replacements have been accumulated to reproduce the human/chimpanzee split the counts were performed on the level of trinucleotides and the results were compared with the results of the human - chimpanzee genomic alignments. The results are presented in Fig. 1, where the logarithm of human/chimpanzee replacement counts are plotted along the horizontal axis and the model values along the vertical axis. The points are scattered along the *y*=*x* line. The four groups of points belong to Δn=0,1,2,3 substitutions per trinucleotide. Each group is dispersed and divided into several subgroups. The Δn=0 group located at the upper right corner of the figure represents the degree of reproduction of the genome composition in terms of trinucleotides. It shows that a two parameter (the C+G:A+T ratio and the degree of CpG depletion) model reproduces reasonably the DNA composition in terms of trinucleotides. The points in the form of full circles are divided into two subgroups on the basis of CpG content. The eight trinucleotides in the form XCG and CGX are separated from the remaining trinucleotides due to their strong depletion. The other three groups (Δn=1,2,3) are further partitioned on the basis of transition/transversion differences and CpG supermutability. The positions of Δn=3 points in the form of empty triangles are systematically deflected below the *y*=*x* line which means that the multiple replacements at the neighboring sites are not as independently occurring as a model of independent mononucleotide events would predict.

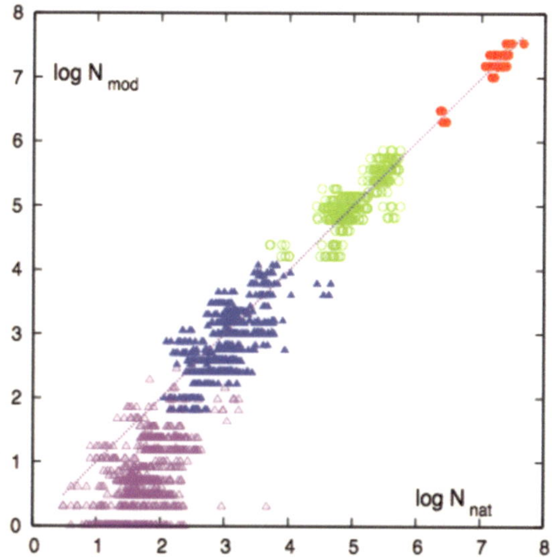

Fig. 1. The comparison between the human - chimpanzee replacement counts based on a simple four parameter model (vertical direction - N_{mod}) and the results based upon the human - chimpanzee genomic alignment (horizontal direction - N_{nat}) in trinucleotides. The four symbols (full circle, empty circle, full triangle, empty triangle) refer to Dn=0, 1, 2 ,3 replacements within a trinucleotide frame.

2.2 Multi-parameter dinucleotide replacement model

In general one can construct a multi-parameter nucleotide replacement model. Hwang and Green (2004) presented the most elaborate model by dividing the genomic sequences in several classes according to their functional role. The context was taken into account with left and right neighbor and the replacement probabilities for all possible pairs of trinucleotides were optimized in order to match the results of multiple genomic alignments. Only those trinucleotide pairs were taken into account where the left and right nucleotides are identical while the middle one is being replaced. Also several other authors (Arndt and Hwa (2005), Baele et al. (2008), Duret and Arndt (2008), Lunter and Hein (2004), Borštnik and Pumpernik (to be published)) were trying to infer the replacement probabilities. It turns out that the results are pretty elusive. There are several circumstances that render the parameterization of the mutational process difficult. It is hard to attain the statistical significance. A particular class of mutational changes can easily be defined in such a way that, when it is sampled within the appropriate database becomes too narrow to guarantee a satisfactory statistics. In this work we would like to present an approach with the classification of the mutational changes that does not follow the standard practice in order to gain a profit in the form of the reduction of statistical fluctuations. We are halving the number of the nucleotides defining the context and perform the analyses in the space of dinucleotides. In this case the number of unknown replacement probability parameters is reduced to the number of the entities defining the context (4 in our case) multiplied with the number of distinct type of replacements (four transitions and 8 transversions, what makes 12 replacements), thus 48 unknowns. In order to further improve the statistics we have chosen the largest set of nucleotide sequences possible: the complete human genome aligned with the counterparts of chimpanzee, orangutan and rhesus genomic sequences. The number of nucleotides aligned was close to one billion.

The simulation procedure was performed in order to determine the elements of the replacement probability matrix and to retrieve the replacement count matrix that is free of superposition errors. This goal was achieved by simulating the replacement process on an artificial starting DNA sequence. The simulation was run along the dendrogram in the form of four branches. The branch representing the outgroup species (rhesus or orangutan) extends from the common root to the present. Its length is denoted by T_r or T_o , respectively. The human/chimpanzee common ancestor branch extends from the common root to the point of human/chimpanzee split and its length is denoted by T_{hp}. The replacements were generated using the random number generator uniformly on all the branches according to the probabilities defined by the mutation probability matrix **W**. The **W** matrix was expressed as

$$W_{ij}=a_{ij}\, A_{ij}/(Nk_j\, f_j) \tag{2}$$

where A_{ij} and f_j elements were taken from the results of the triple alignments and a_{ij} and k_j are the correction coefficients subjected to the optimization procedure. In a hypothetical ideal case when the **A** matrix would represent genuine replacement numbers free of superposition errors, all the a_{ij} and k_j coefficients would be equal to unity. In our case the a_{ij} and k_j coefficients were determined by the following procedure: After each simulation round the three artificial sequences were aligned and the resulting $\mathbf{A}^{(t)}$ matrix was compared with the corresponding $\mathbf{A}^{(t)}$ matrix obtained when aligning the natural sequences. The difference between the two matrices was minimized by optimizing the correction coefficients by a brute force Monte Carlo procedure. Random variations were performed and the variations not improving the matching of the two matrices were discarded. The variational procedure in such an enormous parameter space as it is spanned by the entire set of the correction coefficients is not easy to carry out. It is expected that the main source of the superposition events are the replacements caused by CG dinucleotide decay. Therefore the Monte Carlo procedure was conducted in such a way that the parameter subspace associated with the CG decay was given more attention than the remaining regions of the parameter space. The end result of the simulation procedure were the **W** matrix and the matrix $\mathbf{A}^{(d)}$ of direct counts of the dinucleotide replacements that was free of deformation due to multiple replacements taking place at the same site.

In Fig. 2 the pairs of $\mathbf{A}^{(t)}$ matrix elements are plotted in such a way that the i <= j replacement counts are used as the x coordinate and the j <= i value as the y coordinate. The two points belonging to the same i,j pair are positioned symmetrically with respect to the y=x line and the distance between them represents the measure of the asymmetry. The dinucleotides connected by the strand symmetry are positioned approximately at the same place. The data plotted in Fig. 2 were extracted from the human/chimpanzee/rhesus (*hpr*) alignment. We can see that the majority of the replacements exhibit an appreciable degree of asymmetry. When these data are compared to the human/chimpanee/orangutan (*hpo)* case it turns out that the asymmetry is independent of the choice of the triple alignment sources. Nearly all the pairs of points belonging to *hpr* and *hpo* coincide to a rather high extent. Only the points corresponding to the CG <=> CA/TG replacements are in disagreement. The

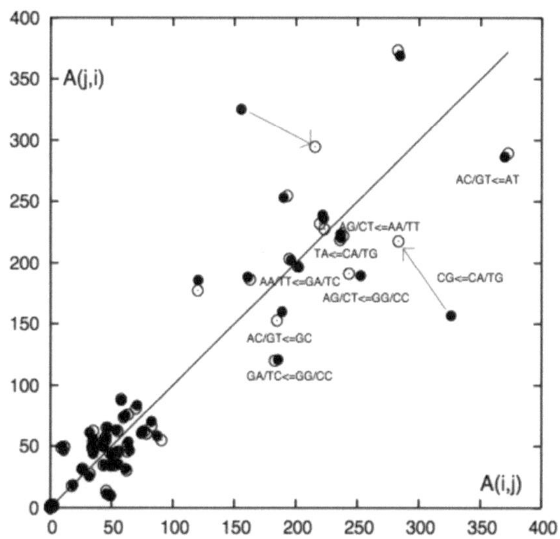

Fig. 2. The dinucleotide replacement counts presented in such a way that each pair of counts running in opposite directions is represented by a point in A_{ij}, A_{ji} plane. If the two counts are equal the corresponding replacement would be located along the y=x line. The distance from y=x line is a measure of the directionality asymmetry. The two replacement pairs connected by the strand symmetry is mapped as a pair of points mirroring across the y=x line. Bullets correspond to the replacement counts obtained from human/chimpanzee/rhesus triple alignments ($\mathbf{A}^{(t)}$) and circles to the direct replacement count ($\mathbf{A}^{(d)}$) generated in the simulation procedure. In nearly all the cases the bullets and circles coincide. A significant discrepancy takes place in the case of CG <=> CA/TG replacements where a pair of arrows indicate the extent of the superposition error inflicted upon the counts retrieved by the triple alignments. Only the replacements of the transition type below the y=x line are interpreted. The interpretation is also valid for the points that are mirrored across the y=x axis, provided that the arrows symbolizing the replacement directions are reversed. The units are arbitrary.

asymmetries of the CG <=> CA/TG replacements are larger in the case of *hpr* than in the case of *hpo*. Such a disagreement leads us to the idea that the CG <=> CA/TG replacement asymmetries are the artifact of the procedure by which they were detected. The process to be blamed is the superposition of multiple replacement events at a single site which was resolved by the simulation of the replacement process.

The optimal agreement between the natural and simulated $\mathbf{A}^{(t)}$ replacement count matrices was achieved with the branch length ratio $T_{hp}/T_r = 0.8$ and $T_{hp}/T_o = 0.53$. The majority of the resulting correction factors emerged from the optimization procedure within the interval 0.96 to 1.04. The following values emerged outside this interval $a_{ij}=1.3$; $a_{ji}=0.9$ and $k_j=1.35$ for j=CG; i=CA/TG. The final correlation coefficient between the two (natural and model) $\mathbf{A}^{(t)}$ matrices was equal to 0.9995 when simulating the *hpr* case. The two direct count matrices $\mathbf{A}^{(d)}$ belonging to the *hpr* and *hpo* case exhibit small differences. The extent of corrections that emerge from the simulation procedure is seen in Fig. 2. The two arrows mark the position of CG<=>CA/TG replacements in the A_{ij}/A_{ji} plane corresponding to the *hpr* case.

The dinucleotide replacement probabilities W_{ij} that resulted from the optimization procedure are presented in Fig. 3 in a similar way as the A_{ij} counts are presented in Fig. 2.

The location of the two points belonging to CG decay are located outside the margins of the figure and their position is indicated by the arrows. The probability of CG decay is for one order of magnitude above the average probability of the transition type replacements. The asymmetries of the dinucleotide replacements do not need to exhibit the same direction in the W_{ij} and A_{ij} cases because the factor f_i/f_j in the relation $W_{ij}/W_{ji} = (A_{ij}/A_{ji})(f_i/f_j)$ can reverse the directionality of the two pairs of i,j values.

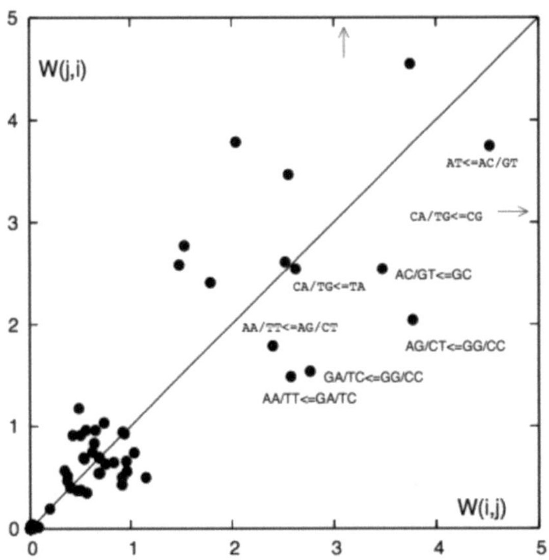

Fig. 3. The dinucleotide replacement probabilities W(i,j) presented in the same way as the A(i,j) counts in Fig. 2. Note that the italicized dinucleotide pairs exhibit the opposite directionalities in comparison with the A(i,j) values. The CA/TG<= CG replacement probabilities are located in the direction indicated by the two arrows at x=21 (horizontal arrow) and and y=21 (vertical arrow). The units are arbitrary.

The deviation from reciprocally equilibrated replacements between the dinucleotide pairs are statistically the most significant in the cases where the two dinucleotides differ at one place - and the difference is of the transition type. The dinucleotide pairs of this type can be grouped into three clusters (Figs. 4 and 5). The first cluster (Fig. 4) comprises the dinucleotides GG/CC that can be replaced by the dinucleotides GA/TC or AG/CT, which can be further replaced by AA/TT dinucleotides. The next two clusters (Fig. 5) comprise the four palindromic nucleotides of which AT and GC can be replaced by AC/GT, while TA and CG can be replaced by CA/TG dinucleotides. Also the asymmetries of the three clusters of the replacements are presented in Figs. 4 and 5. It is evident that the transition components of the fluxes are not equilibrated. In order to see whether the replacement process is running in a steady state or not, one should examine the **A** and **W** matrices in their entirety. Both $\mathbf{A}^{(d)}$ matrices, in the *hpr* and *hpo* case clearly show that in the case of AC/GT, TA and CA/TG dinucleotides are increasing their share in the replacement process, while CC/GG, AG/CT and AT are losing their share in dinucleotide population.

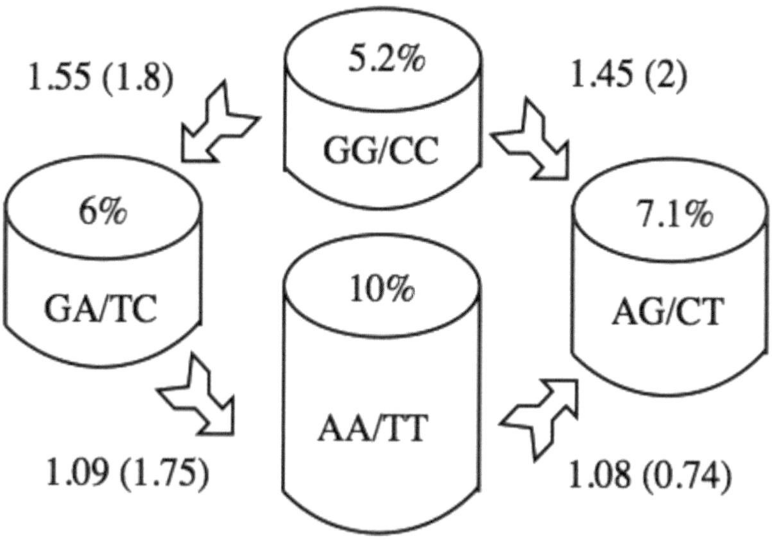

Fig. 4. The asymmetries of the GG/CC, GA/TC, AG/CT replacements. The height of the barrels is proportional to their composition (given in percents at the top). For each replacement the arrow shows the predominant directionality. The numbers beside the arrows give the asymmetry factor - the $A_{ij}^{(d)}/A_{ji}^{(d)}$ ratio. The numbers in parentheses give the corresponding Wij/Wji ratios.

2.3 The density of mutations: Diversity versus divergence comparison

The genetic diversification within the human population appears on the account of two mechanisms – both having essential stochastic component – point mutations and genetic recombination in the process of meiosis. The former process generates new varieties and the latter one generates new combinatorial realizations of the genetic differences. Nucleotide sequencing reveals the differences between the individuals and make them available for bioinformatical processing. Roughly 10^7 single nucleotide polymorphisms are known today what means one to ten polymorphic sites per thousand nucleotides.

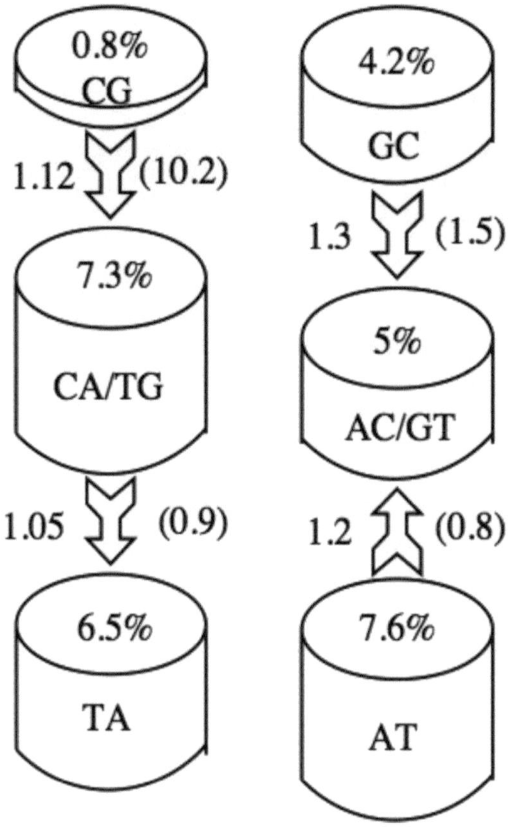

Fig. 5. The asymmetries of the GC, AC/GT, AT, CG, CA/TG and TA replacements. See also the caption of Fig. 4.

Also the differences between the master sequences of closely related diverging primate species exhibit a comparable densities of point mutations as the above mentioned intraspecies diversities. One can compare the two types of mutabilities in several ways. The standard approach is to compare the nucleotide replacement matrices. Our preliminary results (Borštnik and Pumpernik - in preparation) show that there exists a certain difference between the replacement matrices. In this work we focus our attention on the question as to how the two types of mutations are distributed along the chromosomes. In Figure 6 the distribution of genomic and *snp* mutations is presented for a typical segment located on the first chromosome. The density of mutations is proportional to the slope of the line on which lies the sequence of points representing the counts of nucleotide replacements. We can see that, roughly speaking, there exist chromosomal segments with diverse densities of mutations. This is valid for *snp* and for the genomic mutations. However, the densities of the two types of mutations do not necessarily fluctuate in phase. A more detailed information regarding the distribution of the replacement sites is presented in Figure 7. The two horizontal directions in the plot refer to the number of two types of the replacements per 1000 nucleotides. The direction marked with "gen" refers to the density of genomic mutations and the other horizontal coordinate corresponds to the density of the *snp* replacements. The values along the vertical direction represent the number of 1000 bp

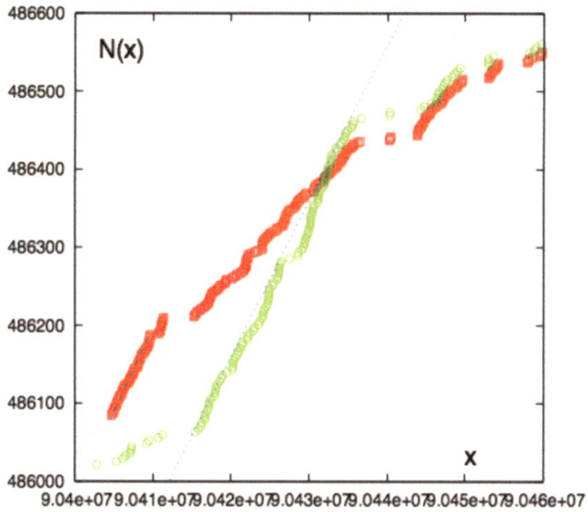

Fig. 6. The comparison of counts of genomic and *snp* type of nucleotide replacements. Horizontal variable x represents the coordinate (running nucleotide number (from 1 to 250 million)) along the first chromosome, N(x) is the cumulative number of human - chimpanzee nucleotide replacements within the interval [0-x] (red square symbols). Green circles represent the *snp* counts as a function of the chromosome coordinate. The *snp* counts are multiplied by a factor 3.827 in order that only one series of values suffice to be displayed along the vertical axis. The nucleotide replacement densities are proportional to the slope of N(x) plot. One can identify segments with well defined densities, that vary from segment to segment. The straight lines are plotted to guide the eye.

segments possessing the characteristics defined by the two horizontal coordinates. The distribution is close to what one would expect. The plot in two dimensions exhibits its highest values close to zero density and not at the average value that is located at higher values of the densities. The essential message of Fig. 7 is the following. In spite of the fact that the genomic and *snp* replacements exhibit strong fluctuations in mutation density and that the fluctuations are apparently out of phase, the two dimensional distribution of the two densities exhibits normal unskewed properties.

Besides the comparison of genomic and *snp* replacements we also performed the comparison between the nucleotide replacement type of point mutations and replication slippage type mutations. Short tandem repeats (*str*) with the monomer lengths 1 and 2 were first located within the human sequence. In the next step the human - chimpanzee *str* counterparts with unequal lengths were detected in the human/chimpanzee alignment. The result was a list of chromosomal coordinates of replication slippage type of mutations. This list can be compared with the list of genomic nucleotide replacement type mutations. The question can be posed again whether there is a noticeable correlation in the distribution of the mutations of various classes. In Figure 8 the mutation counts are plotted as a function of the chromosome coordinate. The densities of three kinds of mutations are presented: mutated *strs* with monomer lengths 1 and 2 and single nucleotide replacement mutations that were already presented in Fig. 6. We can see again that the densities of the three kinds of mutation do not oscillate in phase. The strongest fluctuations are present in the

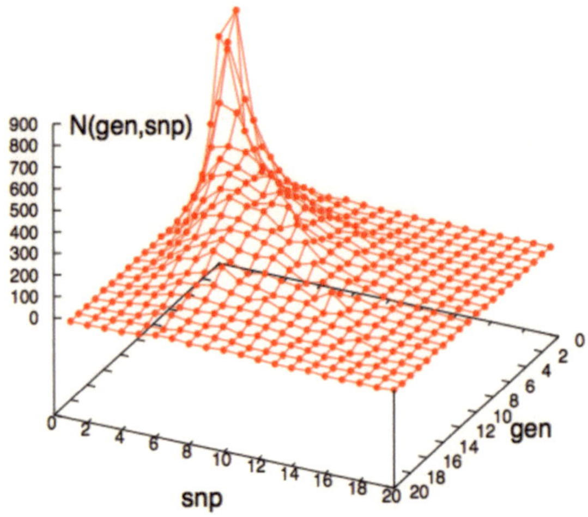

Fig. 7. A three dimensional plot of the genomic and *snp* type nucleotide replacement densities. The coordinates of the points in two horizontal directions have the following meaning: number of genomic replacements per 1000 nucleotides for the "gen" direction and number of *snp* nucleotide replacements per 3800 nucleotides for the "snp" direction. The heights of the points represent the number of segments having the densities specified by the two horizontal coordinates.

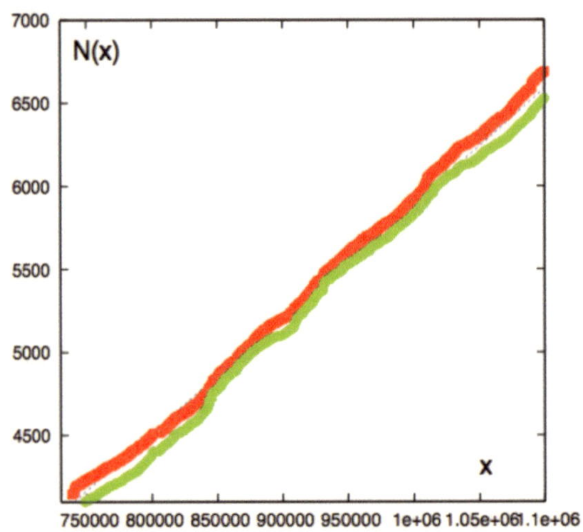

Fig. 8. Red squares, green circles and blue triangles (hidden behind the red squares) represent the counts of nucleotide replacements and repeat elongation/shortening of mononucleotide and dinucleotide repeats, respectively, as a function of the first chromosome coordinate x.

distribution of *strs* composed of dinucleotides. This is to be expected. There is a significant difference between the mononucleotide and dinucleotide repeats. Mononucleotide repeats of the type C_n or G_n are very rare. The majority of mononucleotide repeats are of the form A_n or T_n and more than one half of them have their origin in retroposed segments of retroposons with a polyadenyl tail. After these elements are retroposed they begin with their mutational dynamics. The dinucleotide repeats, on the other hand, are supposed to be the result of a pure replication slippage dynamics and therefore the densities of their mutations exhibit a different pattern than the mononucleotide repeats.

2.4 The density of mutations: Human versus non-human mutations

As the last case, let us present the analysis of the differences between the densities of the mutations that occurred in human lineage on one hand and the densities of the mutations that occurred in other primate species. We analyzed quadruple alignment of human, chimpanzee, orangutan and gorilla genomic sequences. Suppose that a site is populated by x,y,z,w nucleotides at their respective human, chimpanzee, orangutan and gorilla sequence. In the majority of cases all four nucleotides are identical, indicating that the site was not subject to mutation. The cases where the diversity of x,y,z,w goes beyond two unequal nucleotides are rare and were ignored. What remains are the cases where a site is populated by two nucleotides, say x and y. There are 6 realizations of (2x,2y) case and 4 realizations of (3x,y) case. We considered only the cases y,x,x,x and x,y,x,x. In the first case it is plausible to conclude that the mutation took part in human lineage and in the second case chimpanzee lineage can be supposed to be hit by the nucleotide replacement. In our earlier study (Borštnik and Pumpernik - in preparation) we produced the trinucleotide 64x64 replacement matrices for the cases where only the middle nucleotide is allowed to be replaced. Using the above mentioned criterion to determine the directionality of the replacement we have shown that no significant difference exists between the nucleotide 64x64 replacement matrices taking place in human lineage and chimpanzee lineage. Also the results based upon the study of sequential distribution of the nucleotide replacements shown in Fig. 9 corroborate the notion that on average there is no appreciable difference between the mutation densities in the two species. The most important information emerging from Fig. 9 can be extracted by comparing the mutation densities in human and chimpanzee species. To

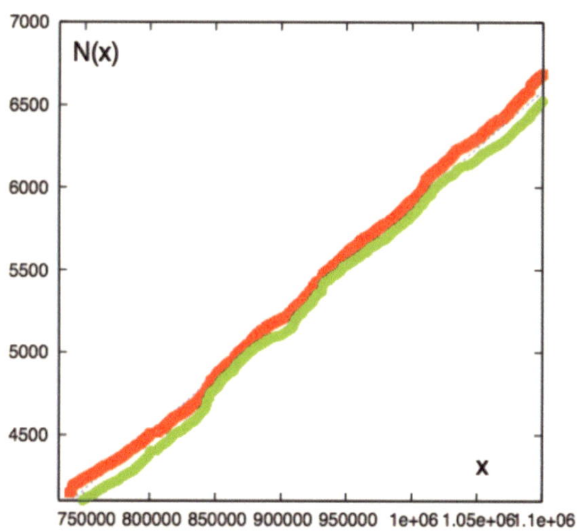

Fig. 9. Red squares and green circles represent the counts of nucleotide replacements taking place in human and chimpanzee species, respectively, as a function of the first chromosome coordinate x.

some extent the two densities go hand in hand, but the deviations of this rule are appreciable. This means that after the human - chimpanzee split the mutational process in each genome ran with comparable pace in orthologous regions. Obviously in the course of time species-specific mutation patterns came into the existence. Detecting and scrutinizing such regions can provide vital information about the human ascent.

3. Discussion

The purpose of this work is to contribute new findings in the field of the studies of point mutations in human lineage. This topics is of paramount importance because at the moment a greater part of questions concerning the correspondence between genotypic and phenotypic mutational changes remain unsolved. A conservative scenario as to how to figure out the meaning of the genomic differences should point towards the 22.000 primate genes and, of course towards their regulatory regions. The differences between the coding regions of the primate genes are known (Jordan et al. 2006, Goldstein and Pollock 2006), but the exact identity of the regulatory sequences is still missing (Tuch et al. 2008) and one does not know exactly what to search for in the genomic comparison between human and other primates. This means that the studies of the genomic differences between human and other great apes are welcome even if the studies are not directed to a specific gene product. One can follow the philosophy due to which one decides to accumulate and analyze mutational data on large scale. Doing this one should carefully evaluate the statistical errors. A simple guideline to estimate the uncertainties can be deduced from the theory of radioactive decay for which we know that if one measures N events the relative uncertainty of the quantities that are deduced from this measurement is 1/sqrt(N). This means that when counting, for instance, the number of replacements of a pair of dinucleotides or trinucleotides and finds N occurrences, the relative uncertainty of the corresponding replacement probability will be again 1/sqrt(N). In order to achieve 1% accuracy N should be of the order of magnitude of 10^4. When determining the dinucleotide mutation probability matrix the number of essential replacement classes is of the order of magnitude of 100. To accumulate 10^4 replacements per replacement class one needs to have at least 10^6 replacement events. Taking into account one percent difference between distinct primate sequences the body of aligned sequences should encompass a sequence length of at least 10^8 bp. Such an amount of aligned sequence material is rarely reported in the literature. Usually the analyses are performed on the samples containing a set of pseudogenes, introns or other sequence samples with low functional constraints (Zhang and Gerstein 2003). Our approach in the studies of dinucleotide replacement was based upon the premise that more than 95% of genetic sequences (Davydov et al. 2010) is subjected to low functional constraints and therefore we decided to align the entire set of genomic sequences.

To return to the question regarding the genetic basis of human phenotypic abilities let us discuss the results presented in Fig. 9. The general picture supports the notion that the two species are pretty equilibrated in the nucleotide replacement densities. The two replacement counts grow nearly at the same pace as a function of chromosome coordinate. However, it is possible to find the difference in details. There are regions where human replacements are more dense than the chimpanzee counterparts. Such regions are the candidates for coding the human specific traits. There is of course a long way to go to attain an in-depth view as to how the human specific traits are coded. One could combine the results of studies of nucleotide replacement densities with the studies of positive or accelerated evolution (Wagner 2007) of protein coding regions. Under normal circumstances the mutabilities of the protein coding regions is an oscillatory function with period 3 - what is the codon length. The third position in a codon is usually, due to the codon degeneracy, subjected to lower constraints than the other two positions and exhibits higher mutability. The replacements taking place at synonymous sites are neutral and the replacements at the nonsynonymous sites produce amino acid changes. It is not easy to detect the deviations of the expected mutational patterns that can indicate the presence of an accelerated evolution. One can envisage the following scenario: The candidates for the accelerated evolution can be sought within the regions where the human genome exhibit mutation densities that exceed the mutation densities of other primate species. Within these regions one would then look for the genetic changes that shaped the properties of human species.

4. Conclusions

The purpose of this work is to contribute new findings in the field of the studies of point mutations in the human genome. We show that the most appropriate approach is to analyze the results of multiple alignments of primate genomic sequences. Several methods are presented how to carry out the analyses. The construction of dinucleotide replacement probabilities provides us with the information about the details of the nucleotide replacements. The role of CpG dinucleotide is unveiled and it is shown how the hypermutability of CpG dinucleotide influences the influx and outflux of all the other dinucleotides. Another aspect of the mutational processes, which is put under scrutiny in this work, is the study of sequential distribution of point mutations. The properties of three types of mutations is compared: nucleotide replacements involved in diversity and divergence processes and replication slippage events. It is also shown how the density of nucleotide replacement events along the chromosome can unveil the sites where human - specific traits can be coded.

5. Acknowledgment

This work was financed by the Slovenian Research Agency.

6. References

Arndt, P F & Hwa T (2004) Regional and time-resolved mutation patterns of the human genome. *Bioinformatics* 20:1482-1485

Borštnik, B & Pumpernik D (2002) Tandem repeats in protein coding regions of primate genes. *Genome Res.* 12:909-915

Borštnik, B & Pumpernik D (2005) Evidence on DNA slippage step-length distribution. *Phys. Rev.* E71:031913;1-7

Borštnik, B; Oblak, B & Pumpernik, D (2008) Replication slippage versus point mutation rates in short tandem repeats of the human genome. *Mol. Genet. Genomics* 279:53-61

Cox, R & Mirkin, S M (1997) Characteristic enrichment of DNA repeats in different genomes. *Proc. Natl. Acad. Sci.* USA 94:5237-5242

Davydov, E; Goode, D; Sirota, M; Cooper, G; Sidow, A; et al. (2010) Identifying a high fraction of the human genome to be under selective constraint using GERP++. *PLoS Comput. Biol.* 6:e1001025 (13pages)

Fryxell, K J & Moon W-J (2005) CpG mutation rates in the human genome are highly dependent on local GC content. *Mol. Biol. Evol.* 22:650-658

Fryxell, K J & Zuckerkandl, E (2000) Cytosine deamination plays a primary role in the evolution of mammalian isochores. *Mol. Biol. Evol.* 17:1371-1383

Gentles, A J & Karlin, S (2001) Genome scale compositional comparisons in eukaryotes. *Genome Res.* 11:540-544

Gibbs, R A; Rogers, J; Katze, M G et al. (181 co-authors) (2007) Evolutionary and biomedical insights from the rhesus macaque genome. *Science* 316:222-234

Goldstein, R A & Pollock, D D (2006) Observations of amino acid gain and loss during protein evolution are explained by statistical bias. *Mol. Biol. Evol.* 23:1444-1449

Jabbari, K & Bernardi, G (2004) Cytosine methylation and CpG, TpG(CpA) and TpA frequencies. *Gene* 333:143-149

Jiang, C & Zhao, Z (2006) Directionality of point mutation and 5-methylcytosine deamination rates in the chimpanzee genome. *BMC Genomics* 7: 316 doi:10.1186/1471-2164-7-316

Jordan, I K; Kondrashov, F A; Adzhubel, I A; Wolf, Y I; Koonin, E V; Kondrashov, A S & Sunjaev S (2006) A universal trend of amino acid gain and loss in protein evolution. *Nature* 433:633-638

Kimura, M (1968) Evolutionary rate at the molecular level. *Nature* 217:624-626

Kuhn, R M; Karolchik, D; Zweig, A S; et al. (22 co-authors) (2009) The UCSC Genome Browser Database: update 2009. *Nucleic Acid Res.* 37:D755–D761

Kumar, S & Subramanian, S (2002) Mutation rates in mammalian genomes. *Proc. Natl. Acad. Sci. USA* 99:803-808

Lander, E S; Linton, L M; Birren, B; et al. (249 co-authors) (2001) Initial sequencing and analysis of the human genome. *Nature* 409:860-921

Michel, C J (2007) Evolution probabilities and phylogenetic distance of dinucleotides. *J. Theor. Biol.* 249:271-277

Mikkelsen, T S; Hillier, L W; Eichler, E E; et al. (67 co-authors) (2005) Initial sequence of the chimpanzee genome and comparison with the human genome. *Nature* 437:69-87

Ollila, J; Lappalainen, I & Vihinen, M (1996) Sequence specificity in CpG mutation hotspots. *FEBS Lett.* 396:119-122

Siepel, A & Haussler D (2004) Phylogenetic estimation of context-dependent substitution rates by maximum likelihood. *Mol. Biol. Evol.* 21:468-488

Tuch, B B; Li, H & Johnson A D (2008) Evolution of eucaryotic transcription circuits. *Science* 319:1797-1799

Wagner, A (2007) Rapid detection of positive selection in genes and genomes through variation clusters. *Genetics* 176:2451-2463

Yampolsky, L Y; Kondrashov, F A & Kondrashov, A S (2005) Distribution of the strength of selection against amino acid replacements in human proteins. *Hum.Mol. Genetics* 14:3191-3201

Zhao, Z & Zhang, F (2006) Sequence context analysis of 8.2 million single nucleotide polymorphisms in the human genome. *Gene* 366:316-324

Zhang, Z & Gerstein, M (2003) Patterns of nucleotide substitution, insertion and deletion in the human genome inferred from pseudogenes. *Nucleic Acid Res.* 31:5338-5348

3

Estimating Human Point Mutation Rates from Codon Substitution Rates

Kazuharu Misawa
*Research Program for Computational Science,
Research and Development Group for Next-Generation
Integrated Living Matter Simulation,
Fusion of Data and Analysis Research and
Development Team, Yokohama City, Kanagawa,
Japan*

1. Introduction

Estimation of point mutation rates is essential for studying molecular evolution and genetics. Point mutation rates are also important for developing tools for genome analyses, such as those used for homology searches (Altschul et al., 1990), sequence alignments (Katoh et al., 2002; Larkin et al., 2007), gene finding (Misawa and Kikuno, 2010), or detecting natural selection (Nei and Gojobori, 1986; Hughes and Nei, 1988; Yang, 2007; Yang and Nielsen, 2008), and for reconstructing phylogenetic trees (Felsenstein, 2004; Sullivan and Joyce, 2005). Patterns of mutations also affects the neutrality test for population genetics (Misawa and Tajima, 1997). According to the neutral theory (Kimura, 1968), new alleles may be produced at the same rate per individual as they are substituted in a population. On the basis of this theory, mutation rates were estimated from neutral substitution rates.

One of the causes of mutations is the error during DNA replication (Pray, 2008). Since cell division is tightly linked to DNA replication, mutation rates are expected to correlate the number of cell divisions so that they are higher in sperms than in egg (Haldane, 1956; Miyata et al., 1987). The phenomenon in which mutation rate are higher in males than in females is called 'male-driven evolution' (Miyata et al., 1987). The previous studies show large discrepancies with regard to the effect of male-driven evolution on mutation rates (Li et al., 2002). To investigate the effect of DNA replication on mutation rates, the effect of male male-driven evolution was also investigated in this study.

Recent studies on mutation rates in human non-coding regions have shown that mutation rates in the human genome are negatively correlated to local GC content (Fryxell and Moon, 2005; Taylor et al., 2006; Tyekucheva et al., 2008; Walser et al., 2008) and to the densities of functional elements (Hardison et al., 2003; Hellmann et al., 2005; Tyekucheva et al., 2008). Mutation rates have also been shown to correlate with the distance of a gene from the telomere (Hellmann et al., 2005; Tyekucheva et al., 2008). A study on mutation rates in human coding regions showed that mutation rates also depend on the chromosome sizes, and this is probably attributed to the distance between the genes and telomeres (Misawa, 2011).

Mutation rates are sometimes dependent of the local context, especially the adjacent nucleotides (Cooper and Youssoufian, 1988; Cooper and Krawczak, 1989; Hobolth et al., 2006; Misawa et al., 2008; Misawa and Kikuno, 2009; Misawa, 2011). CpG hypermutability is a major cause of codon substitution in mammalian genes (Huttley, 2004; Lunter and Hein, 2004; Misawa et al., 2008; Misawa and Kikuno, 2009). CpG hypermutation occurs approximately 10 times or more rapidly than other types of point mutations do (Scarano et al., 1967; Bird, 1980; Lunter and Hein, 2004). Figure 1 shows cytosine (C), methylcytosine (methyl-C), and thymine (T). The notation CpG is used to distinguish a C followed by a guanine (G) from a Watson-Crick pair of C and G. CpG dinucleotides are often methylated at C by DNA methyltransferase (DNMT) (Wu and Zhang, 2011), and methyl-C spontaneously undergoes deamination to generate T. The mutation pressure of CpG hypermutability is so high in organisms with DNMT, that they share a similar pattern of amino acid substitutions (Misawa et al., 2008). This pattern of amino acid substitutions used be called the 'universal' trend (Jordan et al., 2005). Misawa et al. (2008) also showed that organisms who lost DNMT, such as *Buchnera* and *Saccharomyces* do not share the 'universal' trend. In the mouse, the effect of CpG hypermutability on codon preference is stronger than that of tRNA abundance (Misawa and Kikuno, 2011). When mutation rates are estimated, the effect of adjacent nucleotides on mutation rates and the direction of mutation rates should be considered.

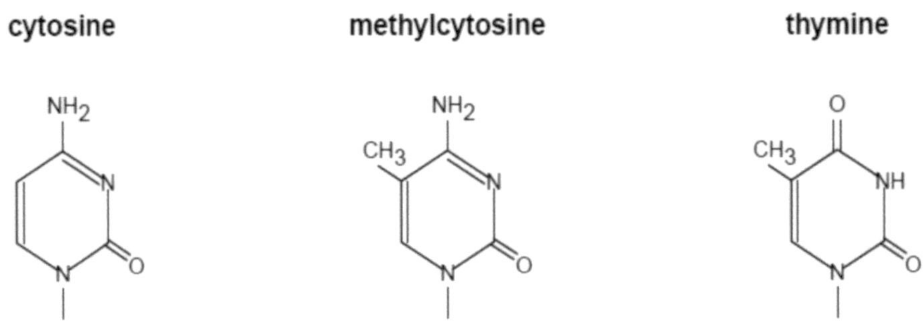

Fig. 1. Cytosine, methylcytosine, and thymine.

Some of previous studies used mutation models that do not consider the effect of adjacent nucleotides; these mutation models were the REV model (Tavare, 1986; Yang, 1994; Whelan et al., 2001) used by Hardison (Hardison et al., 2003), and the JC (Jukes and Cantor, 1969) and HKY models (Hasegawa et al., 1985) used by Tyekucheva (Tyekucheva et al., 2008). Tayler's (Taylor et al., 2006) study was based on two-species comparison, and therefore, the direction of mutation was unclear. Recently, I and my colleagues (Misawa and Kikuno, 2009; Misawa, 2011) estimated the mutation rates in humans by considering the effect of adjacent nucleotides on mutation rates and the direction of mutations. These studies, however, did not consider the effect of the distance of a gene from the telomere on mutation rates.

To understand the effect of DNA replication and the distance of a nucleotide site from the telomere, mutation rates were estimated using the codon substitution rates in the coding regions of thousands of human and chimpanzee genes by using autosomes and X chromosome; further, the ancestral gene sequences were inferred by assuming macaque genes as the outgroup in this study. Regression analyses were conducted to evaluate the effect of GC content, gene density, and CpG island density on the rates of CpG-to-TpG mutations, TpG-to-CpG mutations, and non-CpG transitions and transversions.

2. Methods

2.1 Data set

To estimate the rates of mutation rates, we used 10,372 orthologous gene trios obtained from human, chimpanzee, and macaque genomes (Gibbs et al., 2007). Table 1 shows the sizes of human chromosomes of the NCBI human genome (Build 36) taken from the UCSC genome browser (http://genome.ucsc.edu). Table 1 also shows number of genes on each chromosome used in this study. These genes were binned into a series of 10-Mb windows of human DNA depending on the positions of the midpoint of genes.

Chromosome	Chromosome Size (base pair)	No. of genes used	No. of fourfold sites used
1	247249719	1123	236111
2	242951149	708	158041
3	199501827	644	140972
4	191273063	442	96920
5	180857866	521	120438
6	170899992	623	120260
7	158821424	472	97566
8	146274826	359	70764
9	140273252	420	89507
10	135374737	431	88630
11	134452384	593	121652
12	132349534	567	119251
13	114142980	198	44238
14	106368585	360	78504
15	100338915	321	75640
16	88827254	435	96218
17	78774742	549	119793
18	76117153	192	39089
19	63811651	525	100125
20	62435964	319	62578
21	46944323	127	25595
22	49691432	199	41400
X	154913754	244	41061

Table 1. Summary of data

2.2 Estimation of mutation rates from substitution rate on fourfold sites

To estimate mutation rates from nucleotide substitution rates, it is important to separate substitutions representing neutral evolutionary drift from those influenced by selection. Following Hardison et al.'s study (Hardison et al., 2003), fourfold sites were analyzed in this study. Fourfold sites are sites marked "N" in the codons GCN (Ala), CCN (Pro), TCN (Ser), ACN (Thr), CGN (Arg), GGN (Gly), CTN (Leu), and GTN (Val). is worth noting that nucleotide substitutions at fourfold sites do not change amino acids so that they can be considered as neutral. In the case of mouse, the effect of codon preference on nucleotide substitutions would be smaller than that of mutations (Misawa and Kikuno, 2011). In this study, the mutation rates were estimated from the substitution rates at fourfold sites by assuming that the substitutions at fourfold sites are neutral.

2.3 Classification of sites and mutations

To evaluate the effect of CpG hypermutability on mutation rates, fourfold sites were classified into three categories depending on the adjacent nucleotides, namely, CpG sites, TpG sites, and usual sites. If the nucleotide at fourfold site is C and the first nucleotide of 3'-adjacent codon is G, the site is classified into CpG site. If the nucleotide at fourfold site is T and the first nucleotide of 3'-adjacent codon is G, the site is classified into TpG site. If the nucleotide at fourfold site is C and the first nucleotide of 3'-adjacent codon is A, the site is classified into TpG site, because on the complementary strand T is next to G. The sites that are neither CpG site nor TpG site are classified as usual site.

Mutations were classified into 4 categories: CpG to TpG mutations, TpG to CpG mutations, and non- CpG transitions and transversions. To distinguish CpG to TpG mutations and TpG to CpG mutations from non-CpG transitions, the adjacent nucleotides were also considered. If the observed nucleotide was T, its ancestral nucleotide was C, and the downstream nucleotide was G, the mutation was classified as a CpG to TpG substitution. For example, a mutation from CCC (Pro) to CCT (Pro) is classified into a CpG to TpG mutation only when 3′ adjacent nucleotide of the codon is G. If the observed nucleotide was A, its ancestral nucleotide was G, and the upstream nucleotide was C, the mutation was again classified as a CpG to TpG mutation because a CpG to TpG mutation occurs on the complementary strand of DNA. For example, a mutation from CCG (Pro) to CCA (Pro) corresponds to a CpG to TpG mutation. If the observed nucleotide was C, its ancestral nucleotide was T, and the downstream nucleotide was G, the mutation was classified as a CpG to TpG mutation. If the observed nucleotide was G, its ancestral nucleotide was A, and the upstream nucleotide was C, the mutation was again classified as a CpG to TpG mutation. Other types of mutation are classified into two types: transitions and transversions (Misawa et al., 2008; Misawa and Kikuno, 2009; Misawa, 2011; Misawa and Kikuno, 2011).

2.4 Estimation of mutation rates by using the Maximum Parsimony (MP) method

I determined the codon sequences of the common ancestors of humans and chimpanzees by using the maximum parsimony (MP) method. Next, I counted the number of codon substitutions that had occurred along the human lineage. For some codon trios, the ancestral state between the human and chimpanzee codons appeared ambiguous when estimated by the MP method. In such cases, all possible ancestral states were treated equally. I also calculated the mutation rates by dividing the number of codon substitutions occurring annually by the number of ancestral codons. It was assumed that the human-chimpanzee divergence occurred 5 million years (MY) ago (Horai et al., 1995). Macaque genes were used as the outgroup. To calculate confidence intervals of the estimates, the binomial distribution was assumed. The awk program used in the analysis is available from the author upon request.

2.5 Comparison between mutation rate and the distance from the telomere by using regression analysis

I compared the mutation rates with the distance of a central position of 10-MB windows from the telomere. These values were used in regression analyses, which were performed using the statistical software R (R Development Core Team, 2008).

3. Result

Table 2 shows the mean value of the mutation rate estimates per BY per site and their 99% confidence intervals. The mutation rate of CpG to TpG is similar to that obtained by the previous study, but the rate of other types of mutation is lower than those obtained by the previous study (Misawa, 2011). The mutation rate of CpG to TpG is about 10 times higher than that of transitions and transversions on usual sites. This ratio is similar to previous studies (Scarano et al., 1967; Bird, 1980; Lunter and Hein, 2004). The mutation rates on autosomes were similar to those on X chromosome, except the rates of transversion on usual sites. The rate of transversion on usual sites on autosomes is significantly higher than that of X chromosomes after the Bonferroni correction (P<0.05).

Mutation type	Site type	Autosomes	X chromosome	
CpG to TpG	CpG	3.91 (3.74 - 4.08)	3.96 (2.07 - 4.58)	
Transversion	CpG	0.79 (0.72 - 0.87)	0.44 (0.15 - 1.18)	
TpG to CpG	TpG	0.47 (0.44 - 0.49)	0.47 (0.20 - 0.50)	
non-CpG transition	TpG	0.27 (0.26 - 0.29)	0.09 (0.11 - 0.35)	
Transversion	TpG	0.29 (0.27 - 0.31)	0.30 (0.04 - 0.22)	
non-CpG transition	Usual	0.32 (0.29 - 0.34)	0.41 (0.09 - 0.33)	
Transversion	Usual	0.51 (0.49 - 0.54)	0.24 (0.18 - 0.48)	*

*Significantly lower than autosomes at 5% level

Table 2. Avarage mutation rates per BY per site and their 99% confidence intervals

Figures 2, 3, and 4 are a scatter plot of the mutation rates versus the distances to telomeres. Upper panel of figure 3 is for autosomes and the lower panel is for X chromosome. Figure 3 shows a scatter plot of the mutation rates on TpG sites. Figure 4 shows a scatter plot of the mutation rates on usual sites. These figures show that mutation rates are negatively correlated to the distances from telomeres. These figures also show that a large variation in the rates of mutations exist among genomic regions.

Table 3 shows Pearson's correlation coefficient between mutation rates and the distances from telomeres. Only the mutation rates of TpG to CpG and transversion on TpG sites were significantly correlated to the distance from telomeres ($P < 0.001$ and $P < 0.01$, respectively) after the Bonferroni correction. There were no significant differences of the correlation coefficients between autosomes and X chromosomes.

Mutation type	Site type	Autosomes		X chromosome
CpG to TpG	CpG	-0.06		-0.42
Transversion	CpG	0.18		-0.09
TpG to CpG	TpG	-0.20	***	-0.43
non-CpG transition	TpG	-0.10		-0.05
Transversion	TpG	-0.20	**	0.13
non-CpG transition	Usual	-0.13		-0.61
Transversion	Usual	-0.03		-0.34

*at 1% level of significance; ***at 0.1% level of significance

Table 3. Correlation coefficient between mutation rates and distances to telomeres by regression analysis

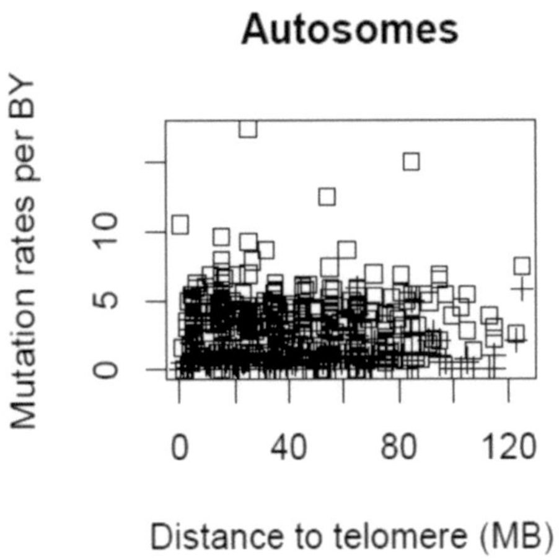

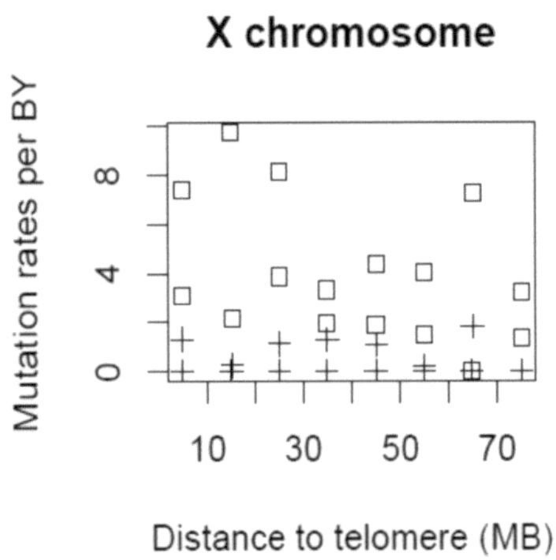

Fig. 2. A scatter plot of the mutation rates on CpG sites versus the distances to telomeres. The open circles (○) show the TpG to CpG mutation rates. The open triangles (Δ) show the rates of non-CpG transition. The crosses (+) show the rates of transition.

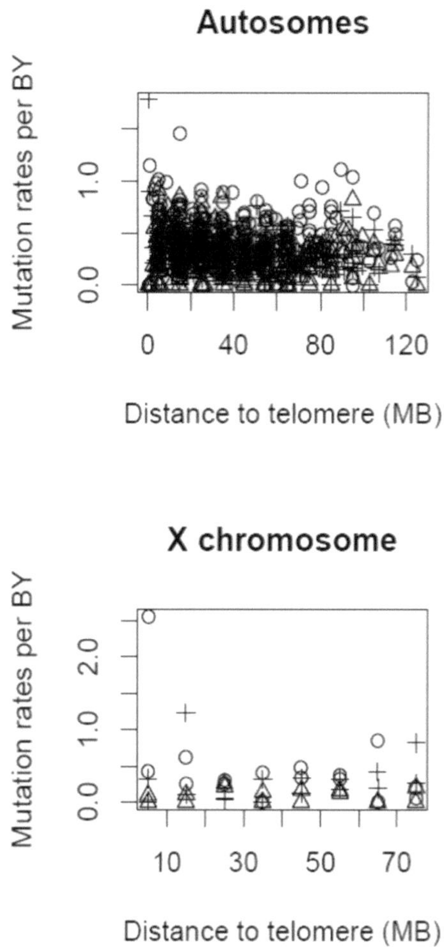

Fig. 3. A scatter plot of the mutation rates on TpG sites versus the distances to telomeres. The open squares (□) show the CpG to TpG mutation rates. The open circles (○) show the TpG to CpG mutation rates. The open triangles (△) show the rates of non-CpG transition. The crosses (+) show the rates of transition.

4. Discussion

In this study, the rates of CpG to TpG mutations, TpG to CpG mutations, and non-CpG transitions and transversions were estimated by comparing the coding regions of thousands of human and chimpanzee genes from entire genome and inferring their ancestral sequences by assuming macaque genes as the outgroup. The mutation rate of CpG to TpG is about 10 times higher than that of transitions and transversions on usual sites. This ratio is similar to previous studies (Scarano et al., 1967; Bird, 1980; Lunter and Hein, 2004). The mutation rate of CpG to TpG is similar to that obtained by the previous study, but the rate of other types of mutation is lower than those obtained by the previous study (Misawa, 2011), probably because previous studies included nonsynonymous substitutions (Misawa, 2011) while only fourfold sites were analyzed in this study.

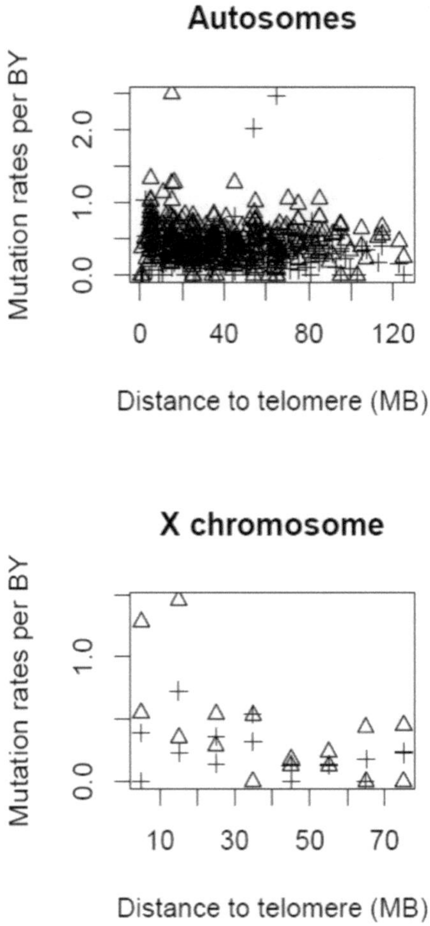

Fig. 4. A scatter plot of the mutation rates on usual sites versus the distances to telomeres. The open squares (□) show the CpG to TpG mutation rates. The open circles (○) show the TpG to CpG mutation rates. The open triangles (△) show the rates of non-CpG transition. The crosses (+) show the rates of transition.

As seen in table 2, a significant difference was not observed between the mutation rates of autosomes and X chromosome, except the rates of transversion on usual sites This result indicates that the effect of "male-driven evolution" (Miyata et al., 1987) is not strong. Figures 2, 3, and 4 show that a large variation in the rates of mutations among genomic regions. These results might be caused by the fact that mutation rates are affected by various factors, such as gene density, GC contents and the density of CpG islands (Misawa, 2011).

Vogel and Motulsky (Vogel and Motulsky, 1997) pointed out that since the deamination of methyl-C occurs spontaneously and is independent of DNA replication, the rate of CpG mutations should be scaled with time and not with the number of cell divisions. Recently, Taylor et al. (Taylor et al., 2006) investigated male mutation bias separately at non-CpG and CpG sites by using human-chimpanzee whole-genome alignments. They concluded that CpG hypermutation is weakly affected by the number of cell divisions. As pointed out by

Misawa (2011), the effect of male-driven evolution on CpG hypermutation is weaker than that of other chromosomal properties. Further study must be necessary.

Figures 2, 3, and 4 indicate that the CpG to TpG substitution rates were negatively correlated to the distances from telomeres. This is consistent with previous studies (Hellmann et al., 2005; Tyekucheva et al., 2008), although their methods for estimating mutation rates were different from this study. However, Table 3 shows that only the mutation rates of TpG to CpG and transversion on TpG sites were significantly correlated to the distance from telomeres after the Bonferroni correction. Tyekucheva et al. (Tyekucheva et al., 2008) suggested the existence of additional mutagenic mechanisms that increase neutral substitution rates in subtelomeric regions. Increased divergence near telomeres has been linked to direct and indirect effects of large-scale chromosomal structure. If the correlation coefficients between mutation rates and the distances from telomeres on X chromosome are different from that on autosomes, cell division and DNA replication might be a part of such mutation mechanisms. Unfortunately, no significant differences of the correlation coefficients between autosomes and X chromosomes were observed in this study.

The numbers data points are not very large; thus, dividing too many bins by the distance from the telomeres may yield weak results. As more data become available, incorporating these additional predictors in the regression analyses may be beneficial.

5. References

Altschul, S.F., Gish, W., Miller, W., Myers, E.W. and Lipman, D.J. Basic local alignment search tool. *J Mol Biol* 215 (1990), pp. 403-10.

Bird, A.P. DNA methylation and the frequency of CpG in animal DNA. *Nucleic Acids Res* 8 (1980), pp. 1499-504.

Cooper, D.N. and Krawczak, M. Cytosine methylation and the fate of CpG dinucleotides in vertebrate genomes. *Hum Genet* 83 (1989), pp. 181-8.

Cooper, D.N. and Youssoufian, H. The CpG dinucleotide and human genetic disease. *Hum Genet* 78 (1988), pp. 151-5.

Felsenstein, J., Inferring phylogenies. Sinauer Associates Sunderland, Mass, USA (2004).

Fryxell, K.J. and Moon, W.J. CpG mutation rates in the human genome are highly dependent on local GC content. *Mol Biol Evol* 22 (2005), pp. 650-8.

Gibbs, R.A., Rogers, J., Katze, M.G., Bumgarner, R., Weinstock, G.M., Mardis, E.R., Remington, K.A., Strausberg, R.L., Venter, J.C., Wilson, R.K., Batzer, M.A., Bustamante, C.D., Eichler, E.E., Hahn, M.W., Hardison, R.C., Makova, K.D., Miller, W., Milosavljevic, A., Palermo, R.E., Siepel, A., Sikela, J.M., Attaway, T., Bell, S., Bernard, K.E., Buhay, C.J., Chandrabose, M.N., Dao, M., Davis, C., Delehaunty, K.D., Ding, Y., Dinh, H.H., Dugan-Rocha, S., Fulton, L.A., Gabisi, R.A., Garner, T.T., Godfrey, J., Hawes, A.C., Hernandez, J., Hines, S., Holder, M., Hume, J., Jhangiani, S.N., Joshi, V., Khan, Z.M., Kirkness, E.F., Cree, A., Fowler, R.G., Lee, S., Lewis, L.R., Li, Z., Liu, Y.S., Moore, S.M., Muzny, D., Nazareth, L.V., Ngo, D.N., Okwuonu, G.O., Pai, G., Parker, D., Paul, H.A., Pfannkoch, C., Pohl, C.S., Rogers, Y.H., Ruiz, S.J., Sabo, A., Santibanez, J., Schneider, B.W., Smith, S.M., Sodergren, E.,

Svatek, A.F., Utterback, T.R., Vattathil, S., Warren, W., White, C.S., Chinwalla, A.T., Feng, Y., Halpern, A.L., Hillier, L.W., Huang, X., Minx, P., Nelson, J.O., Pepin, K.H., Qin, X., Sutton, G.G., Venter, E., Walenz, B.P., Wallis, J.W., Worley, K.C., Yang, S.P., Jones, S.M., Marra, M.A., Rocchi, M., Schein, J.E., Baertsch, R., Clarke, L., Csuros, M., Glasscock, J., Harris, R.A., Havlak, P., Jackson, A.R., Jiang, H., et al. Evolutionary and biomedical insights from the rhesus macaque genome. *Science* 316 (2007), pp. 222-34.

Haldane, J.B.S. The estimation of viabilities. *J. Genet.* 54 (1956), pp. 294-296.

Hardison, R.C., Roskin, K.M., Yang, S., Diekhans, M., Kent, W.J., Weber, R., Elnitski, L., Li, J., O'Connor, M., Kolbe, D., Schwartz, S., Furey, T.S., Whelan, S., Goldman, N., Smit, A., Miller, W., Chiaromonte, F. and Haussler, D. Covariation in frequencies of substitution, deletion, transposition, and recombination during eutherian evolution. *Genome Res* 13 (2003), pp. 13-26.

Hasegawa, M., Kishino, H. and Yano, T. Dating of the human-ape splitting by a molecular clock of mitochondrial DNA. *J Mol Evol* 22 (1985), pp. 160-74.

Hellmann, I., Prufer, K., Ji, H., Zody, M.C., Paabo, S. and Ptak, S.E. Why do human diversity levels vary at a megabase scale? *Genome Res* 15 (2005), pp. 1222-31.

Hobolth, A., Nielsen, R., Wang, Y., Wu, F. and Tanksley, S.D. CpG + CpNpG analysis of protein-coding sequences from tomato. *Mol Biol Evol* 23 (2006), pp. 1318-23.

Horai, S., Hayasaka, K., Kondo, R., Tsugane, K. and Takahata, N. Recent African origin of modern humans revealed by complete sequences of hominoid mitochondrial DNAs. *Proc Natl Acad Sci U S A* 92 (1995), pp. 532-6.

Hughes, A.L. and Nei, M. Pattern of nucleotide substitution at major histocompatibility complex class I loci reveals overdominant selection. *Nature* 335 (1988), pp. 167-70.

Huttley, G.A. Modeling the impact of DNA methylation on the evolution of BRCA1 in mammals. *Mol Biol Evol* 21 (2004), pp. 1760-8.

Jordan, I.K., Kondrashov, F.A., Adzhubei, I.A., Wolf, Y.I., Koonin, E.V., Kondrashov, A.S. and Sunyaev, S. A universal trend of amino acid gain and loss in protein evolution. *Nature* 433 (2005), pp. 633-8.

Jukes, T.H. and Cantor, T.H.: Evolution of protein molecules. In: Munro, H.N. (Munro, H.N.)Munro, H.N.s), *Mammalian Protein Metabolism.* Academic Press, New York (1969).

Katoh, K., Misawa, K., Kuma, K. and Miyata, T. MAFFT: a novel method for rapid multiple sequence alignment based on fast Fourier transform. *Nucleic Acids Res* 30 (2002), pp. 3059-66.

Kimura, M. Evolutionary rate at the molecular level. *Nature* 217 (1968), pp. 624-6.

Larkin, M.A., Blackshields, G., Brown, N.P., Chenna, R., McGettigan, P.A., McWilliam, H., Valentin, F., Wallace, I.M., Wilm, A., Lopez, R., Thompson, J.D., Gibson, T.J. and Higgins, D.G. Clustal W and Clustal X version 2.0. *Bioinformatics* 23 (2007), pp. 2947-8.

Li, W.H., Yi, S. and Makova, K. Male-driven evolution. *Curr Opin Genet Dev* 12 (2002), pp. 650-6.

Lunter, G. and Hein, J. A nucleotide substitution model with nearest-neighbour interactions. *Bioinformatics* 20 Suppl 1 (2004), pp. I216-I223.

Misawa, K. A codon substitution model that incorporates the effect of the GC contents, the gene density and the density of CpG islands of human chromosomes. *BMC Genomics* 12 (2011), p. 397.

Misawa, K., Kamatani, N. and Kikuno, R.F. The universal trend of amino acid gain-loss is caused by CpG hypermutability. *J Mol Evol* 67 (2008), pp. 334-42.

Misawa, K. and Kikuno, R.F. Evaluation of the effect of CpG hypermutability on human codon substitution. *Gene* 431 (2009), pp. 18-22.

Misawa, K. and Kikuno, R.F. GeneWaltz--A new method for reducing the false positives of gene finding. *BioData Min* 3 (2010), p. 6.

Misawa, K. and Kikuno, R.F. Relationship between amino acid composition and gene expression in the mouse genome. *BMC Res Notes* 4 (2011), p. 20.

Misawa, K. and Tajima, F. Estimation of the amount of DNA polymorphism when the neutral mutation rate varies among sites. *Genetics* 147 (1997), pp. 1959-64.

Miyata, T., Hayashida, H., Kuma, K., Mitsuyasu, K. and Yasunaga, T. Male-driven molecular evolution: a model and nucleotide sequence analysis. *Cold Spring Harb Symp Quant Biol* 52 (1987), pp. 863-7.

Nei, M. and Gojobori, T. Simple methods for estimating the numbers of synonymous and nonsynonymous nucleotide substitutions. *Mol Biol Evol* 3 (1986), pp. 418-26.

Pray, L. DNA replication and causes of mutation. *Nature Education* 1 (2008), p. 1.

R Development Core Team, R: A language and environment for statistical computing, Vienna, Austria (2008).

Scarano, E., Iaccarino, M., Grippo, P. and Parisi, E. The heterogeneity of thymine methyl group origin in DNA pyrimidine isostichs of developing sea urchin embryos. *Proc Natl Acad Sci U S A* 57 (1967), pp. 1394-400.

Sullivan, J. and Joyce, P. Model selection in phylogenetics. *Annual Review of Ecology, Evolution, and Systematics* 36 (2005), pp. 445-466.

Tavare, S. Some probabilistic and statistical problems in the analysis of DNA sequences. *Lectures on Mathematics in the Life Sciences* 17 (1986), pp. 57-86.

Taylor, J., Tyekucheva, S., Zody, M., Chiaromonte, F. and Makova, K.D. Strong and weak male mutation bias at different sites in the primate genomes: insights from the human-chimpanzee comparison. *Mol Biol Evol* 23 (2006), pp. 565-73.

Tyekucheva, S., Makova, K.D., Karro, J.E., Hardison, R.C., Miller, W. and Chiaromonte, F. Human-macaque comparisons illuminate variation in neutral substitution rates. *Genome Biol* 9 (2008), p. R76.

Vogel, F. and Motulsky, A.G., Human genetics: problems and approaches. Springer-Verlag, Berlin (1997).

Walser, J.C., Ponger, L. and Furano, A.V. CpG dinucleotides and the mutation rate of non-CpG DNA. *Genome Res* 18 (2008), pp. 1403-14.

Whelan, S., Lio, P. and Goldman, N. Molecular phylogenetics: state-of-the-art methods for looking into the past. *Trends Genet* 17 (2001), pp. 262-72.

Wu, S.C. and Zhang, Y. Active DNA demethylation: many roads lead to Rome. *Nat Rev Mol Cell Biol* 11 (2011), pp. 607-20.

Yang, Z. Estimating the pattern of nucleotide substitution. *J Mol Evol* 39 (1994), pp. 105-11.

Yang, Z. PAML 4: phylogenetic analysis by maximum likelihood. *Mol Biol Evol* 24 (2007), pp. 1586-91.

Yang, Z. and Nielsen, R. Mutation-selection models of codon substitution and their use to estimate selective strengths on codon usage. *Mol Biol Evol* 25 (2008), pp. 568-79.

Part 2

Point Mutation in Viruses: From Drug Resistance to Vaccination

4

Point Mutations and Antiviral Drug Resistance

José Arellano-Galindo[1], Blanca Lilia Barron[2], Yetlanezi Vargas-Infante[3], Enrique Santos-Esteban[4], Emma del Carmen Herrera-Martinez[5], Norma Velazquez-Guadarrama[1] and Gustavo Reyes-Teran[6]

[1]Laboratorios de Virología y Microbiología Hospital Infantil de México Federico Gómez,
[2]Head of laboratory of Virology Escuela Nacional de Ciencias Biologicas, Instituto Politecnico Nacional,
[3]Internal Medicine/Infectious Diseases/HIV, Centro de Investigación en Enfermedades Infecciosas Instituto Nacional de Enfermedades Respiratorias, Nacional de Enfermedades Respiratorias
[4]Departamento de Bioquimica Escuela Nacional de Ciencias Biologicas, Instituto Politecnico Nacional,
[5]Academisian of Facultad de Ciencias de la Salud Universidad Anahuac, Mexico Norte
[6]Head of Department, Centro de Investigación en Enfermedades Infecciosas Instituto Nacional de Enfermedades Respiratorias, México

1. Introduction

Viruses are the most abundant biological entities on the planet and their life cycles include the infection of other organisms. Although the presence of viruses is obvious in host organisms that show signs of disease, many healthy organisms are also hosts of non-pathogenic virus infections, where some are active and others are quiescent. It is doubtless that the known viruses represent only a tiny fraction of the viruses on Earth. There is a strong correlation between how intensively a species is studied and the number of viruses found in that species. Our own species is the subject of the most attention, because we have the greatest interest in learning about agents and processes that affect our health. If other species received the same amount of attention, it is likely that many would be found to be hosts to similar numbers of viruses (Breitbart et al., 2005).

Viruses are important agents of many human diseases ranging from the trivial to the lethal, and they play roles in the development of several other types of disease. The history of viral pathogenesis is intertwined with the history of medicine. Humans were clearly aware of viral diseases in ancient times and, since recognizing viruses as disease agents, have taken on the task of fighting them. This fight entails a need to understand the nature of viruses, how they replicate, and how they cause disease. Having such knowledge would facilitate the development of effective means for prevention, diagnosis, and treatment of viral diseases - medical applications that constitute the main aspects of the science of virology (John et al., 2007).

Currently, the principal strategy for treating viral infections is to use antiviral drugs. For a long time, very few antiviral drugs were available for clinical use compared with the number of anti-bacterial drugs. This was because it was difficult to find compounds that interfere specifically with viral activities without causing significant harm to host cells. However, drugs are now available to treat diseases caused by a variety of viruses and, in some circumstances, to prevent viral infections. The development of these drugs is closely connected with a better understanding of viral life cycles. Chemists are now applying their knowledge of the three-dimensional structure and the molecular function of viral proteins and other structures to the design of molecules that inhibit important functions of viral proteins (De Clercq, 2004; John et al., 2007).

In recent years, the demand for new antiviral strategies has increased markedly. Factors contributing to this growing demand include the ever-increasing prevalence of chronic viral infections and the emergence of new, more infectious viruses (De Clerq, 2004). One of the most dramatic aspects of virology is the emergence of new viral diseases or the re-emergence of viruses with increased pathogenicity (as in the outbreak of swine flu).

In some instances, the emergence of a viral disease represents the original identification of cause of this event (Geisbert et al., 2004). On occasion, a virus that is already widespread in a population can emerge as an endemic or epidemic disease because of an increase in the ratio of infectious cases. Such increases may result from either an increase in host susceptibility or an enhancement in the virulence of a virus. This can lead to large numbers of deaths among human populations, depending on the local social and environmental conditions (Weiss et al., 2004).

When a viral disease becomes pandemic, antiviral drugs are vital in the management of infections (Moscona et al., 2008). However, the emergence of drug-resistant viral strains is of great concern, because these can compromise the effectiveness of treatment, or even lead to its failure. Drug-resistant viruses began to appear soon after antiviral drugs were introduced into clinical practice. This should not have been surprising given that antibiotic-resistant bacteria and insecticide-resistant insects emerged as a result of natural selection. It is now known that viruses can mutate at high frequencies (RNA viruses have a mutation rate estimated at 10^{-4}, i.e., one mutation in 10,000 bases, while DNA viruses have a rate of 10^{-8}) and evolve rapidly, thereby allowing genotypes encoding for drug resistance to arise. Drug-resistant genotypes can be advantageous in hosts where the drug is present and they can become the dominant genotypes in such hosts (Nathanson et al., 2007).

The drug resistance of viruses is relative, rather than absolute. A measure of the degree of resistance can be obtained by determining the IC_{50}. A virus strain is considered to be 'resistant' to a drug if it is able to replicate in the body in the presence of a concentration of the drug that inhibits replication of 'sensitive' strains. Drug-resistant virus isolates are found to have one or more mutations in genes encoding for proteins that are drug targets (John et al., 2007).

Clinical problems arise when drug-resistant virus strains emerge in patients undergoing treatment and when resistant strains are transmitted to other individuals. In such cases, patients may be treated with alternative drugs or a strategy of multidrug therapy can be used, which is the current trend (John et al., 2007; l Nathanson et al., 2007). However, there are fewer therapeutic options when a new drug-resistant viral strain emerges (Tan et al., 2007).

Therefore, there is a great need to continue research programmes aimed at extending the range of drugs available. In particular, it is very important to know and understand the mechanisms by which viral strains can become resistant to existing drugs in order to design new drugs for which the development of resistance will prove more difficult. In this chapter, we focus on the molecular mechanisms involved in the emergence of drug resistance, using different types of virus to describe current knowledge.

2. Influenza virus

Influenza is one of the most prevalent viral diseases, affecting an estimated 10–20% of the world population annually, with 3–5 million cases of severe respiratory illness and up to 500 000 deaths. The aetiological agent is influenza virus (l Nathanson et al., 2007).

Influenza virus belongs to the Orthomyxoviridae family, which is subdivided into three serologically distinct types: A, B, and C. Only influenza viruses A and B appear to be of concern as human pathogens, because influenza C virus does not cause significant disease (Collier et al., 2006).

The virions are 100–200 nm in diameter with a spherical shape. The lipid envelope is covered with projections corresponding to different proteins on the virion surface (Itzstein et al., 2007). These proteins are: haemagglutinin (HA), which is a trimeric protein in the form of a spike; neuraminidase (NA), which is a tetrameric protein with a mushroom-like shape; and the M2 protein, which penetrates the lipid membrane of the virus during replication in the host cells and forms ion channels that allow the entry of protons from the interior of the virus (Figure. 1) (Horimoto et al., 2005).

HA is a glycoprotein with a triangular cross-section, which was first identified based on its ability to agglutinate erythrocytes (hence its name). It is now apparent that it also has important roles in the attachment and entry of the virus into host cells, thereby determining virulence. NA (also called sialidase) removes the neuraminic (sialic) acid from cellular glycoproteins to facilitate viral release and the spread of infection to new cells (Eun-Sun et al., 2011).

The genome of the influenza virus consists of eight discrete fragments of negative single-stranded RNA (approximately 13 kb in size). These fragments form a complex with various proteins (PA, PB1, and PB2) to form a ribonucleoprotein arranged in a helix. The M1 protein forms a shell that provides strength and rigidity to the lipid membrane and it is associated with the NS2 protein. RNA transcriptase, which is found inside the matrix shell, is essential for the transcription of viral RNA to mRNA during replication (Palese et al., 2004).

Influenza A viruses are designated based on the antigenic relationships of their external HA and NA proteins, i.e., they classified based on antibodies to H1–H16 and N1–N9. Only viruses with H1, H2, H3, N1, and N2 are known to infect humans or cause serious disease

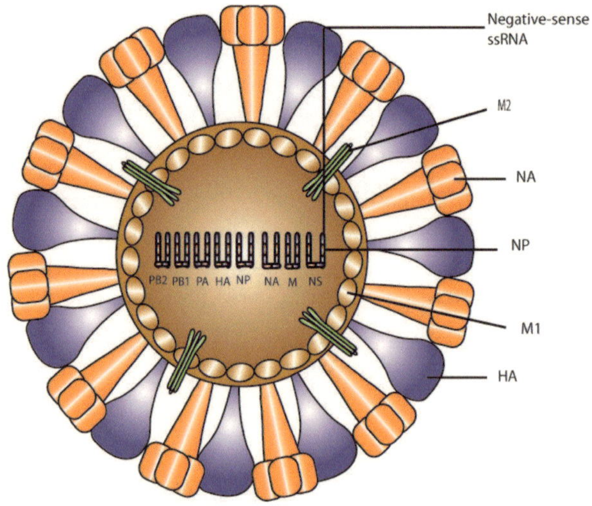

Fig. 1. Schematic diagram of influenza A virus. Two surface glycoproteins, hemagglutinin (HA) and neuraminidase (NA), together with the M2 ion-channel protein, are embedded in the viral envelope, which is derived from the host plasma membrane. The ribonucleoprotein complex comprises a viral RNA segment associated with the nucleoprotein (NP) and three polymerase proteins (PA, PB1 and PB2). The matrix (M1) protein is associated with both ribonucleoprotein and the viral envelope. A small amount of non-structural protein 2 is also presen. (Modified from: Horimoto T, et. al. *Nature Rev. Microbiol.* 2005. 3: 591-600, reproduced with permission of the author)

outbreaks (Collier et al., 2006). Although influenza B viruses cause the same types of disease as influenza A, they do not cause pandemics, because the only hosts are humans and seals (Eun-Sun et al., 2011).

With at least 16 different HA and nine different NA subtypes, there is considerable antigenic variation among influenza viruses (Palese et al., 2004). This variation occurs because RNA viruses (e.g., influenza viruses) are extremely mutable and possess highly efficient strategies for generating viral diversity during evolution. RNA viruses have few or no proofreading mechanisms and many mutations are introduced during replication. Thus, RNA viruses exist as quasispecies, where viruses possess slightly different genetic compositions. Unfortunately, the evolution of viruses is not simply confined to point mutations inserted during replication. Viruses can also undergo leaps in evolution through the processes of recombination and reassortment. These processes produce population heterogeneity in viruses through the acquisition of large sections of genomic material from other viruses (Figure. 2) (Webby et al., 2004).

These same mechanisms of evolution allow viruses to develop resistance to drugs. This is the case with resistance to oseltamivir (Tamiflu®), where mutations confer resistance (mutations in NA) and there might be possible exchange of genetic information between resistant and susceptible viral strains (Janies et al., 2010).

As mentioned earlier, a pandemic can arise because of either an increase in host susceptibility or the enhancement of viral virulence, and antiviral drugs are vital in the

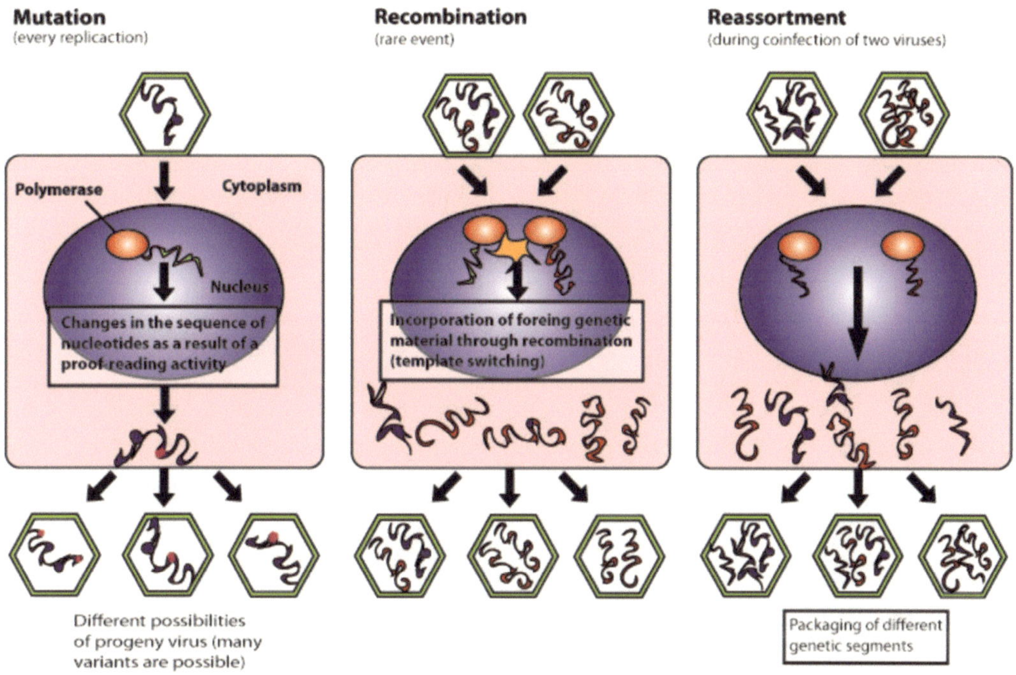

Fig. 2. Molecular mechanisms for generating viral diversity. The viruses have three main mechanisms for generating diversity on replication. (a) Mutation: during replication, single point mutations are incorporated into one or more genomic positions as a result of a lack of proof-reading activity of the viral polymerase. (b) Recombination: foreign genetic material is incorporated into the viral genome through mechanisms such as template switching during replication. (c) Reassortment: occurs on dual infection of a cell with segmented genome viruses, whole gene segments can be swapped. Any of the three mechanisms (which are not exclusive), may result in viruses that have new biological properties, such as new host range and pathogenic potential. (Modified from: Webby R., et. al. *Nature Med. Suppl.* 2005. 10: S77-S81, reproduced with permission of the author)

management of infection when a viral disease becomes pandemic. Therefore, it is important to combat the emergence of drug resistance in seasonal strains (normal) and pandemic strains (Janies et al., 2010).

Antiviral therapeutics can be divided into the following categories: drugs directed against the virus itself (either its genome or its proteins); drugs directed against host cell proteins that are critical for the replication of individual viruses; and therapeutics that mimic or enhance host defence mechanisms (Neal Nathanson et al., 2007). Two classes of antiviral agents are currently in use for the control of influenza infections: M2 ion channel blockers (directed against host cells) and NAIs (antivirus) (Fig. 3) (Palese et al., 2004; Okomo-Adhiambo et al., 2010).

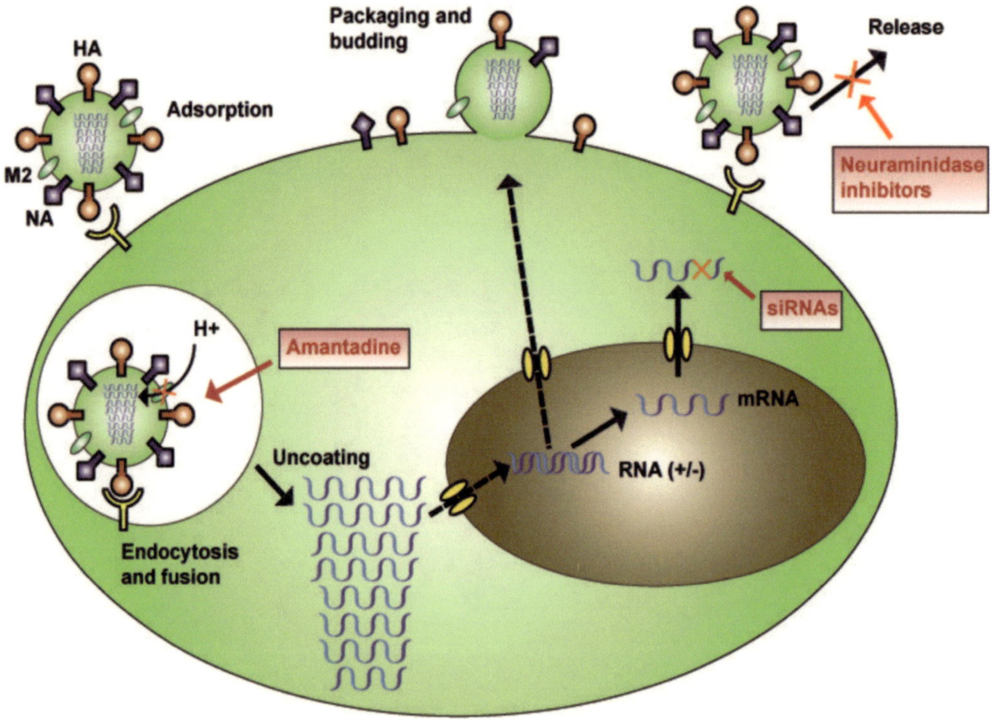

Fig. 3. Inhibition of influenza virus replication cycle by antivirals. After binding to sialic acid receptors, the virus is internalized by receptor-mediated endocytosis. The low pH in the endosome triggers the fusion of viral and endosomal membranes and the influx of H+ ions through the M2 channel releases the viral genes into the cytoplasm. Amantadine blocks this uncoating step. RNA replication and transcription occur in the nucleus. siRNA inhibition may affect the stability of mRNA, preventing translation of viral protein. Packaging and budding of virions occurs at the cytoplasmic membrane. Neuraminidase inhibitors block the release of the virus from the infected cell. Because sialic acid receptors are not removed by the neuraminidase, aggregates of virus stick to the cytoplasmic membrane of the infected cell and cannot move on to infect other cells. (Modified from: Peter P. et al. *Nature Med.* 2004. Supp. 10: S82-S87)

The M2 blockers (amantadine and rimantadine) are effective against influenza A viruses, but not influenza B viruses. However, their effectiveness has been compromised by drug-resistant mutants that are frequently isolated from patients within a few days of therapy (Okomo-Adhiambo et al., 2010).

2.1 Antivirals used to the treatment of influenza

Oseltamivir and zanamivir are neuraminidase inhibitors (NAIs) that are commonly used against type A and type B influenza infections (Fig. 4). Oseltamivir is administered orally, whereas zanamivir is inhaled. Another drug of this type is peramivir, which is currently being studied. NAIs competitively bind to the highly conserved NA active site by mimicking sialic acid (N-acetylneuraminic acid), which is the natural substrate of NA. This inhibits the enzyme's key function by destroying neuraminic acid-containing receptors, which prevents the release of progeny virions from infected cells and any possible dissemination to neighbouring cells (Neal Nathanson et al., 2007).

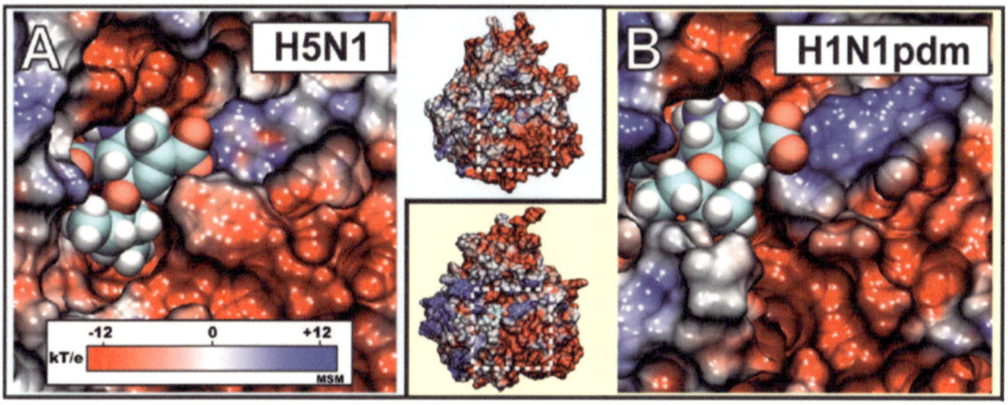

Fig. 4. Electrostatic surface potential of the sialic acid (SA) binding pocket of H1N1pdm and oseltamivir. Shown in A) and B) are closeup views of the SA binding pocket with drug bound H1N1pdm and avian H5N1 neuraminidase, respectively. The region of the binding pocket, where the drug binds, exhibits a negative potential (colored red), whereas the opening of the pocket is surrounded by a highly positive potential ring (colored blue). (Reproduced with permission of the author).

The highly conserved NA enzyme active site is comprised of catalytic amino acid residues that directly interact with the substrate (R118, D151, R152, R224, E276, R292, R371, and Y406) and framework (E119, R156, W178, S179, D198N, I222, E227, H274, E277, N294, and E425) residues that support the catalytic residues (Ferraris et al., 2008; Le et al., 2010).

The influenza A H1N1 virus can develop resistance to oseltamivir because of a point mutation at one of several sites in the NA protein (e.g., D79G, S247G, N294S, or H274Y). Resistance to zanamivir (Relenza®) by the influenza A H1N1 virus can occur because of the NA point mutations H126N or Q136K (Janies et al., 2010).

2.2 Antiviral resistance

Resistance to oseltamivir in pandemic influenza strains can appear in various forms: 1) sporadic evolution in an infected patient in response to treatment; 2) evolution of resistance to oseltamivir in an infected patient and transfer of the strain among personal contacts; 3) maintenance of a genotype that confers resistance to oseltamivir in a viral lineage due to selection pressure; and 4) a reassortment event between oseltamivir-resistant seasonal H1N1 and a pandemic strain (Janies et al., 2010).

The frequency of resistance to oseltamivir was previously low, except in hospitalized children and immunocompromised patients. However, during the 2007-2008 and 2008-2009 influenza seasons, the emergence and transmission of oseltamivir-resistant seasonal influenza A (H1N1) viruses with an H274Y mutation were detected globally in untreated individuals, which emphasized the need for close monitoring of oseltamivir resistance. Mutations at catalytic (R292K) and framework (E119V and N294S) NA residues have been detected in the N2 viral subtype in oseltamivir-treated patients. A four-amino-acid deletion mutation (deletion of residues 245 to 248) was reported to confer oseltamivir resistance in an influenza A (H3N2) virus isolated from an immunocompromised patient treated with the drug (Okomo-Adhiambo et al., 2010). This shows that the clinical use of oseltamivir is associated with the emergence of drug resistance resulting from subtype-specific NA mutations (Janies et al., 2010; Okomo-Adhiambo et al., 2010).

Zanamivir-resistant mutants are less common than oseltamivir-resistant mutants, partly because of differences between how the two drugs bind to the NA active site and possibly because of lower frequency of the prescription and use of zanamivir (Okomo-Adhiambo et al., 2010).

Variant strains with an advantage are quickly amplified when selective conditions are present, such as the conditions after jumping to a new host, and they become the dominant strain by selective pressure, e.g., when a host is treated with a drug that the strain can resist (Webby et al., 2004).

Several mutations in seasonal or pandemic strains confer resistance to oseltamivir, which is currently the most widely used drug. These mutations are found mainly in the framework of the enzyme and they appear to destabilize drug binding to the target enzyme, thereby reducing viral susceptibility to the treatment (Itzstein et al., 2007; Janies et al., 2010; Okomo-Adhiambo et al., 2010).

Mutants in E119 (influenza A H3N2) are known to emerge after oseltamivir treatment. The E119V variant was resistant to oseltamivir, but it did not exhibit reduced susceptibility to peramivir. The E119I variant was resistant to oseltamivir, but it also showed decreased susceptibility to zanamivir, peramivir, and A-315675 (another NAI under study) (Okomo-Adhiambo et al., 2010). Mutants in E119 (influenza A H3N2) were also reported to disrupt E276-R224 salt bridges that accommodate the hydrophobic pentyl group of oseltamivir, although further studies are required to confirm this (Wang et al., 2009). Another very important mutation is H274Y (influenza H5N1 and H1N1), which is a mutation in the framework of the NA.

Despite advances in our understanding of some viruses, we generally know very little about the specific molecular changes that allow many viruses to overcome known barriers (Webby et al., 2004). Therefore, new studies are investigating the molecular mechanisms that allow a virus to become drug resistant. One example is a computer simulation study of the union and disunion of oseltamivir with NA, and the effects that might be caused by known mutations (Le et al., 2010).

These studies rely on the recent elucidation of crystal structures of both wild-type and mutant H5N1 NAs, which have opened the way for the investigation of drug resistance mechanisms and structure-based drug design at the atomic level. These crystal structures represent a frozen-in-time snapshot of a possible conformation during drug-protein interaction. However, drug binding is a dynamic process and computational studies using crystal structures as starting points can shed light on how protein flexibility and point mutations influence drug–protein endpoint interactions (Le et al., 2010).

The major finding with this approach is the discovery that the union of oseltamivir to the NA occurs through charged groups on the protein surface. These interactions through a charged pathway have proved to be very important in the process of interaction between oseltamivir and the NA, because they facilitate binding or stabilize it. It is now known that many mutations prevent or weaken key interactions that allow the union or stabilization between oseltamivir and the NA enzyme (Fig. 5) (Itstein, 2007; Le et al., 2010; Eun-Sun et al., 2011).

This finding opens up a whole new landscape for drug design. Chance and virological screening will continue to play a part in the discovery of new antivirals, but knowledge of viral gene structure and protein functioning is leading to a new generation of drugs (Collier et al., 2006). The insights gained so far should assist in the rational design of NAIs and other types of drugs, while avoiding drug resistance (Le et al., 2010).

Given the results of simulations of the interaction between oseltamivir and the NA enzyme, the next generation of drugs for the treatment of influenza will probably consist of inhibitors with positively charged groups, because these compounds have potential as antiviral therapeutics, although the strain specificity of these inhibitors must be resolved (Eun-Sun et al., 2011).

Alternative drug discovery targets, such as RNA polymerase, HA, or the M2 ion channel protein, which are essential components of the viral life cycle, are also under investigation. This research may lead to a combination therapy approach or the use of sialidase inhibitors alone, to provide new classes of anti-influenza drugs. Combination therapy might also reduce the potential of resistance development (Izstein, 2007).

It is also very important to limit the prescription of antivirals in order to reduce the possibility of the emergence of drug-resistant strains and thus maintain the ability of antivirals to treat high-risk patients (Le et al., 2010).

Finally, a precise diagnosis of influenza A is very important, including the identification of resistant strains and point-of-care pathogen genotyping, because this information can help to identify the appropriate antiviral in each situation. Some studies have indicated that genomics technology, bioinformatics, and geographical information systems can be immediately applicable to help in the treatment of infectious diseases. In addition to data collection, analyses are useful for turning raw data into prospective public health intelligence on drug resistance in a specific region, and into a form that provides easy visualization (Janies et al., 2010).

Is very important a precise diagnosis of influenza A, including the identification of resistant strains and point-of-care pathogen genotyping, because this information can help to identify the appropriate antiviral in each situation. Some studies have indicated that genomics technology, bioinformatics, and geographical information systems can be immediately applicable to help in the treatment of infectious diseases. In addition to data collection, analyses are useful for turning raw data into prospective public health intelligence on drug resistance in a specific region, and into a form that provides easy visualization

3. HIV drug-resistance related point mutations

3.1 Introduction

The advent of highly active antiretroviral therapy [HAART] has changed the natural history of human immunodeficiency virus infection [HIV], extending the survival of carrier subjects and reducing progression to human immunodeficiency syndrome. The success in the combination of antiretroviral treatments to suppress viral replication depends on several factors, including the host, the virus and medications. Nowadays, therapeutic options against HIV-1 include more than 20 drugs, classified according to their action mechanism and targeted to four different points of the viral replication cycle: the entry of the virus into the cell, inverse transcription, the integration of viral genetic material into the cell nucleus, and maturation of virions [Fig. 5] (Altman et al., 2007). Since its introduction, ARV therapy showed marginal and short-duration benefits when drug combinations did not achieve a satisfactory control of viral replication. This phenomenon has been associated with the high replicative capacity of the virus and the high error rate in the transcription of its genetic material, but also with a Darwinian phenomenon of quasispecies selection and accumulation exhibiting resistance due to the presence of specific mutations resulting from pharmacological pressure and suboptimal viral suppression under a treatment scheme (Johnson et al, 2010). That is to say, both the preexistence and selection of resistance mutations are important failure predictors for an ARV therapy (Hatano, 2006; Perno, 2002; Poveda, 2010; Shafer, 2006).

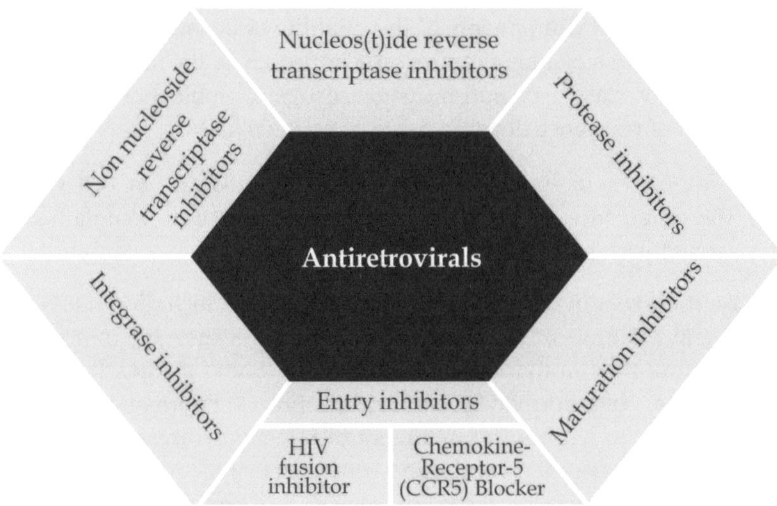

Fig. 5. Antirretroviral drug classes

Retroviruses use the reverse transcription of viral RNA into linear double-stranded DNA, with subsequent integration into the host genome. The characteristic enzyme used for this process is known as reverse transcriptase (Arnold & Sarafianos, 2008). This enzyme is error-prone; with the massive turnover of virions in the infected host, these errors accumulate in the viral DNA, accounting for the relatively high mutability of HIV-1. Retroviruses have the survival advantage of great genetic diversity, and latency, because the DNA provirus is integrated into the chromosomal DNA of the infected cell (Reitz & Gallo, 2009).

3.2 HIV biology and resistance point mutations

Pathogenic human retroviruses include lentiviruses [HIV-1 and -2] and oncoviruses [HTLV-I and –II]. Current knowledge places retroviral infection of humans as zoonoses that originated in primate-to-human species-jumping events. For HIV-1 and HIV-2, these events occurred in Central and West Africa. All retroviral genomes consist of at least 4 *genes: gag, pro, pol and env*. The *gag* gene encodes the major structural polyprotein Gag. The viral protease is encoded by the *pro* gene and is responsible for facilitating the maturation of viral particles. Products of the *pol* gene include reverse transcriptase, RNase H and integrase, while *env* is responsible for the viral surface glycoprotein and transmembrane proteins that mediate cellular receptor binding and membrane fusion. In addition, complex retroviruses such as HIV-1 encode accessory proteins that enhance replication and infectivity (Reitz & Gallo, 2009).

Resistance to ARV therapy implies the selection and accumulation of mutations in one or more HIV genes [mainly *gag* and *pol*], which reduce the antiviral activity of one or more ARV drugs. It can be "primary" when occurring in individuals not previously and directly exposed to these drugs and whose transmission of resistant strains is presumed or "secondary" when there is history of previous exposure. Interestingly, the frequency in the selection and transmission of mutations conferring resistance can also vary according to the adaptive and reproductive capacity preserved by the mutant virus in a given environment [viral fitness], and to the greater or lower ability of the drug to retain its antiviral activity despite the presence of specific resistance mutations [genetic barrier] (De Luca, 2006).Table 1 shows the mutations suggested for the monitoring of resistance transmitted to the HIV by the World Health Organization [WHO] for the three primary classes of antiretroviral treatment (Bennett et al, 2009).

NRTI	**M41L, K65R, D67N/G/E, T69D/Ins, K70R/E, L74V/I, V75M/T/A/S, F77L, Y115F, F116Y, Q151M, M184V/I, L210W, T215Y/F/I/S/C/D/V/E, K219Q/E/N/R**
NNRTI	L100I, K101E/P, K103N/S, V106M/A, V179F, Y181C/I/V, Y188L/H/C, G190A/S/E, P225H, M230L
PI	L23I, L24I, D30N, V32I, M46I/L, I47V/A, G48V/M, I50V/L, F53L/Y, I54V/L/M/A/T/S, G73S/T/C/A, L76V, V82A/T/F/S/C/M/L, N83D, I84V/A/C, I85V, N88D/S, L90M

Table 1. List of mutations for surveillance of transmitted drug resistant HIV, World Health Organization 2009.NRTI: nucleotide reverse transcriptase inhibitors, NNRTI: non-nucleotide reverse transcriptase inhibitors, PI: protease inhibitors

3.3 Impact of resistance on clinical response to antiretroviral treatment

The main purpose of antiretroviral therapy is to achieve a sustained control of HIV replication. Virological failure is defined as the inability to achieve or maintain the viral replication suppression at levels below 200 copies/mL.

An incomplete virological response refers to the presence of two consecutive readings of HIV RNA higher than 200 copies/mL in plasma, after 24 weeks on continuous ARV therapy; and viral rebound is a detectable viral load [VL] higher than 200 copies/mL after achieving viral suppression (Department of Health and Human Services [DHHS], 2011). Usually, once the ARV therapy is initiated and constantly administered, the HIV VL in plasma is quantitatively reduced in two phases, a fast initial phase during the first weeks, and a slower late phase that can extend up to 6 months. There are multiple factors involved in the viral response to the ARV therapy, such as evolutionary issues of the virus (Esté & Telenti, 2009; Parkin et al, 2005; Rivas et al, 2006), host immunology (Gragsted et al, 2004; Telenti & Goldstein, 2006), compliance of the individual with the treatment (Muller et al, 2011; Protopopescu et al, 2009), pharmacogenetics (Clifford et al, 2009; Telenti et al, 2002), pharmacologic interactions (Zhu et al, 2001), and the occurrence of comorbidities. Table 2 shows examples for the abovementioned issues.

Item	Example
Virus	- In some non-B strains, the accumulation of certain polymorphisms and secondary mutations in the enzyme protease has been associated with a reduction in susceptibility in vitro to protease inhibitors, even in absence of primary mutations. - Primary mutations associated with resistance are the same regardless the viral group and subtype. However, some clearly appear more frequently in some groups or subtypes than in others.
Host immunity	- The adequate response to antiretroviral treatment is inversely proportional to the number of basal CD4+ cells.
Adherence to treatment	- The satisfactory virological suppression depends on the adherence to the antiretroviral treatment. On the other hand, social factors such as stigmatization, the fear of knowing the diagnosis and the attitude of health providers to the patient can also affect response to treatment.
Pharmacogenetics	- Study ACTG 5097s found that clearance of efavirenz from the body was increased by 32% in non-hispanic whites compared to blacks and Hispanics. There was a slight association between higher blood levels of efavirenz and study discontinuations. In a subsequent study, the authors found that a single nucleotide polymorphism (SNP) that changed the DNA code from a "G" to a "T" at position 516 of the gene for the CYP2B6 metabolic enzyme was associated with slower clearance of efavirenz, higher blood levels of the drug and more CNS-related side effects.
Pharmacologic interactions	- The pharmacologic interaction between antiretroviral drugs and other drugs can cause a reduction in the minimum and maximum levels, as well as the area under the curve of one or more antiretroviral agents. This can be associated with the exposure to suboptimal doses of these agents and treatment failures (atazanavir-omeprazole, protease inhibitors-rifamycins). - Additionally, the pharmacologic interaction between certain drugs can also increase the level of co-administered agents generating adverse effects to such drugs (protease inhibitors-phosphodiesterase inhibitors, protease inhibitors-statins).
Comorbidity	- The association between the HIV and other pathologies is capable to deteriorate the response to treatment (e.g. absorption issues at intestinal level), or to increase adverse effects of the antiretroviral agent. This is the case of co-infection with the Hepatitis B and C viruses.

Table 2. Determinants of response to antiretroviral treatment.

Blips are transient episodes of low-level viremia [from 51 a 1,000 copies/mL]. Some of their causes are: sample processing artefacts due to the use of collection tubes with PPT™ versus ethylenediaminetetraacetic acid [EDTA], frequency of 70% and 5.4%, respectively (Lee et al, 2006); immunizations, acute infections or viral release from cell compartments known as "reservoirs". A recent report determined that annual frequency of a viral rebound was 85%, two events in 13% and three or more in 1.9%, defined as a VL detectable between 50 and 400 copies/mL in previously undetectable in individuals. The persistent rebounds (identified in two or more readings) behaved as an independent risk factor increasing from 1.4 to 2.18 times the relative risk of viral failure compared to individuals with transient viremia [blips] (Geretti et al, 2008).

On the other hand, it has been found that the incidence of persistent low-level viremia is more frequent than high-level viremia when evaluating the virological response in subjects with HIV infection and HAART, reporting incidences of 29% and 6.7% for readings > 50 copies/mL and > 1,000 copies/mL, respectively (Van Sighem et al, 2008). Likewise, the UK-CHIC study reported that the cumulative risk for resistance mutation detection for two of the three primary classes of ARV therapy within a population increases in time, passing from 6% to 14% and 20% after a follow-up period of 2, 4, and 6 years for each period (Phillips et al, 2005).

3.4 Resistance assessment

There are, at least, four types of assays to identify the resistance or viral susceptibility to drugs available in clinical practice: genotype, actual phenotype, virtual phenotype, and viral tropism tests.

3.4.1 Genotype

Standard genotypic assays are primarily based on the amplification of the inverse transcriptase and protease genes in order to identify resistance mutations already known for their ability to reduce viral susceptibility to certain drugs. Generally, these studies only provide data on the substitutions associated with resistance to NRTI, NNRTI and protease inhibitors [PI]. Usually, these substitutions reduce the susceptibility to the drug compared with that of the wild-type viral strain through changes in the molecular target of the therapy or in other viral proteins that indirectly interfere with the drug activity. There are also resistance detection tests for fusion inhibitors [FI] and INI, but their access is more limited and they are not performed routinely (Fransenet al, 2009; Long et al, 2009; Perno & Mertoli, 2006).

Genotype is indicated in the following situations:

- Confirmed viral failure and VL > 1,000 copies/mL [considered in individuals with VL > 500 but < 1,000 copies/mL if there are available special techniques to easy ultrasensitive amplification].
- Suboptimal response to treatment [e.g. fall of HIV VL < 1 log^{10} during the first four weeks of therapy].
- ARV therapy naive subjects in whom transmitted resistance is suspected.

- In populations with prevalence of transmitted resistance > 5% in chronically ill individuals, its execution is recommended on all the cases at diagnosis, and its repetition before initiating the HAART when the decision is to change the treatment (Hirsch et al, 2003).

The search of resistance mutations for FI and INI must be performed in subjects with virological failure to these drugs. However, in the absence of an adequate compliance, the lack of pharmacologic pressure reduces the possibility of identifying situations associated with resistance [due to the predominance of the wild-type strain]. This is more frequent in individuals with increased HIV VLs [more than 100,000 copies/mL], notwithstanding the type of ARV scheme administered (Geretti et al, 2008).

On the other hand, ultrasensitive genotypic tests have a very high probability to identify resistance mutations [even in individuals with VL < 500 copies/mL], although their clinical utility has not been reliably demonstrated. This is explained because at present it is considered that the resistant mutant viral strain must represent at least 2-3% of the existing population in order to have an impact on the response to a given drug, and the diagnostic sensitivity of such tests is higher than this cut-off [up to 0.1%] (Mackie et al, 2004; Villahermosa et al, 2000). There are two commercial methods approved by the Food and Drug Administration [FDA] and the European CE Notified Bodies: the TruGene HIV-1 genotypic assay and the ViroSeq assay. For both, the sequence is determined by amplifying the interest genes using the reverse transcriptase-polymerase chain reaction [RT-PCR] with primers in conserved regions capable to align most M strains of HIV-1. The mutations that have been associated with a reduction in the antiretroviral susceptibility as of today are included in Table 3.

3.4.2 Phenotype

This test measures the ability of the virus to multiply under different ARV concentrations in comparison with a wild-type reference strain. It is based in the HIV-1 isolation in plasma or serum mononuclear cells, and the measurement of its susceptibility to ARV drugs *in vitro*. This is performed through the insertion of genetic sequences of reverse transcriptase and protease obtained from the HIV under study [recently also from integrase and viral envelope], which are inserted into a laboratory viral clone. Thus, the recombinant HIV carries the genetic characteristics of the test virus, regarding the genes involved in resistance expression. The viral strain is effectively replicated *in vitro* and exposed to different ARV drug concentrations. That is how the mean inhibitory concentration [IC50] is calculated, which represents the drug concentration capable of limiting the viral replication by 50%. The ratio difference between IC50 of the HIV under study and the reference strain is reported as the change in the IC50 ratio [fold-change] and the significance is determined according to clinical or biological cut-off values (Perno & Mertoli, 2006).

In a few words, the fold-change represents the similarity or loss of partial or total susceptibility of the test strain versus the reference strain. It is important, however, to point out that there are multiple technical difficulties for these procedures and that the integrated proviruses are not necessarily representative of the circulating virus, but they can constitute stored viruses or residual, free virions in plasma.

	Antiretroviral	Mutations potentially associated with high-level resistance	Other significant mutations
Nucleotide reverse transcriptase inhibitors	Abacavir	K65R, L74V	Y115F, M184V, TAMs, Q151M complex
	Didanosine	K65R, L74V	TAMs, Q151M complex
	Emtricitabine, Lamivudine	M184V	K65R, Q151M complex
	Stavudine	M41L, K65R, D67N, L210W, T215 Y/F, K219Q/E	Q151M complex
	Tenofovir	K65R	K70E, TAMs
	Zidovudine	M41L, D67N, K70R, L210W, T215Y/F, K219Q/E	Q151M complex
Non-nucleotide reverse transcriptase inhibitors	Efavirenz	L100I, K103N/S/T, V106A/M, Y181C/I/V/S, Y188L, G190A/C/E/Q/S/V/T, P225H, M230L	K103I/P, V108I, V179F, Y181S, Y188C/H, F227C
	Nevirapine	L100I, K103N/S/T, V106A/M, V179F, Y181C/I/V/S, Y188C/L, G190A/C/E/Q/S/V/T, F227C, M230L, K238T/N, Y318F	K101E/P, V108I, Y188H
	Etravirine	Y181I/V, E138K	V90I, A98G, L100I, K101E/H/P, V106I, E138A, V179D/F/T, Y181C/I/V, G190S/A, M230L
Protease inhibitors	Atazanavir	I50L, G73S/T, I84A/C/V, N88S, L90M	G48V/M, F53L, I54A/L/M/T/V, V82A/F/S/T, N88D
	Darunavir	I50V/I	V11I, V32I, L33F, I47A/V, I54L/M, G73S/T, L76V, V82A/F/S/T,I84A/C/V, L90M
	Fosamprenavir	V32I, I47A/V, I50V, I54L/M, L76V, I84A/C/V, L90M	L24I, L33F, M46I/L, I54L/T/V, G73ST, V82A/F/S/T
	Indinavir	V82A/F/S/T, I84A/C/V	L24I, V32I, M46I/L, I47V, F53L, I54A/L/M/T/V, G73S/T, L76V, N88S, L90M
	Lopinavir	I47A	L10F/I/R/V, K20M/N/R,L24I, V32I, L33F, M36I, M46I/L, I47V,G48M/V, I50V, I54A/L/M/T/V, L76V, V82A/F/S/T, I84A/C/V, L90M
	Nelfinavir	L23I, D30N, M46I/L, G48M/V, I84A/C/V,	L24I, L33F, I47/V, F53L, I54A/L/M/T/V, G73S/T,

	Antiretroviral	Mutations potentially associated with high-level resistance	Other significant mutations
		N88D/S, L90M	V82A/F/S/T
	Saquinavir	G48M/V, L90M	L24I, F53L, I54A/L/M/T/V, G73S/T, V82A/T, I84A/C/V, N88S
	Tipranavir	V82L/T, N83D	L10V,V32I, L33F, M36I/L/V,K43T,M46I/L, I47V, I54A/M/V, Q58E, T74P, V82A/F/S, I84A/C/V, L89I/M/V, L90M
Fusion inhibitors	Enfuvirtide	G36D/S, I37V, V38A/M/E, Q39R, Q40H, N42T, N43D	
Integrase inhibitors	Raltegravir	Q148R	E92Q, E138A/K,G140A/S,Y143R/H/C, Q148H/K, N155H

Table 3. Overview of drug resistance mutations in HIV-1. TAMs: Thymidine analog mutations (M41L, D67N, K70R, L210W, T215Y/F and K219Q/E). Q151M complex: A62V, V75I, F77L, F116Y and Q151M.

Phenotype is considered as supplementary to genotype, and it is reserved for cases where a complex mutation pattern is suspected, in which resistance-associated mutations and hypersusceptibility have been selected, and that specially involves multiple PI o more than two classes of ARV drugs. Virco and Monogram laboratories currently offer the technology to develop commercial phenotypes.

3.4.3 Virtual phenotype

Virtual phenotype combines the knowledge generated by both resistance assays: genotype and phenotype. In the virtual phenotype, the investigational virus is sequenced and the identified changes are compared with the information of a great database that contains genotype-phenotype paired data for viruses previously sequenced. That is how the fold-change of a HIV under study is inferred, calculated based on the mean of all the results of the actual phenotype obtained for virus existing in the database and with genotypic characteristics similar to those of the test virus. Generally, concordance of results obtained for NNRTIs and PIs is very good, although that observed with NRTIs is very lower. This is laid to a poor representation of certain genotypes in the system and it is expected that this issue be corrected (Mazzotta et al, 2003; Torti et al, 2003; Loutfy et al, 2004). Virtual phenotype shares the same advantages and disadvantages as that the genotype. The indications, advantages and disadvantages of the viral genotype and phenotype are included in Table 4.

3.4.4 Tropism test

The assay for the identification of the type of tropism to co-receptors that the HIV exhibits [CCR5 or CXCR4] must be performed when considering the initiation of a co-receptor antagonist and there is viral replication. The purpose of these tests is to identify the receptor molecules CCR5 and CXCR4 in the host cell membranes. Phenotypic and, to a lesser extent, genotypic studies have been developed to determine co-receptors of the dominant viral population in each case.

Viruses can be monotropic [CCR5 or CXCR4], or can exhibit a mixed tropism or D/M dual tropism. Prevalence of tropic CCR5 viruses in heavily treated individuals or with CD4 < 100 cells/mm^3 has been reported of 50% (Hunt et al, 2006; Wilkin, 2007). Currently, Trofile [Monogram Biosciences, Inc.], Phenoscript assay, [VIRalliance], Xtrack C/Phen X-R [inPheno] and Virco, provide phenotypic tropism assays.

This study is expensive and requires an average time of 3-4 weeks to have the results. Detection of minority variants is the primary limitation and varies from 1% to 10%, depending on the assay used. Likewise, it is difficult to establish the cut-off points for the minority species X4, and this is affected by multiple variables such as sample quality, collected volume, HIV-1 VL, detection limits and and PCR variations (Braun & Wiesmann, 2007).

3.4.5 Genotropism test

Several bioinformatic tools have been proposed to predict co-receptor usage by interpretation of genotypic data—mainly through the use of V3 loop sequencing. Nevertheless, there are important differences between algorithms in detection sensitivity of X4 isolates. In one report, the most sensitive bioinformatic tools were PSSM and Geno2pheno, with sensitivities of about 60%. Moreover, more studies will be needed to further the study on the prediction of co-receptor use in HIV-1 non-B subtypes and throughout different stages of the HIV infection (Recordon-Pinson et al, 2010; Coakley et al, 2011).

Changes on the treatment supported in resistance assays have a greater potential impact on the virological response, especially when an expert in the interpretation of the results is available (Palella et al, 2009; Sax et al, 2005; Tural et al, 2002).

3.4.6 Integration of the rescue scheme

There is a high risk that every new rescue may offer less possibilities to maintain a long-term virological control as a result of stored mutations underestimated when implementing the rescue treatment. Currently, there are interpretation algorithms facilitating the physician to select the ARV therapy, to predict the activity of a drug or its potential virological response. There are computing platforms that function through different methodological rules and which are populated from the results of clinical studies or *in vitro* assays concentrated in big databases. Some of the best known are the ANRS HIV-1 genotypic drug resistance interpretation algorithms and the Stanford HIV Drug Resistance database [both with on-line free access].

The selection of point mutations in HIV infection is a complex event, frequency and causes of which vary notoriously depending on different factors. Some of such factors are associated to the socioeconomic characteristics of the studied population, the antiretroviral drugs used, prevalent viral groups and subtypes, etc. These mutations have a great relevance in HIV infection because of their negative impact on the response to antiretroviral treatment, which induces a suboptimal or transient viral suppression, immune deterioration and clinical progression to the acquired immune deficiency syndrome.

	Genotype	Phenotype
Advantages	- It is the most inexpensive resistance assay. - Detects changes in the viral genome associated with resistance faster than the phenotypic assay. - Technically less complex. - Results are obtained in 1-2 weeks. - Preferred assay to guide rescue strategies in naïve individuals, with suboptimal response, or after the first and second HAART failure. - The occurrence of mutations may precede to the development of phenotypic resistance.	- Higher sensitivity to identify viral susceptibility to PIs. - Direct and quantitative measurement of viral susceptibility. - It is capable to measure the accumulated impact of different viral mutations (resistance and hypersusceptibility mutations).
Disadvantages	- Qualitative result. - Low sensitivity to detect resistance mutations in patients with viral replication lower than 1000 copies/mL. - Indirect measurement of resistance. - Incapable to quantify the interaction between mutations. - It cannot be used to detect the residual activity of some drugs. - Its capacity to detect resistance mutations falls drastically in absence of pharmacologic pressure; it has to be performed preferably before discontinuing the HAART and not beyond the firsts 4 weeks after its discontinuation. - Low sensitivity to identify resistance in viral strains with representativeness lower than 20% of the circulating population (minorities). - Requires specific training for its interpretation. - It cannot be used to identify resistance mutations that have not been previously associated with loss of viral susceptibility.	- Supplementary to genotype. - Very limited availability. - Expensive. - *In vitro* assay. - The results are available in 3-4 weeks when performed through automated assays. - Interpretation is complex and not completely standardized. - Lack of information clinically correlating to fold-change of some available ARV with suboptimal response or viral failure. - Its capacity to detect resistance mutations falls drastically in absence of pharmacologic pressure; it has to be performed preferably before discontinuing the HAART and not beyond the firsts 4 weeks after its discontinuation. - Low sensitivity to identify resistance in viral strains with representativeness lower than 10% or 20% of the circulating population (minorities). - Mutant viral strains with higher viral fitness may reduce the identification of strains with superior resistance profile but lower replicative capacity. - Requires specific training for its interpretation.

Table 4. Resistance tests, genotype and phenotype: advantages and disadvantages.

The prescription of new agents with better pharmacologic profiles and a higher genetic barrier does not replace the need of a comprehensive approach, a narrow clinical follow-up and an appropriate diagnosis of the viral failure. There are still multiple subjects for basic and clinical investigation, such as to specify the role of minority populations who express resistance to antiretroviral drugs in the clinical settings, to evaluate the importance of resistance assays and genotropism tests in proviral DNA, to implement strategies optimizing the pharmacokinetics and pharmacodynamics of the current antiretroviral agents, to identify new agents with a higher genetic barrier and with different action mechanisms. All of the above with the main objective of extending the productive life of subjects infected with the HIV.

4. Point mutations and herpes virus resistance to antivirals

4.1 Introduction

Herpesviruses comprise a large group of enveloped DNA-containing viruses infecting a wide range of vertebrate hosts, such as humans, horses, cattle, mice, pigs, chickens, turtles, lizards, fish, and even in some invertebrates, such as oyster. According to the International Committee on Taxonomy of Viruses, these viruses are classified in the Order *Herpesvirales,* with three families: *Alloherpesviridae, Herpesviridae* and *Malacoherpesviridae.* The human herpesviruses are included in the *Herpesviridae* family (Fauquet et al., 2005). All of them share four biological properties: 1) they express a large number of enzymes involved in metabolism of nucleic acid (e.g. thymidine kinase), DNA synthesis (e.g. DNA helicase/primase) and processing of proteins (e.g. protein kinase). 2) The synthesis of viral genomes and assembly of capsids occurs in the nucleus. 3) The success of herpes virus infection depends upon viral inhibition of several cell functions, such as turning off host protein synthesis, inhibition of mRNA splicing, blocking presentation of antigenic peptides on the cell surface and apoptosis. 4) They have the ability to hide their bare, circularized genome in the nucleus of lymphocytes and neuron cells and return to productive infection months, even years later. These latent herpes virus infections are often benign, but can be devastating especially to newborns and immuno-suppressed individuals (Roizman et al., 2007).

Human herpeviruses infections are a leading cause of human viral disease, second only to influenza and cold viruses (Murray et al., 2009). There are eight known human herpesviruses (Table 5): herpes simplex virus 1 (HSV-1), herpes simplex virus 2 (HSV-2), varicella-zoster virus (VZV), Epstein-Barr virus (EBV), human cytomegalovirus (HCMV), human herpesvirus 6 (HHV-6), human herpesvirus 7 (HHV-7), and Kaposi's sarcoma-associated herpesvirus (KSHV) (Pellett & Roizman, 2007). Herpesvirus infections are endemic and sexual contact is a significant method of transmission for HSV-1, HSV-2, also HCMV and likely KSHV. The increasing prevalence of genital herpes and corresponding rise of neonatal infection and the implication of EBV and KSHV as cofactors in human cancers are of great public health concern (Anzivino et al, 2009, Shiley & Blumberg, 2011). But also, the association between herpes genital and susceptibility to HIV infection has clearly emerged in the last years (Van de Perre et al., 20008).

Table 6 shows a summary of the most common anti-herpes drugs and their inhibition mechanism. It is important to mention that antiviral therapy is available for HSV, VZV and HMCV infections. Therefore the other herpesviruses infections will not be discussed further.

Virus	Main disease(s)
Herpes simplex virus type 1 or human herpesvirus 1 (HSV-1 or HHV-1) Herpes simplex virus type 2or human herpesvirus 2 (HSV-2 or HHV-2)	The causal agents of oral and genital herpes, respectively (Roizman et al., 2007).
Varicella-zoster virus or human herpesvirus 3 (VZV or HHV-3)	The causal agent of chickenpox and shingles (Cohen et al., 2007).
Human cytomegalovirus or human herpesvirus 5 (HCMV or HHV-5)	The major cause of infectious morbidity and mortality in immunocompromised individuals and developing fetuses, and HCMV-caused disease is called cytomegalovirus inclusion disease (CID) (Mocarski et al., 2007).
Human herpes virus 6A (HHV6A) Human herpesvirus 6B (HHV-6B)	Associated with roseola (Yamanishi et al., 2007).
Human herpesvirus (HHV-7)	HHV-7 has not been definitively documented to cause a specific disease and has been associated to pityriasis rosea (Blauvelt, 2001)
Epstein-Barr virus or human herpesvirus 4 (EBV or HHV-4)	Associated with several diseases, most notably infectious mononucleosis (colloquially known as *mono* or *kissing disease*) and Burkitt's lymphoma (Rickinson & Kief, 2007).
Kaposi's sarcoma herpesvirus or Human herpesvirus 8 (KSHV or HHV-8)	Associated with Kaposi's sarcoma , but KSHV can also cause B-cell lymphoma (Ganem 2007)

Table 5. Human herpesviruses and their main diseases

EBV is a gammaherpes virus responsible for several clinical entities, is the causative agent of infectious mononucleosis, Burkitt lymphoma, and nasopharyngeal carcinoma, and accounts for 90% of the cases of posttransplant lymphoproliferative disorder (PTLD). The cornerstone of therapy is decreasing the level of immunosuppression whenever is possible. Some antiviral drugs as acyclovir and ganciclovir have been used as a prophylactic measure but their efficacy has not showed clear results. HHV-6, the causative agent of the common childhood disease roseola infantum (exanthema sabitum), has received attention in the past several years as an opportunistic infection in the posttransplant population.

4.2 Antiviral agents for herpesvirus infections

In vitro data has shown that HHV-6 is inhibited by ganciclovir, foscarnet, and cidofovir, but no prospective clinical trials have evaluated the use of antiviral-drugs in the treatment of HHV-6 associated disease.

KSHV is responsible for the malignant entities of Kaposi sarcoma (KS) and primary effusion lymphoma (PEL), as well as some forms of multicentric Castleman disease (MCD). As the case with EBV-associated PTLD, reduction in immunosuppression is the first-line therapy for KS and is often curative (Shiley & Blumberg, 2011). Herpesvirus primary infections are followed by latency and subsequent periodic reactivations in most patients. Both primary and recurrent infections may require therapeutic or prophylactic interventions. Individuals at particularly high risk of developing severe consequences from HSV infection include immunocompromised hosts, such as transplant recipients, patients who receive cytotoxic drugs, HIV-infected individuals, and pregnant women and their newborns.

Drug	Chemical formula[A]	Name[A]	Antiviral mechanism	Active against	Uses
Idoxuridine	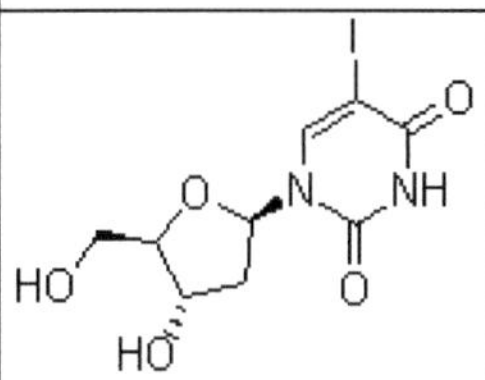	2'-Deoxy-5-iodouridine CAS # 54-42-2	Thymidine analog	HSV-1, HSV-2, VZV, and CMV	Limited to topical ophthalmic treatment of herpes simplex keratoco-njunctivitis.
Vidarabine (adenine arabinoside, ara-A)	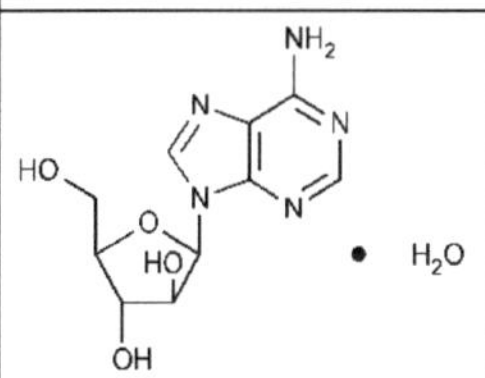	9-beta-D-Arabinosyla-denine CAS # 5536-17-4	Adenine arabinoside	HSV-1, HSV-2	Ophthalmic preparations: Effective for acute keratoco-njunctivitis and recurrent superficial keratitis.
Trifluridine (trifluorothym idine)	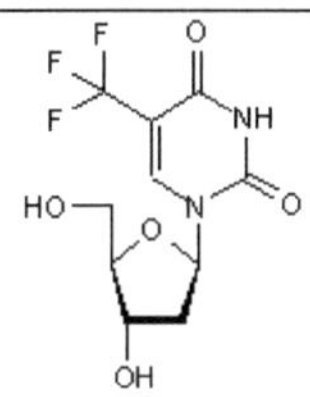	2'-Deoxy-5-(trifluoromethy l) uridine CAS # 70-00-8	Thymidine analog	HSV-1, HSV-2	Topical: Ophthalmic treatment of primary keratoco-njunctivitis and recurrent keratitis or ulceration caused by herpes simplex 1 and 2.
Acyclovir	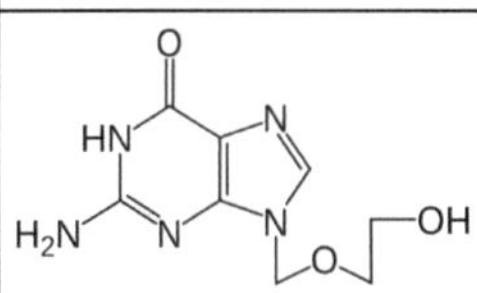	9-[(2-Hydroxyethoxy)methyl]guanine CAS # 59277-89-3	Guanosine analog	HSV-1, HSV-2, VZV, and EBV Minimal activity against CMV	Oral or IV (IV indicated when a higher serum drug level is required, as for herpes simplex encephalitis).
Ganciclovir	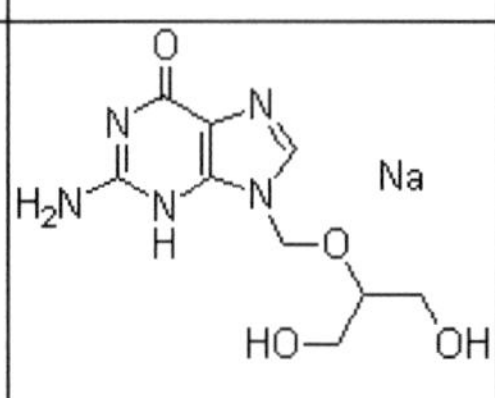	2-Amino-1,9-dihydro-9-[[2-hydroxy-1-(hydroxymethyl)ethoxy]methyl]-6H-purin-6-one sodium salt CAS #107910-75-8	Guanosine analog	A homologue of acyclovir,	Effective in the treatment of HCMV. It inhibits all the herpesviruses and transformation of normal cord-blood

Drug	Chemical formula[A]	Name[A]	Antiviral mechanism	Active against	Uses
					lymphocytes by EBV.
Famciclovir	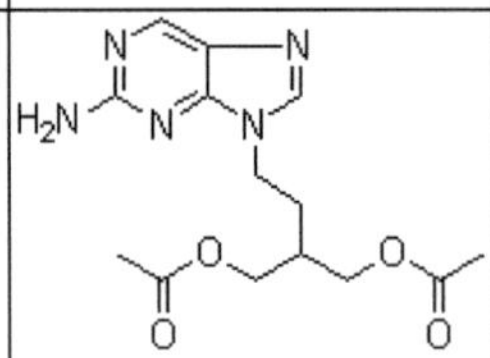	2-[(acetyloxy) methyl]-4-(2-amino-9H-purin-9-yl)butyl acetate CAS # 104227-87-4	Guanosine analog	Antiviral spectrum similar to acyclovir	As effective as acyclovir for genital herpes and herpes zoster and more bioavailable after oral administration.
Penciclovir	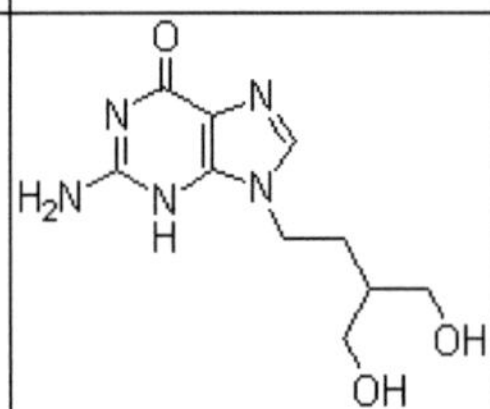	2-amino-9-[4-hydroxy-3-(hydroxymethyl)butyl]-6,9-dihydro-3*H*-purin-6-one CAS # 39809-25-1	Guanosine analog	Potent activity against CMV (inhibits CMV protein synthesis)	Intravitreal injection: For patients with HIV infection and CMV retinitis that is resistant to other therapies
Valacyclovir	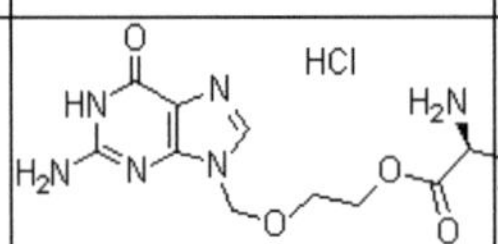	L-Valine 2-(guanin-9-ylmethoxy)ethyl ester CAS # 124832-26-4	Guanosine analog	HSV, VZV	Management of herpes simplex and herpes zoster (shingles). It is a prodrug, being converted *in vivo* to acyclovir.
Foscarnet	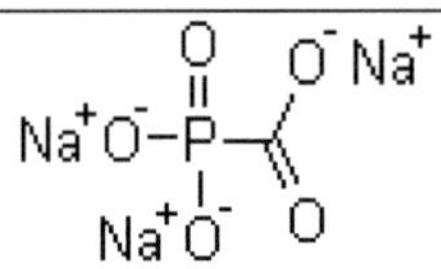	Trisodium phosphonoformate CAS # 63585-09-1	Pyrophosphate analog	EBV, HHV-8, HHV-6, HSV and VZV, CMV	Efficacy similar to that of ganciclovir for treating and delaying progression of CMV retinitis.
Cidofovir	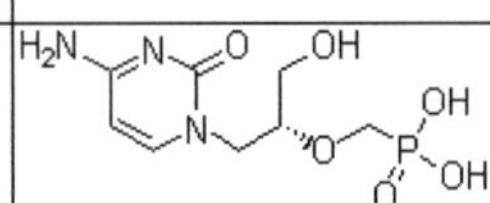	[1-(4-Amino-2-oxo-pyrimidin-1-yl)-3-hydroxy-propan-2-yl]oxymethylphosphonic acid CAS # 113852-37-2	Cytosine analog	HSV-1, HSV-2, VZV, CMV, EBV, KSHV,	Generally used for CMV, but use limited by renal toxicity.
Fomivirsen	5'-GCG TTT GCT CTT CTT CTT GCG-3'	Oligonucleotide with phosphorothioate linkages	The first antisense antiviral approved by the FDA	CMV	CMVretinitis in immunocompromised patients.

*Adapted from Porter & Kaplan, 2004; Shors, 2009; [A]Online Database of Chemicals from Around the World

Table 6. FDA-Approved antiherpesvirus drugs*.

4.2.1 Acyclovir and analogs

The first report detailing the selective antiviral activity of acyclovir against herpesviruses was published in 1977 (Elion et al., 1977). Penciclovir, a structurally related compound identified in the 1980s (Boyd et al., 1993), is also a potent and selective inhibitor of many human herpesviruses. Both compounds are analogues of the natural nucleoside deoxyguanosine. Oral prodrugs of penciclovir (famciclovir) and acyclovir (valaciclovir) were subsequently developed to improve their oral bioavailability (Beauchamp et al., 1992).

Acyclovir (ACV), valacyclovir and famciclovir have a similar mechanism of antiviral action against HSV (Corey et al., 2004; Mertz et al., 1997; Sacks, 2004). Acyclovir is a purine nucleoside analogue with inhibitory activity against HSV-1, HSV-2 and VZV. It has a highly selective inhibitory activity due to its affinity for the thymidine kinase enzyme (TK) encoded by HSV and VZV. The TK converts ACV into ACV-monophasphate, a nucleotide analogue. This monophosphate is further converted into diphosphate by cellular guanylate kinase and into triphosphate by a number of cellular enzymes. The ACV-triphosphate stops viral replication by competitive inhibition of viral DNA polymerase, incorporation and termination of the growing viral DNA chain, and inactivation of the viral DNA polymerase (GlaxoSmithKline).

4.2.2 Foscarnet

Foscarnet is a pyrophosphate analogue with activity against herpesviruses, human immunodeficiency virus (HIV), and other RNA and DNA viruses. Foscarnet and its analogues achieve their antiviral effects via inhibition of viral polymerases. Current evidence indicates that foscarnet interferes with exchange of pyrophosphate from deoxynucleoside triphosphate during viral replication by binding to a site on the herpesvirus DNA polymerase or HIV reverse transcriptase (Crumpacker, 1992).

4.2.3 Cidofovir

Cidofovir is a monophosphate nucleotide analogue of deoxycytidine (dCTP), which does not require a viral activation. After undergoing cellular phosphorylation, it competitively inhibits the incorporation of dCTP into viral DNA by viral DNA polymerase, disrupting further chain elongation (Lea & Bryson, 1996, De Clercq, 2004).

4.3 Herpesvirus-resistance to antiviral drugs

Treatment of HSV-infections with nucleoside analogs has been used for more than 20 years, and the isolation of drug-resistant virus from immunocompetent patients has been an infrequent event, from 0.1 to 0.7% (James et al., 2009; Kriesel et al., 2005; Reyes et al., 2003; Shin et al., 2003; Bacon et al., 2002; Blower et al., 1998; Christophers et al., 1998; Crumpacker et al., 1982). However, herpes-resistance to antiviral drugs is well established (7-14%) in imunocompromised patients (Griffiths, 2009; Chen et al., 2000; Levin et al., 2004; Safrin et al., 1994) and neonates (Levin et al., 2001; Nyquist et al., 1994; Oram et al., 2000). It has been found that the most significant risk factors to developing antiviral-resistance are the degree of immunosuppression and prolonged exposure to the antiviral agent (Levin et al., 2004). Nowadays, the drug-resistant viruses have become a very important issue, since the immunocompromissed population has been increasing around the world, either due to viral infections such as AIDS, or immunosuppression for cancer treatment, organ transplant, and chronic diseases treatment, among others. It's estimated that about 10 million people in the United States (3.6 percent of the population) are immunocompromised. But that's likely an underestimate because it only includes those with HIV/AIDS, organ transplant recipients, and cancer patients; but there's a sizable population that takes immunosuppressive drugs for other disorders such as rheumatoid arthritis and inflammatory bowel disease (Kahn, 2008).

4.3.1 Resistance to acyclovir

It is known that HSV has a low inherent propensity to develop mutations within its genome because its polymerase has a proof reading mechanism, therefore many replication cycles are required statistically to generate a virus that has resistance to ACV or similar drugs, and also due to the potency of these drugs to inhibit viral replication, the chance that this may occur in practice is decreased. Nevertheless, mutations of the viral Thymidine kinase (TK) and DNA polymerase (DNApol) can occur and both are intimately involved in mechanisms of resistance to acyclovir and penciclovir (Bacon et al., 2003; Boyd et al., 1993; Coen and Schaffer 1980; Schnipper & Crumpacker, 1980; Schmit & Boivin, 1999). Among ACV-resistant HSV, 95% are due to mutations in the TK gene and 5% in the DNA pol gene (Frobert et al., 2008), and resistance mutations are located mainly in catalytic or conserved domains of TK and DNA polymerase (Chibo et al., 2002; Gibs et al., 1988; Schmit & Boivin, 1999; Stránská et al., 2004; Sauerbrei et al., 2010).

4.3.1.1 Mutations in the TK gene

HSV TK is a 376-amino-acid protein, encoded by the UL23 gene. Known primarily as a TK, this enzyme is a wide spectrum nucleoside kinase capable of phosphorylating both purine and pyrimidine nucleosides and their analogues (Roizman et al., 2007). It contains an ATP binding site (codons 51 to 63), a nucleoside binding site (codons 168 to 176 for HSV-1 and 169 to 177 for HSV-2), and a highly conserved cysteine residue at position 336 for HSV-1 and 337 for HSV-2 (Balasubramaniam et al., 1990; Kit et al., 1983). TK utilizes ATP to phosphorylate deoxythymidine (dT) in the formation pathway of deoxythymidine triphosphate for DNA synthesis.

Three distinct classes of acyclovir resistant TK mutants have been identified:

1. TK-negative (TKN) mutants. They lack of TK activity. These phenotypes are the consequence of either single-base insertions/deletions occurring in guanosine (G) or cytidine (C) homopolymer repeats, leading to the shift of the translational reading frame of UL23 TK, or missense point mutations (Gaudreau et al., 1998; Morfin et al., 2000; Sarisky et al., 2001). Therefore, a deletion, insertion or point mutation, often within a hotspot, of the viral UL23 gene, originates a premature stop codon at one of several different places within the gene (Sasadeusz et al., 1997), resulting in a truncated TK protein, which does not have enzymatic activity (Gilbert et al., 2002; Summers et al., 1975). The TKN strains replicate very slowly because they lack the activity of the viral TK gene, which is required to synthetize deoxythymidine triphosphate for DNA synthesis, and these negative mutants have shown to be impaired in their pathogenicity, establishment of latency and low reactivation efficiency (Piret et al.,

2011). In immunocompetent individuals the immune response can rapidly dealt with the viral mutants before they can become clinically apparent (Coen, 1994). However, it is not always the case, it has been published that acyclovir-resistant HSV-2 mutants can be developed rapidly in neonatal infection and cause clinically significant disease, in spite of the *in vitro* decreased replication and attenuated virulence in an animal model showed by the viral strain (Oram, 2000).

2. TK-partial (TKP), express reduced levels of TK activity. Rare mutations can produce a virus which maintains the ability to reactivate as well as some virulence for an immunocompetent animal host, and some residual TK activity is present (Collins & Darby, 1991; Bacon et al., 2003; Coen, 1994).
3. TK-altered (TKA) mutants are substrate specificity mutants, which phosphorylate thymidine but not acyclovir and/or penciclovir, due to a specific mutation in the TK gene such, that it recognizes acyclovir/penciclovir poorly, but can still phosphorylate the natural nucleosides required by the virus for replication (Darby et al., 1981).

Approximately 95 to 96% of acyclovir-resistant HSV isolates are TK deficient (TKN or TKP), and the remaining isolates are usually TKA. It has been generally shown that acyclovir-resistant mutants do not appear to be capable of initiating a latent infection that can subsequently be reactivated (Pottage & Kessler, 1995). Gaudreu et al., 1998 analyzed 30 acyclovir-resistant HSV isolates from immunocopromissed patients, finding 17 TKN, 12TKP and 1TK undefined. Half of them had an insertion or deletion of one or two nucleotides, within homopolymers of G or C, which are considered resistance hot spots. The two longest homopolymers, one composed of 7 Gs and one of 6 Cs, are the sites of the most frequently reported mutations in ACV-resistant clinical isolates; other resistance cases are due to nucleotide substitutions usually in the conserved sites of the UL23 gene (Piret et al., 2011) (Figure 6)

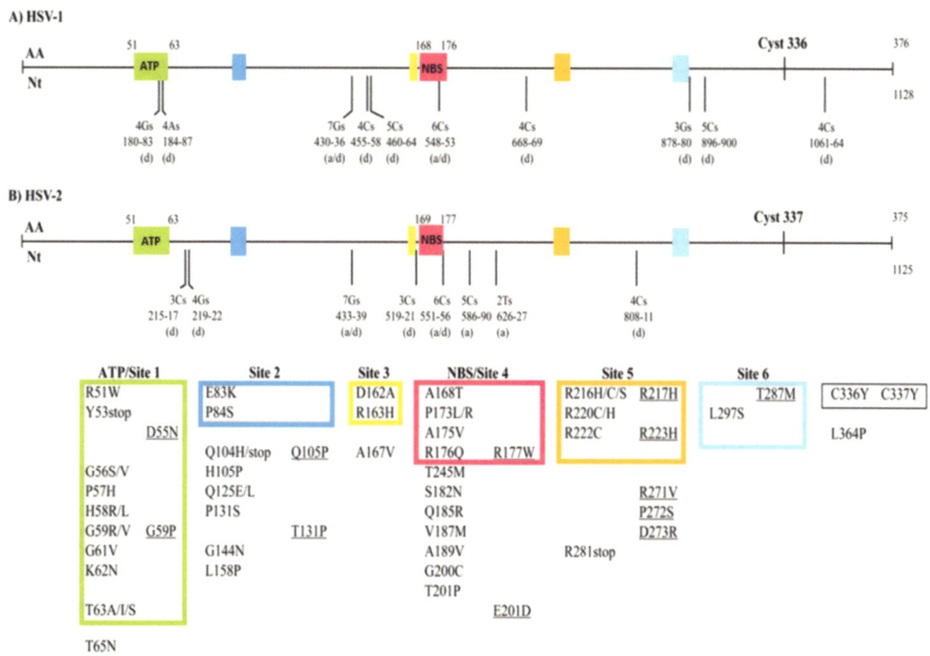

C

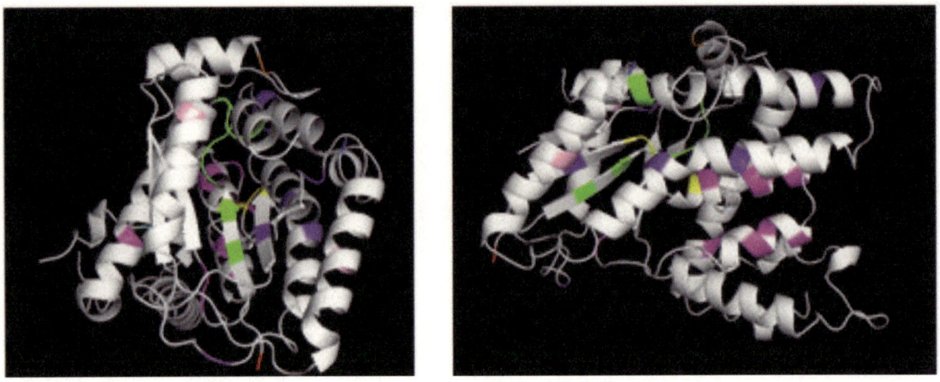

Fig. 6. Mutations identified in the UL23 gene of HSV isolates resistant to ACV. A) and B) maps of mutations of HSV-1 and HSV-2 isolates resistant to ACV, respectively. The ATP-binding site (ATP), the nucleoside-binding site (NBS), and the six regions of the *UL23* gene that are conserved among *Herpesviridae* are shown by the color boxes. The six highly conserved regions are located at amino acids (AA) 56 to 62 (site 1), 83 to 88 (site 2), 162 to 164 (site 3), 171 to 173 (site 4), 216 to 222 (site 5), and 284 to 289 (site 6) for HSV-1 and 56 to 62, 83 to 88, 163 to 165, 172 to 174, 217 to 223, and 285 to 290 for HSV-2. The additions (a), deletions (d), or both additions and deletions (a/d) reported in homopolymer runs, as well as the nucleotides (Nt) involved, are indicated below vertical bars. Substitutions of amino acids reported in the *UL23* gene that are included in the boxes correspond to those identified in conserved regions, and those outside the boxes are located in nonconserved regions. Underlined mutations correspond to the HSV-2 mutations (Adapted from Piret & Boivin, 2011; reproduced with permission of the American Society for Microbiology). **C**) Two views of the 3D structure of the TK protein (PDB:1KI2) of HSV-1 in ribbon diagram. The TK protein is in white, the NH2 end in red, the carboxyl end in blue, and the HSV-1 mutations published by Piret & Boivin 2011 are shown in different colors: Site 1 mutations are in green (R51W, Y53Stop, G56S/V, P57H, H58R/L, G59R/V, G61V, K62N, T63A/I/S, T65N; Site 2 mutations in pale blue (E83K, P84S, Q104H, H105P, Q125E/L, P131S, G144N, L158P); Site 3 mutations in yellow (D162A, R163H, A167V); Site 4 mutations in magenta (A168T, P173L/R, A175V, R176Q, T245M, S182N, Q185R, V187M, A189V, G200C, T201P); Site 5 mutations in orange (R216H/C/S, R220C/H, R222C, R281STOP); Site 6 mutations in cyan (L297S); mutations in the carboxyl end are in pink (C336Y, C337Y, L364P).

No consistent differences have been identified in the mutations associated to acyclovir-resistant isolates from immunocompetent and immunocompromised patients (Levin et al., 2004). Genotyping of the UL23 TK gene of HSV-1 has confirmed its uncommonly high polymorphism, in comparison to the TK gene of HSV-2 isolates, which was considerably less polymorphic. These findings are in agreement with the fact that the variability of the HSV-1 genome is about fourfold higher than that of HSV-2 (Sauerbrei et al., 2010; Chiba et al., 1998).

Recent work by Burrel et al., 2010 analyzing the natural polymorphism of UL23 TK and UL30 DNA pol among HSV-1 and HSV-2 strains to identify the amino acids changes potentially associated to antivirals HSV-resistance, identified 15 and 51 new natural polymorphisms within the TK and DNA pol, respectively (Fig. 7). Several amino acid changes among drug-resistant HSV were identified in the TK (S29A for HSV-2) or in the

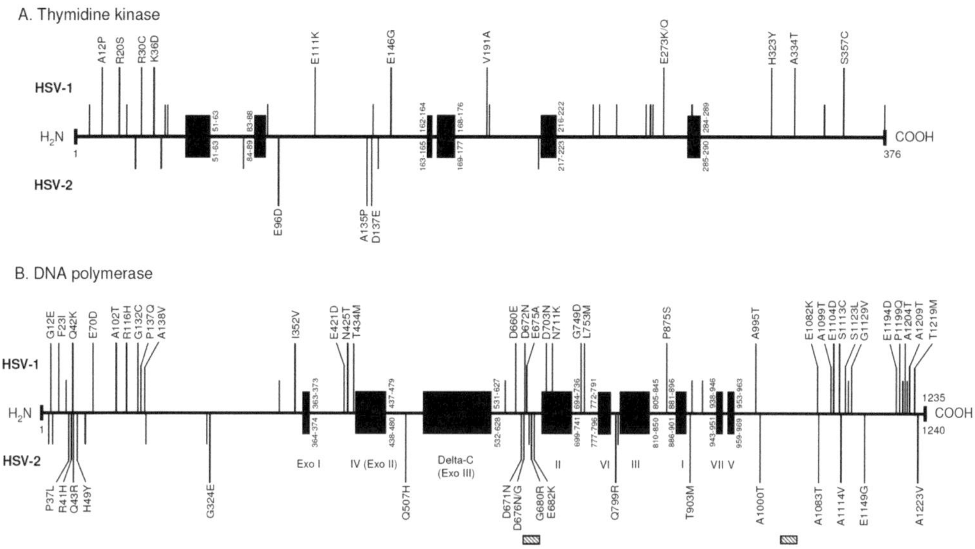

Fig. 7. Natural polymorphism map (to scale) of thymidine kinase (TK) (A) and DNA polymerase (B) among HSV-1 and HSV-2 strains. For each viral enzyme, conserved regions and functional domains are indicated by the black boxes, and natural polymorphisms are represented separately for HSV-1 (top) and HSV-2 (bottom). Amino acid changes related to natural polymorphism are indicated by vertical bars: short vertical bars correspond to changes previously reported, long vertical bars labeled with amino acid change correspond to changes newly described in this study. Regarding HSV-2 DNA polymerase, hatched boxes indicate amino acid insertions or deletions related to natural polymorphism (Burrel and Boutolleau, 2010; reproduced with permission of the American Society for Microbiology).

DNA pol (H98Y, V117L, L267M, A870G, L1188F, and R1229I for HSV-1; I291V, V544A, Y823C, and H837R for HSV-2) proteins. Moreover, the genotypic characterization of 25 drug-resistant HSV isolates revealed 8 new amino acid changes located in TK, potentially accounting for acyclovir-resistance (Y53D, I101S, L170P, and A207P for HSV-1; and S66P, A72S, R176W, and M183I for HSV-2). Wang et al., 2011 analyzed 68 ACV-resistant HSV-1 isolated from children, and identified 21 mutations in the TK gene, 11 of them have not been previously reported (D14H, Q15L, A28V, Q67R, .E95A, I203L, A207S, D215N, Q275P, A365T, Q342K). It is known that viruses with TK mutations are normally-resistant to other drugs which require the viral TK for activation, such as penciclovir; but generally remain susceptible to antiviral agents that act directly on DNA polymerase, such as foscarnet and cidofovir (Bacon et al., 2003).

In summary there is not a unique mutation pattern to explain HSV ACV-resistance, and further work is necessary to construct a more complete mutations data base of the TK gene.

4.3.1.2 Mutations in the DNA pol gene

The herpes simplex virus-1 DNA polymerase is a heterodimer, which consists of the products of the *UL30 (Pol)* and *UL42* genes. The *UL30* gene encodes the catalytic subunit, while the *UL42* gene encodes a phosphoprotein that possesses double-stranded DNA-binding activity. DNA pol is a multifunctional enzyme which possesses a polymerase activity for the extension of DNA primer chains, an intrinsic 3-5´ exonuclease proofreading activity, and an RNase H activity that could be removed the RNA primers to initiate the synthesis of Okazaki fragments at a replication fork during herpes DNA replication (Crute & Lehman, 1989). HSV DNA pol belongs to the family of α-like DNA polymerases. It is formed by 6 structural domains; **1)** A pre-NH2 domain, from NH2-terminal to aa 140; **2)** An NH2-terminal domain, from aa 141–362 and 594–639; **3)** A 3´-5´ exonuclease domain, from aa 363–593, contains three highly conserved sequence motifs: Exo I, Exo II, and Exo III; **4)** polymerase palm domain (catalytic site), from aa 701–766 and 826–956, contains the conserved regions I, II, and VII; **5)** Fingers domain, from aa 767–825, contains the conserved regions III and VI, and the base subdomain may play a role in positioning the template and primer strands ; **6)**Thumb domain, from aa 957–1197, contains the conserved region V (Liu et al., 2006). In clinical isolates, mutants with altered DNA polymerase conferring resistance to nucleoside analogues are less frequent detected (Sacks et al., 1989). The mutations are single amino acid substitutions located in regions which are directly or indirectly involved in the recognition and binding of nucleotides or pyrophosphate, as well as in catalysis. Fig 8 shows several identified mutations in the UL30 gene of HSV-1 and HSV-2 (Piret, et al., 2011).

4.3.2 Foscarnet-resistance

Foscarnet (FOS) is a pyrophosphate analogue that inhibits the viral DNA pol by mimicking the structure of pyrophosphate produced during the elongation of DNA, and it acts as a noncompetitive inhibitor of DNA pol activity. FOS does not require phosphorylation by viral and cellular kinases and binds to the pyrophosphate binding site on the viral DNA pol and blocks the release of pyrophosphate. It is only available as an intravenous formulation, and is indicated as a second-line therapy for HSV infections.

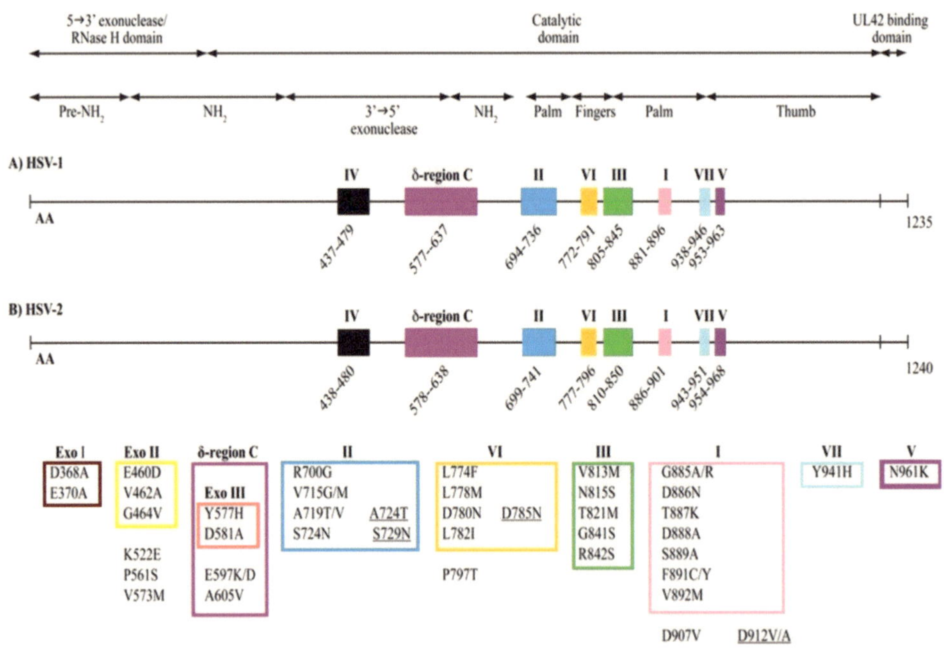

C

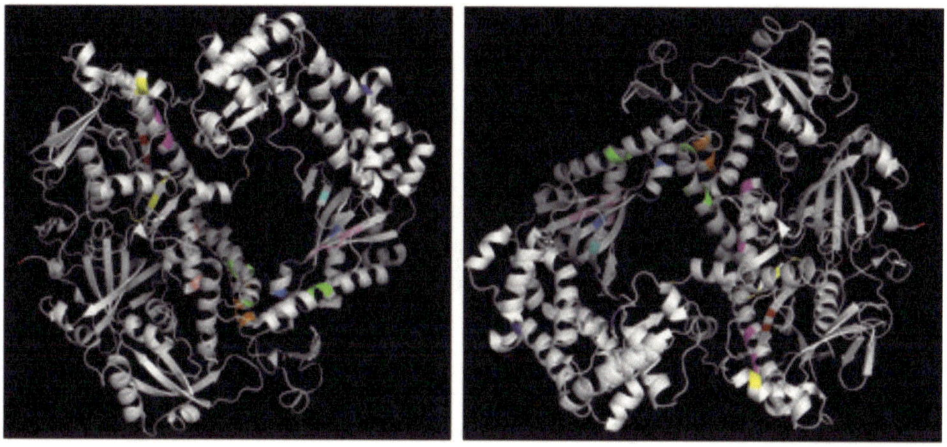

Fig. 8. Mutations identified in the UL30 gene of HSV isolates resistant to ACV. A) and B) maps of mutations of HSV-1 and HSV-2 isolates resistant to ACV, respectively. Regions conserved among Herpesviridae genes are shown by the color boxes. The roman numbers (I to VII and δ-region C) corresponding to each of these regions are indicated above the boxes. Amino acid (AA) locations are noted below each of these regions for HSV-1 and HSV-2. Substitutions reported in the UL30 gene that are included in the boxes correspond to those identified in conserved regions, and those outside the boxes are located in nonconserved regions. Underlined mutations correspond to the HSV-2 mutations. Mutations E460D, G464V, K522E, and P561S in and outside Exo II are lethal to the virus; mutations Y577H and D581A in the Exo III motif in δ-region C are associated with hypersusceptibility to ACV; and none of the mutations in region I are spontaneously induced (Adapted from Piret & Boivin 2011; reproduced with permission of the American Society for Microbiology). **C**) Two views of 3D structure of the DNA pol protein (PDB 2GV9) of HSV-1 in ribbon diagram. The DNA pol is in white, the NH2 end in red, the carboxyl end in blue, and the HSV-1 mutations from the conserved regions published by Piret & Boivin 2011 are shown in different color: in the region 1 are in pink (G885A/R, D886N, T887K, D888A, S889A, F891C/Y and V892M); in the region II in pale blue (R700G, V715G/M, A719T/V and S724N); in the region III in green (V813M, N815S, T821M, G841S and R842S); in the region V in purple (N961K); in the region VI in orange (L774F, L778M, D780N and L782I); in the region VII en cyan (Y941H); in the Exo I motif in dark red (D368A and E370A); in the Exo II in yellow (E460D, V462A and G464V); in the Exo III in salmon pink (Y577H and D581A); in the δ-region C, in magenta (E597K/D ad A605V)

Most FOS-resistant clinical HSV isolates contain single base substitutions in conserved regions and in a non-conserved region of the DNA pol gene. Some of these isolates retained their susceptibility or, at the most, borderline levels of susceptibility to ACV and cidofovir. However, some mutations conferring resistant to both ACV and FOS have been found in clinical isolates: V715G, S724N/S729N and Y941H (HSV-1/HSV-2). Mutants with alterations in both HSV TK and DNA pol can also occur, resulting in double resistance to both ACV and FOS (Piret et al., 2011).

4.3.3 Cidofovir and adefovir

These drugs are acyclic nucleoside phosphonates derivatives of cytosine (cidofovir) and adenine (adefovir), which are converted into active ANP-diphosphates by cellular kinases. Thus, do not require the activation by the viral TK enzyme, and act as competitive inhibitors of the viral DNA pol, and chain terminators. Cidofovir is indicated for HCMV infections, including ganciclovir-resistant strains, and also against HSV and VZV strains. Several mutations linked to cidofovir resistance have mapped in HSV DNA pol gene: R700M, G841C and G850I, L773M, Y941H and V573M, and in laboratory-derived HSV strains resistant to cidofovir, L1007M and I1028T (Piret et al., 2011).

4.4 VZV-resistant to antiviral drugs

The current drug of choice for the antiviral treatment of VZV infections in patients at risk is ACV (De Clercq, 2004). VZV-resistant to ACV or foscarnet has only been reported in rare cases of immunocompromised patients, and the resistance to ACV is associated to alterations in the TK activity as it happens with HSV. One of the problems to study the antiviral-resistance of VZV, is the low rate of VZV isolations in cell culture, usually between 20% and 43% from vesicle samples; and even more, there is a restricted spectrum of permissive cell cultures and a long time (up to a few weeks) is required to developing cytopathic effect (Cohen et al., 2007). On the other hand, there is not enough information about the natural polymorphism or resistance associated to the TK and DNA pol genes. Sauerbrei et al., 2011 analyzed genotypically 16 VZV strains with clinical diagnosis of ACV-resistance, finding seven strains with alterations in the TK gene: three were associated to amino acid substitutions (L73I, W225R, T256M), three with stop codon generation (A163-, Q303-, N334-) and one frameshift due to a deletion of nucleotides 19–223. All of them were not previously reported, except the Q303- mutation, which has been reported in two patients with AIDS treated with ACV to control persistent zoster (Fillet et al., 1998; Saint-Léger et al., 2001).

Even though herpes viruses have a low rate of mutations, it is clear that apparition of viral strains resistant to the current antivirals drugs is a serious problem, especially for the immunocompromised patients. The resistance is associated with a wide range of mutations located mainly in catalytic or conserved domains of the viral TK and DNA pol enzymes, enzymes that play a critical role to achieve herpes viruses inhibition by the current antiviral drugs. Therefore it is necessary to monitor the efficacy of the antiviral therapy administered to the patients, but also to develop new antiviral drugs against different viral targets.

5. Point mutations and antiviral resistance in cytomegalovirus: Molecular basis and clinical implications

Despite progress in the diagnosis and management of cytomegalovirus (CMV) infections in different groups of immunosuppressed patients, this virus continues to be an important pathogen that can establish acute and chronic infections (Snydman et al., 2011) with high morbidity and mortality in immunosuppressed individuals and/or the immunologically immature. The main risk groups are: a) newborns; b) individuals receiving organ transplants; c) patients with cancer; and d) AIDS patients, although the incidence in this group has declined with the advent of HAART (Emery et al., 2001; Snydman et al., 2011).

Drugs approved by the Food Drug Administration FDA for treating CMV infection include ganciclovir (GCV), foscarnet (FOS), cidofovir (CDV), and valganciclovir (VGV). The characteristics of these drugs are described in Table 6

5.1 Viral proteins targeted by the antivirals

5.1.1 UL97 protein

A protein encoded by the UL97 gene. The natural role of this protein in viral replication is not fully known, but recent studies suggest it is involved in the regulation of viral replication (Wolf et al., 2001) and other studies highlight the involvement of UL97 in viral envelope assembly (Goldberg et al., 2011). This protein has a kinase activity, so it may be involved in the monophosphorylation of GCV. This feature has been widely studied and is exploited in the pharmacokinetics of GCV.

5.1.2 UL54 protein

The viral polymerase UL54 is encoded by the UL54 gene. Several functional regions have enzyme activity. They are divided into I to VII with polymerization activity and EXO I to EXO III with exonuclease activity. The first function allows polymerization activity, while the second provides an editing function that significantly reduces the rate of mutation and leads to high fidelity (Picard-Jean, 2007).

5.2 Drugs and their mechanism of action

5.2.1 Ganciclovir

This drug is an analogue of guanosine. It was the first drug approved by the FDA for the treatment of CMV infection. GCV is a pro-drug that is inactive until phosphorylated. This process is carried out by a viral protein kinase encoded by the UL97 gene, which phosphorylates GCV. The product from this biochemical reaction is ganciclovir monophosphate, which is further phosphorylated twice more by cellular kinases to produce ganciclovir triphosphate. This form is recognized by the polymerase and it competes with deoxyguanosine triphosphate (dGTP) to block chain elongation (Figure. 9) (Faulds et al., 1990; Sullivan et al., 1992).

5.2.2 Valganciclovir

Although GCV has proved to be an efficient CMV induction therapy in various groups of patients, such patients also require maintenance therapy with oral GCV. This therapy is limited because oral GCV has low bioavailability (Markham et al., 1994; Anderson et al., 1995). By contrast, the pro-drug VGV has the advantage of a high oral bioavailability. VGV is hydrolysed by esterases in the gut and liver in a first step; the product is GCV, which can be phosphorylated to block viral replication (Sugawara et al., 2000).

5.2.3 Foscarnet

This drug is a conjugate base of phosphonoformic acid that has the advantage that it does not need to be phosphorylated. It is capable of inhibiting the activity of the viral polymerase, because it binds to a site that recognizes pyrophosphates on bases. It interferes with the exchange of pyrophosphates and phosphates by dideoxynucleosides and inhibits viral replication (Crumpacker et al., 1992) (Fig. 9).

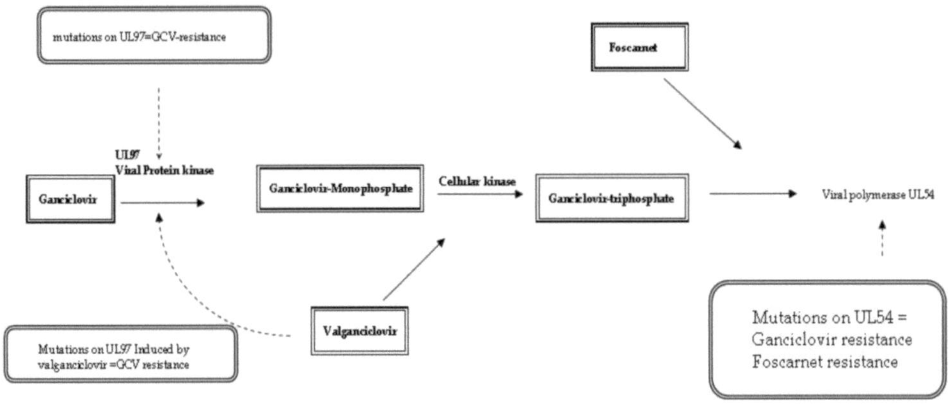

Fig. 9. Mechanism of action to ganciclovir, valganciclovir and foscarnet. GCV and valganciclovir, need phosphorilation while foscarnet recognize the UL54 without previous phosphorilation. Ganciclovir is initially phoshorilated by a viral protein kinase UL97. Mutations on UL97 confer them ganciclovir resistance, valganciclovir can induce ganciclovir resistance. Mutations on UL54 gene can confer ganciclovir and/or foscarnet resistance.

5.2.4 Cidofovir

This drug is the acyclic nucleotide analogue 1-(3-hydroxy-2-phosphonomethoxyethyl) cytosine and it competes with cytosine. Several cellular enzymes are involved in the phosphorylation of this compound. These include pyrimidine nucleoside monophosphate kinase, pyruvate kinase, creatine kinase, and nucleoside diphosphate kinase (Cihlar et al., 1996). This antiviral is not dependent on UL97 phosphorylation and it inhibits viral polymerase activity through a similar mechanism to GCV (Fig. 9) (De Clercq, 2003).

5.2.5 Fomivirsen

This drug is an antisense nucleotide phosphorothioate that contains 21 nucleotides. It is resistant to cellular nucleases and binds to transcripts of the immediate early viral proteins (6) (Azad et al., 1993). Studies show that this oligonucleotide can specifically block viral genes without interfering with cellular translation.

5.3 Point mutations and antiviral drug resistance

Strains resistant to antivirals emerged following the treatment of active infections, with this emergence linked to the prolonged and intermittent administration of drugs to immunocompromised patients. The most studied drug in this context is GCV. Several point mutations in viral phosphotransferase sequences (UL97) or DNA polymerase sequences

(UL54) are involved. The role of UL97 in the CMV life cycle is not clear, but its participation in the phosphorylation of GCV is well known. The mechanism occurs as follows. The GCV domain is recognized by the UL97 protein kinase. The deoxyguanosine analogue (9-[1,3-dyhydroxy-2-propoxymethyl]guanine) or monophosphate deoxyguanosine are the products of GCV phosphorylation. Two subsequent phosphorylations are mediated by cellular phosphate kinases. Triphosphorylated GCV is the active molecule for the inhibition of viral replication, because it competes with the natural substrate deoxyguanosine triphosphate for the viral DNA polymerase.

5.3.1 Resistance to ganciclovir

GCV resistance is most frequently a result of amino acid substitutions due to mutations in the codons 460, 594, and 595, which are in the coding sequence of the protein UL97. These mutational changes reduce the affinity for GCV without affecting polymerase activity (Chou et al., 1995). GCV resistance was first reported in isolates obtained from blood samples of immunosuppressed hospitalized patients. Two had been diagnosed with AIDS, while another had lymphoblastic leukaemia. These strains showed poor response to GCV with *in vitro* cell cultures (Erice et al., 1989). Resistance to GCV was previously obtained *in vitro* by the selective pressure of low doses of GCV on the strain AD169 (Biron et al., 1986). Subsequently, Lurain et al. reported the isolation of three mutants resistant to GCV with a reduced ability to phosphorylate GCV. Resistance was associated with the emergence of a mutation in the exonuclease function of polymerase (Lurain et al., 1992). The same authors later reported isolates with a point mutation at position 460 in region IV of the UL97 gene, where a change of methionine for isoleucine (M460I) was involved (Lurain et al., 1994).

Several mutations that are known to change the active site of UL97 and prevent the phosphorylation of GCV have been described and characterized. More than 25 mutations are associated with this process. The most common are at codons 460 (methionine to valine), 594 (methionine to isoleucine), and 595 (aspartic acid to serine). In some cases, there is more than one mutation.

UL54 mutations are also involved with resistance to GCV. These mutations produce changes in the amino acid sequence of the viral polymerase, which affects the affinity for a guanosine triphosphate analogue (GCV triphosphate). More than 20 mutations have been described, and combinations of mutations are also found in UL97 and UL54. Strains with mutations in UL97 alone are resistant to GCV but susceptible to FOS and CDV, strains with mutations in UL54 show a pattern of resistance to GCV and CDV, and strains with double mutations in UL97 and UL54 are highly resistant to GCV.

5.3.2 Induction of resistance with valganciclovir

This antiviral is a GCV pro-drug, so its prolonged administration may be a factor in developing resistance to GCV. This effect has a low incidence, but greater use of this antiviral is now encouraged. Reports have described mutations in UL97 as V466G, V466M, and V466G, and these were obtained after treatment with VGV (Boivin et al., 2001; Foulongne et al., 2004; Martin et al., 2010).

5.3.3 Foscarnet

Mutations involved with FOS resistance are located on the UL54 gene. A great diversity of point mutations can change the amino acid sequence of the viral polymerase and lead to FOS resistance. These mutations are located in regions II and III (codons 696–845). The presence of these mutations changes the reading frame of the sequence leading to blocking of antiviral recognition by the polymerase (Lurain et al., 2010).

5.3.4 Cidofovir

As with GCV, most mutations that confer resistance to CDV are concentrated in the exonuclease domain of the polymerase (codons 301, 408–413, and 501–545) and region V (codons 981–987) (Bowen et al., 1999).

5.3.5 Fomivirsen

An antisense nucleotide inhibits viral replication by two different mechanisms that are either dependent on or independent of the sequence. The antiviral mechanism was analysed *in vitro* using fibroblasts, and it was shown that the oligonucleotide recognizes the mRNA sequence of the viral Immediate Early Protein IE2 following internalization. This results in reduced expression levels of the IE proteins. Mulabampa et al. obtained an *in vitro* mutant with fomivirsen resistance. It was expected that the mutation leading to resistance would be located on the complementary region to fomivirsen. However, no mutation was found when the region was sequenced. Despite this result, the induction of fomivirsen resistance induced antiviral and the clinical impact is not clear.(Mulamba et al., 1998, Anderson et al., 2004).

5.4 Multidrug resistance

Mutations can provide different levels of resistance or cross-resistance to antivirals. Occasionally, mutations in both UL97 and UL54 occur, resulting in multidrug resistance. For example, Eckle et al. reported a paediatric patient undergoing bone marrow transplantation with a disseminated infection during the conditioning procedure and encephalitis on day +100. FOS was started, which was followed by combination therapy and subsequently GCV, FOS, and CDV on day +167. Multidrug resistance with multiple mutations was observed seven months later (Eckle et al., 2000). Rodriguez et al. reported on a 58-year-old patient undergoing a liver transplant. On day +86, they isolated a possible mutation at A594V in UL97 and six point mutations that potentially affected the amino acid sequence of the UL54 protein. The resistance to GCV and FOS in this patient was apparently associated with multiple factors, but prolonged therapy with GCV and co-infection may have produced at least two strains (Rodríguez et al., 2007).

5.5 Laboratory methods for the detection of antiviral drugs

Based on *in vitro* analysis, antiviral resistance can be classified as phenotypic or genotypic.

Phenotypic resistance is tested using a cell culture assay to determine an antiviral's ability to reduce viral replication. This technique is considered the gold standard. The AD169 strain is used as a reference where the profile drug susceptibility is already known. The reference values for the drugs are 6 μM for GCV, 2 μM for CDV, and 400 μM for FOS. The *in vitro* assay determines the antiviral's ability to reduce the number of lytic plaques, which quantifies the cytopathic effect induced by the virus. This can be determined as a 50% inhibitory concentration (IC_{50}) (Chou et al., 1999; Landry et al., 2000). This is a difficult method that requires trained personnel and standard antiviral concentrations. Simplified techniques have been developed that can be applied to a large number of samples, which significantly reduces the workload (Prix et al., 1998). However, this is still a laborious technique and it is difficult to apply it routinely. Nevertheless, these are necessary tests that are required to confirm potential drug resistance to a new drug or new mutations found by genotypic assays (Lurain et al., 2010).

Phenotypic resistance tests are perhaps the most widely used, because a number of mutations associated with resistance are already known. Thus, the presence of a mutation can be inferred if the strain is resistant. Several molecular methods have been proposed for the detection of mutations that are known to be associated with resistance to antiviral drugs. These methods are described below.

5.5.1 Polymerase chain reaction coupled to restriction fragment length polymorphism (PCR–RFLP)

This method has been used for several years, because it is easy to perform and it requires no sophisticated equipment. However, it cannot identify new mutations associated with resistance. This method is more applicable to routine detection of the most common mutations, particularly those in codons 520, 460, 594, 595, 591, and 592 that confer GCV resistance (Hanson et al., 1995; Prix, 1999).

5.5.2 Real-time PCR

Several studies report the use of real-time PCR as a tool for the detection of mutations associated with resistance. Yeo et al. (2005) used a strategy of molecular beacons for the detection of mutations in codon 460 in UL97. Liu et al. developed a method based on SYBR green for the detection of mutations at position 460 in UL97. Liu et al. (2008) and Göhring et al. (2008) developed a method based on real-time PCR for the detection of mutations in codons 594, 595, 603, and 607.

5.5.3 PCR sequencing

This is the gold standard method for detecting the presence of mutations known to be involved in resistance. It also allows the genotypic detection of new mutations that are correlated with phenotypic tests to determine whether they are associated with resistance.

5.6 Clinical impact of cytomegalovirus drug resistance

Published evidence indicates the emergence of resistance and severe complications in patients. For example, Jabs et al. (2010) observed that the emergence of resistance associated with mutations was closely linked to high mortality in a study of 266 patients with AIDS who were treated with GCV or FOS for CMV retinitis. We observed a fatal outcome with viral pneumonitis and graft rejection in a paediatric patient undergoing bone marrow transplant, where two resistance mutations (M460V and M460I) appeared following non-response to treatment with GCV. We attributed these complications to the lack of response to the treatment, which apparently allowed high viral replication coupled with strong resistance while toxic damage induced by the antiviral therapy led to rejection of the graft. (Arellano-Galindo et al., 2011).

6. Conclusions

At present, it is clear that mutations conferring resistance to the currently approved antiviral drugs is a growing problem , so it is very important to continue research in various areas that would allow better resolution of the problem:

First, the knowledge of mutation's type that allows virus avoid the action of drugs, will allow an understanding as to how these mutations arise and how we must avoid them. Also, this knowledge, will allow a better design of new drugs.

It is also, very important to establish definitive criteria for the diagnosis of resistance and specific treatment, mainly in immunocompromised population, where several factors are involved.

Also, there are still multiple subjects for basic and clinical investigation, such as specify the role of minority populations who express resistance to the antiviral drugs in the clinical settings, implement strategies optimizing the pharmacokinetics and pharmacodynamics either of the current or of the new antiviral agents. All with the main objective to improve the action of drugs, reduce the likelihood of emergence of resistant strains and have under control those which are already presented.

On the other hand, we must not forget the monitoring of the efficacy of the antiviral therapy which is administered to the patients, to avoid the appearance of point mutations conferring drug resistance. Finally, it is also important to bear in mind that clinical centres attending immunosuppressed patients should implement special techniques for the detection of genotypic viral resistance.

7. Acknowledges

The author are grateful with the support of CONACyT México: CB2008-99164 and FOSSIS 2008-01-87920

8. References

Altmann, A., Beerenwinkel, N., Sing, T., et al (2007). Improved prediction of response to antiretroviral combination therapy using the genetic barrier to drug resistance. *Antiviral Therapy,* Vol. 12, pp. 169-178.

Anderson, K., Fox, M., Beown-Driver, V., Martin, M. & Azad R. (1996). Inhibition of Human Cytomegalovirus Immediate-Early Gene. Expression by an antisense oligonucleotide complementary to immediate-early RNA. *Antimicrobial Agents and Chemotherapy.* Vol. 40, No. 9 (September 1996), pp. 1767-1773.

Anderson, RD., Griffy, KG., Jung D, Dorr, A., Hulse JD. & Smith RB.(1995) Ganciclovir absolute bioavailability and steady-state pharmacokinetics after oral administration of two 3000-mg/d dosing regimens in human immunodeficiency virus- and cytomegalovirus-seropositive patients. *Clinical Therapeutics.* Vol. 17, No. 3, (May-June 1995), pp. 425-432

Anzivino, E., Fioriti D., Mischitelli M., Bellizzi A., Barucca V., et al. (2009). Herpes simplex virus infection in pregnancy and in neonate: status of art of epidemiology, diagnosis, therapy and prevention. *Virology Journal.* Vol. 6, No. 40, (April 2009), pp 1-40.

Arellano-Galindo ,J., Vázquez-Meraz, E., Jiménez-Hernández, E., Velazquez-Guadarrama, N., Mikeler, E., et al. (2011). The role of cytomegalovirus infection and disease in pediatric bone marrow transplant recipients in Mexico City in the context of viral drug resistance. Pediatric Transplantion. Vol. 15, No. 1, (February 2011), pp. 103-111.

Arnold, E. & Sarafianos SG (2008). An HIV secret uncovered. *Nature,* Vol. 453, pp. 169-170. Available in: http://www.nature.com/nature/journal/v453/n7192/pdf/453169b.pdf.

Azad, R., Driver, V. & Tanaka, K. (1993). Antiviral activity of a phosphorothioate oligonucleotide complementary to RNA of the human cytomegalovirus major immediate-early region. *Antimicrobial Agents and Chemotherapy.* Vol. 37, No. 9, (September 1993), pp. 1945-1954.

Bacon, T. H.,. Boon R. J,. Schultz M, & Hodges-Savola C. (2002). Surveillance for antiviral-agent-resistant herpes simplex virus in the general population with recurrent herpes labialis. *Antimicrobial Agents Chemotheraphy.* Vol. 46, No. 9, (September 2002), pp. 3042–3044.

Bacon, T.H., Levin M.J., Leary J.J., Sarisky R.T. & Sutton D. (2003). Herpes simplex virus resistance to acyclovir and penciclovir after two decades of antiviral therapy. *Clinical Microbiology Reviews.* Vol.16, No. 1, (January), pp. 114-28.

Balasubramaniam, N. K., Veerisetty V. & Gentry G. A. (1990). Herpesviral deoxythymidine kinases contain a site analogous to the phosphoryl-binding arginine-rich region of porcine adenylate kinase; comparison of secondary structure predictions and conservation. *Journal of General Virology.* Vol. 71, No. 12, (December 1990), 2979–2987.

Balfour, H.H., Chace B.A., Stapleton J.T., Simmons R.L. & Fryd D.S. (1989). A randomized, placebo-controlled trial of oral acyclovir for the prevention of cytomegalovirus disease in recipients of renal allografts. *New England Jorunal of Medicine.* Vol. 320, No. 21, (May 1989), 1381–1387.

Beauchamp, L. M., Orr G. F., de Miranda P., Burnette T. & Krenitsky T. A. (1992). Amino acid ester prodrugs of acyclovir. *Antiviral Chemistry and Chemotherapy.* Vol. 3, No. 3, pp. 157–164.

Bennett, DE., Camacho, RJ., Otelea. D., et al (2009). Drug resistance mutations for surveillance of transmitted HIV-1 drug-resistance: 2009 Update. *PLoS One,* Vol. 4, No. 3, pp. e4724.

Biron, K., Fyfe J, Stanat S, Leslie L, Sorrell J, Lambe C, et al. (1986). A human cytomegalovirus mutant resistant to the nucleoside analog 9-([2-hydroxy-1-(hydroxymethyl)ethoxy]methyl)guanine (BW B759U) induces reduced levels of BW B759U triphosphate. *Proceedings of the National Academy of Sciences USA* Vol. 83, No. 22 (November 1986), pp. 8769–8773.

Blauvelt, A. (2001). Skin diseases associated with human herpesvirus 6, 7, and 8 infection. *The journal of investigative dermatology. Symposium proceedings.* Vol. 6 No.3, (December 2001), pp.197-202.

Blower, S. M., Porco T. C. & Darby G. (1998). Predicting and preventing the emergence of antiviral drug resistance in HSV-2. *Nature Medicine* Vol.4, No. 6, (June 1998), pp. 673–678

Boivin, G., Gilbert, C., Gaudreau, A., Greenfield, I., Sudlow, R. & Roberts NA. (2001). Rate of emergence of cytomegalovirus (CMV) mutations in leukocytes of patients with acquired immunodeficiency syndrome who are receiving valganciclovir as induction and maintenance therapy for CMV retinitis. *Journal of Infectious Diseases* Vol. 184, No. 12, (December 2001), pp.1598–602.

Bowen, E., Cherrington, J., Lamy, P., Griffiths, P., Johnson, M., et al. (1999) Quantitative changes in cytomegalovirus DNAemia and genetic analysis of the UL97 and UL54 genes in AIDS patients receiving cidofovir following ganciclovir therapy. *Journal of Medical Virology.* Vol. 58, No. 4, pp. 402-407.

Boyd, M. R., Safrin S. & Kern E. R. (1993). Penciclovir: a review of its spectrum of activity, selectivity, and cross-resistance pattern. *Antiviral Chemistry & Chemotherapy* Vol 4, No. 1 Suppl, pp. 3–11.

Braun, P. & Wiesmann F (2007). Phenotypic assays for the determination of co-receptor tropism in HIV-1 infected individuals. *European Journal of Medical Research,* Vol. 12, No. 9, pp. 463-472.

Breitbart, M. & Rohwer, F. (2005). Here a virus, there a virus, everywhere the same virus?. *Trends in Microbiology.* Vol. 13, No: 6, (june 2006), pp. 278-284.

Burrel, S, Deback C., Agut H. & Boutolleau D. (2010). Genotypic characterization of UL23 thymidine kinase and UL30 DNA polymerase of clinical isolates of herpes simplex virus: natural polymorphism and mutations associated with resistance to antivirals. *Antimicrobial Agents and Chemotherapy.* Vol. 54, No. 11, (November 2010), pp. 833-842

Chen, Y., Scieux C., Garrait V., Socie G., Rocha V., et al. (2000). Resistant herpes simplex virus type 1 infection: an emerging concern after allogeneic stem cell transplantation. *Clinical Infecious. Diseases* Vol. 31, No 4 (October 2000), pp. 927–935.

Chiba, A., Suzutani T., Sajo M., Koyano S. & Azuma M. (1998). Analysis of nucleotide sequence variations in herpes simplex virus types 1 and 2, and varicella-zoster virus. *Acta Virologica* Vol. 42, No. 6, (December 1998), pp. 401-407.

Chibo, D., Mijch A., Doherty R. & Birch C. (2002). Novel mutations in the thymidine kinase and DNA polymerase genes of acyclovir and foscarnet resistant herpes simplex viruses infecting an immunocompromised patient. *Journal of Clinical Virology* Vol. 25, No. 2 (August 2002), pp. 165–170.

Chou, S. (1999). Antiviral drug resistance in human cytomegalovirus. *Transplant Infectious Disease* . Vol. 1, No. 2, (June 1999), pp. 105–114.

Chou, S., Erice, A., Jordan, MC., Vercellotti, GM., Michels, KR., Talarico CL, et al. (1995). Frequency of UL97 Phosphotransferase Mutations Related to Ganciclovir Resistance in Clinical Cytomegalovirus Isolates *Journal of Infectious Diseases.* Vol. 172, No. 1, (July 1995), pp. 239-242.

Christophers J., Clayton J., Craske J., Ward R., Collins P., et al. (1998). Survey of resistance of herpes simplex virus to acyclovir in Northwest England. *Antimicrobial Agents and Chemotherapy.* Vol. 42, No. 4, (April 1998), pp. 868–872.

Cihlar T, Chen M. (1996). Identification of enzymes catalyzing two-step phosphorylation of cidofovir and the effect of cytomegalovirus infection on their activities in host cells. *Mol Pharmacol.* Vol. 50, No. 6, (December 1996), pp. 1502-1510.

Clifford, DB., Evans, S., Yang, Y., et al (2009). Long-term impact of efavirenz on neuropsychological performance and symptoms in HIV-infected individuals (ACTG 5097s). *HIV Clinical Trials*, Vol. 10, No. 6, pp. 343-355.

Coakley, E., Stawiski, E., Toma, J., et al (2011). HIV-1 Disease Stage Significantly Correlates with Sensitivity of V3 Sequence-based Predictions of CXCR4 Use. *18th Conference of Retroviruses and Opportunistic Infections*, ISBN 0-9793191-9-6, Boston, Mass, February 2011 [abstract 592].

Coen, DM., & Schaffer PA. (1980). Two distinct loci confer resistance to acycloguanosine in herpes simplex virus type 1. *Proceedings of the National Academy of Sciences USA* Vol. 77, No. 4, (April), pp. 2265–2269.

Coen, DM., (1994). Acyclovir-resistant, pathogenic herpesviruses. *Trends in Microbiology* Vol. 2, No. 12, (December 1994), pp. 481–485.

Cohen, JI., Straus S. E. & Arvin, A. (2007), Varicella-zoster, virus replication, pathogenesis, and management, In *Field's Virology*, D. M. Knipe and P. M. Howley, Eds., pp.2773-218, Lippincott Williams &Wilkins, ISBN 978-0-7817-6060-7, Philadelphia, Pa, USA, 5th edition.

Collier, L, (2006). *Human virology*, ISBN 978-0-19-957088-1 Oxford University Press. New York, USA.

Collins, P. & Darby, G. (1991). Laboratory studies of herpes simplex virus strains resistant to acyclovir. *Reviews in Medical Virology* Vol. 1, No. 1, (May 1991), pp. 19–28.

Corey, L. & Ashley, R. (2004).Valaciclovir HSV Transmission Study Group. Prevention of herpes simplex virus type 2 transmission with antiviral therapy. *Herpes*. Suppl 3, (August 2004), pp. 170A-174A.

Crumpacker, CS. (1992). Mechanism of action of foscarnet against viral polymerases. *The American Journal of Medicine* Vol. 92, No. 2A (February 1992), pp. 3S-7S.

Crumpacker, CS. (1992). Mechanism of action of foscarnet against viral polymerases. *The American Journal of Medicine*. Vol 92, No. 2A, (February 1992), pp. 3S-7S.

Crumpacker, CS., Schnipper, LE., Marlowe, SI., Kowalsky PN., Hershey BJ., et al. (1982). Resistance to antiviral drugs of herpes simplex virus isolated from a patient treated with acyclovir. *New England Journal of Medicine*. Vol. 306, No. 6, (February 1982), pp:343–346.

Crute, JJ. & Lehman, IR. (1989). Herpes simplex-1 DNA polymerase. Identification of an intrinsic 5'----3' exonuclease with ribonuclease H activity. The Journal of Biological Chemistry. Vol. 264, No. 32, (November 1989), pp. 19266-19270.

Darby, G., Field, HJ. & Salisbury SA. (1981). Altered substrate specificity of herpes simplex virus thymidine kinase confers acyclovir-resistance. *Nature*. Vol. 289, No. 5793, (January 1981), pp. 81–83.

De Clercq E. (2002). Strategies in the design of viral drugs. *Nature Review Drug Discovery*. Vol 1(January 2002), pp.13-25.

De Clercq E. (2004). Antivirals and antiviral strategies. *Nature Review Microbiology*. Vol. 2, No. 9, (September 2004), pp. 704-720.

De Clercq, E. (2003). Clinical potential of the acyclic nucleoside phosphonates cidofovir, adefovir, and tenofovir in treatment of DNA virus and retrovirus infections. *Clinical Microbiology Reviews*. Vol. 16, No. 3 (October 2003), pp. 569–596.

De Clercq, E. (2004). Antivirals and antiviral strategies. Nature Reviews Microbiology Vol. 2, No. 9, (September 2004), pp. 704-720.

De Luca, A. (2006). The impact of resistance on viral fitness and its clinical implications, In: *Antiretroviral resistance in clinical practice.* Geretti M, Londres: Mediscript Ltd, Retrieved from http://www.ncbi.nlm.nih.gov/books/NBK2244/

Department of Health and Human Services [DHHS] (2011). *Panel on Antiretroviral Guidelines for Adult and Adolescents: Guidelines for the use of antiretroviral agents in HIV-1-infected adults and adolescents.* In: AIDSinfo, January 2011, pp. 68-85, Access 03 July 2011, Available from: http://aidsinfo.nih.gov/contentfiles/AdultandAdolescentGL.pdf.

Eckle, T., Prix, L., Jahn, G., Klingebiel, T., Handgretinger, R., et al. (2000). Drug-resistant human cytomegalovirus infection in children after allogeneic stem cell transplantation may have different clinical outcomes. *Blood.* Vol. 96 No. 9, (November 2000), pp. 3286-3289.

Elion, GB., Furman PA., Fyfe JA., De Miranda, P., Beauchamp L., et al. (1977). Selectivity of action of an antiherpetic agent, 9-(2-hydroxyethoxymethyl) guanine. *Proceedings of the National Academy of Sciences USA* Vol. 74, No. 12, (December 1977), pp. 5716-5720.

Emery, VC. (2001). Progress in understanding cytomegalovirus drug resistance. Journal of Virology. Vol 21, No. 3, (June 2001), pp. 223-228.

Erice, A., Chou, S., Biron, K., Stanat, C., Balfour, H.& Jordan, M. (1989). Progressive, disease due to ganciclovir-resistant cytomegalovirus in immunocompromised patients. *The New England Journal of Medicine.* Vol. 320, No. 5 (February 1989), pp. 289–293.

Esté, JA., Telenti, A. (2007). HIV entry inhibitors. *Lancet,* Vol. 370, No. 9581, pp. 81-88.

Eun-Sun, Y. (2011). Study of specific oligosaccharide structures related with swine flu (H1N1) and avian flu, and Tamiflu as their remedy. *Journal Microbiology Biotechnology.* Vol. 21, No. 5 (May 2011), pp. 449-454.

Faulds, D. & Heel, C. (1990).Ganciclovir. A review of its antiviral activity, pharmacokinetic properties and therapeutic efficacy in cytomegalovirus infections. *Drugs.* Vol. 39, No.4 (April 1990); 39:597–638.

Fauquet, C.M., Mayo M.A., Maniloff J., Desselberger U. & Ball L.A. (2005). *Virus taxonomy,* Elsevier Academic Press, ISBN 0-12-249951-4, Chian.

Ferraris, O. & Lina, B. (2008). Mutations of neuraminidase implicated in neuraminidase inhibitors resistance. *Journal Clinical Virology.* Vol. 41, No. 1, (January 2008), pp.13–19.

Field, H.J. & Biswas S. (2011). Antiviral drug resistance and helicase-primase inhibitors of herpes simplex virus. *Drug Resistance Updates.* Vol. 14, No. 1, (February 2011), pp. 45-51.

Fillet, AM., Dumont, B., Caumes, E., Visse, B., Agut, H., et al. (1998). Acyclovir-resistant varicella-zoster virus: phenotypic and genotypic characterization. *Journal of Medical Virology.* Vol. 55, No. 3, (July 1998), pp. 250–254.

Foulongne, V., Turriere, C., Diafouka, F., Abraham, B., Lastere, S., et al. (2004). Ganciclovir resistance mutations in UL97 and UL54 genes of human cytomegalovirus isolates resistant to ganciclovir. *Acta Virologica* Vol 48 No. 1, pp. 51–55.

Fransen, S., Karmochkine, M., Huang, W., et al (2009). Longitudinal analysis of raltegravir susceptibility and integrase replication capacity of human immunodeficiency virus type 1 during virologic failure. *Antimicrobial Agents Chemotherapy,* Vol. 53, No. 10, pp.4522-4524.

Frobert, E., Cortay JC., Ooka T., Najioullah F., Thouvenot D., et al. (2008). Genotypic detection of acyclovir-resistant HSV-1: characterization of 67 ACV-sensitive and 14 ACV-resistant viruses. *Antiviral Research.* Vol. 79, No.1, (July 2008), pp. 28–36.

Ganem, D. (2007), Kaposi's sarcoma-associated herpesvirus, In *Field's Virology*, D. M. Knipe and P. M. Howley, Eds., pp.2847-2888, Lippincott Williams &Wilkins, ISBN 978-0-7817-6060-7, Philadelphia, Pa, USA, 5th edition.

Gaudreau, A., Hill E., Balfour H. H., Erice A. & Boivin G.. (1998). Phenotypic and genotypic characterization of acyclovir-resistant herpes simplex viruses from immunocompromised patients. *Journal of Infectious Diseases*. Vol.178, No. 2, (August 1998), pp. 297–303.

Geisbert, T. & Jahrling, P. (2004). Exotic emerging viral diseases: progress and challenges. *Nature Medicine Supplement*. Vol.10, No. 12, (December 2004), S110-S21.

Geretti, AM., Smith C., Haberl, A., et al (2008). Determinants of virological failure after successful viral load suppression in first-line highly active antiretroviral therapy. *Antiviral Therapy*, Vol. 13, pp.927-936.

Gibbs, JS., Chiou HC., Bastow KF., Cheng YC. & Coen DM. (1988). Identification of amino acids in herpes simplex virus DNA polymerase involved in substrate and drug recognition. *Proceedings of the National Academy of Sciences U. S. A.* Vol. 85, No. 1, (September 1988), pp. 6672–6676

Gilbert, C., Bestman-Smith J. & Boivin G. (2002). Resistance of herpesviruses to antiviral drugs: clinical impactsand molecular mechanisms. *Drug resistance updates* Vol. 5, No. 2, pp. 88–114

GlaxoSmithKline. (November 2007). Zovirax in: ZOVIRAX® (acyclovir) Capsules, 11.07, Available from http://us.gsk.com/products/assets/us_zovirax.pdf.

Göhring, K., Mikeler, E., Jahn, G., Rohde, F. & Hamprecht K. (2008). Rapid semiquantitative real-time PCR for the detection of human cytomegalovirus UL97 mutations conferring ganciclovir resistance. *Antiviral Therapy*. Vol. 13, No. 3, pp. 461-466.

Goldberg, M., Honigman, A., Weinstein, J., Chou, S., Taraboulos, A., Rouvinski, A., et al. (2011). Human cytomegalovirus UL97 kinase and nonkinase functions mediate viral cytoplasmic secondary envelopment. *Journal of Virology*. Vol. 85, No.7, (April 2011), pp. 3375-84.

Gragsted, UB., Mocroft, A., Vella, S., et al (2004). Predictors of immunological failure after initial response to highly active antiretroviral therapy in HIV-1 infected adults: an EuroSIDA study. *Journal of Infectious Diseases*, Vol. 190, No. 1, pp.148-155.

Griffiths, PD. (2009). A perspective on antiviral resistance. *Journal of clinical virology*. Vol. 46, No. 1, (September 2009). pp. 3-8.

Hanson, M., Preheim, L., Chou, S., Talarico, C., Biron, K., et al. (1995) A. Novel mutation in the ul97 gene of a clinical cytomegalovirus strain conferring resistance to ganciclovir. *Antimicrobial Agents Chemother.* Vol 39, No 5, (May 1995), pp. 1204–1205.

Hatano, H., Hunt, P., Weidler, J., et al (2006). Rate of Viral Evolution and Risk of Losing Future Drug Options in Heavily Pretreated, HIV-Infected Patients Who Continue to Receive a Stable, Partially Suppressive Treatment Regimen. *Clinical Infectious Diseases*, Vol. 43, No. 10, pp.1329-1336.

Hirsch, MS., Brun-Vezinet, F., Clotet, B., et al (2003). Antiretroviral drug resistance testing in adults infected with human immunodeficiency virus type 1: 2003 recommendations of an International AIDS Society-USA Panel. *Clinical Infectious Diseases*, Vol. 37, No. 1, pp.113-128.

Horimoto, T. & Kawaoka, Y. (2005). Influenza: lessons from past pandemics, warnings from current incidents. *Nature Review Microbioogy.* Vol 3, No.8, (August 2005), pp: 591-600.

Hunt, PW., Harrigan, PR., Huang, W., et al (2006). Prevalence of CXCR4 tropism among antiretroviral-treated HIV-1-infected patients with detectable viremia. *Journal of Infectious Diseases,* Vol. 194, No. 7, pp.926-930.

Itzstein, M. (2007). The war against influenza: discovery and development of sialidase inhibitors. *Nature Review Drug Discovery.* Vol. 6, No.12, (December 2007), pp. 967-974.

Jabs, D., Martin, B. & Forman, M. (2010). Cytomegalovirus Retinitis and Viral Resistance Research Group. Mortality associated with resistant cytomegalovirus among patients with cytomegalovirus retinitis and AIDS. *Ophthalmology.* Vol. 117, No.1 (January 2010), pp.128-132.

Jabs, DA., Enger C., Dunn JP. & Forman M. (1998). Cytomegalovirus retinitis and viral resistance: ganciclovir resistance. CMV Retinitis and Viral Resistance Study Group. *Journal of Infectious Diseases* Vol. 177 No. 3 (March 1998), pp. 770–773.

James, SH, Kimberlin DW. & Whitley RJ. (2009). Antiviral therapy for herpesvirus central nervous system infections: neonatal herpes simplex virus infection, herpes simplex encephalitis, and congenital cytomegalovirus infection. *Antiviral Research.* Vol. 83, No. 3, (September 2009), pp.207-13.

Janies, DA., Voronkin, IO., Studer, J., Hardman, J., Alexandrov, BB., et al. (2010). Selection of resistance to oseltamivir in seasonal and pandemic H1N1 influenza and widespread co-circulation of the lineages. *International Journal of Health Gepgraphics.* Vol. 24, No. 9, (February 2010), pp. 13-18.

John, C. & Saunders, V. (2007). *Virology. Principles and applications,* ISBN 978-0470023877, John Wiley & Sons, Ltd. England.

Johnson, VA., Brun-Vézinet, F., Clotet, B., et al (2010). Update of the drug resistance mutations in HIV-1: 2010. *Topics in HIV Medicine,* Vol. 18, No. 5, pp.156-163.

Kahn L (January 2008). The growing number of immunocompromised in: The growing number of immunocompromised, 01.06.2008, Available from http://
http://www.thebulletin.org/web-edition/columnists/laura-h-kahn/the-growing-number-of-immunocompromised

Kit, S., Kit M., Qavi H., Trkula D. & Otsuka H.. (1983). Nucleotide sequence of the herpes simplex virus type 2 (HSV-2) thymidine kinase gene and predicted amino acid sequence of thymidine kinase polypeptide and its comparison with the HSV-1 thymidine kinase gene. *Biochimica et biophysica acta* Vol. 741, No. 2 (November 1983), pp. 158–170.

Kriesel, J.D., Spruance S.L., Prichard M., Parker J.N. & Kern E.R. (2005). Recurrent antiviral-resistant genital herpes in an immunocompetent patient. *Journal of Infectious Diseases.* Vol. 192, No. 1, (July 2005), pp. 156-161.

Landry, ML., Stanat, S., Biron, K., Brambilla, D., Britt, et al.(2000). A standardized plaque reduction assay for determination of drug susceptibilities of cytomegalovirus clinical isolates. *Antimicrobial Agents &Chemotherapy.* Vol. 44, No. 3, (March 2000), pp. 688–692.

Le, L., Lee, EH., Hardy, DJ., Truong, TN. & Schulten K. (2010) Molecular dynamics simulations suggest that electrostatic funnel directs binding of Tamiflu to influenza N1 neuraminidases. PLoS Computational Biology. Vol. 6, No. 9, (September 2010), pp. e1000939.

Lea, AP. & Bryson HM.(1996). Cidofovir. *Drugs* Vol. 52, No. 2, (August 1996), pp. 225-230.

Lee, PK., Kieffer, TL., Siliciano, RF & Nettles, RE. (2006). HIV-1 viral load blips are of limited clinical significance. *Journal of Antimicrobial Chemotherapy,* Vol. 57, No. 5, pp.803-805.

Levin, M.J., Bacon T.H. & Leary J.J. (2004). Resistance of herpes simplex virus infections to nucleoside analogues in HIV-infected patients. *Clinical Infectious diseases*. Vol 39, Suppl 5, (November 2004), pp. S248-57.

Levin, MJ., Weinberg A., Leary JJ. & Sarisky R.T. (2001). Development of acyclovir-resistant herpes simplex virus early during the treatment of herpes neonatorum. *Pediatric Infectious Diseases Journal*. Vol. 20, No. 11, (November 2001), pp. 1094-1097.

Liu, JB. & Zhang, Z. (2008). Development of SYBR Green I-based real-time PCR assay for detection of drug resistance mutations in cytomegalovirus. *Journal of Virology Methods. Vol.* 149 No. 1, (April 2008), pp. 129-35.

Liu, S., Knafels JD., Chang JS., Waszak G.A., Baldwin E.T., et al. (2006).Crystal structure of the herpes simplex virus 1 DNA polymerase. *The Journal of biological chemistry*. Vol. 281, No. 26 (June 2006). pp. 18193-18200.

Long, MC., King, JR. & Acosta, EP. Pharmacologic aspects of new antiretroviral drugs. *Current Infectious Diseases Reports* 2008; Vol. 10, No. 6, pp. 522-529.

Loutfy, MR., Raboud, JM., Walmsley, SL., et al (2004). Predictive value of HIV-1 protease genotype and virtual phenotype on the virological response to lopinavir/ritonavir-containing salvage regimens. *Antiviral Therapy*, Vol. 9, pp. 595-602.

Lowance, D., Neumayer HH., Legendre CM., Squifflet J.P., Kovarik J., et al. (1999). Valacyclovir for the prevention of cytomegalovirus disease after renal transplantation. *The New England Journal of Medicine*. Vol 340, No. 19, (May 1999), pp. 1462–1470.

Lurain, N. & Chou, S. (2010) Antiviral drug resistance of human cytomegalovirus. *Clinical Microbiology Reviews*. Vol. 23, No. 44, (October 2010), pp. 689-712.

Lurain, N., Spafford., E. & Thompson, K. (1994). Mutation in the UL97 Open Reading Frame of Human Cytomegalovirus Strains Resistant to Ganciclovir. *Journal of Virology*. Vol. 68, No. 7, (July 1994), pp.4427-4431.

Lurain, N., Thompson, K., Holmes, E. & Sullivan, G. (1992)Point Mutations in the DNA Polymerase Gene of Human. *Journal of Virology* Vol. 66, No. 12 (December 1992), pp. 7146-7152.

Mackie, N., Dustan, S., McClure, MO., et al (2004). Detection of HIV-1 antiretroviral resistance from patients with persistently low but detectable viraemia. *Journal of Virological Methods*, Vol. 119, No. 2, pp.73-78.

Markham A, Faulds D. (1994). Ganciclovir: an update of its therapeutic use in cytomegalovirus infection. *Drugs*; Vol 48 No. 3 (September 1994), pp. 455-484.

Martin, M., Goyette, N., Ives, J. & Boivin, G. (2010). Incidence and characterization of cytomegalovirus resistance mutations among pediatric solid organ transplant patients who received valganciclovir prophylaxis. *Journal of clinical virology*. Vol. 47, No. 4 (April 2010), pp. 321–324.

Mazzotta, F., Lo Caputo, S., Torti C., et al (2003). Real versus virtual phenotype to guide treatment in heavily pretreated patients: 48-week follow-up of the Genotipo-Fenotipo di Resistenza (GenPheRex) trial. *Journal of Acquired Immune Deficiency Syndrome*, Vol. 32, No. 3, pp.268-280.

Mertz, G.J., Loveless M.O., Levin M.J., Kraus S.J., Fowler S.L., et al. (1997). Oral famciclovir for suppression of recurrent genital herpes simplex virus infection in women. A multicenter, double-blind, placebo-controlled trial. Collaborative Famciclovir Genital Herpes Research Group. *Archives of Internal Medicine*.. Vol. 157, No. 3, (February 1997), pp. 343-349.

Mocarski, E. S., Shenk T. & Pass R. F. (2007). Cytomegaloviruses, In *Field's Virology,* D. M. Knipe and P. M. Howley, Eds., pp.2701-2772, Lippincott Williams &Wilkins, ISBN 978-0-7817-6060-7, Philadelphia, Pa, USA, 5th edition.

Morfin, F., G. Souillet, K. Bilger, T. Ooka, M. Aymard, et al. (2000). Genetic characterization of thymidine kinase from acyclovir-resistant and -susceptible herpes simplex virus type 1 isolated from bone marrow transplant recipients. *Journal of Infectious Diseases*. Vol. 182, No. 1 (July 2000), pp. 290–293.

Moscona A. (2008). Medical management of influenza infection. *Annual Review Medicine.* Vol.59, (February 2008), pp. 397-413.

Mulamba, G., Hu, A., Azad, R., Anderson, K. & Coen, D. (1998). Human cytomegalovirus mutant with sequence-dependent resistance to the phosphorothioate oligonucleotide fomivirsen (ISIS 2922). *Antimicrobial Agents and Chemotherapy.* Vol 42, No. 4, (April 1998), pp. 971-973.

Muller, AD., Bode, S., Myer, L., et al (2011). Predictors of adherence to antiretroviral treatment and therapeutic success among children in South Africa. *AIDS Care,* Vol. 23, No. 2, pp. 129-138.

Murray, P.R., Rosenthal K.S. & Pfaller M.A. (2009). Human Herpesviruses. In *Medical Microbiology,* Mosby, ISBN 978-0-323-0570-6, St. Louis, Mo, USA.

Neal Nathanson (ed). (2007). *Viral pathogenesis and immunity.* ISBN 13:978-0-12-369464-5 Academic Press. London UK.

Nyquist, A.C., Rotbart H.A., Cotton M., Robinson C., Weinberg A., et al. (1994). Acyclovir-resistant neonatal herpes simplex virus infection of the larynx. *J Pediatr.* Vol. 124, No. 6 (June 1994), pp. 967-71.

Okomo-Adhiambo, M., Demmler-Harrison, GJ., Deyde, VM., Sheu, TG., Xu X., et al. (2010). Detection of E119V and E119I Mutations in influenza A (H3N2) viruses isolated from an immunocompromised patient: Challenges in diagnosis of oseltamivir resistance. *Antimicrobial Agents and Chemoteraphy.* Vol. 54, No. 5, (May 2010), pp. 1834-1841

Chemiblink database (2011). In: acyclovir, valacyclovir Ganciclovir, penciclovir, famciclovir, foscarnet, cidofovir. 2011, Available from http://www.chemblink.com/asp/searching.asp

Oram, R.J., Marcellino D., Strauss D., Gustafson E., Talarico C.L., et al.(2000). Characterization of an acyclovir-resistant herpes simplex virus type 2 strain isolated from a premature neonate. *Journal of Infectious Diseases.* Vol 181, No.4 (July 2000), pp. 1458-1461.

Palella, FJ Jr., Armon, C., Buchacz, K., et al (2009). The association of HIV susceptibility testing with survival among HIV-infected patients receiving antiretroviral therapy: a cohort study. *Annals of Internal Medicine,* Vol. 151, No. 2, pp.73-84.

Palese, P. (2004). Influenza: old and new threats. *Nature Medicine.* Vol.10, No. 12 Suppl, (December 2004), pp: S82-S87.

Parkin, N., Chappey, C., Lam, E. & Petropoulos, C. (2005). Reduced susceptibility to protease inhibitors in the abscence of primary PI-resistance-associated mutations. *Antiviral Therapy,* Vol. 10, pp. S118.

Pellett, PE & Roizman B. (2007). The family Herpesviridae: a brief introduction, In *Field's Virology,* D.M. Knipe and P. M. Howley, Eds., pp. 2479-2500, Lippincott Williams & Wilkins, ISBN 978-0-7817-6060-7, Philadelphia, Pa, USA, 5th edition

Perno, CF., Ceccherini-Silberstein, F., De Luca, A., et al (2002). Virologic correlates of adherence to antiretroviral medications and therapeutic failure. *Journal of Acquired Immune Deficiency Syndrome*, Vol. 31, Suppl. 3, pp.S118-S122.

Perno, CF. & Mertoli, A. (2006). Clinical cut-offs in the interpretation of phenotypic resistance, In: *Antiretroviral resistance in clinical practice.* Geretti M, Londres: Mediscript Ltd, Retrieved from: http://www.ncbi.nlm.nih.gov/books/NBK2254/

Phillips, AN., Dunn, D., Sabin, C., et al (2005). Long term probability of detection of HIV-1 drug resistance after starting antiretroviral therapy in routine clinical practice. *AIDS*, Vol. 19, No. 5, pp. 487-494.

Picard-Jean, F., Bougie, I. & Bisaillon, M. (2007).Characterization of the DNA- and dNTP-binding activities of the human cytomegalovirus DNA polymerase catalytic subunit UL54. *Biochemical Journal.* Vol 407, No. 3 (November 2007), pp. 331-41.

Piret, J. & Boivin G. (2011). Resistance of herpes simplex viruses to nucleoside analogues: mechanisms, prevalence, and management. *Antimicrobial Agents and Chemotherapy.* Vol. 55, No. 2, (February 2011), pp. 459-472.

Porter, RS & Kaplan JL. (2004). Overview of Herpesvirus Infections. In The Merck Manual for health care professionals. 19th edition, Merck Sharp & Dohme Corp., a subsidiary of Merck & Co., Inc., Whitehouse Station, N.J., U.S.A. Copyright © 2004-2011 Merck Sharp & Dohme Corp. (Http://www.merckmanuals.com/professional/index.html.

Pottage, JC. & Kessler H. A. (1995). Herpes simplex virus resistance to acyclovir: clinical relevance. *Infectious agents and disease.* Vol. 4, No. 3, (September 1995), pp. 115-124.

Poveda, E., Anta, L., Blanco, JL., et al (2010). Drug resistance mutations in HIV-infected patients in the Spanish drug resistance database failing tipranavir and darunavir therapy. *Antimicrobial Agents Chemotherapy*, Vol. 54, No. 7, pp. 3018-3020.

Prix, L., Hamprecht, K., Holzhüter, B., Handgretinger, R., Klingebiel, T. & Jahn, G. (1999), Comprehensive restriction analysis of the UL97 region allows early detection of ganciclovir-resistant human cytomegalovirus in an immunocompromised child. *Journal of Infectious Diseases.* Vol. 180 No.2 (August 1999), pp. 491-495.

Prix, L., Maierl, J., Jahn, G. & Hamprecht, K. (1998). A simplified assay for screening of drug resistance of cell-associated cytomegalovirus strains. *Journal of clinical virology.* Vol. 11, No. 1 (July 1998), pp. 29-37.

Protopopescu, C., Raffi, F., Roux, P., et al (2009). Factors associated with non-adherence to long-term highly active antiretroviral therapy: a 10 year followup analysis with correction for the bias induced by missing data. *Journal of Antimicrobial Chemotherapy*, Vol. 64, No. 3, pp. 599-606.

Recordon-Pinson, P., Soulié, C., Flandre, P., et al (2010). Evaluation of the genotypic prediction of HIV-1 coreceptor use versus a phenotypic assay and correlation with the virological response to maraviroc: the ANRS geno tropism study. *Antimicrobial Agents Chemotherapy*, Vol. 54, No. 8, pp. 3335-3340.

Reitz, MS. & Gallo, R (2009). Human Immunodeficiency Viruses. In: *Principles and Practice of Infectious Diseases*, Mandell GL, Bennet JE, Dolin R, pp. 2323-2335, Churchill Livingstone, Elsevier, ISBN 978-0-4430-6839-3, Philadelphia, PA.

Reyes, M., Shaik NS., Graber JM., Nisenbaum R., Wetherall NT., et al. (2003). Task Force on Herpes Simplex Virus Resistance. Acyclovir-resistant genital herpes among persons attending sexually transmitted disease and human immunodeficiency virus clinics. *Archives of internal medicine.* Vol. 163, No.1, (January 2003), pp. 76-80.

Rickinson, A. B, Kieff E. (2007), Epstein-Barr virus, In *Field's Virology*, D. M. Knipe and P. M. Howley, Eds., pp. 2655-2700, Lippincott Williams & Wilkins, ISBN 978-0-7817-6060-7, Philadelphia, Pa, USA, 5th edition.

Rivas, P., Holguin, A., Ramirez de Arellano, E., et al (2006). Tratamiento antirretroviral según tipos and subtipos del virus de la inmunodeficiencia humana. *Enfermedades Infecciosas y Microbiología Clínica*; Vol. 24, Supl. 2, pp. 29-33.

Rodriguez, J., Casper, K., Smallwood, G., Stieber, A., Fasola, C., et al.(2007). Resistance to Combined Ganciclovir and Foscarnet Therapy in a Liver Transplant Recipient with Possible Dual-Strain Cytomegalovirus Coinfection. *Liver Transplant*. Vol. 13, No.10, (October 2007), pp. 1396-1400.

Roizman, B., Knipe D. M., Whitley R. (2007). Herpes simplex viruses, In *Field's Virology*, D. M. Knipe and P. M. Howley, Eds., pp. 2501-2602 Lippincott Williams & Wilkins, ISBN 978-0-7817-6060-7, Philadelphia, Pa, USA, 5th edition.

Sacks, SL., Griffiths PD., Corey L., Cohen C., Cunningham A., et al. (2004). HSV-2 transmission. *Antiviral Research*. Vol. 63, Suppl 1 (August 2004), S27-35.

Sacks, SL.,. Wanklin RJ, Reece DE., Hicks KA., Tyler KL., et al.. (1989). Progressive esophagitis from acyclovir-resistant herpes simplex virus. Clinical roles for DNA polymerase mutants and viral heterogeneity? *Annals of Internal Medicine*. Vol. 111, No. 11, (December 1989), pp. 893–899.

Safrin, S., Elbeik T., Phan L., Robinson D., Rush J., et al.. (1994). Correlation between response to acyclovir and foscarnet therapy and in vitro susceptibility result for isolates of herpes simplex virus from human immunodeficiency virus-infected patients. *Antimicrob. Agents Chemother*. Vol. 38, No. 6, (June), pp.1246–1250.

Saint-Léger, E., Caumes, E., Breton, G., Douard, D., Saiag, P., et al. (2001). Clinical and virologic characterization of acyclovir resistant varicella-zoster viruses isolated from 11 patients with acquired immunodeficiency syndrome. *Clin. Infect. Dis*. Vol. 33, No. 12, (December 2001), pp. 2061–2067.

Sarisky, RT., Quail MR., Clark PE., Nguyen TT., Halsey WS., et al. (2001). Characterization of herpes simplex viruses selected in culture for resistance to penciclovir or acyclovir. *Journal of Virology*. Vol. 75, No. 4, (February 2001), pp. 1761–1769.

Sasadeusz, JJ., Tufaro F., Safrin S., Schubert, K., Hubinette MM., et al. (1997). Homopolymer mutational hot spots mediate herpes simplex virus resistance to acyclovir. *Journal of Virology*. Vol. 71, No. 5, (May 1997), pp. 872–878.

Sauerbrei, A., Deinhardt S., Zell R., Wutzler P. (2010). Testing of herpes simplex virus for resistance to antiviral drugs. *Virulence* Vol. 1, No. 6, (November-December), pp. 555-557

Sauerbrei, A., Taut J., Zell R. & Wutzler P. (2011). Resistance testing of clinical varicella-zoster virus strains. *Antiviral Research*. Vol. 90, No.3, (June 2011), pp. 242-247.

Sax, PE., Islam, R., Walensky, RP., et al (2005). Should resistance testing be performed for treatment-naïve HIV-infected patients? A cost-effectiveness analysis. *Clinical Infectious Diseases*, Vol. 41, No. 9, pp. 1316-1323.

Schang, L.M. (2004). Effects of pharmacological cyclin-dependent kinase inhibitors on viral transcription and replication. *Biochimica et biophysica acta*. Vol. 1697, No. 1-2, (March 2004), pp. 197-209.

Schmit, I., Boivin, G., (1999). Characterization of theDNApolymerase and thymidinekinase genes of herpes simplex virus isolates from AIDS patients in whom acyclovir and foscarnet therapy sequentially failed. *Journal of Infectious Diseases*. Vol. 180, No. 2, (August 1999), pp. 487–490

Schnipper, LE., Crumpacker CS. (1980). Resistance of herpes simplex virus to acycloguanosine: role of viral thymidine kinase and DNA polymerase loci. *Proceedings of the National Academy of Sciences USA* Vol. 77, No.4, (April 1980), pp. 2270–2273.

Shafer, RW. (2006). Rationale and uses of a public HIV drug-resistance database. *Journal of Infectious Diseases*, Vol. 194, Suppl. 1, pp. S51-S58.

Shiley, K., & Blumberg, E. (2011). Herpes viruses in transplant recipients: HSV, VZV, human herpes viruses, and EBV. *Hematology/Oncology Clinics of North America*. Vol. 25 No. 1, (June 2011), pp. 171-191.

Shin, YK., Weinberg A., Spruance S., Bernard M., Bacon TH., et al. (2003). Susceptibility of herpes simplex virus isolates to nucleoside analogues and the proportion of nucleoside-resistant variants after repeated topical application of penciclovir to recurrent herpes labialis. *Journal of Infectious Diseases*. Vol. 187, No.8, (April 2003), pp. 1241-1245.

Shors, T. (2009). *Understanding viruses*. Jones and Bartlett Publishers, Sudbury, Massachusetts, ISBN 13-978-0-7637-2932-5.

Singh, N. (2006). Antiviral drugs for cytomegalovirus in transplant recipients: advantages of preemptive therapy. *Reviews in Medical Virology*. Vol. 16, No. 5, (Sep-Oct), pp.281–287.

Snydman, D., Limaye, A., Potena, L & Zamora M. (2011). Update and review: state-of-the-art management of cytomegalovirus infection and disease following thoracic organ transplantation. *TTransplantation Proceedings*. Vol. 43, Suppl 3, (April), pp. S1-S17.

Stránská, R., Van Loon AM., Polman, M., Beersma MF., Bredius, RG., et al. (2004). Genotypic and phenotypic characterization of acyclovir-resistant herpes simplex viruses isolated from haematopoietic stem cell transplant recipients. *Antiviral Therapy*. Vol. 9, No. 4, (August 2004), pp. 565–575.

Sugawara, M., Huang, W., Fei, Y-J., et al. Transport of valganciclovir a ganciclovir prodrug, via peptide transporters PEPT1 and PEPT2. (2000). *Journal of Pharmaceutical Sciences*. Vol. 89, No. 6, (June 2000), pp. 781-789

Sullivan, V., Talarico, C., Stanat, S., Davis, M., Coen, M. &Biron, K. (1992). A protein kinase homologue controls phosphorylation of ganciclovir in human cytomegalovirus-infected cells. *Nature*. Vol. 358, No. 6382, (July 1992), pp. 162-164.

Summers, W.P., Wagner M. & Summers WC. (1975). Possible peptide chain termination mutants in thymide kinase gene of a mammalian virus, herpes simplex virus. *Proc Natl Acad Sci USA*. Vol. 72, No. 10, (October 2010),:4081–4084.

Tan, SL., Ganji, G., Paeper, B., Proll, S. & Katze, MG. (2007). Systems biology and the host response to viral infection. *Nature Biotechnology*. Vol. 25, No. 12 (December 2007), pp. 1383-1389.

Telenti, A. & Goldstein DB. (2006). Genomics meets HIV-1. *Nature Reviews Microbiology*, Vol. 4, pp. 865-873.

Telenti, A., Aubert, V., Spertini, F. (2002). Individualising HIV treatment-pharmacogenetics and immunogenetics. *Lancet*, Vol. 359, No. 9308, pp. 722-723.

Torti, C., Quiros-Roldan, E., Keulen, W., et al (2003). Comparison between rules-based human immunodeficiency virus type 1 genotype interpretations and real or virtual phenotype: concordance analysis and correlation with clinical outcome in heavily treated patients. *Journal of Infectious Diseases*, Vol. 188, No. 2, pp.194-201.

Tural, C., Ruiz, L., Holtzer, C., et al (2002). Clinical utility of HIV-1 genotyping and expert advice: the Havana trial. *AIDS*, Vol. 16, No. 2, pp. 209-218.

Van de Perre, P., Segondy, M., Foulongne, V., Ouedraogo A., Konate I., et al. (2008). Herpes simplex virus and HIV-1: deciphering viral synergy. *Lancet Infectious Diseases*. Vol. 8, No. 8, (August 2008), pp. 490-497.

Van Sighem, A., Zhang. S., Reiss, P., et al (2008). Immunologic, virologic, and clinical consequences of episodes of transient viremia during suppressive combination antiretroviral therapy. *Journal of Acquired Immune Deficiency Syndrome*, Vol. 48, No. 1, pp. 104-108.

Villahermosa, ML., Thomson, M., Vazquez de Parga, E., et al (2000). Improved conditions for extraction and amplification of human immunodeficiency virus type 1 RNA from plasma samples with low viral load. *Journal of Human Virology*, Vol. 3, No. 1, pp. 27-34.

Wang NX., Zheng JJ. (2009). Computational studies of H5N1 influenza virus resistance to oseltamivir. *Protein Sciences*. Vol. 18 No. 4 (April 2009), pp 707–715.

Wang, Y., Wang Q., Zhu Q., Zhou R., Liu J., et al. (2011). Identification and characterization of acyclovir-resistant clinical HSV-1 isolates from children. *Journal of Virology*. [Epub ahead of print] PubMed PMID: 21778105.

Webby, R., Hoffman, E. & Webster R. (2004). Molecular constraints to interspecies transmission of viral pathogens. *Nature Medicine Supplement*. Vol. 10, No. 12 Suppl, (December 2004), pp: S77-S81.

Weiss, RA. & McMichael, AJ. (2004). Social and environmental risk factors in the emergence of infectious diseases. *Nature Medicine* Vol. 10, No.12 Suppl, (December 2004), pp. S70-S76.

Wilkin, TJ., Su, Z., Kuritzkes, DR., et al (2007). HIV type 1 chemokine coreceptor use among antiretroviral-experienced patients screened for a clinical trial of a CCR5 inhibitor: AIDS Clinical Trial Group A5211. *Clinical Infectious Diseases*, Vol. 44, No. 4, pp. 591-595.

Wolf, G., Courcelle, C., Prichard, M. & Mocarski, E. (2001). Distinct and separate roles for herpesvirus-conserved UL97 kinase in cytomegalovirus DNA synthesis and encapsidation. *Proceedings of the National Academy of Sciences* U. S. A. Vol 98, No. 4, (February 2001), pp. 1895–1900.

Yamanishi, K, Mori Y., Pellett P. E, (2007), Human herpesviruses, In *Field's Virology*, D. M. Knipe and P. M. Howley, Eds., pp. 22819-2846, Lippincott Williams & Wilkins, ISBN 978-0-7817-6060-7, Philadelphia, Pa, USA, 5th edition.

Yeo, A., Chan, K., Kumarasinghe, G. & Yap, H. (2005). Rapid detection of codon 460 mutations in the UL97 gene of ganciclovir-resistant cytomegalovirus clinical isolates by real-time PCR using molecular beacons. *Mol Cell Probes*. Vol.19, No. 6, (December 2005), pp. 389-93.

Zhu, L., Persson, A., Mahnke, L., et al (2001). Effect of low-dose omeprazole (20 mg daily) on the pharmacokinetics of multiple-dose atazanavir with ritonavir in healthy subjects. Journal of Clinical Pharmacology, Vol. 51, No. 3, pp. 368-377.

5

Point Mutations Associated with HIV-1 Drug Resistance, Evasion of the Immune Response and AIDS Pathogenesis

Makobetsa Khati[1,2] and Laura Millroy[1]
[1]*Council for Scientific and Industrial Research, Biosciences,*
[2]*Department of Medicine,*
Groote Schuur Hospital and University of Cape Town, Cape Town,
South Africa

1. Introduction

Point mutations within the human immunodeficiency virus-type 1 (HIV-1) genome confer resistance to antiretroviral drugs. The mutations also help the virus to evade the immune system response and influence transmission and progression of the disease, collectively called acquired immune deficiency syndrome (AIDS) pathogenesis. This chapter presents an up-to-date critical review of the literature and provides a synthesis of the current understanding of HIV-1 point mutations in relation to drug resistance, evasion of the immune system and AIDS pathogenesis. First, to prime the reader, the chapter briefly describes organization and function of the HIV-1 genes. It then pinpoints salient point mutations within specific HIV-1 genes associated with resistance to current antiretroviral drugs. In particular, it pays attention to the *env* gene and its product, the surface envelope (Env) glycoprotein because the Env protein mediates viral entry, tropism and disease progression. Thus the role and frequencies of point mutations within the *env* gene is related to HIV-1 transmission dynamics and progression to AIDS. The *env* gene and Env protein are further unpacked to provide a better understanding of the role point mutations within this gene play in helping the virus to evade antibody mediated immune response. Finally, drawing mainly from our recent research work, the chapter proposes an aptamer-based strategy for the design of desirable approaches that can help circumvent HIV-1 point mutations and delay or diminish drug resistance.

2. Organization and function of the HIV-1 genes

The genome of HIV-1, unlike other retroviruses is made up of a single coding RNA strand of 9.2 kb in length and is far more complex than those of other retroviruses. The genome of most retroviruses is diploid. It is made up of two identical RNA strands with a plus (+) polarity. All retroviruses have the *env, gag* and *pol* genes, but HIV-1 has 6 additional regulatory and accessory genes (Figure 1), which produces 14 proteins (Table 1). The *env* gene encodes the envelope (Env) protein. The Env protein is made up of two polypeptides derived from a gp160 single precursor; the transmembrane (TM) gp41 and the outer surface

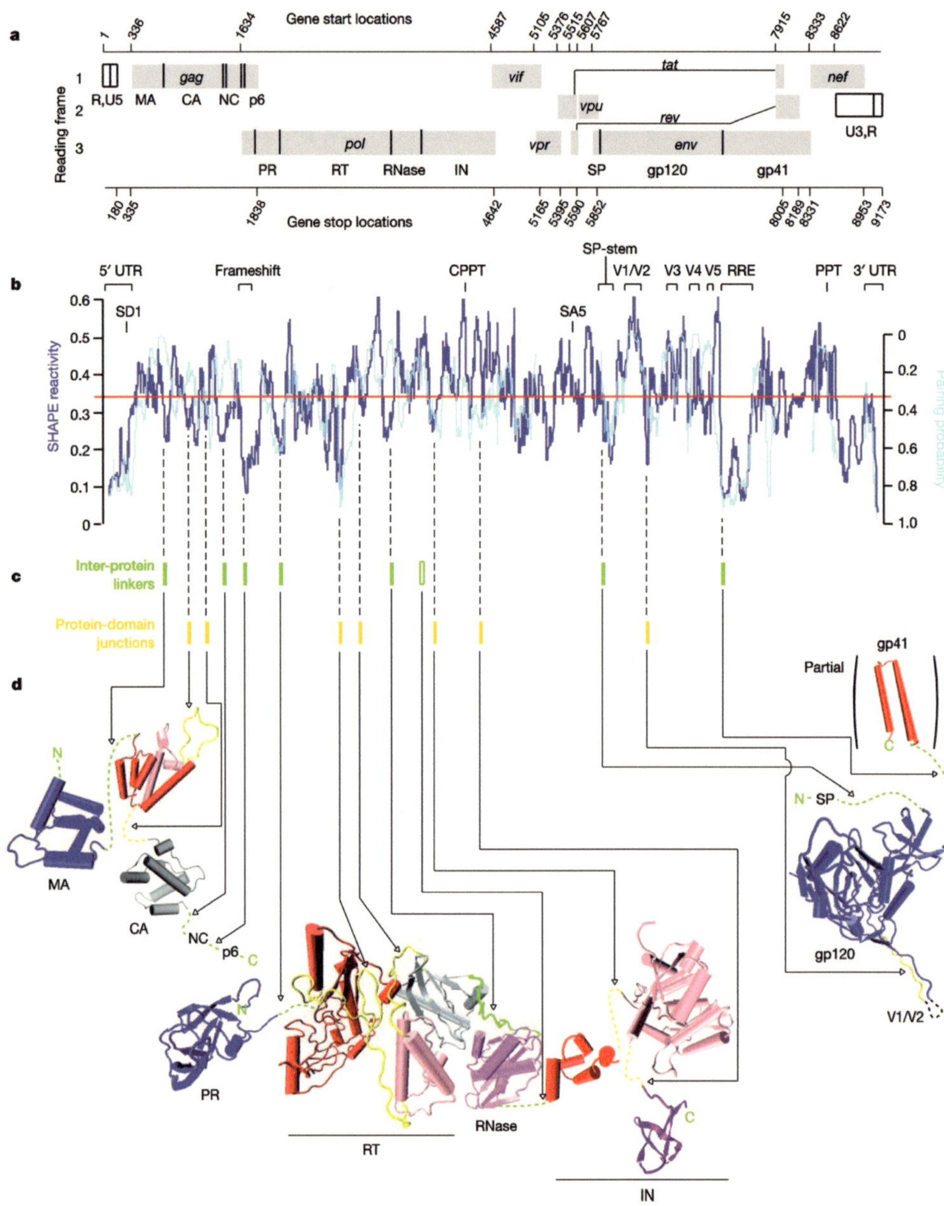

Fig. 1. Organization and function of the HIV-1 genome in relation to the proteins coded. (**a**) Protein coding region are shown as grey boxes. (**b**) Comparison of the pairing probability of nucleotides in the overall HIV-1 structure using 2′-hydroxyl acylation analysed by primer extension (SHAPE) reactivity. (c) Inter-protein linkers and unstructured peptide loops that link protein domains. (d) Three-dimensional structures of large and key HIV-1 proteins encoded by *env* and *pol* genes, respectively. Reproduced from (Watts et al., 2009) with permission from Nature Publishing Group (Copyright Clearance Centre License Number: 2754150202433)

(SU) gp120 (Figure 1). For a mature virion, on the inner leaflet of the envelope there are proteolytically processed *gag* gene products: a p17 matrix (MA) protein and a p24 capsid (CA) protein that form the core of the particle and an RNA-binding p7 nucleocapsid (NC) protein (Figure 1 and Table 1). Other proteins present in the core of the virion particle are derived from the *pol* gene and perform enzymatic functions. HIV-1 gp120 and gp41 (*env* gene products) and *pol* gene products, reverse transcriptase (RT) and integrase (IN) are involved in early stages of the HIV life cycle and are primary targets of therapeutic drugs. Env, RT and IN are targets of antiretroviral drugs called entry inhibitors (EI), reverse transcriptase inhibitors (RTI) and integrase inhibitors (INI), respectively. Another *pol* gene product called protease (PR) is involved in later stages of the HIV life cycle and it is also a target of a class of antiretroviral drugs called protease inhibitors. Other HIV-1 genes encode auxiliary proteins (Figure 1).

Gene	Protein encoded	Function
gag	Gag MA	Membrane anchoring; env interaction; nuclear transport of viral core
gag	Gag CA	Core capsid
gag	Gag NC	Binds RNA and Vpr, respectively
pol	Protease (PR)	gag/pol cleavage
pol	Reverse Transcriptase (RT)	Reverse transcription
pol	RNase H	RNase H activity
pol	Integrase (IN)	DNA provirus integration
env	Env (gp120 and gp41)	gp120 binds CD4 receptor and CXCR4/CCR5 co-receptors , gp41 mediates fusion
tat	Tat	Viral transcription activator
rev	Rev	RNA transport, stability and utilization factor (phosphoprotein)
vif	Vif	Promotes virion maturation and infectivity
vpr	Vpr	Promotes nuclear localization of preintegration complex, inhibits cell division, arrest infected cells at G2/M
vpu	Vpu	Promotes extracellular release of viral particles. Important for viral assembly and budding
nef	Nef	CD4 and class I downregulation

Table 1. HIV-1 genes, proteins coded by the respective genes and their functions

3. Point mutations and HIV-1 drug resistance

Antiretroviral drugs are currently the cornerstone of controlling HIV-1 in infected individuals. To date, 24 antiretroviral drugs have been approved and licensed for the treatment of HIV-1 infection. Thirteen of these drugs are reverse transcriptase inhibitors (nine nucleoside and four non-nucleoside RT inhibitors); nine are protease inhibitors; a fusion inhibitor; a CCR5 inhibitor and an integrase inhibitor. However, despite the use of current antiretroviral drugs, HIV-1 can still persists in infected individuals by accumulating mutations, which make it resistant to one or more drugs. The antiretroviral drug resistant mutations can be identified by one or more of the following: (a) *in vitro* passage experiments or site directed mutagenesis studies (Clark et al., 2006); (b) mutagenically separated PCR (Frater et al., 2001); (c) drug susceptibility testing (Petropoulos *et al.*, 2000; Svicher *et al.*, 2011); (d) nucleotide sequencing of viruses from patients failing a specific drug (McNicholas et al., 2011; Shulman et al., 2004); (e) correlation studies between genotype at baseline and virologic response in patients exposed to a specific antiretroviral drug (Demeter et al., 2008). Currently, more than 200 mutations in the HIV-1 *pol* and *env* genes associated with resistance to current antiretroviral drugs, which include reverse transcriptase inhibitors (RTIs), protease inhibitors (PIs), integrase inhibitors (INI), fusion inhibitors and attachment inhibitors respectively, have been identified (V. A. Johnson *et al.*, 2010; Shafer & Schapiro, 2008).

3.1 Point mutations associated with resistance to NRTIs

HIV-1 RT is a heterodimer made up of two subunits, p66 and p51 (di Marzo Veronese et al., 1986) and its crystal structure has been solved (Arnold *et al.*, 1992; Kohlstaedt *et al.*, 1992b). RT is important in the HIV-1 life cycle because it orchestrates synthesis of a linear double-stranded DNA copy of a viral single-stranded RNA genome. The knowledge that HIV-1 is a retrovirus immediately pinpointed RT synthesis of proviral DNA as a target for a class of antiretroviral drugs called RTIs. Indeed, RTIs including the prototype azidothymidine (AZT) also known as zidovudine (ZDV), were the first to be approved for clinical use (Fischl et al., 1987), and remains the mainstay of HIV-1 therapy. Nearly half of current antiretroviral drugs target the polymerase activity of RT. RTIs belong to one of the two broad categories: nucleoside RT inhibitors (NRTIs) and non-nucleoside RT inhibitors (NNRTIs).

NRTIs are structural analogues of natural substrate of DNA synthesis. They lack the 3′-hydroxyl group (3′-OH) and hence they block HIV-1 replication by acting as chain terminators when incorporated into a viral DNA by RT. Two basic NRTI resistance mechanisms are exclusion and excision. The exclusion mechanism involves enhanced discrimination at the time the NRTI tri-phosphate is incorporated in the nascent DNA strand. The M184V/I point mutation (Figure 2 and Table 2), which selectively reduces incorporation of abacavir (ABC); emtricitabine (FTC) and lamivudine (3TC) NRTIs into a nascent DNA chain by steric hindrance (Gao et al., 2000; Sarafianos et al., 1999) is a common example of the exclusion mechanism. M184V point mutation causes a median 1.5-fold and 3.0-fold reduction in susceptibility to didanosine (ddI) and ABC, respectively in the PhenoSenseGT™ assay (Petropoulos *et al.*, 2000; Rhee *et al.*, 2004). However several clinical trials have shown that ABC and ddI retain clinical activity in the presence of M184V point mutation (Brun-Vezinet *et al.*, 2003; J. J. Eron, Jr. *et al.*, 2007; Lanier *et al.*, 2004a; Marcelin *et al.*, 2005; Molina *et al.*, 2005; M. A. Winters *et al.*, 2003). The phenotypic and clinical significance of M184V is influenced by the presence or absence of other NRTI resistance mutations (Shafer & Schapiro, 2008). For instance, the presence of K65R or L74V (J. Eron, Jr. *et al.*, 2006; Gallant *et al.*, 2006; Moyle *et al.*, 2005) point mutations (Figure 2 and Table 2) in addition to the M184V is sufficient for high level resistance to ddI and ABC (Rhee *et al.*, 2004), particularly in patients with non-subtype B clades (Harrigan *et al.*, 2000; Lanier *et al.*, 2004a; Svarovskaia *et al.*, 2007; M. A. Winters *et al.*, 1997). K65R has emerged more rapidly during the *in vitro* passage of subtype C compared with subtype B isolates in the presence of increasing concentrations of TDF (Brenner *et al.*, 2006). The emergence of K65R mutation is suppressed maximally in regimens containing AZT compared with d4T (Roge *et al.*, 2003). Thus, the K65R point mutation commonly causes intermediate resistance to tenofovir (TDF), ABC, ddI, 3TC and FTC (Table 2), low level resistance to d4T, and increased susceptibility to AZT (Antinori *et al.*, 2007; Lanier *et al.*, 2004b). There is a body of evidence suggesting that K65R mutation occurs more commonly in low-income countries when patients with non-subtype B HIV-1 strains are treated with d4T/ddI and d4T/3TC (Doualla-Bell *et al.*, 2006; Hawkins *et al.*, 2009) or TDF/3TC (Rey *et al.*, 2009). In comparison to K65R, L74V point mutation causes intermediate resistance to ddI and ABC, and a slight increase in susceptibility to AZT and TDF (Rhee *et al.*, 2006b). L74V and K65R mutations rarely occur in the same viruses (Shafer & Schapiro, 2008). However, several patients harbouring HIV-1 species containing the L74V point mutation while receiving a regimen containing ABC or ddI have been found to have minor variants containing K65R (Descamps *et al.*, 2006; Svarovskaia *et al.*, 2007). On the other hand, K65R and M184V mutations are primarily found in patients receiving the NRTI backbone TDF/3TC (Gallant *et al.*, 2004; Margot *et al.*, 2006) and less commonly ABC/3TC (Moyle *et al.*, 2005) or TDF/FTC (Gallant *et al.*, 2006; Smith *et al.*, 2008). L74V and M184V mutations primarily occur in patients receiving ABC/3TC or ddI/3TC/FTC NRTI backbones (Descamps *et al.*, 2006; Moyle *et al.*, 2005; Sosa *et al.*, 2005). In addition to the M184V, K65R and L74V mutations, which between them cause resistance to ABC, 3TC, FTC, TDF and ddI by the exclusion mechanism; there is a complex set of several mutations that involves Q151M causing multi-NRTI resistant (Figure 2 and Table 2). All of the amino acids involved in the NRTIs resistance by the exclusion mechanism are in the fingers or the palm of RT (Figure 2) and could potentially affect the binding of an incoming deoxy-nucleotide triphosphate (dNTP).

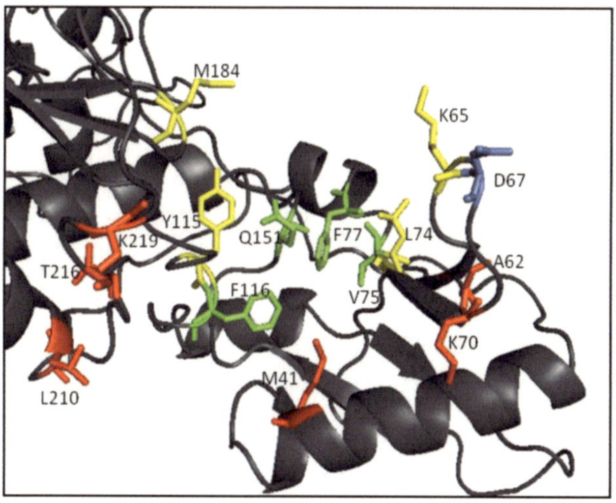

Fig. 2. Ribbon representation of the NRTI-binding site (palm and fingers of RT) showing residues that confer resistant when mutated as illustrated in Table 2. Red show amino acid residues that confer multi-NRTI resistance (all the FDA approved drugs). Green show residues that affect all the FDA approved NRTIs except for TDF. Mutations of blue residues are associated with TAMs. Yellow shows residues that confer resistance to certain NRTIs (Table 2) by the exclusion mechanism.

NRTI	TAMs (excision)						Non-TAMs (exclusion)					Multi-NRTI resistance mutations						
*	M41	D67	K70[a]	I210	T215	K219	K65	K70[a]	L74	V75[b]	Y115	M184	T69	Q151	A62	V75[b]	F77	F116
3TC	-	-	-	-	-	-	RN	EG	-	-	-	**VI**	Ins	M	V	-	-	-
ABC	L	N	-	W	FY	-	**RN**	EG	**VI**	TM	F	VI	Ins	**M**	V	I	L	Y
D4T	**L**	N	R	W	**FY**	QE	RN	-	-	**TM**	-	-	Ins	**M**	V	I	L	Y
ddI	L	N	-	W	FY	-	**RN**	EG	-	TM	-	VI	Ins	**M**	V	I	L	Y
FTC	-	-	-	-	-	-	RN	EG	-	-	-	**VI**	Ins	M	V	-	-	-
TDF	**L**	N		W	FY	-	**RN**	EG	-	M	F	-	Ins	M	V	-	-	-
ZDV	**L**	N	R	W	**FY**	QE	-	-	-	-	-	-	Ins	**M**	V	I	L	Y

*Denotes position of consensus amino acids that confer resistance to NRTIs when mutated. Dashes (-) indicate that the respective NNRTIs are not affected by the mutation(s). All amino acids are denoted by the single letter annotation, except for "Ins", which stands for one or more amino acid insertions. Mutations in bold are associated with high levels of phenotypic resistance or reduced virologic response. [a]K70R occur in HIV-1 isolates from patients receiving thymidine analogs. [b]V75I occurs in combination with Q151M. Modified from (Shafer & Schapiro, 2008).

Table 2. Mutations in the RT gene associated with resistance to NRTIs

In contrast to the exclusion mechanism discussed above; the excision mechanism involves selective removal of the NRTI from the end of the viral DNA after it has been incorporated by RT (Arion *et al.*, 1998; Boyer *et al.*, 2001; Meyer *et al.*, 1999; Meyer *et al.*, 1998). This is ATP-dependent excision and polymerization run in reverse, where an AZT resistant RT efficiently incorporates AZT triphosphate but has the enhanced ability to remove the incorporated AZT-monophosphate from the 5'-end of the template strand (Arion *et al.*, 1998; Meyer *et al.*, 1998). The first and well studied example of excision mechanism involves a set of AZT resistant mutations such as M41L, D67N, K70R, L210W, T215F/Y and K219E (Figure 1 and Table 1). These AZT resistant mutations are also called thymidine-analog mutations (TAMs) or excision-enhancing mutations (EEMs). In addition to AZT, the TAMs decrease susceptibility to d4T and to a lesser extent ABC, ddI and TDF (Whitcomb *et al.*, 2003). TAMs are common in low income countries in which the fixed-dose combinations containing thymidine analogues are the mainstay of therapy (Ross *et al.*, 2001). TAMs are also common in HIV-1 isolates from patients who began therapy in the pre-highly active antiretroviral therapy (HAART) era (De Luca *et al.*, 2006; Rhee *et al.*, 2005). The mutations accumulate in two distinct but overlapping patterns (De Luca *et al.*, 2006; Gonzales *et al.*, 2003; Marcelin *et al.*, 2004b; Yahi *et al.*, 1999). The type I pattern includes the M41L, L210W and T15Y mutations, respectively (De Luca *et al.*, 2006; Miller *et al.*, 2004). Type II patterns includes D67N, K70R, T215F and K219Q/E (Figure 2). D67N point mutation also occurs commonly with type I TAMs (Cozzi-Lepri *et al.*, 2005; Rhee *et al.*, 2007). However, K70R and L210W rarely occur together (Yahi *et al.*, 2000). Type I TAMs cause higher levels of phenotypic and clinical resistance to the thymidine analogs and cross resistance to ABC, ddI and TDF than do the type II TAMs (Cozzi-Lepri *et al.*, 2005; De Luca *et al.*, 2007; Lanier *et al.*, 2004a; Miller *et al.*, 2004). The clinical significance of the type II TAMs is not well understood.

3.2 Point mutations associated with resistance to NNRTIs

The NNRTIs block RT activity allosterically by binding to a hydrophobic pocket close to but not contiguous with the polymerase active site (Figure 3). The NNRTI-binding pocket

(NNIBP), which exists only in bound RT (Kohlstaedt *et al.*, 1992a; Ren *et al.*, 1995a), consists of the following amino acid residues: L100; K101; K013; V106; T107; V108; V179, Y181; Y188; V189; G190; F227; W229; L234; Y318 and E138 (Figure 3). Nearly all the of the NNRTI resistance mutations are within the NNIBP or adjacent to residues in the pocket (Ren *et al.*, 2008; Ren & Stammers, 2008; Sarafianos *et al.*, 2004). The NNRTI resistant mutations are broadly classified as: (a) primary mutations that cause high-level resistance to one or more NNRTIs and are the first to develop during the therapy; (b) secondary mutations that usually occur in combination with primary NNRTI resistance mutations (c) minor non-polymorphic mutations that may occur alone or in combination with other NNRTI resistance mutations and (d) polymorphic accessory mutations that modulate the effects of other NNRTI resistance mutations (Shafer & Schapiro, 2008). There is low genetic barrier to NNRTI resistance. Only one or two mutations are required for high level resistance.

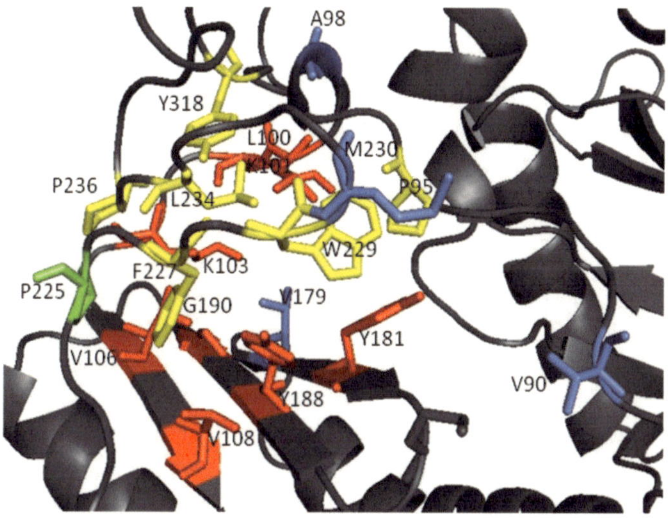

Fig. 3. Ribbon representation of the NNIBP showing the residues where NNRTI-resistance mutations occur. Red shows residues where primary point mutations which cause resistance to nearly all the current NNRTIs occur. Green shows a residue where a major secondary mutation which causes resistance to EFV occurs. Blue shows unique residues which confers resistance to ETR when mutated. Yellow shows residues where miscellaneous mutations that cause resistance to at least one of the NNRTI may occur.

The most frequently observed primary point mutations in patients treated with approved NNRTIs are K103N and Y181C (Table 3). Each of the primary NNRTI resistance mutations, namely, K103N/S; V106A/M; Y181C/I/V, Y188L/C/H and G190A/S/E (Figure 3 and Table 3) cause high level resistance to nevirapine (NVP) and variable resistance to efavirenz (EFV), ranging from about 2-fold for V106A and Y181C; 6-fold for G190A; 20-fold for K103N; and more than 50-fold for Y188L and G190S (Bacheler *et al.*, 2001; Rhee *et al.*, 2006b). Transient virologic responses to EFV-based salvage therapy regimen occur in some NNRTI-experienced patients but a sustained response is not common (Antinori *et al.*, 2002; Delaugerre *et al.*, 2001; Shulman *et al.*, 2000; Walmsley *et al.*, 2001). On the other hand, patients with any of the NNRTI resistance primary point mutations (Figure 3 and Table 3) may benefit from etravirine (ETR) salvage therapy (Lazzarin *et al.*, 2007; Madruga *et al.*, 2007). However, point mutations at Y181 and to a lesser extent G190 compromise ETR response and may provide the foundation for the development of high-level ETR resistance (Lazzarin *et al.*, 2007; Madruga *et al.*, 2007). Major secondary and minor/miscellaneous mutations that usually occur in combination with one of the primary NNRTI resistance point mutations are depicted in Figure 3 and their respective effects on NNRTIs is summarized in Table 3.

Current understanding suggests that there are at least three classes of NNRTI-resistance mechanisms (Sarafianos *et al.*, 2009). The first mechanism involves loss or change of key hydrophobic amino acid residues in the NNIBP such as Y181, Y188 and F227 (Figure 3). Specific point mutations in one of these hydrophobic residues cause significant resistance through the loss of the aromatic ring interactions with NNRTIs (Das *et al.*, 1996; Kohlstaedt *et al.*, 1992a; Ren *et al.*, 1995b; Ren *et al.*, 2001; Ren *et al.*, 2004). This causes high levels of resistance to the first generation NNRTIs, which are relatively rigid (Sarafianos *et al.*, 2009). Second generation and more advanced NNRTI are designed with an inherent flexibility. This intrinsic flexibility called the wiggling and jiggling makes the second and subsequent generation NNRTIs to have compensatory interactions with RT that has mutations causing resistance to first generation NNRTIs (Das *et al.*, 2008; Das *et al.*, 2004). The second mechanism of NNRTI-resistance point mutations involves steric hindrance by amino acid residues in the central region of the NNIBP such as L100 and G190 (Figure 3). The L100I point mutation confers high-level resistance to all the current NNRTIs (Table 3) by changing the shape of the pocket (Ren *et al.*, 2004). In contrast G190A point mutation, which also confers high-level resistance to almost all the current NNRTIs (Table 3), causes a bulge (Sarafianos *et al.*, 2004). The third and last mechanism of NNRTI-resistance point mutation involves pocket entrance mutations at the rim of the NNIBP such as K103N and K101E (Figure 3). These point mutations cause resistance to first generation NNRTIs by interfering with the entry of NNRTIs into the NNIBP pocket (Hsiou *et al.*, 2001; Ren *et al.*, 2007). Second generation NNRTIs were designed to circumvent this problem. For instance, diarylpyrimidine NNRTIs such as ETR are able to inhibit HIV-1 isolates with K103N point mutation because they interact with the side chain of the mutated N103 residue (Das *et al.*, 2004; Janssen *et al.*, 2005).

NRTI	Primary mutations					Major secondary mutations					Minor and miscellaneous mutations				
*	K103	V106	Y181	Y188	G190	L100	K101	P225	F227	M230	A98	V108	V179	P236	K238
DLV	**NS**	**AM**	**CIV**	**LHC**	E	**I**	**EP**	-	C	**L**	G	I	DEF	**L**	**NT**
EFV	**NS**	AM	CIV	LHC	**ASE**	**I**	EP	H	C	**L**	G	I	DEF	-	NT
ETR	-	-	**CIV**	**LHC**	**ASE**	**I**	EP	-	**C**	**L**	G	-	DEF	-	-
NVP	**NS**	**AM**	**CIV**	LHC	**ASE**	**I**	**EP**	-	LC	**L**	G	I	DEF	-	**NT**

*Denotes position of consensus amino acids that confer resistance to NNRTIs when mutated. Dashes (-) indicate that the respective NNRTIs are not affected by the mutation(s). All amino acids are denoted by the single letter annotation. Mutations in bold are associated with high levels of phenotypic resistance or reduced virologic response. Modified from (Shafer & Schapiro, 2008).

Table 3. Mutations in the RT gene associated with resistance to NNRTIs

3.3 Point mutations associated with resistance to protease inhibitors

Resistance mutations in the protease genes are classified as major or minor (V. A. Johnson *et al.*, 2010). Major mutations are defined as those selected first in the presence of the protease inhibitor (PI) antiretroviral drug or those substantially reducing drug susceptibility. These mutations tend to be the primary contact residues for drug binding (Figure 4). Major PI resistance mutations that are of the most clinical significance occur at 17 largely non-polymorphic positions (Figure 4). Mutations at 13 of these 17 positions, including mutations at the substrate cleft positions L23, D30, V32, I47, G48, I50, V82 and I84; the flap positions M46 and I54; and the interior enzyme positions L76, N88 and L90 (Figure 4), reduce susceptibility to at least one PI (Table 4). Mutations at the other 4 positions (L24, L33, F53 and G73) are also important because they are common, non-polymorphic and cause resistance to several PI (Rhee *et al.*, 2006b).

Many major mutations reduce susceptibility to nelfinavir. In particular, L31I, D30N, M46I/L, G48V/M, I84V, N88D/S and L90M mutations are associated with high levels of phenotypic resistance to nelfinavir because they cause inferior virologic response to therapy relative to that obtainable with most other PI (Johnston *et al.*, 2004; Patick *et al.*, 1996; Vray *et al.*, 2003; B. Winters *et al.*, 2008). Similarly; I50L, I84 and N88S mutations are associated with high levels of phenotypic resistance to atazanavir/r (Colonno *et al.*, 2004; Pellegrin *et al.*, 2006; Rhee *et al.*, 2006b; Vermeiren *et al.*, 2007; Vora *et al.*, 2006; B. Winters *et al.*, 2008). G48V/M, 184V and L90M mutations are relative contraindications to the use of saquinavir/r (Marcelin *et al.*, 2004a; Marcelin *et al.*, 2007; Zolopa *et al.*, 1999). V32I, I47V/A, I54L/M and I84V mutations are relative contraindications to the use of fosamprenavir/r (Dandache *et al.*, 2007; Masquelier *et al.*, 2008; Pellegrin *et al.*, 2007; B. Winters *et al.*, 2008). V82A/F/T and I84V mutations are relative contraindications to the use of indinavir/r (Table 4). V47A and V82L/T major mutations are relative contraindications to the use of lopinavir/r (Dandache *et al.*, 2007; Friend *et al.*, 2004; Kagan *et al.*, 2005) and tipranavir/r (Baxter *et al.*, 2006). Table 4 lists the 17 major PI resistance mutations that are of clinical significance.

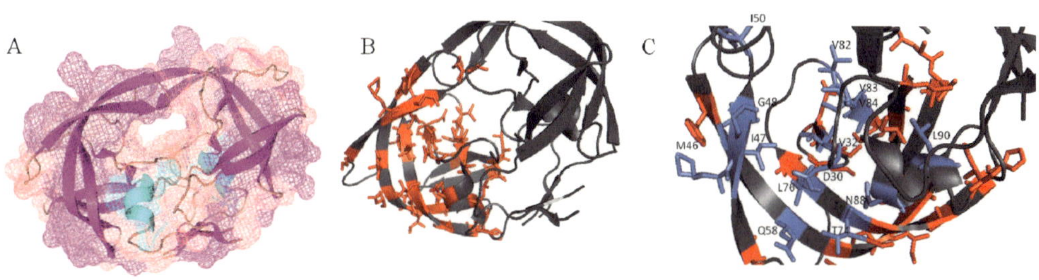

Fig. 4. Bound crystal structure of HIV-1 protease showing the residues where major PI-resistance mutations occur. (A) Mesh illustration of HIV-1 protease in bound state with saquinavir. (B) Illustration of amino acid residues (colour coded red) where PI-resistance point mutations occurs. (C) Zoomed-in illustration showing in detail residues (colour coded blue) where major PI-resistance mutations occur.

In contrast to the major PI resistance mutation discussed above; minor PI resistance mutations generally emerge later than major mutations and they do not have substantial effect on drug resistance phenotype by themselves. Instead, they improve replication of viruses containing major mutations (V. A. Johnson *et al.*, 2010). For instance, minor mutations at amino acid residues L10, K20, M36, L63 and A71 up-regulates protease processivity to compensate for the decreased fitness associated with the major PI resistance mutations (Hoffman *et al.*, 2003; Mammano *et al.*, 1998; Martinez-Picado *et al.*, 1999; Nijhuis *et al.*, 1999; van Maarseveen *et al.*, 2006). Residues L10, M36 and L63 are highly polymorphic. Baseline mutations at residues L10 and M36 are associated with an increased risk of virologic failure in patients receiving first generation PI such as nelfinavir (Perno *et al.*, 2001; Perno *et al.*, 2004). L10V and A71V/T minor mutations respectively occur in 5% and 10% of PI-naïve patients, and in much higher proportion of PI-experienced patients (Rhee *et al.*, 2003). In comparison, L10F/R and A711/L minor mutations do not occur in the absence of PI therapy (Rhee *et al.*, 2003). Additional PI-selected mutations include the highly polymorphic mutations I13V, D60E, I62V, V77I and I93L as well as several uncommon mutations including V11I, E34Q, E35G, K43T, K45I, K55R, Q58E, T74P/A/S, V75I, N83D, P79A/S, I85V, L89V, T91S, Q92K and C95F (Ceccherini-Silberstein *et al.*, 2004; Parkin *et al.*, 2003; Rhee *et al.*, 2005; Svicher *et al.*, 2005; Vermeiren *et al.*, 2007; T. D. Wu *et al.*, 2003).

The mechanism of some PI resistance mutations seems subtype-specific. For example, the accessory PI resistance mutations I13V, K20I, M36I and I93L represent the consensus variant in one or more non-subtype B isolates (Rhee *et al.*, 2006a). Furthermore, although both D30N and L90M mutations occur in non-subtype B viruses during nelfinavir therapy, D30N point mutation occurs more commonly in subtype B viruses; while L90M occurs more commonly in subtypes C, F, G and circulating recombinant form-AE (CRF-AE) viruses (Abecasis *et al.*, 2005; Calazans *et al.*, 2005; Cane *et al.*, 2001; Grossman *et al.*, 2004; Sugiura *et al.*, 2002). The increased predilection for a certain subtype to develop L90M may relate to the presence of variants other than L, which is subtype B consensus, at position 89 (Abecasis *et al.*, 2005; Calazans *et al.*, 2005; Gonzalez *et al.*, 2004). Similarly, T74S, which is a polymorphism that occurs in 8% of subtype C sequences, but rarely in other subtypes, is associated with reduced susceptibility to nelfinavir (Deforche *et al.*, 2007; Deforche *et al.*, 2006; Rhee *et al.*, 2006b). Notwithstanding, with notable aforementioned exceptions, the genetic mechanisms of PI resistance are highly similar among different subtypes (Kantor *et al.*, 2005).

3.4 Point mutations associated with resistance to integrase inhibitors

The HIV-1 integrase catalyses the ligation of the viral 3′-OH end to the 5′-DNA of host chromosomal DNA through a process called the strand transfer (A. A. Johnson *et al.*, 2006; Pommier *et al.*, 2005). The current generation of clinically relevant INI drugs such as the recently USA Food and Drug Administration (FDA) approved raltegravir (FDA, 2007) and elvitegravir, currently undergoing phase III clinical trials (Gilead Sciences, 2008), preferentially inhibit strand transfer by binding to the target DNA site of the enzyme. Most INI resistance mutations are in the vicinity of the putative INI binding pocket (Figure 5). Some of the INI resistance mutations decrease susceptibility by themselves, whereas others compensate for the decrease fitness associated with other INI resistance mutations (Lataillade *et al.*, 2007). There is a high level of cross-resistance between raltegravir and elvitegravir, as well as between these INI and the first generation of strand-transfer inhibitors, suggesting that the development of non cross-resistant INI will be challenging (Hombrouck *et al.*, 2008; Shimura *et al.*, 2008).

Common INI resistance point mutations are N155H and Q148H/R/K (Table 5), each of which can reduce raltegravir susceptibility by up to 25-fold (Cooper *et al.*, 2008). Higher levels of raltegravir resistance occur with accumulation of additional mutations. E92Q mutation and the two polymorphic mutations L74M and G163R generally occur with N155H, while G140A/S generally occurs with Q148H/R/K (Cooper *et al.*, 2008). Additional mutations (listed in Table 4) have been reported as being selected either *in vitro* or *in vivo* by raltegravir and include the non-polymorphic L74R, E138A/K, Y143R/C/H, N155S, H183P, Y226D/F/H, S230R, and D232N and the polymorphic mutations T97A and V151I (Delelis *et al.*, 2011; Malet *et al.*, 2008; Mouscadet *et al.*, 2009). For both raltegravir and elvitegravir, virologic failure has generally been accompanied by 100-fold or greater decreases in susceptibility and the development of two or more INI resistance mutations. Mutations at amino acid residues E92, F121, G140, Q148 and N155 are associated with more than 10-fold decrease in susceptibility to both INI, whereas mutations at amino acid residues T66 and S147 are associated with marked decreases in susceptibility only to elvitegravir (Figure 5 and Table 5).

PI	**Major mutations**																
*	L23	L24	D30	V32	L33	M46	I47	G48	I50	F53	I54	G73	L76	V82	I84	N88	L90
ATVr	-	I	-	-	F	IL	V	**VM**	**L**	L	VTALM	**ST**	-	**ATFS**	**VAC**	DS	**M**
DRVr	-	-	-	**I**	F	-	VA	-	V	-	**LM**	ST	**V**	-	VAC	-	M
FPVr	-	-	-	**I**	F	**IL**	**VA**	-	**V**	-	VTA**LM**	ST	**V**	ATFS	**VAC**	-	**M**
INDVr	-	**I**	-	V	-	**IL**	V	-	-	L	**VTALM**	ST	V	**AFTS**	**VAC**	S	**M**
LPVr	-	I	-	I	F	IL	**VA**	VM	**V**	-	**VTALM**	-	**V**	**AFTS**	VAC	-	M
NFV	**I**	**I**	**N**	-	F	**IL**	V	**VM**	-	L	**VTALM**	**ST**	-	**AFTS**	**VAC**	**DS**	**M**
SQVr	-	I	-	-	-	-	-	**VM**	-	L	**VTALM**	**ST**	-	AT	**VAC**	S	**M**
TPVr	-	-	-	I	F	IL	**V**	-	-	-	**VAM**	-	-	ATFSL	**VAC**	-	M

*Denotes position of consensus amino acids that confer resistance to PI when mutated. Dashes (-) indicate that the respective PI are not affected by the mutation(s). All amino acids are denoted by the single letter annotation. Mutations in **bold** are associated with high levels of phenotypic resistance or reduced virologic response. Mutations in **bold underline** are relative contraindications to the use of specific PI. ATVr (atazanavir/r); DRVr (darunavir/r); FPVr (fosamprevanir); IDVr (indinavir/r); NFV (nelfinavir); SQVr (saquinavir/r); TPVr (tipranavir/r). Modified from (Shafer & Schapiro, 2008).

Table 4. Mutations in the protease gene associated with major resistance to PI

INI	**Mutations**											
*	T66	E92	F121	E138	G140	Y143	S147	Q148	S153	N155	E157	R263
Raltegravir	-	**Q**	**Y**	AK	**AS**	CHR	G	**HRK**	-	**HS**	Q	-
Elvitegravir	**I**	**Q**	**Y**	AK	**AS**	-	**G**	**HRK**	**Y**	**HS**	Q	K

*Denotes position of consensus amino acids that confer resistance to INI when mutated. Dashes (-) indicate that the respective INI are not affected by the mutation(s). All amino acids are denoted by the single letter annotation. Mutations in bold are associated with more than 5-10 fold phenotypic resistance or reduced virologic response. Modified from (Shafer & Schapiro, 2008).

Table 5. Mutations in the integrase gene associated with resistance to INI

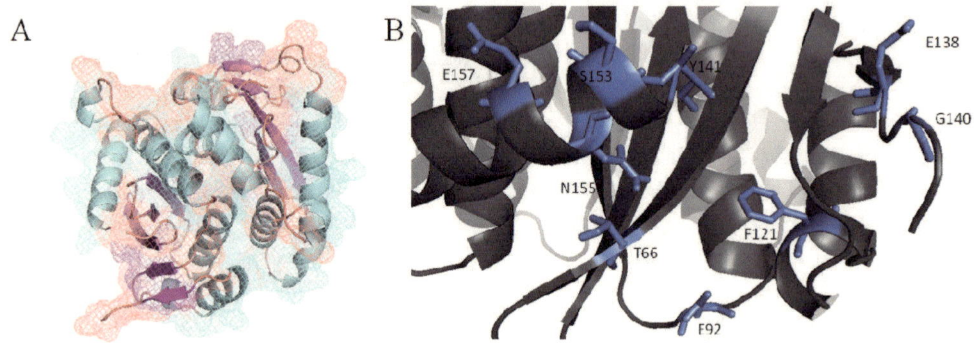

Fig. 5. Crystal structure of HIV-1 integrase showing the residues where major INI-resistance mutations occur. (A) Mesh illustration of bound HIV-1 integrase. (B) Illustration of amino acid residues where INI-resistance point mutations occurs.

3.5 Point mutations associated with resistance to fusion inhibitors

The HIV-1 gp41 mediates the fusion between the virus and host cell membrane. Fusion inhibitors act by a dominant negative mechanism of action, preventing formation of the six-helix bundle that is the driving force for the fusion process. Enfurvirtide, also known as T20 (Kilby et al., 1998; Wild et al., 1994), is the only FDA approved fusion inhibitor to date. Enfurvirtide has antiviral activity similar to most other classes of antiretroviral drugs discussed above; however resistance develop rapidly in patients receiving the drug for salvage therapy who do not receive a sufficient number of RTI, PI and INI drugs such as efavirenz, lopinanir/r and raltegravir, respectively. The emergence of enfurvirtide resistant strains followed by virologic rebound has been observed in some patients within two to four weeks (Cabrera *et al.*, 2006; Lu *et al.*, 2006).

Mutations in gp41 codons 36 to 45 (Figure 6), the region to which enfurvirtide binds, are primarily responsible for resistance to the drug (Marcelin *et al.*, 2004c; Melby *et al.*, 2006; Menzo *et al.*, 2004; Mink *et al.*, 2005; Sista *et al.*, 2004; Su *et al.*, 2006). The most common and potent T20-resistance mutations in this region are G36D/E, V38E/A, Q40H and N43D/K/S (Table 6). A single point mutation is generally associated with about 10-fold decreased susceptibility; whereas double point mutations can decrease susceptibility by more than 100-fold (Charpentier *et al.*, 2011; Su *et al.*, 2006; Xu *et al.*, 2005). The replication fitness of recombinant viruses carrying the enfurvirtide-resistant mutations is relatively poor (Lu *et al.*, 2004) and the mutant viruses rapidly revert to wild type phenotype in patients who discontinue the drug (Deeks *et al.*, 2007). Some enfurvirtide-resistant mutations, particularly V38A/E mutations, are associated with significant CD4 count increases (Aquaro *et al.*, 2006), presumably because mutations at residue V38 decrease HIV-1 replication or render the virus more susceptibility to a subset of neutralizing antibodies that target fusion intermediates (Reeves *et al.*, 2005).

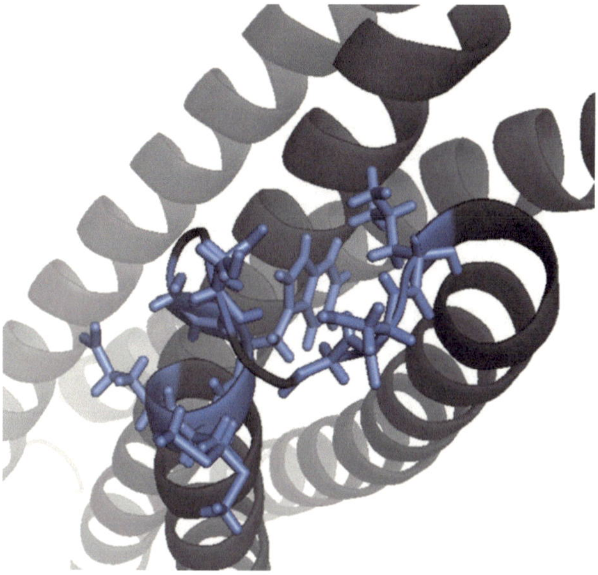

Fig. 6. Ribbon representation of HIV-1 heptad repeat fusogenic domain showing point mutations (colour coded blue) that cause resistance to fusion inhibitors.

Fusion inhibitor	Mutations								
*	G36	I37	V38	Q39	Q40	N42	N43	L44	L45
Enfuvirtide	**DEVS**	V	**EAMG**	R	**H**	T	**DKS**	M	M

*Denotes position of consensus amino acids that confer resistance to enfuvirtide when mutated. All amino acids are denoted by the single letter annotation. Mutations in bold are associated with more 10-fold phenotypic resistance or reduced virologic response in most clinical isolates. Modified from (Shafer & Schapiro, 2008).

Table 6. Mutations in the gp41 *env* gene associated with resistance to fusion inhibitors

3.6 Point mutations associated with resistance to attachment inhibitors

Despite the important role gp120 plays in attachment of HIV-1 to the CD4 receptor and CCR5/CXCR4; maraviroc, which is a CCR5 antagonist, is the only FDA approved attachment inhibitor in clinical use to date. While gp120 binds to the N-terminus and the second extracellular loop region of CCR5 (Hartley *et al.*, 2005), site-directed mutagenesis study suggests that small molecule attachment inhibitors such as maraviroc bind to a CCR5 pocket formed by the transmembrane helices (Dragic *et al.*, 2000). Thus, although gp120 and maraviroc do not bind to the same site of the CCR5 coreceptor, maraviroc allosterically inhibit gp120 binding to the CCR5 coreceptor. Point mutations in gp120 that allow the virus to bind to the maraviroc-bound form of CCR5 in the drug insensitive manner have been described (Westby *et al.*, 2007). Most of these mutations are found in the V3 loop of gp120 (Figure 7A), which determines HIV-1 tropism (discussed in the next section). One study showed that reverse mutations at positions 316 and 323 in the V3 loop of maraviroc-resistant HIV-1 variants to their original sequence restored wild-type susceptibility to maraviroc, while reversion of either mutation resulted in a partially sensitive virus with reduced maximal inhibition (Westby *et al.*, 2007). In another recent study maraviroc-resistant variants were isolated from the V3 loop library virus (HIV-1(V3lib)) containing the T199K and T275M plus 5 mutations in the V3 loop, namely I304V; F312W; T314A; E317D; I318V (Yuan *et al.*, 2011). Furthermore, the same study showed that the profile of HIV-1(JR-FL) pseudotype containing I304V/F312W/T314A/E317D/I318V (Figure 7A) in the V3 loop alone revealed a typical non-competitive resistance to maraviroc (Yuan *et al.*, 2011). Generally, amino acids mutations in the V3 loop may include known polymorphism as well as novel substitutions, insertions, and deletions. Further complicating the genetic basis of maraviroc or CCR5 inhibitor resistance is the observation that the same inhibitor may select for different mutations in different HIV-1 isolates (Westby *et al.*, 2007). The mutations observed in maraviroc-resistant strains isolated from patients are variable and differed for each HIV-1 isolate (Seclen *et al.*, 2011; Tilton *et al.*, 2011).

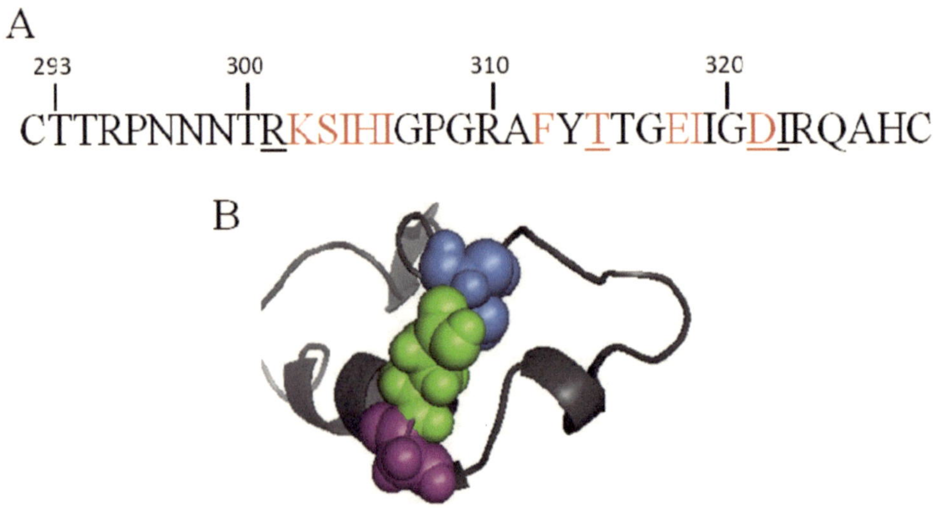

Fig. 7. Illustration of amino acid residues in the V3 loop important for HIV-1 tropism and resistance to maraviroc. (A) The sequence of the V3 variable loop indicating the sites of unique X4 substitution sites when compared to R5 clones (underlined). The red residues indicate the positions where maraviroc resistance mutations occur. Together with T199K and T275M, these mutations confer complete resistance to maraviroc. (B) Ribbon diagram of gp120 V3 variable loop highlighting amino acid residues essential for co-receptor usage. X4 tropism is determined by positively charged residues at position 11, 24 and 25 (colour coded blue, green and magenta respectively). R5 tropism is determined by a negative or neutral residue at any of the three positions.

4. Point mutations associated with HIV-1 tropism, transmission dynamics and AIDS pathogenesis

The identification of CCR5 and CXCR4 chemokine receptors as having critical roles in the cellular entry of HIV-1 allowed development of a more precise system for defining the viral tropism. Prototype T-cell tropic strains use CXCR4, macrophage-tropic strains use CCR5, and dual-tropic strains use both CXCR4 and CCR5 chemokine receptors, culminating in the currently used nomenclature X4, R5 and R5X4 strains, respectively (Berger et al., 1998). The phenotype of HIV-1 that is transmitted *in vivo* is R5 even when the contaminating virus is a mixture of R5, R5X4 and X4. The reason for this selection of viral phenotype during transmission is not well understood. The viraemia present during primary infection consists of oligoclonal R5 virus, and this virus type generally persists during the asymptomatic phase of the infection until the onset of AIDS. Viral transmission and disease progression, collectively called AIDS pathogenesis, corresponds to evolution of coreceptor phenotype. In about half of all HIV-1 infections there is viral evolution towards dual (R5X4) tropism and CXCR4 usage that is prognostic for accelerated progression to AIDS (Collman et al., 1992; Doranz et al., 1996). Thus when the phenotype switch occurs, there is an initial evolution from CCR5 using viruses to those that can use both CCR5 and CXCR4 (Connor et al., 1997). While evolution towards usage of the CXCR4 coreceptor and emergence of X4 viruses coincides with a decline in $CD4^+$ T cells and the onset of AIDS, the dominant theory is that X4 viruses are opportunistic infections that can only appear once the $CD4^+$ T cells have dropped below a certain threshold level. Notwithstanding, in another 50% of individuals infected with HIV-1 there is no viral evolution towards CXCR4 usage or emergence of X4 viruses; R5 viruses persists from primary infection until one succumbs to AIDS. This suggests that R5 viruses are necessary and sufficient to cause AIDS.

The main determinants for coreceptor tropism resides in the V3 loop (Figure 7), although mutations outside of the V3 loop may also influence tropism, either in combination or independently of the V3 mutations (Hartley *et al.*, 2005; W. Huang *et al.*, 2008; Pastore *et al.*, 2007; Pastore *et al.*, 2006). Very few mutations in the V3 loop are sufficient for switching coreceptor use from CCR5 to CXCR4 in most HIV-1 isolates, but in some isolates additional mutations in V1/V2 (Pastore *et al.*, 2006) and gp41 (W. Huang *et al.*, 2008) are observed during coreceptor switching. The presence of positively charged amino acids at positions 11, 24 and 25 in the V3 loop, combined with other V3 sequence characteristics (Figure 7), have specificity of about 90% and sensitivity of 70- 80% for predicting X4 tropism (Hartley *et al.*, 2005; Jensen & van 't Wout, 2003; Sing *et al.*, 2007). However, the number and type of mutations by which an R5 virus switches to X4 is complex and depends on the sequence of the baseline R5 virus (Low *et al.*, 2007; Moncunill *et al.*, 2008; Pastore *et al.*, 2007; Pastore *et al.*, 2006). The frequency and genetic basis for tropism switch is different for different HIV-1 subtypes (Hartley *et al.*, 2005; W. Huang *et al.*, 2007). While differential use of CXCR4 or CCR5 by HIV-1 strains has been observed, the striking differences seen appear to be in how R5 and R5X4 viruses utilize the CCR5 coreceptor. Generally, R5-tropic viruses are particularly well adapted for CCR5 use (Choe et al., 1996; Deng et al., 1996; Dragic et al., 1996), and can tolerate deletion or substitution of the CCR5 amino-terminal domain (Howard *et al.*, 1999; Z. Wang *et al.*, 1999). R5X4 viruses, however, are much more sensitive to mutations in CCR5, particularly in the amino terminal domain (Doranz et al., 1997). Thus, there is a cost associated with the benefit to use dual chemokine receptors as exhibited by R5X4 tropic strains that have more stringent requirements for CCR5 usage (Rana et al., 1997).

Host genetic factors can also influence HIV-1 tropism and transmission. Cohorts of HIV-1 infected individuals have been established based on specific clinical, virological and immunological criteria. One type of cohort contains individuals selected after frequent exposure to HIV-1 without seroconversion. A mutation in the CCR5 gene has been frequently found in this type of cohort (Zimmerman et al., 1997). This mutation is a deletion of 32 base pairs (Δ32), resulting in a defective CCR5 receptor. $CD4^+$ T cells and macrophages carrying the Δ32 mutation are resistant to infection with R5 viruses. Homozygous individuals carrying the mutation on both alleles (1% of Caucasians) are almost completely refractory to infection with R5 HIV-1 strains (Samson et al., 1996; Zimmerman et al., 1997). Very rare examples of infection of these individuals have been reported (O'Brien et al., 1997; Theodorou et al., 1997). In these cases the transmitted R5 viruses appear to use CXCR4. Individuals heterozygous for the Δ32 mutation are not protected from HIV-1 infection, but have slower rate of progression to AIDS. This is because the mutated form of the protein acts as a dominant negative mutant and prevents most of the wild-type CCR5 protein from reaching the cell surface. However, HIV-1 can evolve adaptive mutations on the V3 loop of gp120 that allows it to use defective or mutant CCR5 co-receptor. For instance, it has been shown that a N300Y adaptive point mutation on the V3 loop of gp120 enhances binding of HIV-1 to the mutant CCR5 co-receptor (Platt *et al.*, 2001). A follow-up study from the same group has shown that in addition to the adaptive mutation on the V3 loop of gp120, an S193N point mutation on the V2 stem and loss of N-linked oligosaccharide from position N403 of gp120 help HIV-1 to efficiently use defective CCR5 co-receptor that has a badly damaged amino terminus (Platt *et al.*, 2005). Taken together, these studies have important implications for understanding HIV-1 transmission dynamics and AIDS pathogenesis.

AIDS pathogenesis is multifactorial; it is a mixture of host and pathogen genetics combined with factors such as the immune response and viral adaptation. Viral adaptation include reverting and compensatory mutations such as the recently described T242N point mutation on the *gag* gene associated with progression to AIDS in South African patients (K. H. Huang *et al.*, 2011). However in general, progression from acute infection is often accompanied by depletion of the $CD4^+$ lymphocytes and this depletion is a major component of the eventual failure of the immune system and hence AIDS pathogenesis. Apoptosis is one mechanism that contributes to depletion of HIV-1 infected and uninfected cells, deterioration of the immune system and progression to AIDS, respectively (Cotton *et al.*, 1997; Gougeon & Montagnier, 1993; Herbein *et al.*, 1998; Joshi *et al.*, 2011; C. J. Li *et al.*, 1995; Zhu *et al.*, 2011). HIV-induced apoptosis is triggered by a number of HIV-1 proteins, notably the envelope protein (Herbein *et al.*, 1998; Ishikawa *et al.*, 1998; Joshi *et al.*, 2011; Micoli *et al.*, 2006; Micoli *et al.*, 2000). Four point mutations (A835W, A838W, A838I, and I842R) in the cytoplasm domain of the gp41 subunit of the envelope protein reduces HIV-induced apoptosis of target cells (Micoli *et al.*, 2006). A recent study has shown that induction of bystander apoptosis in CCR5 expressing cells requires the fusogenic activity of gp41; and that V2E and V38A/E point mutation in the second amino acid and the heptad repeat 1 region of gp41 respectively, abrogated fusion activity and hence apoptosis induced by an R5 virus (Joshi *et al.*, 2011). In an earlier study, the same group showed that a V513E point mutation in the fusion domain of gp41 resulted in a fusion-defective envelope protein that failed to induce apoptosis and that a G547D mutation in the gp41 N-terminal helix also reduced cell fusion capacity and apoptosis induced by an X4 virus (Garg *et al.*, 2007).

5. Point mutations associated with evasion of antibody mediated immune response

Point mutations on HIV-1 envelope protein do not only influence HIV-1 tropism and disease progression, but they also help the virus to evade the antibody mediated immune response. The HIV-1 surface gp120 and the trans-membrane gp41 can elicit both virus-neutralizing and non-neutralizing antibodies during natural infection. Antibodies that lack neutralizing activity are often directed against the gp120 regions that are occluded on the assembled trimer, and which are exposed only upon shedding (Moore & Sodroski, 1996). Neutralizing antibodies, by contrast must access the functional envelope glycoprotein complex and typically recognize conserved or variable epitopes near the receptor binding sites (Posner *et al.*, 1991; Sattentau & Moore, 1995; Trkola *et al.*, 1996a; L. Wu *et al.*, 1996). Neutralising antibodies are also elicited by the membrane proximal external region (MPER) of gp41 (Frey *et al.*, 2008; J. Wang *et al.*, 2011; Zwick *et al.*, 2001). The production and characterization of monoclonal antibodies of human and rodent origin have allowed a precise determination of the neutralization epitopes present on the HIV-1 gp120 (Moore & Ho, 1995; Poignard et al., 1996).

Using epitope maps in conjunction with the X-ray crystal structure of gp120 complexed with CD4 and a neutralizing monoclonal antibody (Kwong *et al.*, 1998b), spatial organization of conserved neutralization epitopes on gp120 was determined (Wyatt et al., 1998). More broadly neutralizing antibodies recognize discontinuous, conserved epitopes in three regions of the gp120 (Figure 8). In HIV-1 infected individuals, the most abundant of these are directed against the CD4 binding site (CD4bs), and block gp120-CD4 interaction (Euler *et al.*, 2011; Ho *et al.*, 1991; Y. Li *et al.*, 2011; Posner *et al.*, 1991; Walker *et al.*, 2009; X. Wu *et al.*, 2010; Zhou *et al.*, 2011). Less common are antibodies against epitopes induced or exposed upon CD4 binding (CD4i) (Thali et al., 1993). Both CD4i and V3 antibodies disrupt the binding of gp120-CD4 complexes to chemokine receptors (Trkola *et al.*, 1996a; L. Wu *et al.*, 1996). Notwithstanding, none of the CD4i antibodies discovered to date such as 17b, 48d or X5 are broadly neutralizing. A third gp120 neutralization epitope is defined by a unique monoclonal antibody, 2G12 (Trkola et al., 1996b), which does not efficiently block receptor binding (Trkola et al., 1996a). Table 6 lists broadly neutralising monoclonal antibodies elicited by the HIV-1 gp120 and gp41 envelope proteins. Although high-titer antibodies are sustained in infected individuals throughout the course of infection, these antibodies have very poor neutralizing activity against autologous as well as representative primary HIV-1 isolates (Montefiori et al., 1996; Moog et al., 1997). This observation suggests that neutralizing antibodies that arise in response to HIV-1 infection may not be critical in limiting viral replication.

The escape of HIV-1 from effects of neutralizing antibodies includes mutations in gp120 and/or gp41. One of the seminal studies showed that A582T point mutation in the HIV-1 envelope gene made a laboratory adapted HIV-1 strain called HXB2 to be resistant to HIV-1 neutralizing human serum (Reitz *et al.*, 1988). Another study published ten years later, showed that HIV-1 MN molecular clones which had 294N/K mutation before the V3 loop, 307N/I mutation proximal to the V3 loop, 327I/K mutation within V3 and 336N/I mutation after the V3 loop were resistant to human serum containing neutralizing antibodies directed at the immunodominant V3 loop of gp120 (Park *et al.*, 1998). Point mutations in a highly conserved structural motif within the intracytoplasmic tail of gp41 rendered HIV-1 molecular clones resistant to broadly neutralizing polyclonal human serum antibodies (Kalia *et al.*, 2005).

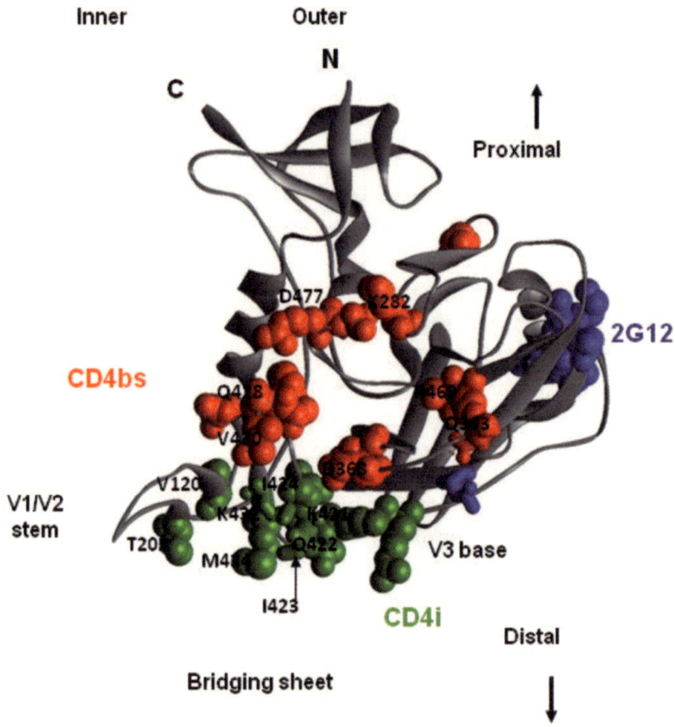

Fig. 8. Ribbon diagram illustrating epitopes of the gp120 core, highlighting some amino acid residues that interact with broadly neutralizing antibodies. The CD4bs (red) and the CD4i co-receptor-binding surface (green) as well as residues implicated in 2G12 binding (blue) are depicted.

In a clinically relevant study, paediatric HIV-1 subtype C clinical isolates with K665S/R/N point mutation were found to be resistant to a 2F5 broadly neutralizing monoclonal antibody (Gray *et al.*, 2006). This study confirmed earlier findings that the amino acid residue K665 is crucial for neutralization by 2F5 (Binley *et al.*, 2004). In the same study, the Lynn Morris' group found out that all the paediatric HIV-1 subtype C clinical isolates analysed had a conserved 4E10 epitope (W672, F673, W680) consistent with their phenotypic sensitivity to the 4E10 monoclonal antibody (Gray et al., 2006). 4E10 recognizes an epitope containing the sequence NWF(D/N)IT (Zwick et al., 2001). Mutagenesis studies have shown that the amino acid residues W672, F673 and W680 are indispensable for recognition by 4E10 (Zwick et al., 2005). Indeed, a recently published study describing four subjects infected with viruses carrying rare MPER polymorphisms associated with resistance to 4E10 neutralization has shown that three subjects had W680 polymorphism, including a W680G point mutation (Nakamura et al., 2011). The study demonstrated that W680G point mutation was necessary to confer 4E10 resistant phenotype (Nakamura et al., 2011). In another subject a W680R point mutation caused variable resistant to 4E10 (Nakamura et al., 2011). A fourth subject possessed a F673L point mutation also associated with 4E10 resistance (Nakamura et al., 2011). Earlier, an independent study conducted in South Africa also showed that an HIV-1 subtype C virus isolated from a 7-year-old perinatally infected child with F673L point mutation was resistant to 4E10 (Gray et al., 2008). These case studies are examples of the challenges presented by point mutations in controlling HIV-1 infection by antibodies. Notwithstanding, recent discovery of additional and more potent broadly neutralizing antibodies such as VRC01 (X. Wu *et al.*, 2010), PG9 and PG16 (Walker et al., 2009) is encouraging and boosts the impetus for HIV-1 vaccine design that may elicit broadly neutralizing antibodies (Burton & Weiss, 2010).

Epitopes	Example of mAb	Mechanism of neutralization	Properties	Selected references
CD4 binding site(CD4bs)	IgGb12, VRC01, HJ16, PG9 and PG16	Interfere with gp120-CD4 binding	CD4bs antibodies compete with CD4 and with antibodies against CD4i epitope. PG9 and PG16 bind to trimer specific glycosylated epitope on the V1/V2 and V3 region.	(Corti *et al.*, 2010; Euler *et al.*, 2011; Ho *et al.*, 1991; Y. Li *et al.*, 2011; Pancera *et al.*, 2010; Posner *et al.*, 1991; Walker *et al.*, 2009; X. Wu *et al.*, 2010; Zhou *et al.*, 2011)
Glycans	2G12	Interfere with binding of gp120 to CCR5 chemokine receptor and DC-SIGN. Also prevent loss of $CD4^{+}$ T cells.	Antibody binding is dependent upon proper N-linked glycosylation. Recognize a mannose rich epitope on the "silent" face of gp120	(Binley *et al.*, 2006; Calarese *et al.*, 2003; Luo *et al.*, 2011; Scanlan *et al.*, 2003; Trkola *et al.*, 1996b)
MPER of gp41	4E10, 2F5	Interfere with HIV-1 fusion and induces shedding of gp120.	Both antibodies bind few crucial residues in the MPER of gp41. HIV-1 2F5 binds both native and fusion-intermediate conformations while 4E10 recognize a predominantly linear and relatively conserved epitope.	(Muster *et al.*, 1994; Muster *et al.*, 1993; Ruprecht *et al.*, 2011; Zwick *et al.*, 2005; Zwick *et al.*, 2001)

Table 8. Broadly neutralizing antibodies that bind gp120 and gp41 HIV-1 envelope proteins

7. Point mutations and anti-gp120 aptamers

Aptamers are synthetic oligonucleotide ligands that can be isolated *in vitro* against diverse targets including HIV-1 gp120 (Khati *et al.*, 2003). Aptamers assume a defined three-dimensional structure and generally bind functional sites on their respective targets. They possess the molecular recognition properties of monoclonal antibodies in terms of their high affinity and specificity (Khati, 2010). Unlike antibodies, aptamers can fold properly and retain activity in the intracellular environment. However, the majority of aptamers with potential therapeutic utility selected to date target extracellular proteins (Chen *et al.*, 2003; Eyetech Study Group, 2002, 2003; Green *et al.*, 1995; Kim *et al.*, 2003; Liu *et al.*, 2009; Lupold *et*

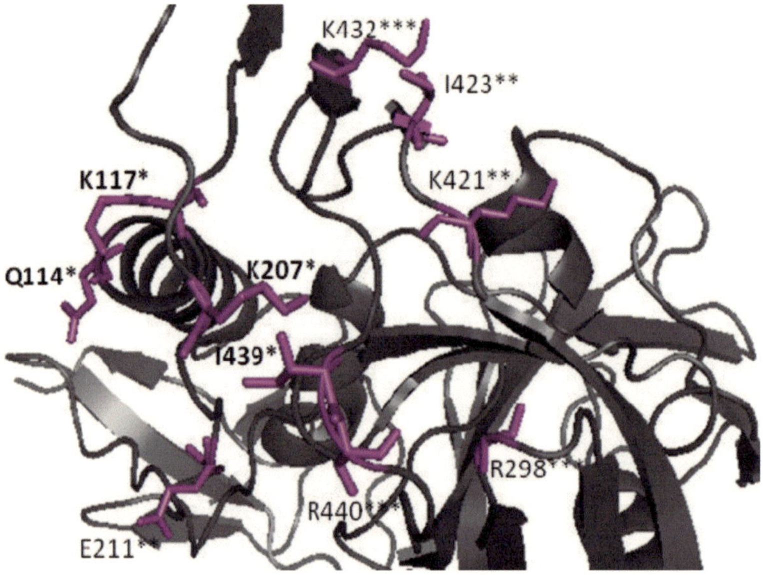

Fig. 9. A ribbon diagram of gp120 highlighting amino acid residues that interact with B40 aptamer. Residues in **bold** and single asterix are highly conserved among all HIV-1 isolates and significantly reduced binding of the aptamer by more than 10-fold when experimentally mutated to alanine, respectively (Joubert *et al.*, 2010). Those residues with double or tripple asterix are moderately and significantly varaiable, respectively, in all HIV isolates and while they make contact with the aptamer they did not significantly affect binding of the aptamer when experimentally mutated to alanine, respectively.

al., 2002; Mi *et al.*, 2009; Nobile *et al.*, 1998; Ruckman *et al.*, 1998; Rusconi *et al.*, 2004; Rusconi *et al.*, 2002; Vinores, 2003; White *et al.*, 2003).

Extracellular therapeutic targets such as HIV-1 gp120 have the advantage of ready access to aptamer intervention without the need for enabling access to cells. The aptamers against HIV-1 gp120 bound the protein with high affinity, high specificity and neutralized a broad range of R5 HIV-1 clinical isolates (Khati *et al.*, 2003). In a recent review, these RNA aptamers were reported to have the most potent in vitro antiviral efficacy of all HIV-1 entry inhibitors described to date (Held *et al.*, 2006), including antibodies. These aptamers prevented entry and suppressed viral replication in cultured human peripheral blood mononuclear cells (PBMC) by up to 10,000-fold (Khati *et al.*, 2003). While the emergence of HIV-1 escape mutants and drug resistance variants appears to be inevitable, our goup and collaborators have recently shown that one extensively studied aptamer called B40 penetrate the highly variable exterior surfaces of gp120 and bind the conserved core at the heart of the CCR5-binding site (Cohen *et al.*, 2008; Dey *et al.*, 2005; Joubert *et al.*, 2010), which the virus may be unable to mutate without compromising its fitness. Four amino acids (Q114, K117, K207, and I439) of gp120 (Figure 9) that weakened binding of gp120 to B40 aptamer by at least 10-fold when experimentally mutated to alanine (Joubert et al., 2010) are naturally conserved among all HIV-1 isolates (Kwong et al., 1998a). This suggests that B40 makes direct contact with at least four conserved core residues on gp120 within the CCR5-binding site, which the virus cannot afford to mutate without losing selective advantage. These data bode well for the future development of aptamers such as B40 as an entry inhibitor drug, which will hopefully help circumvent HIV-1 point mutations and delay or diminish drug resistance. In order to maximally suppress or eradicate the virus; the aptamer or any other anti-HIV molecule in development should be used in combination with current antiretroviral drugs and the envisaged vaccines currently developed to elicit broadly neutralising antibodies.

8. References

Abecasis, A. B., Deforche, K., Snoeck, J., Bacheler, L. T., McKenna, P., Carvalho, A. P., Gomes, P., Camacho, R. J., & Vandamme, A. M. (2005). Protease mutation M89I/V is linked to therapy failure in patients infected with the HIV-1 non-B subtypes C, F or G. *Aids,* 19(16), 1799-1806.

Antinori, A., Trotta, M. P., Lorenzini, P., Torti, C., Gianotti, N., Maggiolo, F., Ceccherini-Silberstein, F., Nasto, P., Castagna, A., De Luca, A., Mussini, C., Andreoni, M., & Perno, C. F. (2007). Virological response to salvage therapy in HIV-infected persons carrying the reverse transcriptase K65R mutation. *Antivir Ther,* 12(8), 1175-1183.

Antinori, A., Zaccarelli, M., Cingolani, A., Forbici, F., Rizzo, M. G., Trotta, M. P., Di Giambenedetto, S., Narciso, P., Ammassari, A., Girardi, E., De Luca, A., & Perno, C. F. (2002). Cross-resistance among nonnucleoside reverse transcriptase inhibitors limits recycling efavirenz after nevirapine failure. *AIDS Res Hum Retroviruses,* 18(12), 835-838.

Aquaro, S., D'Arrigo, R., Svicher, V., Perri, G. D., Caputo, S. L., Visco-Comandini, U., Santoro, M., Bertoli, A., Mazzotta, F., Bonora, S., Tozzi, V., Bellagamba, R., Zaccarelli, M., Narciso, P., Antinori, A., & Perno, C. F. (2006). Specific mutations in HIV-1 gp41 are associated with immunological success in HIV-1-infected patients receiving enfuvirtide treatment. *J Antimicrob Chemother,* 58(4), 714-722.

Arion, D., Kaushik, N., McCormick, S., Borkow, G., & Parniak, M. A. (1998). Phenotypic mechanism of HIV-1 resistance to 3'-azido-3'-deoxythymidine (AZT): increased polymerization processivity and enhanced sensitivity to pyrophosphate of the mutant viral reverse transcriptase. *Biochemistry,* 37(45), 15908-15917.

Arnold, E., Jacobo-Molina, A., Nanni, R. G., Williams, R. L., Lu, X., Ding, J., Clark, A. D., Jr., Zhang, A., Ferris, A. L., Clark, P., & et al. (1992). Structure of HIV-1 reverse transcriptase/DNA complex at 7 A resolution showing active site locations. *Nature,* 357(6373), 85-89.

Bacheler, L., Jeffrey, S., Hanna, G., D'Aquila, R., Wallace, L., Logue, K., Cordova, B., Hertogs, K., Larder, B., Buckery, R., Baker, D., Gallagher, K., Scarnati, H., Tritch, R., & Rizzo, C. (2001). Genotypic correlates of phenotypic resistance to efavirenz in virus isolates from patients failing nonnucleoside reverse transcriptase inhibitor therapy. *J Virol,* 75(11), 4999-5008.

Baxter, J. D., Schapiro, J. M., Boucher, C. A., Kohlbrenner, V. M., Hall, D. B., Scherer, J. R., & Mayers, D. L. (2006). Genotypic changes in human immunodeficiency virus type 1 protease associated with reduced susceptibility and virologic response to the protease inhibitor tipranavir. *J Virol,* 80(21), 10794-10801.

Berger, E. A., Doms, R. W., Fenyo, E. M., Korber, B. T., Littman, D. R., Moore, J. P., Sattentau, Q. J., Schuitemaker, H., Sodroski, J., & Weiss, R. A. (1998). A new classification for HIV-1 [letter]. *Nature,* 391(6664), 240.

Binley, J. M., Ngo-Abdalla, S., Moore, P., Bobardt, M., Chatterji, U., Gallay, P., Burton, D. R., Wilson, I. A., Elder, J. H., & de Parseval, A. (2006). Inhibition of HIV Env binding to cellular receptors by monoclonal antibody 2G12 as probed by Fc-tagged gp120. *Retrovirology,* 3, 39.

Binley, J. M., Wrin, T., Korber, B., Zwick, M. B., Wang, M., Chappey, C., Stiegler, G., Kunert, R., Zolla-Pazner, S., Katinger, H., Petropoulos, C. J., & Burton, D. R. (2004). Comprehensive cross-clade neutralization analysis of a panel of anti-human immunodeficiency virus type 1 monoclonal antibodies. *J Virol,* 78(23), 13232-13252.

Boyer, P. L., Sarafianos, S. G., Arnold, E., & Hughes, S. H. (2001). Selective excision of AZTMP by drug-resistant human immunodeficiency virus reverse transcriptase. *J Virol,* 75(10), 4832-4842.

Brenner, B. G., Oliveira, M., Doualla-Bell, F., Moisi, D. D., Ntemgwa, M., Frankel, F., Essex, M., & Wainberg, M. A. (2006). HIV-1 subtype C viruses rapidly develop K65R resistance to tenofovir in cell culture. *Aids,* 20(9), F9-13.

Brun-Vezinet, F., Descamps, D., Ruffault, A., Masquelier, B., Calvez, V., Peytavin, G., Telles, F., Morand-Joubert, L., Meynard, J. L., Vray, M., & Costagliola, D. (2003). Clinically relevant interpretation of genotype for resistance to abacavir. *Aids,* 17(12), 1795-1802.

Burton, D. R., & Weiss, R. A. (2010). AIDS/HIV. A boost for HIV vaccine design. *Science,* 329(5993), 770-773.

Cabrera, C., Marfil, S., Garcia, E., Martinez-Picado, J., Bonjoch, A., Bofill, M., Moreno, S., Ribera, E., Domingo, P., Clotet, B., & Ruiz, L. (2006). Genetic evolution of gp41 reveals a highly exclusive relationship between codons 36, 38 and 43 in gp41 under long-term enfuvirtide-containing salvage regimen. *Aids,* 20(16), 2075-2080.

Calarese, D. A., Scanlan, C. N., Zwick, M. B., Deechongkit, S., Mimura, Y., Kunert, R., Zhu, P., Wormald, M. R., Stanfield, R. L., Roux, K. H., Kelly, J. W., Rudd, P. M., Dwek, R. A., Katinger, H., Burton, D. R., & Wilson, I. A. (2003). Antibody domain exchange is an immunological solution to carbohydrate cluster recognition. *Science,* 300(5628), 2065-2071.

Calazans, A., Brindeiro, R., Brindeiro, P., Verli, H., Arruda, M. B., Gonzalez, L. M., Guimaraes, J. A., Diaz, R. S., Antunes, O. A., & Tanuri, A. (2005). Low accumulation of L90M in protease from subtype F HIV-1 with resistance to protease inhibitors is caused by the L89M polymorphism. *J Infect Dis,* 191(11), 1961-1970.

Cane, P. A., de Ruiter, A., Rice, P., Wiselka, M., Fox, R., & Pillay, D. (2001). Resistance-associated mutations in the human immunodeficiency virus type 1 subtype c protease gene from treated and untreated patients in the United Kingdom. *J Clin Microbiol,* 39(7), 2652-2654.

Ceccherini-Silberstein, F., Erba, F., Gago, F., Bertoli, A., Forbici, F., Bellocchi, M. C., Gori, C., D'Arrigo, R., Marcon, L., Balotta, C., Antinori, A., Monforte, A. D., & Perno, C. F. (2004). Identification of the minimal conserved structure of HIV-1 protease in the presence and absence of drug pressure. *Aids,* 18(12), F11-19.

Charpentier, C., Jenabian, M. A., Piketty, C., Karmochkine, M., Tisserand, P., Laureillard, D., Belec, L., Si-Mohamed, A., & Weiss, L. (2011). Dynamics of enfuvirtide resistance mutations in enfuvirtide-experienced patients remaining in virological failure under salvage therapy. *Scand J Infect Dis,* 43(5), 373-379.

Chen, C. H., Chernis, G. A., Hoang, V. Q., & Landgraf, R. (2003). Inhibition of heregulin signaling by an aptamer that preferentially binds to the oligomeric form of human epidermal growth factor receptor-3. *Proc Natl Acad Sci U S A,* 100(16), 9226-9231.

Choe, H., Farzan, M., Sun, Y., Sullivan, N., Rollins, B., Ponath, P. D., Wu, L., Mackay, C. R., LaRosa, G., Newman, W., Gerard, N., Gerard, C., & Sodroski, J. (1996). The beta-chemokine receptors CCR3 and CCR5 facilitate infection by primary HIV-1 isolates. *Cell,* 85(7), 1135-1148.

Clark, S. A., Shulman, N. S., Bosch, R. J., & Mellors, J. W. (2006). Reverse transcriptase mutations 118I, 208Y, and 215Y cause HIV-1 hypersusceptibility to non-nucleoside reverse transcriptase inhibitors. *Aids,* 20(7), 981-984.

Cohen, C., Forzan, M., Sproat, B., Pantophlet, R., McGowan, I., Burton, D., & James, W. (2008). An aptamer that neutralizes R5 strains of HIV-1 binds to core residues of gp120 in the CCR5 binding site. *Virology,* 381(1), 46-54.

Collman, R., Balliet, J. W., Gregory, S. A., Friedman, H., Kolson, D. L., Nathanson, N., & Srinivasan, A. (1992). An infectious molecular clone of an unusual macrophage-tropic and highly cytopathic strain of human immunodeficiency virus type 1. *J Virol,* 66(12), 7517-7521.

Colonno, R., Rose, R., McLaren, C., Thiry, A., Parkin, N., & Friborg, J. (2004). Identification of I50L as the signature atazanavir (ATV)-resistance mutation in treatment-naive HIV-1-infected patients receiving ATV-containing regimens. *J Infect Dis,* 189(10), 1802-1810.

Connor, R. I., Sheridan, K. E., Ceradini, D., Choe, S., & Landau, N. R. (1997). Change in coreceptor use coreceptor use correlates with disease progression in HIV-1--infected individuals. *J Exp Med,* 185(4), 621-628.

Cooper, D. A., Steigbigel, R. T., Gatell, J. M., Rockstroh, J. K., Katlama, C., Yeni, P., Lazzarin, A., Clotet, B., Kumar, P. N., Eron, J. E., Schechter, M., Markowitz, M., Loutfy, M. R., Lennox, J. L., Zhao, J., Chen, J., Ryan, D. M., Rhodes, R. R., Killar, J. A., Gilde, L. R., Strohmaier, K. M., Meibohm, A. R., Miller, M. D., Hazuda, D. J., Nessly, M. L., DiNubile, M. J., Isaacs, R. D., Teppler, H., & Nguyen, B. Y. (2008). Subgroup and resistance analyses of raltegravir for resistant HIV-1 infection. *N Engl J Med,* 359(4), 355-365.

Corti, D., Langedijk, J. P., Hinz, A., Seaman, M. S., Vanzetta, F., Fernandez-Rodriguez, B. M., Silacci, C., Pinna, D., Jarrossay, D., Balla-Jhagjhoorsingh, S., Willems, B., Zekveld, M. J., Dreja, H., O'Sullivan, E., Pade, C., Orkin, C., Jeffs, S. A., Montefiori, D. C., Davis, D., Weissenhorn, W., McKnight, A., Heeney, J. L., Sallusto, F., Sattentau, Q. J., Weiss, R. A., & Lanzavecchia, A. (2010). Analysis of memory B cell responses and isolation of novel monoclonal antibodies with neutralizing breadth from HIV-1-infected individuals. *PLoS One,* 5(1), e8805.

Cotton, M. F., Ikle, D. N., Rapaport, E. L., Marschner, S., Tseng, P. O., Kurrle, R., & Finkel, T. H. (1997). Apoptosis of CD4+ and CD8+ T cells isolated immediately ex vivo correlates with disease severity in human immunodeficiency virus type 1 infection. *Pediatr Res,* 42(5), 656-664.

Cozzi-Lepri, A., Ruiz, L., Loveday, C., Phillips, A. N., Clotet, B., Reiss, P., Ledergerber, B., Holkmann, C., Staszewski, S., & Lundgren, J. D. (2005). Thymidine analogue mutation profiles: factors associated with acquiring specific profiles and their impact on the virological response to therapy. *Antivir Ther,* 10(7), 791-802.

Dandache, S., Sevigny, G., Yelle, J., Stranix, B. R., Parkin, N., Schapiro, J. M., Wainberg, M. A., & Wu, J. J. (2007). In vitro antiviral activity and cross-resistance profile of PL-100, a novel protease inhibitor of human immunodeficiency virus type 1. *Antimicrob Agents Chemother,* 51(11), 4036-4043.

Das, K., Bauman, J. D., Clark, A. D., Jr., Frenkel, Y. V., Lewi, P. J., Shatkin, A. J., Hughes, S. H., & Arnold, E. (2008). High-resolution structures of HIV-1 reverse transcriptase/TMC278 complexes: strategic flexibility explains potency against resistance mutations. *Proc Natl Acad Sci U S A,* 105(5), 1466-1471.

Das, K., Clark, A. D., Jr., Lewi, P. J., Heeres, J., De Jonge, M. R., Koymans, L. M., Vinkers, H. M., Daeyaert, F., Ludovici, D. W., Kukla, M. J., De Corte, B., Kavash, R. W., Ho, C. Y., Ye, H., Lichtenstein, M. A., Andries, K., Pauwels, R., De Bethune, M. P., Boyer,

P. L., Clark, P., Hughes, S. H., Janssen, P. A., & Arnold, E. (2004). Roles of conformational and positional adaptability in structure-based design of TMC125-R165335 (etravirine) and related non-nucleoside reverse transcriptase inhibitors that are highly potent and effective against wild-type and drug-resistant HIV-1 variants. *J Med Chem,* 47(10), 2550-2560.

Das, K., Ding, J., Hsiou, Y., Clark, A. D., Jr., Moereels, H., Koymans, L., Andries, K., Pauwels, R., Janssen, P. A., Boyer, P. L., Clark, P., Smith, R. H., Jr., Kroeger Smith, M. B., Michejda, C. J., Hughes, S. H., & Arnold, E. (1996). Crystal structures of 8-Cl and 9-Cl TIBO complexed with wild-type HIV-1 RT and 8-Cl TIBO complexed with the Tyr181Cys HIV-1 RT drug-resistant mutant. *J Mol Biol,* 264(5), 1085-1100.

De Luca, A., Di Giambenedetto, S., Romano, L., Gonnelli, A., Corsi, P., Baldari, M., Di Pietro, M., Menzo, S., Francisci, D., Almi, P., & Zazzi, M. (2006). Frequency and treatment-related predictors of thymidine-analogue mutation patterns in HIV-1 isolates after unsuccessful antiretroviral therapy. *J Infect Dis,* 193(9), 1219-1222.

De Luca, A., Giambenedetto, S. D., Trotta, M. P., Colafigli, M., Prosperi, M., Ruiz, L., Baxter, J., Clevenbergh, P., Cauda, R., Perno, C. F., & Antinori, A. (2007). Improved interpretation of genotypic changes in the HIV-1 reverse transcriptase coding region that determine the virological response to didanosine. *J Infect Dis,* 196(11), 1645-1653.

Deeks, S. G., Lu, J., Hoh, R., Neilands, T. B., Beatty, G., Huang, W., Liegler, T., Hunt, P., Martin, J. N., & Kuritzkes, D. R. (2007). Interruption of enfuvirtide in HIV-1 infected adults with incomplete viral suppression on an enfuvirtide-based regimen. *J Infect Dis,* 195(3), 387-391.

Deforche, K., Camacho, R., Grossman, Z., Silander, T., Soares, M. A., Moreau, Y., Shafer, R. W., Van Laethem, K., Carvalho, A. P., Wynhoven, B., Cane, P., Snoeck, J., Clarke, J., Sirivichayakul, S., Ariyoshi, K., Holguin, A., Rudich, H., Rodrigues, R., Bouzas, M. B., Cahn, P., Brigido, L. F., Soriano, V., Sugiura, W., Phanuphak, P., Morris, L., Weber, J., Pillay, D., Tanuri, A., Harrigan, P. R., Shapiro, J. M., Katzenstein, D. A., Kantor, R., & Vandamme, A. M. (2007). Bayesian network analysis of resistance pathways against HIV-1 protease inhibitors. *Infect Genet Evol,* 7(3), 382-390.

Deforche, K., Silander, T., Camacho, R., Grossman, Z., Soares, M. A., Van Laethem, K., Kantor, R., Moreau, Y., & Vandamme, A. M. (2006). Analysis of HIV-1 pol sequences using Bayesian Networks: implications for drug resistance. *Bioinformatics,* 22(24), 2975-2979.

Delaugerre, C., Rohban, R., Simon, A., Mouroux, M., Tricot, C., Agher, R., Huraux, J. M., Katlama, C., & Calvez, V. (2001). Resistance profile and cross-resistance of HIV-1 among patients failing a non-nucleoside reverse transcriptase inhibitor-containing regimen. *J Med Virol,* 65(3), 445-448.

Delelis, O., Thierry, S., Subra, F., Simon, F., Malet, I., Alloui, C., Sayon, S., Calvez, V., Deprez, E., Marcelin, A. G., Tchertanov, L., & Mouscadet, J. F. (2011). Impact of Y143 HIV-1 integrase mutations on resistance to raltegravir in vitro and in vivo. *Antimicrob Agents Chemother,* 54(1), 491-501.

Demeter, L. M., DeGruttola, V., Lustgarten, S., Bettendorf, D., Fischl, M., Eshleman, S., Spreen, W., Nguyen, B. Y., Koval, C. E., Eron, J. J., Hammer, S., & Squires, K. (2008). Association of efavirenz hypersusceptibility with virologic response in ACTG 368, a randomized trial of abacavir (ABC) in combination with efavirenz (EFV) and indinavir (IDV) in HIV-infected subjects with prior nucleoside analog experience. *HIV Clin Trials,* 9(1), 11-25.

Deng, H., Liu, R., Ellmeier, W., Choe, S., Unutmaz, D., Burkhart, M., Di Marzio, P., Marmon, S., Sutton, R. E., Hill, C. M., Davis, C. B., Peiper, S. C., Schall, T. J., Littman, D. R., &

Landau, N. R. (1996). Identification of a major co-receptor for primary isolates of HIV-1 [see comments]. *Nature,* 381(6584), 661-666.

Descamps, D., Ait-Khaled, M., Craig, C., Delarue, S., Damond, F., Collin, G., & Brun-Vezinet, F. (2006). Rare selection of the K65R mutation in antiretroviral-naive patients failing a first-line abacavir/ lamivudine-containing HAART regimen. *Antivir Ther,* 11(6), 701-705.

Dey, A. K., Khati, M., Tang, M., Wyatt, R., Lea, S. M., & James, W. (2005). An aptamer that neutralizes R5 strains of human immunodeficiency virus type 1 blocks gp120-CCR5 interaction. *J Virol,* 79(21), 13806-13810.

di Marzo Veronese, F., Copeland, T. D., DeVico, A. L., Rahman, R., Oroszlan, S., Gallo, R. C., & Sarngadharan, M. G. (1986). Characterization of highly immunogenic p66/p51 as the reverse transcriptase of HTLV-III/LAV. *Science,* 231(4743), 1289-1291.

Doranz, B. J., Lu, Z. H., Rucker, J., Zhang, T. Y., Sharron, M., Cen, Y. H., Wang, Z. X., Guo, H. H., Du, J. G., Accavitti, M. A., Doms, R. W., & Peiper, S. C. (1997). Two distinct CCR5 domains can mediate coreceptor usage by human immunodeficiency virus type 1. *J Virol,* 71(9), 6305-6314.

Doranz, B. J., Rucker, J., Yi, Y., Smyth, R. J., Samson, M., Peiper, S. C., Parmentier, M., Collman, R. G., & Doms, R. W. (1996). A dual-tropic primary HIV-1 isolate that uses fusin and the beta- chemokine receptors CKR-5, CKR-3, and CKR-2b as fusion cofactors. *Cell,* 85(7), 1149-1158.

Doualla-Bell, F., Avalos, A., Brenner, B., Gaolathe, T., Mine, M., Gaseitsiwe, S., Oliveira, M., Moisi, D., Ndwapi, N., Moffat, H., Essex, M., & Wainberg, M. A. (2006). High prevalence of the K65R mutation in human immunodeficiency virus type 1 subtype C isolates from infected patients in Botswana treated with didanosine-based regimens. *Antimicrob Agents Chemother,* 50(12), 4182-4185.

Dragic, T., Litwin, V., Allaway, G. P., Martin, S. R., Huang, Y., Nagashima, K. A., Cayanan, C., Maddon, P. J., Koup, R. A., Moore, J. P., & Paxton, W. A. (1996). HIV-1 entry into CD4+ cells is mediated by the chemokine receptor CC- CKR-5 [see comments]. *Nature,* 381(6584), 667-673.

Dragic, T., Trkola, A., Thompson, D. A., Cormier, E. G., Kajumo, F. A., Maxwell, E., Lin, S. W., Ying, W., Smith, S. O., Sakmar, T. P., & Moore, J. P. (2000). A binding pocket for a small molecule inhibitor of HIV-1 entry within the transmembrane helices of CCR5. *Proc Natl Acad Sci U S A,* 97(10), 5639-5644.

Eron, J., Jr., Yeni, P., Gathe, J., Jr., Estrada, V., DeJesus, E., Staszewski, S., Lackey, P., Katlama, C., Young, B., Yau, L., Sutherland-Phillips, D., Wannamaker, P., Vavro, C., Patel, L., Yeo, J., & Shaefer, M. (2006). The KLEAN study of fosamprenavir-ritonavir versus lopinavir-ritonavir, each in combination with abacavir-lamivudine, for initial treatment of HIV infection over 48 weeks: a randomised non-inferiority trial. *Lancet,* 368(9534), 476-482.

Eron, J. J., Jr., Bosch, R. J., Bettendorf, D., Petch, L., Fiscus, S., & Frank, I. (2007). The effect of lamivudine therapy and M184V on the antiretroviral activity of didanosine. *J Acquir Immune Defic Syndr,* 45(2), 249-251.

Euler, Z., Bunnik, E. M., Burger, J. A., Boeser-Nunnink, B. D., Grijsen, M. L., Prins, J. M., & Schuitemaker, H. (2011). Activity of broadly neutralizing antibodies, including PG9, PG16, and VRC01, against recently transmitted subtype B HIV-1 variants from early and late in the epidemic. *J Virol,* 85(14), 7236-7245.

Eyetech Study Group (2002). Preclinical and phase 1A clinical evaluation of an anti-VEGF pegylated aptamer (EYE001) for the treatment of exudative age-related macular degeneration. *Retina,* 22(2), 143-152.

Eyetech Study Group (2003). Anti-vascular endothelial growth factor therapy for subfoveal choroidal neovascularization secondary to age-related macular degeneration: phase II study results. *Ophthalmology,* 110(5), 979-986.

FDA (2007). FDA approves raltegravir tablets. *AIDS Patient Care STDS,* 21(11), 889.

Fischl, M. A., Richman, D. D., Grieco, M. H., Gottlieb, M. S., Volberding, P. A., Laskin, O. L., Leedom, J. M., Groopman, J. E., Mildvan, D., Schooley, R. T., & et al. (1987). The efficacy of azidothymidine (AZT) in the treatment of patients with AIDS and AIDS-related complex. A double-blind, placebo-controlled trial. *N Engl J Med,* 317(4), 185-191.

Frater, A. J., Chaput, C. C., Beddows, S., Weber, J. N., & McClure, M. O. (2001). Simple detection of point mutations associated with HIV-1 drug resistance. *J Virol Methods,* 93(1-2), 145-156.

Frey, G., Peng, H., Rits-Volloch, S., Morelli, M., Cheng, Y., & Chen, B. (2008). A fusion-intermediate state of HIV-1 gp41 targeted by broadly neutralizing antibodies. *Proc Natl Acad Sci U S A,* 105(10), 3739-3744.

Friend, J., Parkin, N., Liegler, T., Martin, J. N., & Deeks, S. G. (2004). Isolated lopinavir resistance after virological rebound of a ritonavir/lopinavir-based regimen. *Aids,* 18(14), 1965-1966.

Gallant, J. E., DeJesus, E., Arribas, J. R., Pozniak, A. L., Gazzard, B., Campo, R. E., Lu, B., McColl, D., Chuck, S., Enejosa, J., Toole, J. J., & Cheng, A. K. (2006). Tenofovir DF, emtricitabine, and efavirenz vs. zidovudine, lamivudine, and efavirenz for HIV. *N Engl J Med,* 354(3), 251-260.

Gallant, J. E., Staszewski, S., Pozniak, A. L., DeJesus, E., Suleiman, J. M., Miller, M. D., Coakley, D. F., Lu, B., Toole, J. J., & Cheng, A. K. (2004). Efficacy and safety of tenofovir DF vs stavudine in combination therapy in antiretroviral-naive patients: a 3-year randomized trial. *Jama,* 292(2), 191-201.

Gao, H. Q., Boyer, P. L., Sarafianos, S. G., Arnold, E., & Hughes, S. H. (2000). The role of steric hindrance in 3TC resistance of human immunodeficiency virus type-1 reverse transcriptase. *J Mol Biol,* 300(2), 403-418.

Garg, H., Joshi, A., Freed, E. O., & Blumenthal, R. (2007). Site-specific mutations in HIV-1 gp41 reveal a correlation between HIV-1-mediated bystander apoptosis and fusion/hemifusion. *J Biol Chem,* 282(23), 16899-16906.

Gilead Sciences (2008). Phase III trial begins for elvitegravir. *AIDS Patient Care STDS,* 22(9), 762-763.

Gonzales, M. J., Wu, T. D., Taylor, J., Belitskaya, I., Kantor, R., Israelski, D., Chou, S., Zolopa, A. R., Fessel, W. J., & Shafer, R. W. (2003). Extended spectrum of HIV-1 reverse transcriptase mutations in patients receiving multiple nucleoside analog inhibitors. *Aids,* 17(6), 791-799.

Gonzalez, L. M., Brindeiro, R. M., Aguiar, R. S., Pereira, H. S., Abreu, C. M., Soares, M. A., & Tanuri, A. (2004). Impact of nelfinavir resistance mutations on in vitro phenotype, fitness, and replication capacity of human immunodeficiency virus type 1 with subtype B and C proteases. *Antimicrob Agents Chemother,* 48(9), 3552-3555.

Gougeon, M. L., & Montagnier, L. (1993). Apoptosis in AIDS. *Science,* 260(5112), 1269-1270.

Gray, E. S., Meyers, T., Gray, G., Montefiori, D. C., & Morris, L. (2006). Insensitivity of paediatric HIV-1 subtype C viruses to broadly neutralising monoclonal antibodies raised against subtype B. *PLoS Med,* 3(7), e255.

Gray, E. S., Moore, P. L., Bibollet-Ruche, F., Li, H., Decker, J. M., Meyers, T., Shaw, G. M., & Morris, L. (2008). 4E10-resistant variants in a human immunodeficiency virus type

1 subtype C-infected individual with an anti-membrane-proximal external region-neutralizing antibody response. *J Virol,* 82(5), 2367-2375.
Green, L. S., Jellinek, D., Bell, C., Beebe, L. A., Feistner, B. D., Gill, S. C., Jucker, F. M., & Janjic, N. (1995). Nuclease-resistant nucleic acid ligands to vascular permeability factor/vascular endothelial growth factor. *Chem Biol,* 2(10), 683-695.
Grossman, Z., Paxinos, E. E., Averbuch, D., Maayan, S., Parkin, N. T., Engelhard, D., Lorber, M., Istomin, V., Shaked, Y., Mendelson, E., Ram, D., Petropoulos, C. J., & Schapiro, J. M. (2004). Mutation D30N is not preferentially selected by human immunodeficiency virus type 1 subtype C in the development of resistance to nelfinavir. *Antimicrob Agents Chemother,* 48(6), 2159-2165.
Harrigan, P. R., Stone, C., Griffin, P., Najera, I., Bloor, S., Kemp, S., Tisdale, M., & Larder, B. (2000). Resistance profile of the human immunodeficiency virus type 1 reverse transcriptase inhibitor abacavir (1592U89) after monotherapy and combination therapy. CNA2001 Investigative Group. *J Infect Dis,* 181(3), 912-920.
Hartley, O., Klasse, P. J., Sattentau, Q. J., & Moore, J. P. (2005). V3: HIV's switch-hitter. *AIDS Res Hum Retroviruses,* 21(2), 171-189.
Hawkins, C. A., Chaplin, B., Idoko, J., Ekong, E., Adewole, I., Gashau, W., Murphy, R. L., & Kanki, P. (2009). Clinical and genotypic findings in HIV-infected patients with the K65R mutation failing first-line antiretroviral therapy in Nigeria. *J Acquir Immune Defic Syndr,* 52(2), 228-234.
Held, D. M., Kissel, J. D., Patterson, J. T., Nickens, D. G., & Burke, D. H. (2006). HIV-1 inactivation by nucleic acid aptamers. *Front Biosci,* 11, 89-112.
Herbein, G., Mahlknecht, U., Batliwalla, F., Gregersen, P., Pappas, T., Butler, J., O'Brien, W. A., & Verdin, E. (1998). Apoptosis of CD8+ T cells is mediated by macrophages through interaction of HIV gp120 with chemokine receptor CXCR4. *Nature,* 395(6698), 189-194.
Ho, D. D., McKeating, J. A., Li, X. L., Moudgil, T., Daar, E. S., Sun, N. C., & Robinson, J. E. (1991). Conformational epitope on gp120 important in CD4 binding and human immunodeficiency virus type 1 neutralization identified by a human monoclonal antibody. *J Virol,* 65(1), 489-493.
Hoffman, N. G., Schiffer, C. A., & Swanstrom, R. (2003). Covariation of amino acid positions in HIV-1 protease. *Virology,* 314(2), 536-548.
Hombrouck, A., Voet, A., Van Remoortel, B., Desadeleer, C., De Maeyer, M., Debyser, Z., & Witvrouw, M. (2008). Mutations in human immunodeficiency virus type 1 integrase confer resistance to the naphthyridine L-870,810 and cross-resistance to the clinical trial drug GS-9137. *Antimicrob Agents Chemother,* 52(6), 2069-2078.
Howard, O. M., Shirakawa, A. K., Turpin, J. A., Maynard, A., Tobin, G. J., Carrington, M., Oppenheim, J. J., & Dean, M. (1999). Naturally occurring CCR5 extracellular and transmembrane domain variants affect HIV-1 Co-receptor and ligand binding function. *J Biol Chem,* 274(23), 16228-16234.
Hsiou, Y., Ding, J., Das, K., Clark, A. D., Jr., Boyer, P. L., Lewi, P., Janssen, P. A., Kleim, J. P., Rosner, M., Hughes, S. H., & Arnold, E. (2001). The Lys103Asn mutation of HIV-1 RT: a novel mechanism of drug resistance. *J Mol Biol,* 309(2), 437-445.
Huang, K. H., Goedhals, D., Carlson, J. M., Brockman, M. A., Mishra, S., Brumme, Z. L., Hickling, S., Tang, C. S., Miura, T., Seebregts, C., Heckerman, D., Ndung'u, T., Walker, B., Klenerman, P., Steyn, D., Goulder, P., Phillips, R., van Vuuren, C., & Frater, J. (2011). Progression to AIDS in South Africa is associated with both reverting and compensatory viral mutations. *PLoS One,* 6(4), e19018.

Huang, W., Eshleman, S. H., Toma, J., Fransen, S., Stawiski, E., Paxinos, E. E., Whitcomb, J. M., Young, A. M., Donnell, D., Mmiro, F., Musoke, P., Guay, L. A., Jackson, J. B., Parkin, N. T., & Petropoulos, C. J. (2007). Coreceptor tropism in human immunodeficiency virus type 1 subtype D: high prevalence of CXCR4 tropism and heterogeneous composition of viral populations. *J Virol,* 81(15), 7885-7893.

Huang, W., Toma, J., Fransen, S., Stawiski, E., Reeves, J. D., Whitcomb, J. M., Parkin, N., & Petropoulos, C. J. (2008). Coreceptor tropism can be influenced by amino acid substitutions in the gp41 transmembrane subunit of human immunodeficiency virus type 1 envelope protein. *J Virol,* 82(11), 5584-5593.

Ishikawa, H., Sasaki, M., Noda, S., & Koga, Y. (1998). Apoptosis induction by the binding of the carboxyl terminus of human immunodeficiency virus type 1 gp160 to calmodulin. *J Virol,* 72(8), 6574-6580.

Janssen, P. A., Lewi, P. J., Arnold, E., Daeyaert, F., de Jonge, M., Heeres, J., Koymans, L., Vinkers, M., Guillemont, J., Pasquier, E., Kukla, M., Ludovici, D., Andries, K., de Bethune, M. P., Pauwels, R., Das, K., Clark, A. D., Jr., Frenkel, Y. V., Hughes, S. H., Medaer, B., De Knaep, F., Bohets, H., De Clerck, F., Lampo, A., Williams, P., & Stoffels, P. (2005). In search of a novel anti-HIV drug: multidisciplinary coordination in the discovery of 4-[[4-[[4-[(1E)-2-cyanoethenyl]-2,6-dimethylphenyl]amino]-2-pyrimidinyl]amino]benzonitrile (R278474, rilpivirine). *J Med Chem,* 48(6), 1901-1909.

Jensen, M. A., & van 't Wout, A. B. (2003). Predicting HIV-1 coreceptor usage with sequence analysis. *AIDS Rev,* 5(2), 104-112.

Johnson, A. A., Santos, W., Pais, G. C., Marchand, C., Amin, R., Burke, T. R., Jr., Verdine, G., & Pommier, Y. (2006). Integration requires a specific interaction of the donor DNA terminal 5'-cytosine with glutamine 148 of the HIV-1 integrase flexible loop. *J Biol Chem,* 281(1), 461-467.

Johnson, V. A., Brun-Vezinet, F., Clotet, B., Gunthard, H. F., Kuritzkes, D. R., Pillay, D., Schapiro, J. M., & Richman, D. D. (2010). Update of the drug resistance mutations in HIV-1: December 2010. *Top HIV Med,* 18(5), 156-163.

Johnston, E., Winters, M. A., Rhee, S. Y., Merigan, T. C., Schiffer, C. A., & Shafer, R. W. (2004). Association of a novel human immunodeficiency virus type 1 protease substrate cleft mutation, L23I, with protease inhibitor therapy and in vitro drug resistance. *Antimicrob Agents Chemother,* 48(12), 4864-4868.

Joshi, A., Nyakeriga, A., Ravi, R., & Garg, H. (2011). HIV ENV glycoprotein mediated bystander apoptosis is dependent on CCR5 cell surface expression levels as well as env fusogenic activity. *J Biol Chem.*

Joubert, M. K., Kinsley, N., Capovilla, A., Sewell, B. T., Jaffer, M. A., & Khati, M. (2010). A modeled structure of an aptamer-gp120 complex provides insight into the mechanism of HIV-1 neutralization. *Biochemistry,* 49(28), 5880-5890.

Kagan, R. M., Shenderovich, M. D., Heseltine, P. N., & Ramnarayan, K. (2005). Structural analysis of an HIV-1 protease I47A mutant resistant to the protease inhibitor lopinavir. *Protein Sci,* 14(7), 1870-1878.

Kalia, V., Sarkar, S., Gupta, P., & Montelaro, R. C. (2005). Antibody neutralization escape mediated by point mutations in the intracytoplasmic tail of human immunodeficiency virus type 1 gp41. *J Virol,* 79(4), 2097-2107.

Kantor, R., Katzenstein, D. A., Efron, B., Carvalho, A. P., Wynhoven, B., Cane, P., Clarke, J., Sirivichayakul, S., Soares, M. A., Snoeck, J., Pillay, C., Rudich, H., Rodrigues, R., Holguin, A., Ariyoshi, K., Bouzas, M. B., Cahn, P., Sugiura, W., Soriano, V., Brigido, L. F., Grossman, Z., Morris, L., Vandamme, A. M., Tanuri, A., Phanuphak, P., Weber, J. N., Pillay, D., Harrigan, P. R., Camacho, R., Schapiro, J. M., & Shafer, R. W. (2005).

Impact of HIV-1 subtype and antiretroviral therapy on protease and reverse transcriptase genotype: results of a global collaboration. *PLoS Med,* 2(4), e112.

Khati, M. (2010). The future of aptamers in medicine. *J Clin Pathol,* 63(6), 480-487.

Khati, M., Schuman, M., Ibrahim, J., Sattentau, Q., Gordon, S., & James, W. (2003). Neutralization of infectivity of diverse R5 clinical isolates of human immunodeficiency virus type 1 by gp120-binding 2'F-RNA aptamers. *J Virol,* 77(23), 12692-12698.

Kilby, J. M., Hopkins, S., Venetta, T. M., DiMassimo, B., Cloud, G. A., Lee, J. Y., Alldredge, L., Hunter, E., Lambert, D., Bolognesi, D., Matthews, T., Johnson, M. R., Nowak, M. A., Shaw, G. M., & Saag, M. S. (1998). Potent suppression of HIV-1 replication in humans by T-20, a peptide inhibitor of gp41-mediated virus entry. *Nat Med,* 4(11), 1302-1307.

Kim, Y. M., Choi, K. H., Jang, Y. J., Yu, J., & Jeong, S. (2003). Specific modulation of the anti-DNA autoantibody-nucleic acids interaction by the high affinity RNA aptamer. *Biochem Biophys Res Commun,* 300(2), 516-523.

Kohlstaedt, L. A., Wang, J., Friedman, J. M., Rice, P. A., & Steitz, T. A. (1992a). Crystal structure at 3.5 A resolution of HIV-1 reverse transcriptase complexed with an inhibitor. *Science,* 256(5065), 1783-1790.

Kohlstaedt, L. A., Wang, J., Friedman, J. M., Rice, P. A., & Steitz, T. A. (1992b). Crystal structure at 3.5 A resolution of HIV-1 reverse transcriptase complexed with an inhibitor. *Science,* 256(5065), 1783-1790.

Kwong, P. D., Wyatt, R., Robinson, J., Sweet, R. W., Sodroski, J., & Hendrickson, W. A. (1998a). Structure of an HIV gp120 envelope glycoprotein in complex with the CD4 receptor and a neutralizing human antibody. *Nature,* 393(6686), 648-659.

Kwong, P. D., Wyatt, R., Robinson, J., Sweet, R. W., Sodroski, J., & Hendrickson, W. A. (1998b). Structure of an HIV gp120 envelope glycoprotein in complex with the CD4 receptor and a neutralizing human antibody [see comments]. *Nature,* 393(6686), 648-659.

Lanier, E. R., Ait-Khaled, M., Scott, J., Stone, C., Melby, T., Sturge, G., St Clair, M., Steel, H., Hetherington, S., Pearce, G., Spreen, W., & Lafon, S. (2004a). Antiviral efficacy of abacavir in antiretroviral therapy-experienced adults harbouring HIV-1 with specific patterns of resistance to nucleoside reverse transcriptase inhibitors. *Antivir Ther,* 9(1), 37-45.

Lanier, E. R., Givens, N., Stone, C., Griffin, P., Gibb, D., Walker, S., Tisdale, M., Irlbeck, D., Underwood, M., St Clair, M., & Ait-Khaled, M. (2004b). Effect of concurrent zidovudine use on the resistance pathway selected by abacavir-containing regimens. *HIV Med,* 5(6), 394-399.

Lataillade, M., Chiarella, J., & Kozal, M. J. (2007). Natural polymorphism of the HIV-1 integrase gene and mutations associated with integrase inhibitor resistance. *Antivir Ther,* 12(4), 563-570.

Lazzarin, A., Campbell, T., Clotet, B., Johnson, M., Katlama, C., Moll, A., Towner, W., Trottier, B., Peeters, M., Vingerhoets, J., de Smedt, G., Baeten, B., Beets, G., Sinha, R., & Woodfall, B. (2007). Efficacy and safety of TMC125 (etravirine) in treatment-experienced HIV-1-infected patients in DUET-2: 24-week results from a randomised, double-blind, placebo-controlled trial. *Lancet,* 370(9581), 39-48.

Li, C. J., Friedman, D. J., Wang, C., Metelev, V., & Pardee, A. B. (1995). Induction of apoptosis in uninfected lymphocytes by HIV-1 Tat protein. *Science,* 268(5209), 429-431.

Li, Y., O'Dell, S., Walker, L. M., Wu, X., Guenaga, J., Feng, Y., Schmidt, S. D., McKee, K., Louder, M. K., Ledgerwood, J. E., Graham, B. S., Haynes, B. F., Burton, D. R., Wyatt, R. T., & Mascola, J. R. (2011). Mechanism of neutralization by the broadly neutralizing HIV-1 monoclonal antibody VRC01. *J Virol,* 85(17), 8954-8967.

Liu, Y., Sun, Q. A., Chen, Q., Lee, T. H., Huang, Y., Wetsel, W. C., Michelotti, G. A., Sullenger, B. A., & Zhang, X. (2009). Targeting inhibition of GluR1 Ser845 phosphorylation with an RNA aptamer that blocks AMPA receptor trafficking. *J Neurochem,* 108(1), 147-157.

Low, A. J., Dong, W., Chan, D., Sing, T., Swanstrom, R., Jensen, M., Pillai, S., Good, B., & Harrigan, P. R. (2007). Current V3 genotyping algorithms are inadequate for predicting X4 co-receptor usage in clinical isolates. *Aids,* 21(14), F17-24.

Lu, J., Deeks, S. G., Hoh, R., Beatty, G., Kuritzkes, B. A., Martin, J. N., & Kuritzkes, D. R. (2006). Rapid emergence of enfuvirtide resistance in HIV-1-infected patients: results of a clonal analysis. *J Acquir Immune Defic Syndr,* 43(1), 60-64.

Lu, J., Sista, P., Giguel, F., Greenberg, M., & Kuritzkes, D. R. (2004). Relative replicative fitness of human immunodeficiency virus type 1 mutants resistant to enfuvirtide (T-20). *J Virol,* 78(9), 4628-4637.

Luo, X. M., Lei, M. Y., Feidi, R. A., West, A. P., Jr., Balazs, A. B., Bjorkman, P. J., Yang, L., & Baltimore, D. (2011). Dimeric 2G12 as a potent protection against HIV-1. *PLoS Pathog,* 6(12), e1001225.

Lupold, S. E., Hicke, B. J., Lin, Y., & Coffey, D. S. (2002). Identification and characterization of nuclease-stabilized RNA molecules that bind human prostate cancer cells via the prostate-specific membrane antigen. *Cancer Res,* 62(14), 4029-4033.

Madruga, J. V., Cahn, P., Grinsztejn, B., Haubrich, R., Lalezari, J., Mills, A., Pialoux, G., Wilkin, T., Peeters, M., Vingerhoets, J., de Smedt, G., Leopold, L., Trefiglio, R., & Woodfall, B. (2007). Efficacy and safety of TMC125 (etravirine) in treatment-experienced HIV-1-infected patients in DUET-1: 24-week results from a randomised, double-blind, placebo-controlled trial. *Lancet,* 370(9581), 29-38.

Malet, I., Delelis, O., Valantin, M. A., Montes, B., Soulie, C., Wirden, M., Tchertanov, L., Peytavin, G., Reynes, J., Mouscadet, J. F., Katlama, C., Calvez, V., & Marcelin, A. G. (2008). Mutations associated with failure of raltegravir treatment affect integrase sensitivity to the inhibitor in vitro. *Antimicrob Agents Chemother,* 52(4), 1351-1358.

Mammano, F., Petit, C., & Clavel, F. (1998). Resistance-associated loss of viral fitness in human immunodeficiency virus type 1: phenotypic analysis of protease and gag coevolution in protease inhibitor-treated patients. *J Virol,* 72(9), 7632-7637.

Marcelin, A. G., Dalban, C., Peytavin, G., Lamotte, C., Agher, R., Delaugerre, C., Wirden, M., Conan, F., Dantin, S., Katlama, C., Costagliola, D., & Calvez, V. (2004a). Clinically relevant interpretation of genotype and relationship to plasma drug concentrations for resistance to saquinavir-ritonavir in human immunodeficiency virus type 1 protease inhibitor-experienced patients. *Antimicrob Agents Chemother,* 48(12), 4687-4692.

Marcelin, A. G., Delaugerre, C., Wirden, M., Viegas, P., Simon, A., Katlama, C., & Calvez, V. (2004b). Thymidine analogue reverse transcriptase inhibitors resistance mutations profiles and association to other nucleoside reverse transcriptase inhibitors resistance mutations observed in the context of virological failure. *J Med Virol,* 72(1), 162-165.

Marcelin, A. G., Flandre, P., de Mendoza, C., Roquebert, B., Peytavin, G., Valer, L., Wirden, M., Abbas, S., Katlama, C., Soriano, V., & Calvez, V. (2007). Clinical validation of saquinavir/ritonavir genotypic resistance score in protease-inhibitor-experienced patients. *Antivir Ther,* 12(2), 247-252.

Marcelin, A. G., Flandre, P., Pavie, J., Schmidely, N., Wirden, M., Lada, O., Chiche, D., Molina, J. M., & Calvez, V. (2005). Clinically relevant genotype interpretation of resistance to didanosine. *Antimicrob Agents Chemother,* 49(5), 1739-1744.

Marcelin, A. G., Reynes, J., Yerly, S., Ktorza, N., Segondy, M., Piot, J. C., Delfraissy, J. F., Kaiser, L., Perrin, L., Katlama, C., & Calvez, V. (2004c). Characterization of genotypic determinants in HR-1 and HR-2 gp41 domains in individuals with persistent HIV viraemia under T-20. *Aids,* 18(9), 1340-1342.

Margot, N. A., Lu, B., Cheng, A., & Miller, M. D. (2006). Resistance development over 144 weeks in treatment-naive patients receiving tenofovir disoproxil fumarate or stavudine with lamivudine and efavirenz in Study 903. *HIV Med,* 7(7), 442-450.

Martinez-Picado, J., Savara, A. V., Sutton, L., & D'Aquila, R. T. (1999). Replicative fitness of protease inhibitor-resistant mutants of human immunodeficiency virus type 1. *J Virol,* 73(5), 3744-3752.

Masquelier, B., Assoumou, K. L., Descamps, D., Bocket, L., Cottalorda, J., Ruffault, A., Marcelin, A. G., Morand-Joubert, L., Tamalet, C., Charpentier, C., Peytavin, G., Antoun, Z., Brun-Vezinet, F., & Costagliola, D. (2008). Clinically validated mutation scores for HIV-1 resistance to fosamprenavir/ritonavir. *J Antimicrob Chemother,* 61(6), 1362-1368.

McNicholas, P. M., Mann, P. A., Wojcik, L., Phd, P. Q., Lee, E., McCarthy, M., Shen, J., Black, T. A., & Strizki, J. M. (2011). Mapping and characterization of vicriviroc resistance mutations from HIV-1 isolated from treatment-experienced subjects enrolled in a phase II study (VICTOR-E1). *J Acquir Immune Defic Syndr,* 56(3), 222-229.

Melby, T., Sista, P., DeMasi, R., Kirkland, T., Roberts, N., Salgo, M., Heilek-Snyder, G., Cammack, N., Matthews, T. J., & Greenberg, M. L. (2006). Characterization of envelope glycoprotein gp41 genotype and phenotypic susceptibility to enfuvirtide at baseline and on treatment in the phase III clinical trials TORO-1 and TORO-2. *AIDS Res Hum Retroviruses,* 22(5), 375-385.

Menzo, S., Castagna, A., Monachetti, A., Hasson, H., Danise, A., Carini, E., Bagnarelli, P., Lazzarin, A., & Clementi, M. (2004). Genotype and phenotype patterns of human immunodeficiency virus type 1 resistance to enfuvirtide during long-term treatment. *Antimicrob Agents Chemother,* 48(9), 3253-3259.

Meyer, P. R., Matsuura, S. E., Mian, A. M., So, A. G., & Scott, W. A. (1999). A mechanism of AZT resistance: an increase in nucleotide-dependent primer unblocking by mutant HIV-1 reverse transcriptase. *Mol Cell,* 4(1), 35-43.

Meyer, P. R., Matsuura, S. E., So, A. G., & Scott, W. A. (1998). Unblocking of chain-terminated primer by HIV-1 reverse transcriptase through a nucleotide-dependent mechanism. *Proc Natl Acad Sci U S A,* 95(23), 13471-13476.

Mi, Z., Guo, H., Russell, M. B., Liu, Y., Sullenger, B. A., & Kuo, P. C. (2009). RNA aptamer blockade of osteopontin inhibits growth and metastasis of MDA-MB231 breast cancer cells. *Mol Ther,* 17(1), 153-161.

Micoli, K. J., Mamaeva, O., Piller, S. C., Barker, J. L., Pan, G., Hunter, E., & McDonald, J. M. (2006). Point mutations in the C-terminus of HIV-1 gp160 reduce apoptosis and calmodulin binding without affecting viral replication. *Virology,* 344(2), 468-479.

Micoli, K. J., Pan, G., Wu, Y., Williams, J. P., Cook, W. J., & McDonald, J. M. (2000). Requirement of calmodulin binding by HIV-1 gp160 for enhanced FAS-mediated apoptosis. *J Biol Chem,* 275(2), 1233-1240.

Miller, M. D., Margot, N., Lu, B., Zhong, L., Chen, S. S., Cheng, A., & Wulfsohn, M. (2004). Genotypic and phenotypic predictors of the magnitude of response to tenofovir disoproxil fumarate treatment in antiretroviral-experienced patients. *J Infect Dis,* 189(5), 837-846.

Mink, M., Mosier, S. M., Janumpalli, S., Davison, D., Jin, L., Melby, T., Sista, P., Erickson, J., Lambert, D., Stanfield-Oakley, S. A., Salgo, M., Cammack, N., Matthews, T., &

Greenberg, M. L. (2005). Impact of human immunodeficiency virus type 1 gp41 amino acid substitutions selected during enfuvirtide treatment on gp41 binding and antiviral potency of enfuvirtide in vitro. *J Virol,* 79(19), 12447-12454.

Molina, J. M., Marcelin, A. G., Pavie, J., Heripret, L., De Boever, C. M., Troccaz, M., Leleu, G., & Calvez, V. (2005). Didanosine in HIV-1-infected patients experiencing failure of antiretroviral therapy: a randomized placebo-controlled trial. *J Infect Dis,* 191(6), 840-847.

Moncunill, G., Armand-Ugon, M., Pauls, E., Clotet, B., & Este, J. A. (2008). HIV-1 escape to CCR5 coreceptor antagonism through selection of CXCR4-using variants in vitro. *Aids,* 22(1), 23-31.

Montefiori, D. C., Pantaleo, G., Fink, L. M., Zhou, J. T., Zhou, J. Y., Bilska, M., Miralles, G. D., & Fauci, A. S. (1996). Neutralizing and infection-enhancing antibody responses to human immunodeficiency virus type 1 in long-term nonprogressors. *J Infect Dis,* 173(1), 60-67.

Moog, C., Fleury, H. J., Pellegrin, I., Kirn, A., & Aubertin, A. M. (1997). Autologous and heterologous neutralizing antibody responses following initial seroconversion in human immunodeficiency virus type 1-infected individuals. *J Virol,* 71(5), 3734-3741.

Moore, J. P., & Ho, D. D. (1995). HIV-1 neutralization: the consequences of viral adaptation to growth on transformed T cells. *Aids,* 9(Suppl A), S117-136.

Moore, J. P., & Sodroski, J. (1996). Antibody cross-competition analysis of the human immunodeficiency virus type 1 gp120 exterior envelope glycoprotein. *J Virol,* 70(3), 1863-1872.

Mouscadet, J. F., Arora, R., Andre, J., Lambry, J. C., Delelis, O., Malet, I., Marcelin, A. G., Calvez, V., & Tchertanov, L. (2009). HIV-1 IN alternative molecular recognition of DNA induced by raltegravir resistance mutations. *J Mol Recognit,* 22(6), 480-494.

Moyle, G. J., DeJesus, E., Cahn, P., Castillo, S. A., Zhao, H., Gordon, D. N., Craig, C., & Scott, T. R. (2005). Abacavir once or twice daily combined with once-daily lamivudine and efavirenz for the treatment of antiretroviral-naive HIV-infected adults: results of the Ziagen Once Daily in Antiretroviral Combination Study. *J Acquir Immune Defic Syndr,* 38(4), 417-425.

Muster, T., Guinea, R., Trkola, A., Purtscher, M., Klima, A., Steindl, F., Palese, P., & Katinger, H. (1994). Cross-neutralizing activity against divergent human immunodeficiency virus type 1 isolates induced by the gp41 sequence ELDKWAS. *J Virol,* 68(6), 4031-4034.

Muster, T., Steindl, F., Purtscher, M., Trkola, A., Klima, A., Himmler, G., Ruker, F., & Katinger, H. (1993). A conserved neutralizing epitope on gp41 of human immunodeficiency virus type 1. *J Virol,* 67(11), 6642-6647.

Nakamura, K. J., Gach, J. S., Jones, L., Semrau, K., Walter, J., Bibollet-Ruche, F., Decker, J. M., Heath, L., Decker, W. D., Sinkala, M., Kankasa, C., Thea, D., Mullins, J., Kuhn, L., Zwick, M. B., & Aldrovandi, G. M. (2011). 4E10-resistant HIV-1 isolated from four subjects with rare membrane-proximal external region polymorphisms. *PLoS One,* 5(3), e9786.

Nijhuis, M., Schuurman, R., de Jong, D., Erickson, J., Gustchina, E., Albert, J., Schipper, P., Gulnik, S., & Boucher, C. A. (1999). Increased fitness of drug resistant HIV-1 protease as a result of acquisition of compensatory mutations during suboptimal therapy. *Aids,* 13(17), 2349-2359.

Nobile, V., Russo, N., Hu, G., & Riordan, J. F. (1998). Inhibition of human angiogenin by DNA aptamers: nuclear colocalization of an angiogenin-inhibitor complex. *Biochemistry,* 37(19), 6857-6863.

O'Brien, T. R., Winkler, C., Dean, M., Nelson, J. A., Carrington, M., Michael, N. L., & White, G. C., 2nd (1997). HIV-1 infection in a man homozygous for CCR5 delta 32 [letter] [see comments]. *Lancet,* 349(9060), 1219.

Pancera, M., McLellan, J. S., Wu, X., Zhu, J., Changela, A., Schmidt, S. D., Yang, Y., Zhou, T., Phogat, S., Mascola, J. R., & Kwong, P. D. (2010). Crystal structure of PG16 and chimeric dissection with somatically related PG9: structure-function analysis of two quaternary-specific antibodies that effectively neutralize HIV-1. *J Virol,* 84(16), 8098-8110.

Park, E. J., Vujcic, L. K., Anand, R., Theodore, T. S., & Quinnan, G. V., Jr. (1998). Mutations in both gp120 and gp41 are responsible for the broad neutralization resistance of variant human immunodeficiency virus type 1 MN to antibodies directed at V3 and non-V3 epitopes. *J Virol,* 72(9), 7099-7107.

Parkin, N. T., Chappey, C., & Petropoulos, C. J. (2003). Improving lopinavir genotype algorithm through phenotype correlations: novel mutation patterns and amprenavir cross-resistance. *Aids,* 17(7), 955-961.

Pastore, C., Nedellec, R., Ramos, A., Hartley, O., Miamidian, J. L., Reeves, J. D., & Mosier, D. E. (2007). Conserved changes in envelope function during human immunodeficiency virus type 1 coreceptor switching. *J Virol,* 81(15), 8165-8179.

Pastore, C., Nedellec, R., Ramos, A., Pontow, S., Ratner, L., & Mosier, D. E. (2006). Human immunodeficiency virus type 1 coreceptor switching: V1/V2 gain-of-fitness mutations compensate for V3 loss-of-fitness mutations. *J Virol,* 80(2), 750-758.

Patick, A. K., Mo, H., Markowitz, M., Appelt, K., Wu, B., Musick, L., Kalish, V., Kaldor, S., Reich, S., Ho, D., & Webber, S. (1996). Antiviral and resistance studies of AG1343, an orally bioavailable inhibitor of human immunodeficiency virus protease. *Antimicrob Agents Chemother,* 40(2), 292-297.

Pellegrin, I., Breilh, D., Coureau, G., Boucher, S., Neau, D., Merel, P., Lacoste, D., Fleury, H., Saux, M. C., Pellegrin, J. L., Lazaro, E., Dabis, F., & Thiebaut, R. (2007). Interpretation of genotype and pharmacokinetics for resistance to fosamprenavir-ritonavir-based regimens in antiretroviral-experienced patients. *Antimicrob Agents Chemother,* 51(4), 1473-1480.

Pellegrin, I., Breilh, D., Ragnaud, J. M., Boucher, S., Neau, D., Fleury, H., Schrive, M. H., Saux, M. C., Pellegrin, J. L., Lazaro, E., & Vray, M. (2006). Virological responses to atazanavir-ritonavir-based regimens: resistance-substitutions score and pharmacokinetic parameters (Reyaphar study). *Antivir Ther,* 11(4), 421-429.

Perno, C. F., Cozzi-Lepri, A., Balotta, C., Forbici, F., Violin, M., Bertoli, A., Facchi, G., Pezzotti, P., Cadeo, G., Tositti, G., Pasquinucci, S., Pauluzzi, S., Scalzini, A., Salassa, B., Vincenti, A., Phillips, A. N., Dianzani, F., Appice, A., Angarano, G., Monno, L., Ippolito, G., Moroni, M., & d' Arminio Monforte, A. (2001). Secondary mutations in the protease region of human immunodeficiency virus and virologic failure in drug-naive patients treated with protease inhibitor-based therapy. *J Infect Dis,* 184(8), 983-991.

Perno, C. F., Cozzi-Lepri, A., Forbici, F., Bertoli, A., Violin, M., Stella Mura, M., Cadeo, G., Orani, A., Chirianni, A., De Stefano, C., Balotta, C., & d'Arminio Monforte, A. (2004). Minor mutations in HIV protease at baseline and appearance of primary mutation 90M in patients for whom their first protease-inhibitor antiretroviral regimens failed. *J Infect Dis,* 189(11), 1983-1987.

Petropoulos, C. J., Parkin, N. T., Limoli, K. L., Lie, Y. S., Wrin, T., Huang, W., Tian, H., Smith, D., Winslow, G. A., Capon, D. J., & Whitcomb, J. M. (2000). A novel phenotypic drug susceptibility assay for human immunodeficiency virus type 1. *Antimicrob Agents Chemother,* 44(4), 920-928.

Platt, E. J., Kuhmann, S. E., Rose, P. P., & Kabat, D. (2001). Adaptive mutations in the V3 loop of gp120 enhance fusogenicity of human immunodeficiency virus type 1 and enable use of a CCR5 coreceptor that lacks the amino-terminal sulfated region. *J Virol,* 75(24), 12266-12278.

Platt, E. J., Shea, D. M., Rose, P. P., & Kabat, D. (2005). Variants of human immunodeficiency virus type 1 that efficiently use CCR5 lacking the tyrosine-sulfated amino terminus have adaptive mutations in gp120, including loss of a functional N-glycan. *J Virol,* 79(7), 4357-4368.

Poignard, P., Klasse, P. J., & Sattentau, Q. J. (1996). Antibody neutralization of HIV-1. *Immunol Today,* 17(5), 239-246.

Pommier, Y., Johnson, A. A., & Marchand, C. (2005). Integrase inhibitors to treat HIV/AIDS. *Nat Rev Drug Discov,* 4(3), 236-248.

Posner, M. R., Hideshima, T., Cannon, T., Mukherjee, M., Mayer, K. H., & Byrn, R. A. (1991). An IgG human monoclonal antibody that reacts with HIV-1/GP120, inhibits virus binding to cells, and neutralizes infection. *J Immunol,* 146(12), 4325-4332.

Rana, S., Besson, G., Cook, D. G., Rucker, J., Smyth, R. J., Yi, Y., Turner, J. D., Guo, H. H., Du, J. G., Peiper, S. C., Lavi, E., Samson, M., Libert, F., Liesnard, C., Vassart, G., Doms, R. W., Parmentier, M., & Collman, R. G. (1997). Role of CCR5 in infection of primary macrophages and lymphocytes by macrophage-tropic strains of human immunodeficiency virus: resistance to patient-derived and prototype isolates resulting from the delta ccr5 mutation. *J Virol,* 71(4), 3219-3227.

Reeves, J. D., Lee, F. H., Miamidian, J. L., Jabara, C. B., Juntilla, M. M., & Doms, R. W. (2005). Enfuvirtide resistance mutations: impact on human immunodeficiency virus envelope function, entry inhibitor sensitivity, and virus neutralization. *J Virol,* 79(8), 4991-4999.

Reitz, M. S., Jr., Wilson, C., Naugle, C., Gallo, R. C., & Robert-Guroff, M. (1988). Generation of a neutralization-resistant variant of HIV-1 is due to selection for a point mutation in the envelope gene. *Cell,* 54(1), 57-63.

Ren, J., Chamberlain, P. P., Stamp, A., Short, S. A., Weaver, K. L., Romines, K. R., Hazen, R., Freeman, A., Ferris, R. G., Andrews, C. W., Boone, L., Chan, J. H., & Stammers, D. K. (2008). Structural basis for the improved drug resistance profile of new generation benzophenone non-nucleoside HIV-1 reverse transcriptase inhibitors. *J Med Chem,* 51(16), 5000-5008.

Ren, J., Esnouf, R., Garman, E., Somers, D., Ross, C., Kirby, I., Keeling, J., Darby, G., Jones, Y., Stuart, D., & et al. (1995a). High resolution structures of HIV-1 RT from four RT-inhibitor complexes. *Nat Struct Biol,* 2(4), 293-302.

Ren, J., Esnouf, R., Hopkins, A., Ross, C., Jones, Y., Stammers, D., & Stuart, D. (1995b). The structure of HIV-1 reverse transcriptase complexed with 9-chloro-TIBO: lessons for inhibitor design. *Structure,* 3(9), 915-926.

Ren, J., Nichols, C., Bird, L., Chamberlain, P., Weaver, K., Short, S., Stuart, D. I., & Stammers, D. K. (2001). Structural mechanisms of drug resistance for mutations at codons 181 and 188 in HIV-1 reverse transcriptase and the improved resilience of second generation non-nucleoside inhibitors. *J Mol Biol,* 312(4), 795-805.

Ren, J., Nichols, C. E., Chamberlain, P. P., Weaver, K. L., Short, S. A., Chan, J. H., Kleim, J. P., & Stammers, D. K. (2007). Relationship of potency and resilience to drug resistant mutations for GW420867X revealed by crystal structures of inhibitor complexes for wild-type, Leu100Ile, Lys101Glu, and Tyr188Cys mutant HIV-1 reverse transcriptases. *J Med Chem,* 50(10), 2301-2309.

Ren, J., Nichols, C. E., Chamberlain, P. P., Weaver, K. L., Short, S. A., & Stammers, D. K. (2004). Crystal structures of HIV-1 reverse transcriptases mutated at codons 100, 106 and 108 and mechanisms of resistance to non-nucleoside inhibitors. *J Mol Biol,* 336(3), 569-578.

Ren, J., & Stammers, D. K. (2008). Structural basis for drug resistance mechanisms for non-nucleoside inhibitors of HIV reverse transcriptase. *Virus Res,* 134(1-2), 157-170.

Rey, D., Hoen, B., Chavanet, P., Schmitt, M. P., Hoizey, G., Meyer, P., Peytavin, G., Spire, B., Allavena, C., Diemer, M., May, T., Schmit, J. L., Duong, M., Calvez, V., & Lang, J. M. (2009). High rate of early virological failure with the once-daily tenofovir/lamivudine/nevirapine combination in naive HIV-1-infected patients. *J Antimicrob Chemother,* 63(2), 380-388.

Rhee, S. Y., Fessel, W. J., Zolopa, A. R., Hurley, L., Liu, T., Taylor, J., Nguyen, D. P., Slome, S., Klein, D., Horberg, M., Flamm, J., Follansbee, S., Schapiro, J. M., & Shafer, R. W. (2005). HIV-1 Protease and reverse-transcriptase mutations: correlations with antiretroviral therapy in subtype B isolates and implications for drug-resistance surveillance. *J Infect Dis,* 192(3), 456-465.

Rhee, S. Y., Gonzales, M. J., Kantor, R., Betts, B. J., Ravela, J., & Shafer, R. W. (2003). Human immunodeficiency virus reverse transcriptase and protease sequence database. *Nucleic Acids Res,* 31(1), 298-303.

Rhee, S. Y., Kantor, R., Katzenstein, D. A., Camacho, R., Morris, L., Sirivichayakul, S., Jorgensen, L., Brigido, L. F., Schapiro, J. M., & Shafer, R. W. (2006a). HIV-1 pol mutation frequency by subtype and treatment experience: extension of the HIVseq program to seven non-B subtypes. *Aids,* 20(5), 643-651.

Rhee, S. Y., Liu, T., Ravela, J., Gonzales, M. J., & Shafer, R. W. (2004). Distribution of human immunodeficiency virus type 1 protease and reverse transcriptase mutation patterns in 4,183 persons undergoing genotypic resistance testing. *Antimicrob Agents Chemother,* 48(8), 3122-3126.

Rhee, S. Y., Liu, T. F., Holmes, S. P., & Shafer, R. W. (2007). HIV-1 subtype B protease and reverse transcriptase amino acid covariation. *PLoS Comput Biol,* 3(5), e87.

Rhee, S. Y., Taylor, J., Wadhera, G., Ben-Hur, A., Brutlag, D. L., & Shafer, R. W. (2006b). Genotypic predictors of human immunodeficiency virus type 1 drug resistance. *Proc Natl Acad Sci U S A,* 103(46), 17355-17360.

Roge, B. T., Katzenstein, T. L., Obel, N., Nielsen, H., Kirk, O., Pedersen, C., Mathiesen, L., Lundgren, J., & Gerstoft, J. (2003). K65R with and without S68: a new resistance profile in vivo detected in most patients failing abacavir, didanosine and stavudine. *Antivir Ther,* 8(2), 173-182.

Ross, L., Scarsella, A., Raffanti, S., Henry, K., Becker, S., Fisher, R., Liao, Q., Hirani, A., Graham, N., St Clair, M., & Hernandez, J. (2001). Thymidine analog and multinucleoside resistance mutations are associated with decreased phenotypic susceptibility to stavudine in HIV type 1 isolated from zidovudine-naive patients experiencing viremia on stavudine-containing regimens. *AIDS Res Hum Retroviruses,* 17(12), 1107-1115.

Ruckman, J., Green, L. S., Beeson, J., Waugh, S., Gillette, W. L., Henninger, D. D., Claesson-Welsh, L., & Janjic, N. (1998). 2'-Fluoropyrimidine RNA-based aptamers to the 165-amino acid form of vascular endothelial growth factor (VEGF165). Inhibition of receptor binding and VEGF-induced vascular permeability through interactions requiring the exon 7-encoded domain. *J Biol Chem,* 273(32), 20556-20567.

Ruprecht, C. R., Krarup, A., Reynell, L., Mann, A. M., Brandenberg, O. F., Berlinger, L., Abela, I. A., Regoes, R. R., Gunthard, H. F., Rusert, P., & Trkola, A. (2011). MPER-specific antibodies induce gp120 shedding and irreversibly neutralize HIV-1. *J Exp Med,* 208(3), 439-454.

Rusconi, C. P., Roberts, J. D., Pitoc, G. A., Nimjee, S. M., White, R. R., Quick, G., Jr., Scardino, E., Fay, W. P., & Sullenger, B. A. (2004). Antidote-mediated control of an anticoagulant aptamer in vivo. *Nat Biotechnol,* 22(11), 1423-1428.

Rusconi, C. P., Scardino, E., Layzer, J., Pitoc, G. A., Ortel, T. L., Monroe, D., & Sullenger, B. A. (2002). RNA aptamers as reversible antagonists of coagulation factor IXa. *Nature,* 419(6902), 90-94.

Samson, M., Libert, F., Doranz, B. J., Rucker, J., Liesnard, C., Farber, C. M., Saragosti, S., Lapoumeroulie, C., Cognaux, J., Forceille, C., Muyldermans, G., Verhofstede, C., Burtonboy, G., Georges, M., Imai, T., Rana, S., Yi, Y., Smyth, R. J., Collman, R. G., Doms, R. W., Vassart, G., & Parmentier, M. (1996). Resistance to HIV-1 infection in caucasian individuals bearing mutant alleles of the CCR-5 chemokine receptor gene [see comments]. *Nature,* 382(6593), 722-725.

Sarafianos, S. G., Das, K., Clark, A. D., Jr., Ding, J., Boyer, P. L., Hughes, S. H., & Arnold, E. (1999). Lamivudine (3TC) resistance in HIV-1 reverse transcriptase involves steric hindrance with beta-branched amino acids. *Proc Natl Acad Sci U S A,* 96(18), 10027-10032.

Sarafianos, S. G., Das, K., Hughes, S. H., & Arnold, E. (2004). Taking aim at a moving target: designing drugs to inhibit drug-resistant HIV-1 reverse transcriptases. *Curr Opin Struct Biol,* 14(6), 716-730.

Sarafianos, S. G., Marchand, B., Das, K., Himmel, D. M., Parniak, M. A., Hughes, S. H., & Arnold, E. (2009). Structure and function of HIV-1 reverse transcriptase: molecular mechanisms of polymerization and inhibition. *J Mol Biol,* 385(3), 693-713.

Sattentau, Q. J., & Moore, J. P. (1995). Human immunodeficiency virus type 1 neutralization is determined by epitope exposure on the gp120 oligomer. *J Exp Med,* 182(1), 185-196.

Scanlan, C. N., Pantophlet, R., Wormald, M. R., Saphire, E. O., Calarese, D., Stanfield, R., Wilson, I. A., Katinger, H., Dwek, R. A., Burton, D. R., & Rudd, P. M. (2003). The carbohydrate epitope of the neutralizing anti-HIV-1 antibody 2G12. *Adv Exp Med Biol,* 535, 205-218.

Seclen, E., Gonzalez Mdel, M., Lapaz, M., Rodriguez, C., del Romero, J., Aguilera, A., de Mendoza, C., Soriano, V., & Poveda, E. (2011). Primary resistance to maraviroc in a large set of R5-V3 viral sequences from HIV-1-infected patients. *J Antimicrob Chemother,* 65(12), 2502-2504.

Shafer, R. W., & Schapiro, J. M. (2008). HIV-1 drug resistance mutations: an updated framework for the second decade of HAART. *AIDS Rev,* 10(2), 67-84.

Shimura, K., Kodama, E., Sakagami, Y., Matsuzaki, Y., Watanabe, W., Yamataka, K., Watanabe, Y., Ohata, Y., Doi, S., Sato, M., Kano, M., Ikeda, S., & Matsuoka, M. (2008). Broad antiretroviral activity and resistance profile of the novel human immunodeficiency virus integrase inhibitor elvitegravir (JTK-303/GS-9137). *J Virol,* 82(2), 764-774.

Shulman, N. S., Bosch, R. J., Mellors, J. W., Albrecht, M. A., & Katzenstein, D. A. (2004). Genetic correlates of efavirenz hypersusceptibility. *Aids,* 18(13), 1781-1785.

Shulman, N. S., Zolopa, A. R., Passaro, D. J., Murlidharan, U., Israelski, D. M., Brosgart, C. L., Miller, M. D., Van Doren, S., Shafer, R. W., & Katzenstein, D. A. (2000). Efavirenz- and adefovir dipivoxil-based salvage therapy in highly treatment-experienced patients: clinical and genotypic predictors of virologic response. *J Acquir Immune Defic Syndr,* 23(3), 221-226.

Sing, T., Low, A. J., Beerenwinkel, N., Sander, O., Cheung, P. K., Domingues, F. S., Buch, J., Daumer, M., Kaiser, R., Lengauer, T., & Harrigan, P. R. (2007). Predicting HIV coreceptor usage on the basis of genetic and clinical covariates. *Antivir Ther,* 12(7), 1097-1106.

Sista, P. R., Melby, T., Davison, D., Jin, L., Mosier, S., Mink, M., Nelson, E. L., DeMasi, R., Cammack, N., Salgo, M. P., Matthews, T. J., & Greenberg, M. L. (2004). Characterization of determinants of genotypic and phenotypic resistance to enfuvirtide in baseline and on-treatment HIV-1 isolates. *Aids,* 18(13), 1787-1794.

Smith, K. Y., Weinberg, W. G., Dejesus, E., Fischl, M. A., Liao, Q., Ross, L. L., Pakes, G. E., Pappa, K. A., & Lancaster, C. T. (2008). Fosamprenavir or atazanavir once daily boosted with ritonavir 100 mg, plus tenofovir/emtricitabine, for the initial treatment of HIV infection: 48-week results of ALERT. *AIDS Res Ther,* 5, 5.

Sosa, N., Hill-Zabala, C., Dejesus, E., Herrera, G., Florance, A., Watson, M., Vavro, C., & Shaefer, M. (2005). Abacavir and lamivudine fixed-dose combination tablet once daily compared with abacavir and lamivudine twice daily in HIV-infected patients over 48 weeks (ESS30008, SEAL). *J Acquir Immune Defic Syndr,* 40(4), 422-427.

Su, C., Melby, T., DeMasi, R., Ravindran, P., & Heilek-Snyder, G. (2006). Genotypic changes in human immunodeficiency virus type 1 envelope glycoproteins on treatment with the fusion inhibitor enfuvirtide and their influence on changes in drug susceptibility in vitro. *J Clin Virol,* 36(4), 249-257.

Sugiura, W., Matsuda, Z., Yokomaku, Y., Hertogs, K., Larder, B., Oishi, T., Okano, A., Shiino, T., Tatsumi, M., Matsuda, M., Abumi, H., Takata, N., Shirahata, S., Yamada, K., Yoshikura, H., & Nagai, Y. (2002). Interference between D30N and L90M in selection and development of protease inhibitor-resistant human immunodeficiency virus type 1. *Antimicrob Agents Chemother,* 46(3), 708-715.

Svarovskaia, E. S., Margot, N. A., Bae, A. S., Waters, J. M., Goodman, D., Zhong, L., Borroto-Esoda, K., & Miller, M. D. (2007). Low-level K65R mutation in HIV-1 reverse transcriptase of treatment-experienced patients exposed to abacavir or didanosine. *J Acquir Immune Defic Syndr,* 46(2), 174-180.

Svicher, V., Balestra, E., Cento, V., Sarmati, L., Dori, L., Vandenbroucke, I., D'Arrigo, R., Buonomini, A. R., Van Marck, H., Surdo, M., Saccomandi, P., Mostmans, W., Aerssens, J., Aquaro, S., Stuyver, L. J., Andreoni, M., Ceccherini-Silberstein, F., & Perno, C. F. (2011). HIV-1 dual/mixed tropic isolates show different genetic and phenotypic characteristics and response to maraviroc in vitro. *Antiviral Res,* 90(1), 42-53.

Svicher, V., Ceccherini-Silberstein, F., Erba, F., Santoro, M., Gori, C., Bellocchi, M. C., Giannella, S., Trotta, M. P., Monforte, A., Antinori, A., & Perno, C. F. (2005). Novel human immunodeficiency virus type 1 protease mutations potentially involved in resistance to protease inhibitors. *Antimicrob Agents Chemother,* 49(5), 2015-2025.

Thali, M., Moore, J. P., Furman, C., Charles, M., Ho, D. D., Robinson, J., & Sodroski, J. (1993). Characterization of conserved human immunodeficiency virus type 1 gp120 neutralization epitopes exposed upon gp120-CD4 binding. *J Virol,* 67(7), 3978-3988.

Theodorou, I., Meyer, L., Magierowska, M., Katlama, C., & Rouzioux, C. (1997). HIV-1 infection in an individual homozygous for CCR5 delta 32. Seroco Study Group [letter] [see comments]. *Lancet,* 349(9060), 1219-1220.

Tilton, J. C., Wilen, C. B., Didigu, C. A., Sinha, R., Harrison, J. E., Agrawal-Gamse, C., Henning, E. A., Bushman, F. D., Martin, J. N., Deeks, S. G., & Doms, R. W. (2011). A maraviroc-resistant HIV-1 with narrow cross-resistance to other CCR5 antagonists depends on both N-terminal and extracellular loop domains of drug-bound CCR5. *J Virol,* 84(20), 10863-10876.

Trkola, A., Dragic, T., Arthos, J., Binley, J. M., Olson, W. C., Allaway, G. P., Cheng-Mayer, C., Robinson, J., Maddon, P. J., & Moore, J. P. (1996a). CD4-dependent, antibody-sensitive interactions between HIV-1 and its co- receptor CCR-5 [see comments]. *Nature,* 384(6605), 184-187.

Trkola, A., Purtscher, M., Muster, T., Ballaun, C., Buchacher, A., Sullivan, N., Srinivasan, K., Sodroski, J., Moore, J. P., & Katinger, H. (1996b). Human monoclonal antibody 2G12 defines a distinctive neutralization epitope on the gp120 glycoprotein of human immunodeficiency virus type 1. *J Virol,* 70(2), 1100-1108.

van Maarseveen, N. M., de Jong, D., Boucher, C. A., & Nijhuis, M. (2006). An increase in viral replicative capacity drives the evolution of protease inhibitor-resistant human immunodeficiency virus type 1 in the absence of drugs. *J Acquir Immune Defic Syndr,* 42(2), 162-168.

Vermeiren, H., Van Craenenbroeck, E., Alen, P., Bacheler, L., Picchio, G., & Lecocq, P. (2007). Prediction of HIV-1 drug susceptibility phenotype from the viral genotype using linear regression modeling. *J Virol Methods,* 145(1), 47-55.

Vinores, S. A. (2003). Technology evaluation: pegaptanib, Eyetech/Pfizer. *Curr Opin Mol Ther,* 5(6), 673-679.

Vora, S., Marcelin, A. G., Gunthard, H. F., Flandre, P., Hirsch, H. H., Masquelier, B., Zinkernagel, A., Peytavin, G., Calvez, V., Perrin, L., & Yerly, S. (2006). Clinical validation of atazanavir/ritonavir genotypic resistance score in protease inhibitor-experienced patients. *Aids,* 20(1), 35-40.

Vray, M., Meynard, J. L., Dalban, C., Morand-Joubert, L., Clavel, F., Brun-Vezinet, F., Peytavin, G., Costagliola, D., & Girard, P. M. (2003). Predictors of the virological response to a change in the antiretroviral treatment regimen in HIV-1-infected patients enrolled in a randomized trial comparing genotyping, phenotyping and standard of care (Narval trial, ANRS 088). *Antivir Ther,* 8(5), 427-434.

Walker, L. M., Phogat, S. K., Chan-Hui, P. Y., Wagner, D., Phung, P., Goss, J. L., Wrin, T., Simek, M. D., Fling, S., Mitcham, J. L., Lehrman, J. K., Priddy, F. H., Olsen, O. A., Frey, S. M., Hammond, P. W., Kaminsky, S., Zamb, T., Moyle, M., Koff, W. C., Poignard, P., & Burton, D. R. (2009). Broad and potent neutralizing antibodies from an African donor reveal a new HIV-1 vaccine target. *Science,* 326(5950), 285-289.

Walmsley, S. L., Kelly, D. V., Tseng, A. L., Humar, A., & Harrigan, P. R. (2001). Non-nucleoside reverse transcriptase inhibitor failure impairs HIV-RNA responses to efavirenz-containing salvage antiretroviral therapy. *Aids,* 15(12), 1581-1584.

Wang, J., Tong, P., Lu, L., Zhou, L., Xu, L., Jiang, S., & Chen, Y. H. (2011). HIV-1 gp41 core with exposed membrane-proximal external region inducing broad HIV-1 neutralizing antibodies. *PLoS One,* 6(3), e18233.

Wang, Z., Lee, B., Murray, J. L., Bonneau, F., Sun, Y., Schweickart, V., Zhang, T., & Peiper, S. C. (1999). CCR5 HIV-1 coreceptor activity. Role of cooperativity between residues in N-terminal extracellular and intracellular domains. *J Biol Chem,* 274(40), 28413-28419.

Watts, J. M., Dang, K. K., Gorelick, R. J., Leonard, C. W., Bess, J. W., Jr., Swanstrom, R., Burch, C. L., & Weeks, K. M. (2009). Architecture and secondary structure of an entire HIV-1 RNA genome. *Nature,* 460(7256), 711-716.

Westby, M., Smith-Burchnell, C., Mori, J., Lewis, M., Mosley, M., Stockdale, M., Dorr, P., Ciaramella, G., & Perros, M. (2007). Reduced maximal inhibition in phenotypic susceptibility assays indicates that viral strains resistant to the CCR5 antagonist maraviroc utilize inhibitor-bound receptor for entry. *J Virol*, 81(5), 2359-2371.

Whitcomb, J. M., Parkin, N. T., Chappey, C., Hellmann, N. S., & Petropoulos, C. J. (2003). Broad nucleoside reverse-transcriptase inhibitor cross-resistance in human immunodeficiency virus type 1 clinical isolates. *J Infect Dis*, 188(7), 992-1000.

White, R. R., Shan, S., Rusconi, C. P., Shetty, G., Dewhirst, M. W., Kontos, C. D., & Sullenger, B. A. (2003). Inhibition of rat corneal angiogenesis by a nuclease-resistant RNA aptamer specific for angiopoietin-2. *Proc Natl Acad Sci U S A*, 100(9), 5028-5033.

Wild, C. T., Shugars, D. C., Greenwell, T. K., McDanal, C. B., & Matthews, T. J. (1994). Peptides corresponding to a predictive alpha-helical domain of human immunodeficiency virus type 1 gp41 are potent inhibitors of virus infection. *Proc Natl Acad Sci U S A*, 91(21), 9770-9774.

Winters, B., Montaner, J., Harrigan, P. R., Gazzard, B., Pozniak, A., Miller, M. D., Emery, S., van Leth, F., Robinson, P., Baxter, J. D., Perez-Elias, M., Castor, D., Hammer, S., Rinehart, A., Vermeiren, H., Van Craenenbroeck, E., & Bacheler, L. (2008). Determination of clinically relevant cutoffs for HIV-1 phenotypic resistance estimates through a combined analysis of clinical trial and cohort data. *J Acquir Immune Defic Syndr*, 48(1), 26-34.

Winters, M. A., Bosch, R. J., Albrecht, M. A., & Katzenstein, D. A. (2003). Clinical impact of the M184V mutation on switching to didanosine or maintaining lamivudine treatment in nucleoside reverse-transcriptase inhibitor-experienced patients. *J Infect Dis*, 188(4), 537-540.

Winters, M. A., Shafer, R. W., Jellinger, R. A., Mamtora, G., Gingeras, T., & Merigan, T. C. (1997). Human immunodeficiency virus type 1 reverse transcriptase genotype and drug susceptibility changes in infected individuals receiving dideoxyinosine monotherapy for 1 to 2 years. *Antimicrob Agents Chemother*, 41(4), 757-762.

Wu, L., Gerard, N. P., Wyatt, R., Choe, H., Parolin, C., Ruffing, N., Borsetti, A., Cardoso, A. A., Desjardin, E., Newman, W., Gerard, C., & Sodroski, J. (1996). CD4-induced interaction of primary HIV-1 gp120 glycoproteins with the chemokine receptor CCR-5 [see comments]. *Nature*, 384(6605), 179-183.

Wu, T. D., Schiffer, C. A., Gonzales, M. J., Taylor, J., Kantor, R., Chou, S., Israelski, D., Zolopa, A. R., Fessel, W. J., & Shafer, R. W. (2003). Mutation patterns and structural correlates in human immunodeficiency virus type 1 protease following different protease inhibitor treatments. *J Virol*, 77(8), 4836-4847.

Wu, X., Yang, Z. Y., Li, Y., Hogerkorp, C. M., Schief, W. R., Seaman, M. S., Zhou, T., Schmidt, S. D., Wu, L., Xu, L., Longo, N. S., McKee, K., O'Dell, S., Louder, M. K., Wycuff, D. L., Feng, Y., Nason, M., Doria-Rose, N., Connors, M., Kwong, P. D., Roederer, M., Wyatt, R. T., Nabel, G. J., & Mascola, J. R. (2010). Rational design of envelope identifies broadly neutralizing human monoclonal antibodies to HIV-1. *Science*, 329(5993), 856-861.

Wyatt, R., Kwong, P. D., Desjardins, E., Sweet, R. W., Robinson, J., Hendrickson, W. A., & Sodroski, J. G. (1998). The antigenic structure of the HIV gp120 envelope glycoprotein [see comments]. *Nature*, 393(6686), 705-711.

Xu, L., Pozniak, A., Wildfire, A., Stanfield-Oakley, S. A., Mosier, S. M., Ratcliffe, D., Workman, J., Joall, A., Myers, R., Smit, E., Cane, P. A., Greenberg, M. L., & Pillay, D. (2005). Emergence and evolution of enfuvirtide resistance following long-term therapy involves heptad repeat 2 mutations within gp41. *Antimicrob Agents Chemother*, 49(3), 1113-1119.

Yahi, N., Tamalet, C., Tourres, C., Tivoli, N., Ariasi, F., Volot, F., Gastaut, J. A., Gallais, H., Moreau, J., & Fantini, J. (1999). Mutation patterns of the reverse transcriptase and protease genes in human immunodeficiency virus type 1-infected patients undergoing combination therapy: survey of 787 sequences. *J Clin Microbiol,* 37(12), 4099-4106.

Yahi, N., Tamalet, C., Tourres, C., Tivoli, N., & Fantini, J. (2000). Mutation L210W of HIV-1 reverse transcriptase in patients receiving combination therapy. Incidence, association with other mutations, and effects on the structure of mutated reverse transcriptase. *J Biomed Sci,* 7(6), 507-513.

Yuan, Y., Maeda, Y., Terasawa, H., Monde, K., Harada, S., & Yusa, K. (2011). A combination of polymorphic mutations in V3 loop of HIV-1 gp120 can confer noncompetitive resistance to maraviroc. *Virology,* 413(2), 293-299.

Zhou, T., Georgiev, I., Wu, X., Yang, Z. Y., Dai, K., Finzi, A., Kwon, Y. D., Scheid, J. F., Shi, W., Xu, L., Yang, Y., Zhu, J., Nussenzweig, M. C., Sodroski, J., Shapiro, L., Nabel, G. J., Mascola, J. R., & Kwong, P. D. (2011). Structural basis for broad and potent neutralization of HIV-1 by antibody VRC01. *Science,* 329(5993), 811-817.

Zhu, D. M., Shi, J., Liu, S., Liu, Y., & Zheng, D. (2011). HIV infection enhances TRAIL-induced cell death in macrophage by down-regulating decoy receptor expression and generation of reactive oxygen species. *PLoS One,* 6(4), e18291.

Zimmerman, P. A., Buckler-White, A., Alkhatib, G., Spalding, T., Kubofcik, J., Combadiere, C., Weissman, D., Cohen, O., Rubbert, A., Lam, G., Vaccarezza, M., Kennedy, P. E., Kumaraswami, V., Giorgi, J. V., Detels, R., Hunter, J., Chopek, M., Berger, E. A., Fauci, A. S., Nutman, T. B., & Murphy, P. M. (1997). Inherited resistance to HIV-1 conferred by an inactivating mutation in CC chemokine receptor 5: studies in populations with contrasting clinical phenotypes, defined racial background, and quantified risk. *Mol Med,* 3(1), 23-36.

Zolopa, A. R., Shafer, R. W., Warford, A., Montoya, J. G., Hsu, P., Katzenstein, D., Merigan, T. C., & Efron, B. (1999). HIV-1 genotypic resistance patterns predict response to saquinavir-ritonavir therapy in patients in whom previous protease inhibitor therapy had failed. *Ann Intern Med,* 131(11), 813-821.

Zwick, M. B., Jensen, R., Church, S., Wang, M., Stiegler, G., Kunert, R., Katinger, H., & Burton, D. R. (2005). Anti-human immunodeficiency virus type 1 (HIV-1) antibodies 2F5 and 4E10 require surprisingly few crucial residues in the membrane-proximal external region of glycoprotein gp41 to neutralize HIV-1. *J Virol,* 79(2), 1252-1261.

Zwick, M. B., Labrijn, A. F., Wang, M., Spenlehauer, C., Saphire, E. O., Binley, J. M., Moore, J. P., Stiegler, G., Katinger, H., Burton, D. R., & Parren, P. W. (2001). Broadly neutralizing antibodies targeted to the membrane-proximal external region of human immunodeficiency virus type 1 glycoprotein gp41. *J Virol,* 75(22), 10892-10905.

6

Recombination and Point Mutations in Type G Rotavirus Strains: The Challenges of Vaccine Development

Abid Nabil Ben Salem[1], Rouis Zyed[1], Buesa Javier[2] and Aouni Mahjoub[1]
[1]Laboratoire des Maladies Transmissibles et Substances Biologiquement Actives LR99-ES27, Faculté de Pharmacie, Université de Monastir,
[2]Dept. de Microbiología, Facultad de Medicina y Hospital Clínico Universitario, Universidad de Valencia, Avda. Blasco Ibañez, Valencia,
[1]Tunisia
[2]Spain

1. Introduction

Active immunity refers to the process of exposing the body to an antigen to generate an adaptive immune response: the response takes days/weeks to develop but may be long lasting—even lifelong. Wild infection with pathogenic agents (eg. Hepatitis A Virus) and subsequent recovery gives rise to a natural active immune response usually leading to lifelong protection. In addition, some infections can be prevented by immunization with vaccines.

The term "vaccine" is derived from the Latin word "vaccinus" which means "pertaining to cows" - a reflection on Jenner's pioneering studies using cowpox vaccinia virus to prevent human smallpox (variola) as discussed previously (Stefan, 2005; Dunn, 1996). Vaccines take advantage of using relatively harmless foreign agents to evoke protective immunity for protection against several important pathogens. Vaccine development has its early roots in the work of Edward Jenner and Louis Pasteur, who discovered how to protect people from smallpox and developed a vaccine to protect from rabies, respectively.

All vaccines contain other substances (termed excipients) that are present because they improve the immune response (an adjuvant), are necessary for ensuring stability of the product (stabilizers and preservatives), are the vehicle for delivering vaccine (carrier) or are a residual of the manufacturing process (for example antibiotics or cell culture components).

Nowadays, many types of vaccines have been proposed and used in vaccine development: Live whole virus vaccines, Killed whole virus vaccines, Subunit vaccines (purified or recombinant viral antigen), Toxoid vaccines, Synthetic vaccines, and DNA vaccines. We will discuss these vaccine types one-by-one.

1.1 Live, attenuated virus vaccines

They are prepared from attenuated strains that are almost or completely devoid of pathogenicity but are capable of inducing a protective immune response. They multiply in the human host and provide continuous antigenic stimulation over a period of time. Primary vaccine failures are uncommon and are usually the result of inadequate storage or administration. Another possibility is interference by related viruses as is suspected in the case of oral polio vaccine in developing countries (Giammanco et al., 1988; Drozdov & Shirman, 1961; Katz & Plotkin, 1968). Several methods have been used to attenuate viruses for vaccine production such as the use of a related virus from another animal (cowpox to prevent smallpox), the administration of pathogenic or partially attenuated virus by an unnatural route, passage of the virus in an "unnatural host" or host cell (e.g. the 17D strain of yellow fever was developed by passage in mice and then in chick embryos (Norrby, 2007) and Polioviruses were passaged in monkey kidney cells (Chezzi et al., 1998) and measles in chick embryo fibroblasts (Katz, 1958), and the development of temperature sensitive mutants (Pringle, 1996).

1.2 Killed/Inactivated vaccines

The term killed generally refers to bacterial vaccines, whereas inactivated relates to viral vaccines (Levine et al., 1997). They were the easiest preparations to use. The preparation was simply inactivated. For viruses, the outer virion coat should be left intact but the replicative function should be destroyed. To be effective, non-replicating virus vaccines must contain much more antigen than live vaccines that are able to replicate in the host. Preparation of killed vaccines may take the route of heat or chemicals (Turner et al., 1970). The chemicals used include formaldehyde or beta-propiolactone (Lo Grippo, 1960; Gard, 1960). The traditional agent for inactivation of the virus is formalin (Weil & Gall, 1940; Kim & Sharp, 1967). Excessive treatment with this detergent can destroy immunogenicity whereas insufficient treatment can leave infectious virus capable of causing disease. Soon after the introduction of inactivated polio vaccine, there was an outbreak of paralytic poliomyelitis in the USA due to the distribution of inadequately inactivated polio vaccine (Prevots et al., 1996). This incident led to a review of the formalin inactivation procedure and other inactivating agents are available, such as beta-propiolactone. Another problem was that SV40 was occasionally found as a contaminant and there were fears of the potential oncogenic nature of the virus (Tam et al., 2004).

1.3 Subunit vaccines

Originally, non-replicating vaccines were derived from crude preparations of virus from animal tissues. As the technology for growing viruses to high titres in cell cultures advanced, it became practical to purify virus and viral antigens. It is now possible to identify the peptide sites encompassing the major antigenic sites of viral antigens, from which highly purified subunit vaccines can be produced. Increasing purification may lead to loss of immunogenicity, and this may necessitate coupling to an immunogenic carrier protein or adjuvant, such as an aluminum salt. Examples of purified subunit vaccines include the HA vaccines for influenza A and B (Bachmayer et al., 1976), and HBsAg derived from the plasma of carriers (Vyas et al., 1984). Subunit vaccines can be further subdivided into those where the antigen is produced using recombinant DNA technology and those based on normal bacteriological growth processes.

Virus proteins have been expressed in bacteria, yeast, mammalian cells, and viruses. *E. Coli* cells were first to be used for this purpose but the expressed proteins were not glycosylated, which was a major drawback since many of the immunogenic proteins of viruses such as the envelope glycoproteins, were glycosylated. Nevertheless, in many instances, it was demonstrated that the non-glycosylated protein backbone was just as immunogenic. Recombinant hepatitis B vaccine is the only recombinant vaccine licensed at present (Yap et al., 1992). An alternative application of recombinant DNA technology is the production of hybrid virus vaccines. The best known example is vaccinia (Smith et al., 1983). The recombinant virus vaccine can then multiply in infected cells and produce the antigens of a wide range of viruses. The genes of several viruses can be inserted, so the potential exists for producing polyvalent live vaccines (Hauser et al., 1988; Hilleman, 1987). HBsAg, rabies, HSV and other viruses have been expressed in vaccinia (Mackett et al., 1985; Panicali et al., 1983; Paoletti et al., 1984; Perkus et al., 1985; Rice et al., 1985; Smith et al., 1983; Kieny et al., 1984; Wiktor et al., 1984).

1.4 Toxoid vaccines

Certain pathogens cause disease by secreting an exotoxin: these include tetanus, diphtheria, botulism and cholera. For these bacteria that secrete toxins, or harmful chemicals, a toxoid vaccine might be the answer. These vaccines are used when a bacterial toxin is the main cause of illness. Scientists have found that they can inactivate toxins by treating them with formalin, a solution of formaldehyde and sterilized water. Such "detoxified" toxins, called toxoids, are safe for use in vaccines. When the immune system receives a vaccine containing a harmless toxoid, it learns how to fight off the natural toxin. The immune system produces antibodies that lock onto and block the toxin. Vaccines against diphtheria and tetanus are examples of toxoid vaccines (Bizzini et al., 1970; Alouf, 1987). These vaccines are: safe because they cannot cause the disease they prevent as there is no possibility of reversion to virulence; the vaccine antigens are not actively multiplying, they cannot spread to unimmunized individuals; they are usually stable and long lasting as they are less susceptible to changes in temperature, humidity and light which can result when vaccines are used out in the community.

1.5 Synthetic peptides

The development of synthetic peptides that might be useful as vaccines depends on the identification of immunogenic sites (Milich, 1990; Hans et al., 2006; Dorothea, 1993; Jonathan, 1987). Synthetic peptide vaccines have been successfully developed for the immunoprophylaxis of infection with foot-and-mouth disease virus (Bittle et al., 1982; Brown, 1990), type A influenza virus (Muller et al., 1982), and poliovirus (Emini et al., 1983). Synthetic peptide vaccines would have many advantages. Their antigens are precisely defined and free from unnecessary components which may be associated with side effects. They are stable and relatively cheap to manufacture. Changes due to natural variation of the virus can be readily accommodated, which would be a great advantage for unstable viruses.

1.6 DNA vaccines

The demonstration by Wolff and colleagues in 1990 (Wolff et al., 1990) that protein could be expressed following direct inoculation of plasmid DNA into muscle tissue unveiled an exciting, new era in vaccinology and gene therapy. DNA-based vaccination offers a number of advantages over other methods of immunization. It is particularly attractive compared to conventional administration of a preformed protein antigen (Ag) because the immunogen is actively synthesized de novo in cells transfected with DNA. The principle of DNA vaccination has been demonstrated for a variety of bacterial, viral and parasitic diseases (Ulmer et al., 1993). Immune responses have been generated by DNA vaccination against a very wide variety of viral, bacterial and protozoal pathogens and toxins (Donnelly et al., 1994; King et al., 1998). Immune responses against influenza viruses have been demonstrated in chickens, mice, ferrets and non-human primates. For humans, the major concern about DNA vaccines is whether the plasmid DNA integrates into the genome randomly, potentially leading to insertional mutagenesis. In addition, the formal acceptance of this novel technology as a new modality of human vaccines depends on the successful demonstration of its safety and efficacy in advanced clinical trials. Several trials evaluated the efficacy of a DNA vaccine targeting human immunodeficiency virus type 1 (HIV-1) for therapeutic and prophylactic applications (MacGregor et al. 1998). However, the results of these early clinical trials were disappointing. The DNA vaccines were safe and well tolerated, but they proved to be poorly immunogenic.

Vaccines may be monovalent (also called univalent) or multivalent (also called polyvalent). A monovalent vaccine is designed to immunize against a single antigen or single microorganism. A multivalent or polyvalent vaccine is designed to immunize against two or more strains of the same microorganism, or against two or more microorganisms. In certain cases a monovalent vaccine may be preferable for rapidly developing a strong immune response.

2. Rotavirus infection and common associated-genotypes

Infectious acute diarrhea is a significant cause of morbidity and mortality of infants in developing and developed countries and constitutes a major public health problem worldwide. It is estimated that in developing countries (in Africa, Asia and Latin America) 744 million to 1 billion cases of diarrhea and 2.4 to 3.3 million deaths occur annually among children less than 5 years of age, corresponding to 6600 to 9000 deaths per day (Linhares & Bresee, 2000). The viruses are the most common aetiology of these diseases, especially in developed countries, where they cause more than 80% of the cases of acute diarrhea. The most common viral causes of gastroenteritis are rotaviruses and calicivirus (norovirus).

Rotavirus, a member of the *Reoviridae* family, is a highly contagious virus that causes severe and acute dehydrating diarrhea in infants and young children as well as other young animals worldwide (Dhama et al., 2009; Kapikian et al., 2001). Mature rotavirus, non-enveloped virions, contains an 11-segmented, double-stranded RNA (dsRNA) genome enclosed in a triple-layered protein capsid (Hoshino & Kapikian, 2000). The segmented nature of the genome allows rotaviruses to reassort *in vitro* and *in vivo* (Greenberg et al., 1981; Kalica et al., 1981; Gombold & Ramig, 1986).

A dual nomenclature has been used to differentiate rotavirus strains based on their serotype specificities, which are carried by the two outer capsid antigens, VP7 and VP4 (Estes & Kapikian, 2007).

The high disease burden motivated major efforts to develop a suitable rotavirus vaccine. However, the vaccine efficacy is being challenged by the extensive strain diversity of the rotaviruses (Estes, 2001; Green et al., 1987, 1988; Hoshino et al., 1994; Kapikian et al., 2001; Linhares et al., 1999).

Reverse-transcription polymerase chain reaction (RT-PCR) is the most widely used method for rotavirus characterization in surveillance studies. Molecular methods have allowed the detection of many rotavirus G-types (Banyai et al., 2003; Cubitt et al., 2000; Cunliffe et al., 1999; Das et al., 1993a, 2003; Gentsch et al., 1996; Gouvea et al., 1994; Pongsuwanna et al., 2002). Because of the natural variation in the rotaviral gene sequences, G-type-specific-primer based RT-PCR led to the genotyping failure (Adah et al., 1997; Iturriza- Gómara et al., 2000, 2004a; Maunula & von Bonsdorff, 1998; Rahman et al., 2005b). In addition, the accumulation of point mutations through genetic drift at the type-specific primer binding sites has resulted in failures to type strains or in mistyping. For example, the accumulation of point mutations at the G9 type-specific primer binding site was reported as having an impact for the efficient genotyping of rotaviruses (Martella et al., 2004; Santos et al., 2003). Moreover, some nucleotide identity between genotypes lead to primer cross-reactivity between rotavirus strains as the case of rotavirus G3 and G10 strains using primers developed by Gouvea et al. (1990) as discussed previously (Iturriza-Gómara et al., 2004b).

In order to overcome this problem, a modified classification system for VP4, VP7, and NSP4, and a novel classification system for VP1, VP2, VP3, VP6, NSP1, NSP2, NSP3, and NSP5/6 were proposed to be used for international standardization and implementation (Matthijnssens et al., 2008a, 2008b).

Actually, VP4 and VP7 are the main targets for vaccine development strategies. In the present review we will focus on the diversity of VP7 among rotavirus strains and the effect of this variability upon vaccine development.

Similar to most of the group A rotaviruses, the VP7 nucleotide sequence is 1062 nucleotides long. The ORF starts at nucleotide 49 with an AUG (ATG) start codon and ends at nucleotide 1029 with a UAG (TAG) termination codon, comprising 981 nucleotides (Estes & Cohen, 1989; Bellamy & Both, 1990).

The gene segment coding for the VP7 glycoprotein is the basis for genotyping group A rotaviruses into at least fifteen G-genotypes. Studies of intragenotype diversity led to subdivision of the G genotypes into several lineages (two major lineages, designated I and II) and sublineages, distinctly identified by unique genomic as well as epidemiological features. Lineage I was further subdivided into four sublineages, Ia–Id.

Genotypes G1, G2, G3, G4 and G9 are the most common G-types in humans (Gentsch et al., 1996; Liprandi et al., 2003; Martella et al., 2003; Okada et al., 2000; Rao et al., 2000; Sereno & Gorziglia, 1994). Nevertheless, over past decades, type G1 rotaviruses have been the most widespread genotype causing acute gastroenteritis in children from many countries covering all continents of the world (Santos & Hoshino, 2005). Type G2 rotavirus represents a different genogroup which appears to have a cyclic pattern of occurrence and yet little information is available about its genetic variability. Type G3 rotavirus have been found in a broad range of host species, including humans, monkeys, dogs, cats, horses, rabbits, mice, sheep and pigs (Martella et al., 2001; Andrej et al., 2008; Hoshino et al., 1984; Paul et al.,

1988; Fitzgerald et al., 1995). The G9 rotavirus was first reported in the United States in the early 1980s (Clark et al., 1987). It represents the fifth most common G genotype of rotavirus infections throughout the world (Gentsch et al., 2005; Santos & Hoshino, 2005, Khamrin et al., 2006).

3. Rotavirus vaccines

3.1 Monovalent animal and human rotavirus vaccines

Monovalent animal rotavirus vaccines. Research to develop a safe, effective rotavirus vaccine began in the mid-1970s, when investigators demonstrated that previous infection with animal rotavirus strains protected laboratory animals from experimental infection with human rotaviruses (Zissis et al., 1983). Researchers thought that live animal strains that were naturally attenuated for humans, when given orally, might mimic the immune response to natural infection and protect children against disease. Three nonhuman rotavirus vaccines, two bovine rotavirus strains, RIT 4237 (P6[1]G6) and WC3 (P7[5]G6), and a simian (rhesus) rotavirus reassortant vaccine (RRV) strain (P[3]G3), were studied (Christy et al., 1988; Clark et al., 1988; Vesikari et al., 1984). These vaccines demonstrated variable efficacy in field trials and gave particularly disappointing results in developing countries (Hanlon et al., 1987; Lanata et al., 1989; Penelope, 2008). Another monovalent, ovine strain vaccine produced by the Lanzhou Institute and licensed in China in 2000 (Lanzhou lamb rotavirus vaccine (LLR); P[12], G10) was available in some parts of China (World Health Organization [WHO], 2000). Few data are available about the effectiveness of this vaccine and it was not included in national immunization programs in China or elsewhere. Finally, monovalent animal strain vaccines have been mostly abandoned.

Monovalent human rotavirus vaccines. Rotarix®, developed by GlaxoSmithKline Biologicals, Belgium, is a monovalent, P1A[8] G1 rotavirus derived from a human G1 strain (89-12) that yielded high efficacy in early trials in the US and Finland (Bernstein et al., 2002). Its Efficacy has been confirmed in many countries (Ruiz-Palacios et al., 2006; De Vos et al., 2004).

RV3 neonatal strain vaccine, a P2A[6] G3 strain, was first isolated from newborns at the Children's Hospital in Melbourne, Australia (Barnes et al., 1997). Neonates infected with this rotavirus strain in hospital nurseries usually were asymptomatic and were later protected against severe disease in early childhood. However, serum immune responses were poor (Das et al., 1993a). Many attempts were undertaken to increase the titer of this vaccine and return to clinical trials.

Another two Indian neonatal strain vaccines 116E and I321 were proposed as candidate vaccines (Das et al., 1993a, 1993b; Iturriza-Gómara et al., 2004a). Both strains are in preclinical development and human trials are being planned in India, but with the new finding of I321-like strains causing disease in children, both careful epidemiological studies and safety monitoring will be essential prior to licensure.

3.2 Polyvalent rotavirus vaccines

In view of the inconsistency of protection from monovalent animal rotavirus-based vaccines, vaccine development efforts began to use either naturally attenuated human rotavirus strains or reassortant rotavirus strains bearing a human rotavirus gene for the VP7 protein together with the other 10 genes from an animal rotavirus strain (Midthun & Kapikian, 1996). The next generation of vaccines was formulated to include more than one rotavirus G serotype to provide heterotypic as well as homotypic immunity. The ability of rotaviruses to reassort during mixed infections in vitro allowed the production of reassortant vaccines, termed the "modified Jennerian" approach (Kapikian et al., 1996b). Reassortant viruses contain some genes from the animal rotavirus parent and some genes from the human rotavirus parent. VP7 was thought to be important for protection; therefore, human-animal reassortant rotaviruses for use as vaccines included human VP7 genes to provide protective immune responses.

Quadrivalent RRV-based rhesus-human reassortant vaccine. A RotaShield was the first multivalent live oral reassortant vaccine (tetravalent, reassortant rhesus-human rotavirus vaccine, [RRV-TV]) contained a mixture of four virus strains representing the most commonly seen G types, G1 to G4: three rhesus-human reassortant strains containing the VP7 genes of human serotypes G1, G2, and G4 strains were substituted for the VP7 gene of the parent RRV, and the fourth strain comprised serotype G3 of rhesus RRV (Kapikian et al., 1996a). RRV-TV was extensively evaluated in field trials in the United States, Finland, and Venezuela and proved highly effective (80 to 100%) in preventing severe diarrhea due to rotavirus in each of these settings (Joensuu et al., 1997; Perez-Schael et al., 1997; Rennels et al., 1996; Santosham et al., 1997). Due to the proven efficacy, the RRV-TV vaccine was licensed in August 1998 for routine use in children in the United States at 2, 4, and 6 months of age (Centers for Disease Control and Prevention [CDCP], 1999b). Later, this vaccine was withdrawn from the market in 1999 as a consequence of vaccine-associated intussusception in several cases of vaccinated infants (CDCP, 1999a).

Pentavalent WC3-based bovine-human reassortant vaccine. Rotateq®, manufactured by Merck, Inc, USA, is a pentavalent vaccine containing five reassortants representing the common human VP7 types, G1-4 and the most common VP4 type, P[8] (CDCP, 2006). A large efficacy trial with Rotateq® has been completed, which found 74 and 98% efficacy against all and severe disease, respectively and has efficacy against each of the common circulating serotypes. Compared with the rhesus reassortants, the bovine-human reassortants appear to cause less fever while maintaining immunogenicity (Clark et al., 2004). A large safety trial found no evidence of an increased risk of intussusceptions among vacinees compared with placebo recipients (Vesikari et al., 2006).

Both RotaTeq and RotaRix have been shown to be effective against rotavirus gastroenteritis, however on March 22, 2010 the Food and Drug Administration (FDA) recommended that the use of the Rotarix vaccine be suspended in the United States because of some DNA from a porcine (pig) virus (porcine circovirus type 1) detected in the vaccine. Subsequently, some DNA from this and another porcine virus were also detected in Rotateq. On May 14, 2010 the FDA updated their recommendations for the use of rotavirus vaccines based on a review of the literature and the input from experts. The RotaTeq vaccine was proven to be effective in many countries such as Finland (Vesikari et al., 2010).

Whatever the type of vaccine and strategy of its development, the introduction of a new vaccine faces many hurdles, including cost, production capabilities, safety, and other programmatic issues. For rotavirus vaccines, while there is clearly a need, there are also additional challenges raised by the emergence of new rotavirus genotypes.

4. The prevalence of uncommon G-type rotaviruses and challenges for vaccine development

Genetic variability has been observed for all RNA viruses examined, and their potential for rapid evolution is increasingly recognized as the basis of their ubiquity and adaptability (Holland et al., 1992; Kilbourne, 1991). The molecular mechanisms underlying RNA virus variations are: mutation, homologous and non homologous recombinations, and genome reassortment in viruses with a segmented genome such as reoviruses. The genetic evolution of viruses is an important aspect of the epidemiology of viral diseases and sometimes causes problems in the development of successful vaccines.

The effectiveness of rotavirus vaccines will be dependent upon the immunity conferred against prevalent and emergent variants causing severe diarrhoeal disease. The global effort toward the prevention of rotavirus disease to be successful, special efforts will be required in countries where new genotypes were detected such as G5, G6, G8, G10, G11, and G12 (Figure 1). Nucleotide analysis using CLUSTAL X (version 1.8) of VP7 gene of these uncommon rotaviruses showed high degree of variability with the common G-type viruses (Figure 2). Genomic similarities between rotaviruses from different animal species are regarded as evidence of interspecies transmission of rotaviruses that may occur as a whole virion or genetic reassortment. The high variability of viral sequences due to genetic reassortment and nucleotide substitution are considered the most important mechanisms of evolution for rotaviruses. The antigenic variation within a serotype was known as a mechanism by which variants of rotavirus emerge to escape host immunity. This variability represents considerable potential for impaired vaccine efficacy.

The available information in literature showed that type G5 rotavirus is an important and commonly detected pathogen of swine and has also been identified in equine (Kapikian et al., 2001). However, in 1994, Gouvea and collaborators first demonstrated the occurrence of rotavirus genotype G5 among Brazilian children with diarrhea (Gouvea et al., 1994; Timenetsky et al., 1997). The detection of rotavirus G5 among children with diarrhea has also been reported in Argentina and Paraguay, indicating the spread of this virus across South America (Coluchi et al., 2002; Bok et al., 2001). In addition, the detection of type G5 rotavirus was reported in Cameroon (Esona et al., 2004). Another genotypes, type G6 and G10 strains have been isolated from humans (Dunn et al., 1993; Gerna et al., 1992, 1994; Armah et al., 2010). Although type G6 is the commonest rotavirus G type found in cows and at low frequency in sheep and goats (Kapikian et al., 2001), it was detected from hospitalized children with acute gastroenteritis in Italy during 1987–1988 (Gerna et al., 1992), Australia (Palombo & Bishop, 1995; Cooney et al., 2001), India (Kelkar & Ayachit, 2000), USA (Griffin et al., 2002), Belgium (Rahman et al., 2003), and Hungary (Banyai et al., 2004; Banyai et al., 2003). Type G8 virus, which can be found in cows at relatively high frequency (Kapikian et al., 2001), was first isolated in a study performed between 1979 and 1981, from stool specimens collected from children with diarrhea in Jakarta and Medan (Indonesia) (Hasegawa et al., 1984), Kenya (Nokes et al., 2010), and other countries such as Finland, Italy, Nigeria, Brazil, Malawi, South Africa, Egypt, Australia, the United States, and the United Kingdom (Adah et al., 1997, 2001; Cunliffe et al., 1999; Cunliffe et al., 2000; Gerna et al., 1990; Holmes et al., 1999; Palombo et al., 2000; Parwani et al., 1993; Rao et al., 2000; Santos et al., 1998; Steele et al., 1999). Type G11 rotaviruses are believed to be circulating in pigs, albeit in low numbers mainly in Mexico in 1983 and in Venezuela in 1989 (Ciarlet et al.,

1994; Ruiz et al., 1988). Later, several reports have described the detection of G11 rotavirus strains from humans in India (Banerjee et al., 2007), Bangladesh (Rahman et al., 2005a; Rahman et al., 2007), Nepal (Uchida et al., 2006), Ecuador (Banyai et al., 2009), and South Korea (Hong et al., 2007). Type G12 rotavirus was detected in stool specimens collected from children with diarrhea in the Philippines (Taniguchi et al., 1990), Thailand (Pongsuwanna et al., 2002), USA (Griffin et al., 2002), India (Das et al., 2003), Japan (Shinozaki et al., 2004), Korea (Cheon et al., 2004), Argentina (Castello et al., 2004), Malawi (Cunliffe et al., 2009), and Saudi Arabia (Kheyami et al., 2008). Type G12 has not been detected in animals other than humans.

Furthermore, recombination between human and animal rotavirus constitutes another challenge for vaccine development. Many G-type rotaviruses are considered to be reassortants between human and bovine viruses such as the case of G8 rotaviruses (Browning et al., 1992; Ohshima et al., 1990; Adah et al., 2003). Reassortment among bovine, porcine and human rotavirus strains was also reported (Park et al., 2011).

Other important issues need to be discussed concerning the potential that the vaccine strains themselves may either cause disease or reassort with wild-type rotavirus to produce a virulent strain as reported for RotaTeq reassortant strain in association with acute gastroenteritis (Payne et al., 2010). In addition, the predominance of G2 rotaviruses in Brazil following the introduction of Rotarix (Gurgel et al., 2007; Nakagomi & Nakagomi, 2009) and the predominance of G3 rotaviruses after vaccine introduction in USA after a Surveillance From 2005 to 2008 (Hull et al., 2011) may enhance the study the effectiveness of the available vaccines and the growing need to evaluate their use.

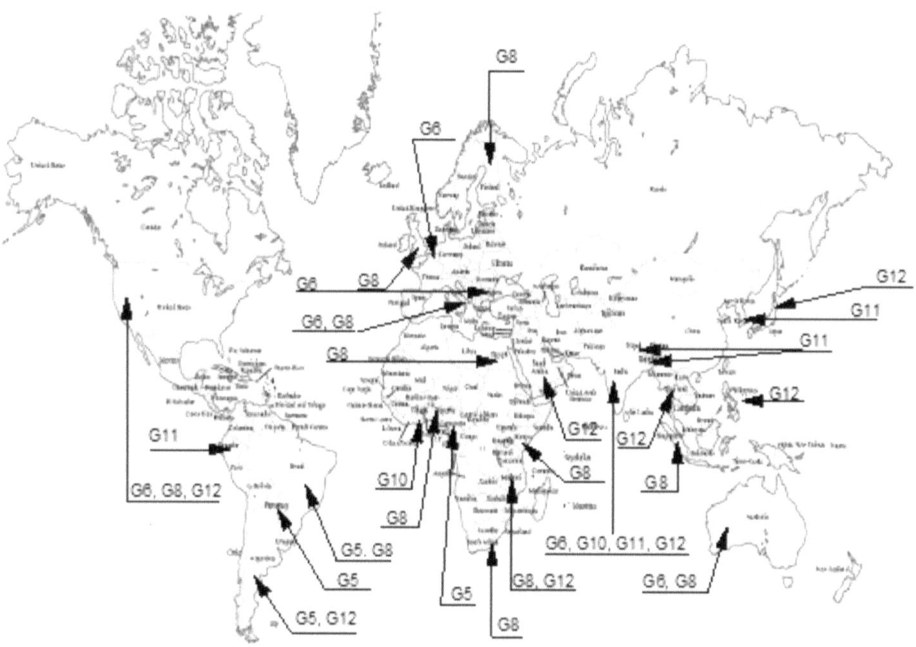

Fig. 1. Distribution of uncommon rotavirus genotypes in the world. The countries where the uncommon rotavirus genotypes were detected are shown by arrows.

```
          ....|....| ....|....| ....|....| ....|....| ....|....| ....|....| ....|....| ....|....| ....|....| ....|....|
                                                                * * * *   * * *   * * *   * * * *   * * *
G1        GGCTTTAAAA GAGAGAATTT CCGTCTGGCT AACGGTTAGC TCCTTTTAAT GTATGGTATT GAATATACCA CAATTCTAAT CTTTCTGATA TCAATCATTC
G2        .......... .......... .......... .G........ ..T....... .......... .......... .......G.C .A..T..... .TT.....AT
G3        .......... .......... .......... .G........ .......... .......... .......... ..G..T...C ....T..... ...G.T..AT
G4        .......... .......... ....T..... .G...A.... .......... .......... .......... ..G.....T. T.A.T..... ..GT..G...
G9        .......... .......... ....T..... .G........ .......... .......... .......... ...C...... ...CT..... .TGC.TG.AT
G6        .......... .......... .......... .T...A.... .......... .......... ....G..... .........C T...T..... ..GC.TG.AT
G8        .......... .......... .......... .G........ .......... .......... .......... .......... ...CT..... .....T.CAT
G10       .......... .......... .......... .G........ .......... .......... .......... .........C .......... .....AG..T
G11       .......... .......... ...A...... .T...A.... .......... .......... .......... .........C T...T..... ...C.TG.AT
G12       .......... .GAG...... .......... .G........ .......... .......... .......... .........C ....T..... .....T....
          ....|....| ....|....| ....|....| ....|....| ....|....| ....|....| ....|....| ....|....| ....|....| ....|....|
           * * *      * * * *    * * *    * * *     * * * *   * * *     * * *     * * * *   * * *     * * *
G1        TACTCAACTA TATATTAAAA TCAGTGACCC AAATAATGGA CTACATCATA TATAGATTTT TGTTAATTTT TGTAGCATTA TTTGCCTTAA CTAAAGCTCA
G2        ..T.G..T.. .......... A.TA.A..TA .T.CG..... ...T..A..T .T...G.... .AC..C.CA. C.CTCTGA.G .CAC.A..TG TG.GGA.G..
G3        .GT.G..T.. CG..C.C... ..CT.A..TA G......... ..TT..T..T ..C......C .T......A. A..TAT.... .CAC.AC.CC T...T..A..
G4        .TG.G.GT.. ...TC.G... A.CA.A.TAA .G........ ...T..T..T ......A.AA CA..TG.GA. .....T.... .CA.TA...T .G..T..A.C
G9        ..T.G..T.. .......... .....A...A G...T..... ...T..AT.G ........C. ..C..T..G. ....ATTG.C ACAC.A..CG TA..CT.A..
G6        .CA....T.. CC........ .....A..TA G......... ..TT..T..C .......... .AA.G...A. AA.TTT.C.T GCAC.AA.T. T...G.....
G8        .G..A..T.. .......... ...A.A..AA G......... ...T..A..T .....G...C .A...G.AG. G...AT.C.G ACCA..G.G. .A..T..G..
G10       ..T.G..... .......... ...C.A..TA GTGCG..... ..TT..A..T .........C .T...C..A. ...TATTGC. .CAT.T..TG T....A.A..
G11       .TA.T..T.. ......G... ...A.A..TA G..C...... ..TTG.T..C .......... ....TG..A. A..T.T.C.. GCAC.A..C. T....A.G..
G12       ..T.A..T.. .......... ...A.A..TA .T..G..... ..TT...... ...C.G.A.. .AC....AG. ...C.TCA.. C.GC.A..T. T.........
          ....|....| ....|....| ....|....| ....|....| ....|....| ....|....| ....|....| ....|....| ....|....| ....|....|
          * * * *     * * *     * * *     * * * *    * * *     * * *     * * * *    * * *     * * *     * * * *
G1        GAACTATGGA CTTAATATAC CAATAACAGG ATCAATGGAT ACTGTATACT CCAACTCTAC TCAAGAAGGA GTATTTCTAA CATCCACATT ATGTTTGTAT
G2        A..T.....T A.GT..T... .......... ....C.A..C GT.......A .A..T..A.. .AGT.G..A. TC........ .T..A..GC. ......A..C
G3        A..T...... A.A...C.T. .G..T..T.. C........C ..ACC...TA .G.....A.. G.G...G.A. .....C.... .T..G..T.. ..........
G4        A..T...... A.A...T.G. ....T..T.. ...T...... ..A.C...TA .T.....A.. A.....CAAT AAT...T..T .T..A..T.. ....C.A...
G9        ...T.....T A.A...C... ....T..T.. ...T...... .TGAAC..TC AG..TGTAT. AACTTCC.AG CCT...T.G. ....G..GC. ....C.A...
G6        .......... A.....T.G. .......T.. ...C...... ..ACC...TA .G..T..A.. AATGAGT.A. ACG....... .T........ ...C......
G8        A..T.....C G.....T.G. .T..T..... ...T...... ..CAC....G .A..T..A.. A...AGT.A. TCT...T... ....A..TC. G.........
G10       A..T...... A.....T... .G..C..T.. T..C...... ..AAC...TG .A..T..AT. A..GC...A. AC....T.G. .T..A..GC. ...C..A...
G11       A......... A.A..CT.G. .G.....T.. T..T...... ..ACC...TA TG..T..A.. AATGAGT.A. AC...CTC.. .T..T..T.. ......A...
G12       A..T...... A.A...C.T. .......... T..T...... ..C.C...TG TA........ A...C...AG AAT...A.G. .T.....T.. ...C..A...
          ....|....| ....|....| ....|....| ....|....| ....|....| ....|....| ....|....| ....|....| ....|....| ....|....|
             * * *    * * *     * * *     * * * *    * * *     * * *     * * * *    * * *     * * *     * * * *
G1        TATCCAACTG AAGCAAGTAC TCAAATCAGT GACGGTGAAT GGAAAGACTC ATTATCACAA ATGTTTCTTA CGAAAGGTTG GCCAACAGGA TCAGTCTATT
G2        ........A. ....T.AA.A .G.G..TTCA ..TAA..... ..G..A.TA. TC....G... T.A...T.A. .T.....A.. ...G..T... .....T....
G3        ..C....... .....GCA.. AG....A.A. ..TAA.TC.. ....G..TA. .C.T..T..G C.A...T.A. TC.....A.. .......... ..TA.T....
G4        ......T.A. ....TCCA.. .......... ...AC..... .......TA. .C....T..G C.....T.A. .C.....A.. ...G.....T .....T....
G9        ......G.A. ....TGAG.. AG.G..TGC. ..TA..TC.. ........A. ...G.....G T.A...T.G. .A.....A.. ......T..T ...A.T..CC
G6        .....G.A.. ....GGC... .G....TGCA ....CCA.G. ...CG..GA. GC.G...... C.......A. .T.....A.. .T........ .....T..C.
G8        ..C...GTC. .....TCG.A .G....AGC. ...ACC.... .....A.TA. T..G...... C.A.....G. .C.....A.. ......T... C.T..G..C.
G10       .....T..A. .....TCA.. ......TG.A ..TACG.... ....G..TA. TC.G..C... T.A..CT.G. .T.....G.. ......T... ..........
G11       ..C..G.AC. ....GGCA.. ...G...GCA ..T.ACA.G. .......TA. TC.C...... C.T.....C. .T.....G.. .......... ..G..T..C.
G12       .......G.T C..TC.CG.. .G....A.C. ..TCCC..C. ...CGA..A. .C.G...... C.T..C..G. .T.....A.. ...G...AAT ..C.....C.
          ....|....| ....|....| ....|....| ....|....| ....|....| ....|....| ....|....| ....|....| ....|....| ....|....|
            * * *     * * *     * * * *    * * *     * * *     * * * *   * * *     * * *     * * * *    * * *
G1        TCAAAGAGTA CTCAAATATT GTTGATTTTT CCGTTGACCC ACAATTATAT TGCGATTATA ATTTAGTACT AATGAAGTAT GATCAAAATC TTGAATTAGA
G2        .T.....C.. .AATG..... AC.ACA.... .TA.GA.T.. ....C..... ..T....... ..G.....T. G....GA... ...A.T.CAT C.........
G3        .T.....T.. TA.TG..... .CCTCG.... .A..C..T.. ....C.G... ..T....... ....G...T. ......A... ..CGCT.CA. .GC..C.G..
G4        .T..T..A.. T.....CG.. T.A..A.... ..A.C..... .A.GC....C ..T....... ..G.T..G.. ...T.GA.TC .C.TCTGG.G AGA.G..G..
G9        .T...AGT.. .GTGG....A .CGATA..C. .AA.AA.T.. T..G..G... ..T....... ..A.....T. .......... A..GCTG..T CA..G.....
G6        ....T.GA.. .G..G..... .CATCA..C. .T..A..A.. ....C....C ..T....... ..A.T..GT. ......A..C ...GC...CT .AC.......
G8        .......A.. .A.TG.C..A .CA.C..... .A..A..T.. T..G..G... ..T.....C. .......C.. ......A... ...TC..C.. .A........
G10       .T.....A.. .A.CG....C .C.TCA..C. .AA....T.. ....C.T... ..T....... ..G.T..... G......... ...TC..CGT .A..GC....
G11       .T.....A.. TA..G..G.. .CATCA.... ....A..T.. ....C..... ..T....... ..A.T...T. ......A... ...GG....T CAC..C....
G12       ....GAGT.. TG.TG....A TCGTCC..C. .T..A..T.. G..GG.G... ..T....... ..A.T..GT. ...AC....C C.AA.TTCAT .A.CG.....
          ....|....| ....|....| ....|....| ....|....| ....|....| ....|....| ....|....| ....|....| ....|....| ....|....|
           * * *      * * * *    * * *     * * *     * * * *    * * *     * * *     * * * *    * * *     * * *
G1        TATGTCAGAA TTAGCTGATT TGATATTGAA TGAATGGTTA TGTAATCCAA TGGATATAAC ATTATATTAT TATCAACAAT CGGGAGAATC AAACAAGTGG
G2        .GCA..G..G .....A...C .T........ C......C.G ..C.....T. ........T. .C.T..C... .....G...A ATA.C..... ...T..A...
G3        C.....C... C....A.... ..T..C.T.. ...G...... .........T. ......AT.. T..G...... .........A .T.AT..GG. ...T..A...
G4        C..A..T... .........C .A...C.... ...G...... .......... .......... .......... .........A .T.....GG. ......A...
G9        ......G... ..G..G..CC .....C.T.. .......... ..C....... ....C..... G..G.....C ........GA ...AC...G. G.....A...
G6        ......T... .........C .A.....A.. C......... ..C....... ....C..... GC.C..C... ..C......A .T.AC..GG. T..T......
G8        ......T... ..G..G..CC .C.....A.. .......C.G ..C....... .......... .........C ..C......A .T.AC...G. ...T..A...
G10       ......T... .......... .A..TC.A.. .......... .....C.... .......... .......... .....G...A .A.AT...G. G..T..A...
G11       ......T... ..G....... .A.....A.. .......... .......... .........G. TC.T..C... .........A .A.AT...G. ...T..A...
G12       .G.C...... C.T....... .A..T..A.. .......... ........G. ....CG.... G..G..C... ........GA .A.AT...G. G..T..A...
          ....|....| ....|....| ....|....| ....|....| ....|....| ....|....| ....|....| ....|....| ....|....| ....|....|
          * * * *     * * *     * * *     * * * *    * * *     * * *     * * * *    * * *     * * *     * * * *
G1        ATATCAATGG GATCATCATG TACTGTGAAA GTGTGTCCAC TGAATACACA AACGTTAGGA ATAGGTTGTC AAACAACGAA TGTAGACTCA TTTGAAACAG
G2        .......... ..A.GGAC.. ...G..A... ..T....... .C........ ...T...... ..T..A..CA ....T...G. C..G..TA.. .......TT.
G3        ..T....... .......T.. ....A.A..G ..A....... .A.....G.. ...A...... ..T..A..C. T......TG. .AC.A..A.G ......GA..
G4        .......... .......... ...C..T... .........T .A.....T.. G..A...... ..T..A.... ....G..A.. .AC..CTA.T ..........
G9        ..TG.G.... ..GAT..... ....A.T... ..A......T .A........ G..A.....T ..T..A.... TT..T..TG. CACTACGA.T ......GA.A
G6        .....T.... .T.....G.. ...GA.T... ........T. .....G.G.. G..CC.T... .....A..CT T...T...G. .ACTA.T... ......GT..
G8        .......... ....GCTTC. C..A..A... ..A......T .A........ ....C.C..T ..C..A.... T..T...TG. .CC.A.TA.. .....G....
G10       .....G.... ..CAG..T.. ...CA.A... ..A......T .......G.. G..T...... .........A TT..C..A.. .AC..CGA.. ......GAG.
G11       .......... .CGAT..... ...GA.A... ..A..C..G. .C........ G..CC.T... .....A...T CG..T..TG. .CC.ACAA.. .....GGA.A
G12       .......... ..GA...... ...A..T... ..A.....CT .A........ ...T...... ..T..A...A CG.....CG. C..CACAA.. ......GAG.
          ....|....| ....|....| ....|....| ....|....| ....|....| ....|....| ....|....| ....|....| ....|....| ....|....|
            * * *     * * *     * * * *    * * *     * * *     * * * *   * * *     * * *     * * * *    * * *
G1        TTGCTGAGAA TGAAAAATTA GCTATAGTAG ACGTCGTTGA TGGGATAAAT CATAAAATAA ATTTGACAAC TACGACATGT ACTATTCGAA ATTGTAAGAA
G2        ....CTC.TC .........G .TA..TACT. .T..T..AA. ...TG.T... .......... ..A.TT...T A.GT..G... .....A..T. .......T..
G3        ....AACAGC .......... .TG..TACT. ....T..A.. ...AG.C... .......T.G. .CG....... A.AC..T... ..G...A... .......A..
G4        .......T.G C........G ..A...A.T. .T..T..C.. CA.CG..... .......T..G ..G.C...T. ...T...... ..A..A..G. .......T..
G9        ....AACAGC ...G.....G ..A...ACG. ....T..... ...AG.G..C T.....G... ..A.C..T.. ...A...... ..C...A... .......A..
G6        .A..CA.T.C .......... ..C...ACT. .T.....C.. ...AG.T... T.....T.GG ..G.A..... G.AT...... .....AA.G. ....C.....
G8        ....AAC..C C.....G... .TG..TACT. .T.....G.. ...ATGCGTA .......T.GG ..G.T..... G..A..T.C. .....A..C. .C........
G10       .G...ACA.G .......... .TA...ACC. .T..T..... ...TG.G..C .......C.TG ..G....T.. A.AT..C... ..A...A.G. ..........
G11       .A...TCTGC A..G.....G .TG...AC.. .T..T..A.. ...AG.T..C ..C...C..G ..G....... CG.T..G... ..A..AA... .C.....A..
G12       .A..AA.TGC G......... .TA...ACT. .......G.. ...AG.C... .....G..T. ..A.T...GT G.AT...... .....A..G. ....C..A..
```

```
          ....|....| ....|....| ....|....| ....|....| ....|....| ....|....| ....|....| ....|....| ....|....| ....|....|
           *  *  *   *  *  *  *   *  *  *   *  *  *  *  *  *  *   *  *  *   *  *  *   *  *  *  *   *  *  *   *  *  *
G1        GTTAGGTCCA AGAGAGAATG TGGCTGTAAT ACAAGTTGGT GGTGCTAATA TATTAGACAT AACAGCGGAT CCAACGACTA ATCCACAAAT TGAGAGAATG
G2        AC....A... C....A.... .T...A.... T......... ..AC.G..CG C.C....T.. C..T..T... .....A..AG T......GG. .C.A.....C
G3        A.....A... ..G..A..C. .A..A..T.. ...G...... ..CC.AG..G ..C.T..... ......T... ........A. TG.......C A..A......
G4        AC....A..G .....A.... .....A.... ...G.....C ..GT...... .......T.. ......T... ..C..A...T C........C A..AC.....
G9        .C.G..A..T ........C. .T..A..T.. C.....A... ...T.A...G .C.....T.. T.....T... ..G.....AG CA.......C ..........
G6        AC.T..A... ........C. .T..A..... T.....A..A ...T.A..C. ..C.T..T.. ......A..C .....T...G CA.......C G..A......
G8        A.....A... .....A..C. .A..A..T.. C.....A..C .....G..C. .TC....... T.....T... .....A...G CG........ A..A......
G10       ......A... .....A.... .A..GA.T.. ......C... ..CT.AG..G .G.....T.. T......... .....T...G CA.......C ...AC.T...
G11       AC.T..A... .....A.... .T..G..... T.....A..A ...T.A.... ..C.C..T.. T.....A... .....T..AG C........C ...A......
G12       A.....A..G .....A.... .A..AA.T.. ......G... A..T..G.CG .CA....... ......A... .....A..G. TC.......C ...A......
          ....|....| ....|....| ....|....| ....|....| ....|....| ....|....| ....|....| ....|....| ....|....| ....|....|
          *  *  *  *   *  *  *  *  *  *   *  *  *  *   *  *  *   *  *  *   *  *  *  *   *  *  *   *  *  *  *  *  *  *
G1        ATGAGAGTGA ATTGGAAAAG ATGGTGGCAA GTGTTCTATA CTATAGTAGA TTATATTAAT CAGATTGTAC AGGTAATGTC CAAAAGATCA AGATCATTAA
G2        ...C....A. .........A .......... .....T.... .AG....T.. C........C ..A...A... .A..T..... T...C.G... .........G
G3        ...C...... .......G.A .......... .....T.... .A.....T.. C..CG.G... ..A.....G. .A.C...... .........G ......C...
G4        ...C.C.... .C.......A .......... ..A....... ..G....T.. .......... .....A.... .A........ .........G .....G...G
G9        ........T. .......G.A .......... ..T..T..C. ..G.T..T.. ....G.A..C .....AA.T. .A.C...... .........T ....TG...G
G6        ...C.CA.A. .......... .......... ..A..T.... .GG.G..T.. ...CG....C ..A.....G. .A..T..... ...GC....G C....TC...
G8        ...C...... .........A .........G ..A....... .AG.C..G.. ...CG.C... .....AA.T. ...C...... .........T ..G..GC...
G10       ...C....A. .......G.A .......... ..T....... .GG....... .......... .........G. .A..T..... .......... C.G.......
G11       ...C.TA.A. .........A .......... ..A..T.... .......C.. ....G..... ..A....... .A..G..... ....C..... C.T..T....
G12       ...C..A.A. .C.......A .........G .....T.... .CG....... ...C..A... ..A..A..T. .......... ....C..... ..........
          ....|....| ....|....| ....|....| ....|....| ....|....| ....|....|
            *  *  *   *  *  *   *  *  *  *   *  *  *   *  *  *   *  *  *  *
G1        ATTCTGCTGC GTTCTATTAT AGAGTATAGA TATATCTTAG ATTAGAATTG TTCGATGTGA CC
G2        .CA.A..... T..T...... ...A.T.... ....G..... .......... .AT....... ..
G3        .......... A..T..C..C .......... ....G..... .......... .AT....... ..
G4        ....GT.AT. T......... .....G.... ......C..A .A.....C.. ..T....... ..
G9        ....A..G.. T..T..C... .....T.GA. ...CAT.G.A ....T.G... GA........ ..
G6        .C..A..... A..T..C... C....T.... .......... .......... .AT....... ..
G8        .C..AT.A.. A.....C..C .....G.... ..C..G.... .......... .AT....... ..
G10       ....A..A.. T..T..C... ..G..T.-.. .......... .......... .AT....... ..
G11       ....C..... T..T...... C....C.... .........A G......... .AT....... ..
G12       ....A..... T..T..C..C ...A.T.... ....G..... .......... AAT....... ..
```

Fig. 2. Nucleotide analysis of rotavirus genotypes. Points indicated no nucleotide change. Nucleotide difference was shown by alphabetical marks. The start codon was underlined at position 49.

In addition, there is evidence of intragenic recombination in rotavirus VP7 genes. The existence of intragenic recombinations between interlineage and intersublineage in G1 rotaviruses was demonstrated (Tung et al., 2007). This variability has led to nucleotide mismatches between the actual VP7 gene and primers and consequently a failure on the detection of the G1 strains (Parra & Espinola, 2006). Other studies have reported the detection of possible new distinct sublineages for G2 genotype (Mascarenhas et al., 2010). Recombination between human rotaviruses and animal rotaviruses were well recognized in G3 rotaviruses (Nishikawa et al., 1989) and the genetic variation in their VP7 gene was reported in China and Japan accompanied with change also on the amino acid level (Wen et al., 1997). In addition, it has been postulated that amino acid substitutions at positions 96 and 213 might be involved in the emergence of G3 rotavirus strains in Japan, China, and Russia from 2001 to 2004 (Trinh et al., 2007). The diversification of rotavirus strains in phylogenetic lineages in G9 strains was reported previously (Santos et al., 2002; Hoshino et al., 2004; Cao et al., 2008; Pattara et al., 2009). Although one amino acid change at position 208 in an antigenic region C of G9 rotaviruses VP7 gene was reported, it is not clear whether this change affected the nature of the viruses in terms of antigenicity, infectivity or pathogenicity.

5. Conclusion

As a conclusion, the use of vaccines with broad and consistent serotype coverage would be important to help decrease the burden of rotavirus in countries with new emergent genotypes. The emergence of new rotavirus strains stresses the importance of a better knowledge of their genotypes and their mechanisms of transmission. Hence the importance of setting up a vaccine design strategy as well as surveillance programs that should detect the diversity of rotavirus strains before, during and after the introduction of a rotavirus vaccine (Palombo, 1999) in order to detect the possible appearance of a mutants escape strains that probably reflect a selective pressure induced by the vaccine and eventually may pose a challenge to vaccine strategies. Further studies need to be carried out in order to elucidate the mechanism(s) behind the genetic recombination of rotaviruses and the emergence of new genotypes.

6. Reference list

Adah, M.I., Rohwedder, A., Olaleyle, O.D., & Werchau, H. (1997). Nigerian rotavirus serotype G8 could not be typed by PCR due to nucleotide mutation at the 3' end of the primer binding site. *Archives of Virology*, Vol.142, No.9, (September 1997), pp. 1881-1887, ISSN 1432-8798

Adah, M.I., Wade, A., & Taniguchi K. (2001). Molecular epidemiology of rotavirus in Nigeria: detection of unusual strains with G2P[6] and G8P[1] specificities. *Journal of Clinical Microbiology*, Vol.39, No.11, (November 2001), pp. 3969-3975, ISSN 0095-1137

Adah, M.I., Nagashima, S., Wakuda, M., & Taniguchi, K. (2003). Close Relationship between G8-Serotype Bovine and Human Rotaviruses Isolated in Nigeria. *Journal of Clinical Microbioloy*, Vol.41, No.8, (August 2003), pp. 3945-3950, ISSN 0095-1137

Alouf, J.E. (1987). From 'diphtheritic' poison to molecular toxicology. *American Society of Microbiology News*, Vol.53, No.10, (n.d.), pp. 547-550, ISSN 0044-7897

Andrej, S., Mateja P-P., Darja B-M., & Jozica M. (2008). Human, porcine and bovine rotaviruses in Slovenia: evidence of interspecies transmission and genome reassortment. *Journal of General Virology*, Vol.89, No.7, (July 2008), pp. 1690-1698, ISSN 1465-2099

Armah, G.E., Hoshino, Y., Santos, N., Binka, F., Damanka, S., Adjei, R., Honma, S., Tatsumi, M., Manful, T., & Anto, F. (2010). The Global Spread of Rotavirus G10 strains: Detection in Ghanaian Children hospitalized with Diarrhoea. *Journal of Infectious Diseases*, Vol.202, Suppl 1, (September 2010), pp. S231–S238, ISSN 0022-1899

Bachmayer, H., Liehl, E., & Schmidt, G. (1976). Preparation and properties of a novel influenza subunit vaccine. *Postgraduate Medical Journal*, Vol.52, No.608, (June 1976), pp. 360-367, ISSN 0032-5473

Banerjee, I., Iturriza-Gómara, M., Rajendran, P., Primrose, B., Ramani, S., Gray, J.J., Brown, D.W., & Kang, G. (2007). Molecular characterization of G11P[25] and G3P[3] human rotavirus strains associated with asymptomatic infection in South India. *Journal of Medical Virology*, Vol.79, No.11, (November 2007), pp. 1768-1774, ISSN 1096-9071

Banyai, K., Gentsch, J.R., Glass, R.I., & Szucs, G. (2003). Detection of human rotavirus serotype G6 in Hungary. *Epidemiology and Infection*, Vol.130, No.1, (February 2003), pp. 107-112, ISSN 1096-9071

Banyai, K., Gentsch, J.R., Glass, R.I., Uj, M., Mihaly, I., & Szucs, G. (2004). Eight-year survey of human rotavirus strains demonstrates circulation of unusual G and P types in Hungary. *Journal of Clinical Microbiology*, Vol.42, No.1, (January 2004), pp. 393-397, ISSN 0095-1137

Banyai, K., Esona, M.D., Kerin, T.K., Hull, J.J., Mijatovic, S., Vasconez, N., et al. (2009). Molecular characterization of a rare, human-porcine reassortant rotavirus strain,

G11P[6], from Ecuador. *Archives of Virology*, Vol.154, No.11, (September 2009), pp. 1823-1829, ISSN 1432-8798

Barnes, G.L., Lund, J.S., Adams, L., Mora, A., Mitchell, S.V., Caples, A., & Bishop R.F. (1997). Phase 1 trial of a candidate rotavirus vaccine (RV3) derived from a human neonate. *Journal of Paediatrics and Child Health*, Vol.33, No.4, (August 1997), pp. 300-304, ISSN 1440-1754

Bittle, J.L., Houghten, R.A., Alexander, H., Shinnick, T.M., Sutcliffe, J.G., Lerner, R.A., Rowlands, D.J., & Brown, F. (1982). Protection against foot-and-mouth disease by immunization with a chemically synthesized peptide predicted from the viral nucleotide sequence. *Nature*, Vol.298, No.5869, (Jul 1982), pp. 30-33, ISSN 0028-0836

Bellamy, A.R. & Both, G.W. (1990). Molecular biology of rotaviruses. *Advances in Virus Research*, Vol.38, (n.d.), pp. 1-43, ISSN 0065-3527

Bernstein, D.I., Sack, D.A., Reisinger, K., Rothstein, E., & Ward, R.L. (2002). Second-year follow-up evaluation of live, attenuated human rotavirus vaccine 89-12 in healthy infants. *Journal of Infectious Diseases*, Vol.186, No.10, (November 2002), pp. 1487–1489, ISSN 0022-1899

Bizzini, B., Blass, J., Turpin, A., & Raynaud, M. (1970). Chemical characterization of tetanus toxin and toxoid. *European Journal of Biochemistry*, Vol.17, (n.d.), pp. 100-105, ISSN 1432-1033

Bok, K., Palacios, G., Sijvarger, K., Matson, D.O., & Gomez, J.A. (2001). Emergence of G9P[6] human rotavirus in Argentina: phylogenetic relationships among G9 strains. *Journal of Clinical Microbiology*, Vol.39, No.11, (November 2001), pp. 4020-4025, ISSN 0095-1137

Brown, F. (1990). Synthetic peptides as potential vaccines against foot-and-mouth disease. *Endeavour*, Vol.14, No.2, (n.d.), pp. 87-94, ISSN 0160-9327

Browning, G.F., Snodgrass, D.R., Nakagomi, O., Kaga, E., Sarasini, A., & Gerna, G. (1992). Human and bovine serotype G8 strains may be derived by reassortment. *Archives of Virology*, Vol.125, No.1-4 , (n.d.), pp. 121-128, ISSN 1432-8798

Cao, D., Santos, N., Jones, R.W., Tatsumi,M., Gentsch, J.R., & Hoshino, Y. (2008). The VP7 genes of two G9 rotaviruses isolated in 1980 from diarrheal stool samples collected in Washington, DC, are unique molecularly and serotypically. *Journal of Virology*, Vol.82, No.8, (April 2008), pp. 4175–4179, ISSN 0022-538X

Castello, A.A., Jiang, B., Glass, R.I., Glikmann, G., & Genstch, J.R. (2004). Rotavirus G and P genotpe prevalence in Argentina 1999–2003: detection of P[9]G12 strains [abstract P37-4]. *Abstract of 23rd Annual Meeting of the American Society for Virology*, Montreal, Canada, (July 2004)

Centers for Disease Control and Prevention. (1999a). In: *MMWR Morbidity and Mortality Weekly Report*, 1999, Available from: http://www.cdc.gov/mmwr/preview/mmwrhtml/mm4827a1.htm, Intussusception among recipients of rotavirus vaccine—United States, 1998–1999

Centers for Disease Control and Prevention. (1999b). In: *MMWR Morbidity and Mortality Weekly Report*, 1999, Available from:Rotavirus vaccine for the prevention of rotavirus gastroenteritis among children. Recommendations of the Advisory Committee on Immunization Practices (ACIP).MMWRMorb. Mortal. Wkly. Rep. 48:1–20.

Centers of disease Control and Prevention. Prevention of Rotavirus Gastroenteritis Among Infants and Children: Recommendations of the Advisory Committee on Immunization Practices (ACIP). MMWR 2006, 55(RR12); 1-13.

Cheon, D.-S., Lee, K., Kim, W., Lee, S., Choi, W., Ahn, J., Jee, Y., Cho, H. Genetic analysis of the VP7 gene of unusual genotypes of human group A rotavirus strains circulating in Korea [abstract P37-3]. *Abstract of 23rd Annual Meeting of the American Society for Virology*, Montreal, Canada, (July 2004).

Chezzi, C., Dornrnann, C.J., Blackburn, N.K., Maselesele, E., McAnerney, J., & Schoub, B.D. (1998). Genetic stability of oral polio vaccine prepared on primary monkey kidney cells or Vero cells-effects of passage in cell culture and the human gastrointestinal tract. *Vaccine*, Vol.16, No.20, (December 1998), pp. 2031-2038, ISSN 0264-410X

Christy, C., Madore, H.P., Pichichero, M.E., Gala, C., Pincus, P., Vosefski, D., Hoshino, Y., Kapikian, A., & Dolin, R. (1988). Field trial of rhesus rotavirus vaccine in infants. *Pediatric Infectious Disease Journal*, Vol.7, No.9, (September 1988), pp. 645-650, ISSN 1532-0987

Ciarlet, M., Hidalgo, M., Gorziglia, M., & Liprandi, F. (1994). Characterization of neutralization epitopes on the VP7 surface protein of serotype G11 porcine rotaviruses. *Journal of General Virology*, Vol.75, No.8, (August 1994), pp.1867-1873, ISSN 1465-2099

Ciarlet, M.L., Hoshino, Y., & Liprandi, F. (1997). Single point mutation may affect the serotype reactivity of G11 porcine rotavirus strains: a widening spectrum? *Journal of Virology*, Vol.71, No.11, (November 1997), pp. 8213-8220, ISSN 0022-538X

Clark, H.F., Hoshino, Y., Bell, L.M., Groff, J., Hess, G., Bachman, P., & Offit, P.A. (1987). Rotavirus isolate WI61 representing a presumptive new human serotype. *Journal of Clinical Microbiology*, Vol.25, No.9, (September 1987), pp. 1757-1762, ISSN 0095-1137

Clark, H.F., Borian F.E., Bell L.M., Modesto K., Gouvea V., & Plotkin S.A. (1988). Protective effect of WC3 vaccine against rotavirus diarrhea in infants during a predominantly serotype 1 rotavirus season. *Journal of Infectious Diseases*, Vol.158, No.3, (September 1988), pp. 570-587, ISSN 0022-1899

Clark, H.F., Bernstein, D.I., Dennehy, P.H., Offit, P., Pichichero, M., Treanor, J., Ward, R.L., Krah, D.L., Shaw, A., Dallas, M.J., Laura, D., Eiden, J.J., Ivanoff, N., Kaplan, K.M., & Heaton, P. (2004). Safety, efficacy and immunogenicity of a live, quadrivalent human-bovine reassortant rotavirus vaccine in healthy infants. *Journal of Pediatrics*, Vol.144, No.2, (February 2004), pp. 184-190, ISSN 0022-3476

Coluchi, N., Munford, V., Manzur, J., Vazquez, C., Escobar, M., Weber, E., Mármol, P., & Rácz, M.L. (2002). Detection, subgroup specificity, and genotype diversity of rotavirus strains in children with acute diarrhea in Paraguay. *Journal of Clinical Microbiology*, Vol.40, No.5, (May 2002), pp. 1709-1714, ISSN 0095-1137

Cooney, M.A., Gorrell, R.J., & Palombo, E.A. (2001). Characterization and phylogenetic analysis of the VP7 proteins of serotype G6 and G8 human rotaviruses. *Journal of Medical Microbiology*, Vol.50, No.5, (May 2001), pp. 462-467, ISSN 0022-2615

Coulson, B., & Kirkwood, C. (1991). Relation of VP7 amino acid sequence to monoclonal antibody neutralization of rotavirus and rotavirus monotype. *Journal of Virology*, Vol.65, No.11, (November 1991), pp. 5968-5974, ISSN 0022-538X

Cubitt, W.D., Steele, A.D., & Iturriza-Gómara, M. (2000). Characterisation of rotaviruses from children treated at a London hospital during 1996: emergence of strains G9P2A[6] and G3P2A[6]. *Journal of Medical Virology*, Vol.61, No.1, (May 2000), pp. 150-154, ISSN 1096-9071

Cunliffe, N.A., Gondwe, J.S., Broadhead, R.L., Molyneux, M.E., Woods, P.A., Bresee, J.S., Glass, R.I., Gentsch, J.R., & Hart, C.A. (1999). Rotavirus G and P types in children with acute diarrhea in Blantyre, Malawi, from 1997 to 1998: predominance of novel P[6]G8 strains. *Journal of Medical Virology*, Vol.57, No.3, (March 1999), pp. 308-312, ISSN 1096-9071

Cunliffe, N.A., Gentsch J.R., Kirkwood C.D., Gondwe J.S., Dove W., Nakagomi O., Nakagomi T., Hoshino Y., Bresee J.S., Glass R.I., Molyneux M.E., & Hart C.A. (2000). Molecular and serologic characterization of novel serotype G8 human rotavirus strains detected in Blantyre, Malawi. *Virology*, Vol.274, No.2, (September 2000), pp. 309-320, ISSN 0042-6822

Cunliffe, N.A., Ngwira, B.M., Dove, W., Nakagomi, O., Nakagomi, T., Perez, A., Hart, C.A., Kazembe, P.N., & Mwansambo, C.C.V. (2009). Serotype G12 Rotaviruses, Lilongwe, Malawi. *Emerging Infectious Diseases*, Vol.15, No.1, (January 2009), pp. 87-90, ISSN 1080-6059

Das, B.K., Gentsch, J.R., Hoshino, Y., Ishida, S., Nakagomi, O., Bhan, M.K., Kumar, R., & Glass, R.I. (1993a). Characterization of the G serotype and genogroup of New Delhi newborn rotavirus strain 116E. *Virology*, Vol.197, No.1, (November 1993), pp. 99-107, ISSN 0042-6822

Das, M., Dunn, S.J., Woode, G.N., Greenberg, H.B., & Rao, C.D. (1993b). Both surface proteins (VP4 and VP7) of an asymptomatic neonatal rotavirus strain (I321) have high levels of sequence identity with the homologous proteins of a serotype 10 bovine rotavirus. *Virology*, Vol.194, No.1, (May 1993), pp. 374-379, ISSN 0042-6822

Das, S., Varghese, V., Chaudhury, S., Barman, P., Mahapatra, S., Kojima, K., Bhattacharya, S.K., Krishnan, T., Ratho, R.K., Chhotray, G.P., Phukan, A.C., Kobayashi, N., & Naik, N.T. (2003). Emergence of novel human group A rotavirus G12 strain in India. *Journal of Clinical Microbiology*, Vol.41, No.6, (June 2006), pp. 2760-2762, ISSN 0095-1137

De Vos, B., Vesikari, T., Linhares, A.C., Salinas, B., Perez-Schael, I., Ruiz-Palacios, G.M., Guerrero, M.L., Phua, K.B., Delem, A., Hardt, K. (2004). A rotavirus vaccine for prophylaxis of infants against rotavirus gastroenteritis. *Pediatric Infectious Disease Journal*, Vol.23, Suppl 10, (October 2004), pp. S179-S182, ISSN 1532-0987

Dhama, K., Chauhan, R.S., Mahendran, M., & Malik, S.V.S. (2009). Rotavirus diarrhea in bovines and other domestic animals. *Veterinary Research Communications*, Vol.33, No.1, (January 2009), pp. 1-23, ISSN 0165-7380

Donnelly, J.J., Ulmer, J.B., Liu, M.A. (1994). Immunization with DNA. *Journal Immunological Methods*, Vol.176, No.2, (December 1994), pp. 145-152, ISSN 0022-1759

Dorothea, S. (1993). Synthetic peptide vaccines. Journal of Medical Microbiology, Vol.39, No.4, (October 1993), pp. 241-242, ISSN 0022-2615

Drozdov, S.G. & Shirman, G.A. (1961). Interaction of viruses in the intestinal tract of man. I. Interference between wild and vaccine poliovirus strains. *Acta virologica*, Vol.5, No., (Jully 1961), pp. 210-219, ISSN 1336-2305

Dunn, S.J., Greenberg, H.B., Ward, R.L., Nakagomi, O., Burns, J.W., Vo, P.T., Pax, K.A., Das, M., Gowda, K., & Rao, C.D. (1993). Serotypic and genotypic characterization of human serotype 10 rotaviruses from asymptomatic neonates. *Journal of Clinical Microbiology*, Vol.31, No.1, (January 1993), pp. 165-169, ISSN 0095-1137

Dunn, P.M. (1996). "Dr Edward Jenner (1749-1823) of Berkeley, and vaccination against smallpox". Archives of disease in childhood-Fetal and neonatal edition, Vol.74, No.1, (January 1996), pp. F77-F78, ISSN 1468-2044

Dyall-Smith, M.L., Lazdins, I., Tregar, G.W., & Holmes, I.H. (1986). Location of major antigenic sites involved in rotavirus serotype-specific neutralization. *Proceedings of the National Academy of Sciences USA*, Vol.83, No.10, (May 1986), pp. 3465-3468, ISSN 0027-8424

Emini, E.A., Jameson, B.A. & Wimmer, E. (1983). Priming for and induction of anti-poliovirus neutralizing antibodies by synthetic peptides. Nature, Vol.304, (August 1983), pp. 699-703, ISSN 0028-0836

Esona, M., Armah, G.E., Geyer, A., & Steele, A.D. (2004). Detection of an unusual human rotavirus strain with G5P[8] specificity in a Cameroonian child with diarrhea. *Journal of Clinical Microbiology*, Vol.42, No.1, (January 2004), pp.441-444, ISSN 0095-1137

Estes, M.K. & Cohen, J. (1989). Rotavirus gene structure and function. *Microbiological Reviews*, Vol.53, No.4, (December 1989), pp.410-449, ISSN 0146-0749

Estes, M.K. (2001). Rotaviruses and their replication, In: *Fields virology*, Howley P.M., pp. 1747-1786, Lippincott Williams & Wilkins, ISBN 0781718325, Philadelphia

Estes, M.K. & Kapikian, A.Z. (2007). Rotaviruses, In: *Fields virology*, Knipe D.M., Howley P.M., Griffin D.E., Lamb R.A., Martin M.A., Roizman B., & Straus S.E., pp. 1917-1974, Lippincott Williams & Wilkins, ISBN 0781718325, Philadelphia

Gard, S. (1960). Theoretical considerations in the inactivation of viruses by chemical means. *Annals of the New York Academy of Sciences*, Vol.83, (January 1960), pp. 638, ISSN 0077-8923

Giammanco, G., De Grandi, V., Lupo, L., Mistretta, A., Pignato, S., Teuween, D., Bogaerts, H., & Andrè F.E. (1988). Interference of Oral Poliovirus Vaccine on RIT 4237 Oral Rotavirus Vaccine. *European Journal of Epidemiology, Vol.*4, No.1, (March 1988), pp. 121-123, ISSN 0392-2990

Gentsch, J.R., Woods, P.A., Ramachandran, M., Das, B.K., Leite, J.P., Alfieri, A., Kumar, R., Bhan, M.K., & Glass, R.I. (1996). Review of G and P typing results from a global collection of rotavirus strains: implications for vaccine development. *Journal of Infectious Diseases*, Vol.174, Supl. 1, (September 1996), pp. S30-S36, ISSN 0022-1899

Gentsch, J.R., Laird, A.R., Bielfelt, B., Griffin, D.D., Banyai, K., Ramachandran, M., Jain, V., Cunliffe, N.A., Nakagomi, O., Kirkwood, C.D., Fischer, T.K., Parashar, U.D., Bresee, J.S., Jiang, B., & Glass, R.I. (2005). Serotype diversity and reassortment between human and animal rotavirus strains: implications for rotavirus vaccine programs. *Journal of Infectious Diseases*, Vol.192, Supl. 1, (September 2005), pp. 146-159, ISSN 0022-1899

Gerna, G., Sarasini, A., Zentilin, L., Di Matteo, A., Miranda, P., Parea, M., Battaglia, M., & Milanesi, G. (1990). Isolation in Europe of 69M-like (serotype 8) human rotavirus strains with either subgroup I or II specificity and a long RNA electropherotype. *Archives of Virolology*, Vol.112, No.1-2, (n.d.), pp. 27-40, ISSN 1432-8798

Gerna, G., Sarasini, A., Parea, M., Arista, S., Miranda, P., Brüssow, H., Hoshino, Y., & Flores, J. (1992). Isolation and characterization of two distinct human rotavirus strains with G6 specificity. *Journal of Clinical Microbiology*, Vol.30, No.1, (January 1992), pp. 9-16, ISSN 0095-1137

Gerna, G., Steele, A.D., Hoshino, Y., Sereno, M., Garcia, D., Sarasini, A., & Flores, J. (1994). A comparison of the VP7 gene sequences of human and bovine rotaviruses. *Journal of General Virology*, Vol.75, No.7, (July 1994), pp. 1781-1784, ISSN 1465-2099

Gombold, J.L. & Ramig, R.F. (1986). Analysis of reassortment of genome segments in mice mixedly infected with rotaviruses SA 11 and RRV. *Journal of Virology*, Vol.57, No.1, (January 1986), pp. 110-116, ISSN 0022-538X

Gouvea, V., Glass, R.I., Woods, P., Taniguchi, K., Clark, H.F., Forrester, B., & Fang, Z.Y. (1990). Polymerase Chain Reaction Amplification and Typing of Rotavirus Nucleic Acid from Stool Specimens. Journal of Clinical Microbiology, Vol.28, No.2, (February 1990), pp. 276-282, ISSN 0095-1137

Gouvea, V., de Castro, L., Timenetsky, M.C., Greenberg, H., & Santos, N. (1994). Rotavirus serotype G5 associated with diarrhea in Brazilian children. *Journal of Clinical Microbiology*, Vol.32, No.5, (May 1994), pp. 1408-1409, ISSN 0095-1137

Green, K.Y., Midthun, K., Gorziglia, M., Hoshino, Y., Kapikian, A.Z., Chanock, R.M., & Flores, J. (1987). Comparison of the amino acid sequences of the major neutralization protein of four human rotavirus serotypes. *Virology*, Vol.161, No.1, (November 1987), pp.153-159, ISSN 0042-6822

Green, K.Y., Sears, J.F., Taniguchi, K., Midthun, K., Hoshino, Y., Gorziglia, M., Nishikawa, K., Urasawa, S., Kapikian, A.Z., & Chanock, R.M. (1988). Prediction of human rotavirus serotype by nucleotide sequence analysis of the VP7 protein gene. *Journal of Virology*, Vol.62, No.5, (May 1988), pp. 1819-1823, ISSN 0022-538X

Greenberg, H.B., Kalica, A.R., Wyatt, R.G., Jones, R.W., Kapikian, A.Z., & Chanock, R.M. (1981). Rescue of noncultivatable human rotavirus by gene reassortment during mixed infection with ts mutants of a cultivatable bovine rotavirus. *Proceedings of the National Academy of Sciences USA*, Vol.78, No.1, (January 1981), pp. 420-424, ISSN 0027-8424

Griffin, D.D., Nakagomi, T., Hoshino, Y., Nakagomi, O., Kirkwood, C.D., Parashar, U.D., Glass, R. I., & Gentsch, J.R. (2002). Characterization of nontypeable rotavirus strains from the United States: identification of a new rotavirus reassortant (P2A[6],G12) and rare P3[9] strains related to bovine rotaviruses. *Virology*, Vol.294, No.2, (March 2002), pp. 256-269, ISSN 0042-6822

Gurgel, R.Q., Cuevas, L.E., Vieira, S.C., Barros, V.C., Fontes, P.B., Salustino, E.F., Nakagomi, O., Nakagomi, T., Dove, W., Cunliffe, N., & Hart, CA. (2007). Predominance of rotavirus P[4]G2 in a vaccinated population, Brazil. *Emerging Infectious Diseases*, Vol.13, No.10, (October 2007), pp. 1571-1573, ISSN 1080-6059

Hanlon, P., Marsh, V., Shenton, F., Jobe, O., Hayes, R., Whittle, H.C., Hanlon, L., Byass, P., Hassan-King, M., Sillah, H., M'Boge, B.H., & Greenwood, B.M. (1987). Trial of an attenuated bovine rotavirus vaccine (RIT 4237) in Gambian infants. *Lancet*, Vol.329, No.8546, (June 1987), pp. 1342-1345, ISSN 0140-6736

Hans, D., Young, P.R., & Fairlie, D.P. (2006). Current status of short synthetic peptides as vaccines. *Journal of Medical Chemistry*, Vol.2, No.6, (November 2006), pp. 627-646, ISSN 0022-2623

Hasegawa, A., Inouye, S., Matsuno, S., Yamaoka, K., Eko, R., & Suharyono, W. (1984). Isolation of human rotavirus with a distinct RNA electrophoretic pattern from Indonesia. *Microbiology and Immunology,* Vol.28, No.6, (n.d.), pp. 719-722, ISSN 1348-0421

Hauser, P., Thomas, H.C., Waters, J., Simoen, E., Voet, P., De Wilde, M., Stephenne, J., & Petre, J. (1988). Induction of neutralising antibodies in chimpanzees and humans by recombinant yeast-derived hepatitis B surface antigen particle, In: *Viral hepatitis and liver disease,* Zuckerman A.J., pp. 1031-1037, Alan R. Liss., ISBN 978-0471612704, New York

Hilleman, M.R. (1987). Yeast recombinant hepatitis B vaccine. *Infection,* Vol.15, No.1, (January 1987), pp. 3-7, ISSN 0300-8126

Holland, J.J., De La Torre, J.C., & Steinhauer, D.A. (1992). RNA virus populations as quasispecies. *Current Topics in Microbiology and Immunology,* Vol.176, (n.d.), pp. 1-20, ISSN 0070-217X

Holmes, J.L., Kirkwood, C.D., Gerna, G., Clemens, J.D., Rao, M.R., Naficy, A.B., Abu-Elyazeed, R., Savarino, S.J., Glass, R.I., & Gentsch, J.R. (1999). Characterization of unusual G8 rotavirus strains isolated from Egyptian children. *Archives of Virology,* Vol.144, No.7, (n.d.), pp. 1381-1396, ISSN 1432-8798

Hong, S.-K., Lee, S.-G., Lee, S.-A., Kang, J.-H., Lee, J.-H., Kim, J.-H., Kim, D.-S., Kim, H.-M., Jang, Y.-T., Ma, S.-H., Kim, S.-Y., & Paik, S.-Y. (2007). Characterization of a G11, P[4] strain of human rotavirus isolated in South Korea. *Journal of Clinical Microbiology,* Vol.45, No.11, (November 2007), pp. 3759-3761, ISSN 0095-1137

Hoshino, Y., Nishikawa, K., Benfield, D.A., & Gorziglia, M. (1994). Mapping of antigenic sites involved in serotype-cross-reactive neutralization on group A rotavirus outercapsid glycoprotein VP7. *Virology,* Vol.199, No.1, (February 1994), pp. 233-237, ISSN 0042-6822

Hoshino, Y., & Kapikian, A.Z. (2000). Rotavirus serotypes: Classification and importance in epidemiology, immunity, and vaccine development. *Journal of Health Population and Nutrition,* Vol.18, No.1, (June 2000), pp. 5-14, ISSN 1606-0997

Hoshino, Y., Jones, R.W., Ross, J., Honma, S., Santos, N., Gentsch, J.R., & Kapikian, A.Z. (2004). Rotavirus serotype G9 strains belonging to VP7 gene phylogenetic sequence lineage 1 may be more suitable for serotype G9 vaccine candidates than those belonging to lineage 2 or 3. *Journal of Virology,* Vol.78, No.14, (July 2004), pp. 7795-7802, ISSN 0022-538X

Hull, J.J., Teel, E.N., Kerin, T.K., Freeman, M.M., Esona, M.D., Gentsch, J.R., Cortese, M.M., Parashar, U.D., Glass, R.I., & Bowen, M.D. (2011). United States Rotavirus Strain Surveillance From 2005 to 2008: Genotype Prevalence Before and After Vaccine Introduction. *Journal of Pediatric Infectious Disease,* Vol.30, No.1, (January 2011), pp. S42-S47, ISSN 1305-7707

Iturriza-Gómara, M., Green, J., Brown, D.W.G, Desselberger, U., & Gray, J. (2000). Diversity within the VP4 gene of rotavirus P[8] strains: implications for reverse transcription-PCR genotyping. *Journal of Clinical Microbiology,* Vol.38, No.2, (February 2000), pp. 898-901, ISSN 0095-1137

Iturriza-Gómara, M., Kang, G., Mammen, A., Jana, A.K., Abraham, M., Desselberger, U., Brown, D., & Gray, J. (2004a). Characterization of G10P[11] rotaviruses causing acute gastroenteritis in neonates and infants in Vellore, India. *Journal of Clinical Microbiology*, Vol.42, No.6, (June 2004), pp. 2541-2547, ISSN 0095-1137

Iturriza-Gómara, M., Kang, G., & Gray, J. (2004b). Rotavirus genotyping: keeping up with an evolving population of human rotaviruses. Journal of Clinical Virology, Vol.31, No.4, (December 2004), pp. 259-265, ISSN

Joensuu, J., Koskenniemi, E., Pang, X.-L., & Vesikari, T. (1997). Randomised placebo-controlled trial of rhesus-human reassortant rotavirus vaccine for prevention of severe rotavirus gastroenteritis. *Lancet*, Vol.350, No.9086, (October 1997), pp. 1205-1209, ISSN 0140-6736

Jonathan, R. (1987). Synthetic peptides as vaccines. *Nature*, Vol.330, (November 1987), pp. 106-107, ISSN 0028-0836

Kalica, A.R., Greenberg, H.B., Wyatt, R.G., Flores, J., Sereno, M.M., Kapikian, A.Z. & Chanock, R.M. (1981). Genes of human (strain Wa) and bovine (strain UK) rotaviruses that code for neutralization subgroup antigens. *Virology*, Vol.112, No.2, (July 1981), pp. 385-390, ISSN 0042-6822

Kapikian, A.Z., Hoshimo, Y., Chanock, R.M., & Perez-Schael, I. (1996a). Efficacy of a quadrivalent rhesus rotavirus-based human rotavirus vaccine aimed at preventing severe rotavirus diarrhea in infants and young children. *Journal of Infectious Diseases*, Vol.174, Suppl. 1, (September 1996), pp. S65-S72, ISSN 0022-1899

Kapikian, A.Z., Hoshino, Y., Chanock, R.M., & Perez-Schael, I. (1996b). Jennerian and modified Jennerian approach to vaccination against rotavirus diarrhea using a quadrivalent rhesus rotavirus (RRV) and human-RRV reassortant vaccine. *Archives of Virology. Supplementum*, Vol.12, (n.d.), pp. 163-175, ISSN 1432-8798

Kapikian, A.Z., Hoshino, Y., & Chanock, R.M. (2001). Rotaviruses, In: *Fields virology*, Howley P.M., pp. 1787-1833, Lippincott Williams & Wilkins, ISBN 0781718325, Philadelphia

Katz, S.L., Milovanovic M.V., & Enders J.F. (1958). Propagation of measles virus in cultures of chick embryo cells. *Proceedings of the Society for Experimental Biology and Medicine*, Vol.97, No.1, (n.d.), pp. 23-29, ISSN 1525-1373

Katz, M. & Plotkin, S.A. (1968). Oral polio immunization of the newborn infant; a possible method for overcoming interference by ingested antibodies. *Journal of Pediatrics*, Vol.73, No.2, (August 1968), pp. 267-270, ISSN 0022-3476

Kim, K.S. & Sharp, D.G. (1967). Influence of the physical state of formalinized vaccinia virus particles on surviving plaque titre: Evidence for multiplicity reactivation. *Journal of Immunology*, Vol.99, No.6, (December 1967), pp. 1221, ISSN 0022-1767

King, C.A., Spellerberg, M.B., Zhu, D.L., Rice, J., Sahota, S.S., Thompsett, A.R., Hamblin, T.J., Radl, J., & Stevenson, F.K. (1998). DNA vaccines with single-chain Fv fused to fragment C of tetanus toxin induce protective immunity against lymphoma and myeloma. *Nature Medicine*, Vol.4, (n.d.), pp. 1281-1286, ISSN 1078-8956

Kelkar, S.D. & Ayachit, V.L. (2000). Circulation of group A rotavirus subgroups and serotypes in Pune, India, 1990–1997. *Journal of Health Population and Nutrition*, Vol.18, No.3, (December 2000), pp. 163-170, ISSN 1606-0997

Khamrin, P., Peerakome, S., Wongsawasdi, L., Tonusin, S., Sornchai, P., Maneerat, V., Khamwan, C., Yagyu, F., Okitsu, S., Ushijima, H., & Maneekarn, N. (2006). Emergence of human G9 rotavirus with an exceptionally high frequency in children admitted to hospital with diarrhea in Chiang Mai, Thailand. *Journal of Medical Virology*, Vol.78, No.2, (February 2006), pp. 273-280, ISSN 1096-9071

Kheyami, A.M., Nakagomi, T., Nakagomi, O., Dove, W., Hart, C.A, & Cunliffe, N.A. (2008). Molecular Epidemiology of Rotavirus Diarrhea among Children in Saudi Arabia: First Detection of G9 and G12 Strains. *Journal of Clinical Microbiology*, Vol.46, No.4, (April 2008), pp. 1185-1191, ISSN 0095-1137

Kieny, M.P., Lathe, R., Drillien, R., Spehner, D., Skory, S., Schmitt, D., Wiktor, T., Koprowski, H., & Lecocq, J.P. (1984). Expression of rabies virus glycoprotein from recombinant vaccinia virus. *Nature*, Vol.312, (November 1984), pp. 163-166, ISSN 0028-0836

Kilbourne, E.D. (1991). New viruses and new disease: mutation, evolution and ecology. *Current Opinion in Immunology*, Vol.3, No.4, (August 1991), pp. 518-524, ISSN 0952-7915

Kirkwood, C., Masendycz, P.J., & Coulson, B.S. (1993). Characteristics and location of cross-reactive and serotype-specific neutralization sites on VP7 of human G type 9 rotaviruses. *Virology*, Vol.196, No.1, (September 1993), pp. 79-88, ISSN 0042-6822

Lanata, C.F., Black, R.E., del Aguila, R., Gil, A., Verastegui, H., Gerna, G., Flores, J., Kapikian, A.Z., & Andre, F.E. (1989). Protection of Peruvian children against rotavirus diarrhea of specific serotypes by one, two, or three doses of the RIT 4237 attenuated bovine rotavirus vaccine. *Journal of Infectious Diseases*, Vol.159, No.3, (March 1989), pp. 452-459, ISSN 0022-1899

Levine, M.M., Woodrow, G.C., Kaper, J.B., & Cobon, G.S. (Eds.). (1997). *New Generation Vaccines*, Marcel Dekker, Inc., ISBN 0-8247-0061-9, New York

Linhares, A.C. & Bresee, J.S. (2000). Rotavirus vaccine and vaccination in Latin America. *Revista Panamericana de Salud Pública*, Vol.8, No.5, (November 2000), pp. 305-331, ISSN 1020-4989

Linhares, A.C., Lanata, C.F., Hausdorff, W.P., Gabbay, W.P., & Black, R.E. (1999). Reappraisal of the Peruvian and Brazilian lower titer tetravalent rhesus-human reassortant rotavirus vaccine efficacy trials: analysis by severity of diarrhea. *Pediatric Infectious Disease Journal*, Vol.18, No.11, (November 1999), pp. 1001-1016, ISSN 1532-0987

Liprandi, F., Gerder, M., Bastidas, Z., Lopez, J.A., Pujol, F.H., Ludert, J.E., Joelsson, D.B., & Ciarlet, M. (2003). Novel Type of VP4 Carried by a Porcine Rotavirus Strain. *Virology*, Vol.315, No.2, (October 2003), pp. 373-380, ISSN 0042-6822

Lo Grippo, G.A. (1960). Investigations of the use of *β*-propiolactone in virus inactivation. *Annals of the New York Academy of Sciences*, Vol.83, (January 1960), pp. 578-594, ISSN 0077-8923

MacGregor, R.R., Boyer, J.D., Ugen, K.E., Lacy, K.E., Gluckman, S.J., Bagarazzi, M.L., Chattergoon, M.A., Baine, Y., Higgins, T.J., Ciccarelli, R.B., Coney, L.B., Ginsberg, R.S., & Weiner D.B. (1998) . First human trial of a DNA-based vaccine for treatment of human immunodeficiency virus type 1 infection: safety and host response. *Journal Infectious Diseases*, Vol.178, (July 1998), pp. 92-100, ISSN 0022-1899

Mackett, M., Yilma, T., Rose, J.K. & Moss, B. (1985). Vaccinia virus recombinants: expression of VSV genes and protective immunization of mice and cattle. Science, Vol.227, No.4685, (January 1985), pp. 433-435, ISSN 0036-8075

Martella V., Pratelli, A., Greco, G., Gentile, M., Fiorente, P., Tempesta, M., & Buonavoglia, C. (2001). Nucleotide sequence variation of the VP7 gene of two G3-type rotaviruses isolated from dogs. Virus Research, Vol.74, No.1-2, (April 2001), pp. 17-25, ISSN 0168-1702

Martella, V., Ciarlet, M., Camarda, A., Pratelli, A., Tempesta, M., Greco, G., Cavalli, A., Elia, G., Decaro, N., Terio, V., Bozzo, G., Camero, M., & Buonavoglia, C. (2003). Molecular characterization of the VP4, VP6, VP7, and NSP4 genes of lapine rotaviruses identified in Italy: emergence of a novel VP4 genotype. *Virology,* Vol.314, No.1, (September 2003), pp. 358-370, ISSN 0042-6822

Martella, V., Terio, V., Arista, S., Elia, G., Corrente, M., Madio, A., Pratelli, A., Tempesta, M., Cirani, A., & Buonavoglia, C. (2004). Nucleotide variation in the VP7 gene affects PCR genotyping of G9 rotaviruses identified in Italy. Journal of Medical Virology, Vol.72, No.1, (January 2004), pp.143-148, ISSN 1096-9071

Mascarenhas, J.D., Lima, C.S., de Oliveira, D.S., Guerra Sde, F., Maestri, R.P., Gabbay, Y.B., de Lima, I.C., de Menezes, E.M., Linhares Ada, C., & Bensabath, G. (2010). Identification of Two Sublineages of Genotype G2 Rotavirus Among Diarrheic Children in Parauapebas, Southern Para State, Brazil. *Journal of Medical Virology,* Vol.82, No.4, (April 2010), pp. 712–719, ISSN 1096-9071

Matthijnssens, J., Ciarlet, M., Heiman, E., Arijs, I., Delbeke, T., McDonald, S.M., Palombo, A.E., Iturriza-Gómara, M., Maes, P., Patton, J.T., Rahman, M., & Van Ranst, M. (2008a). Full genome-based classification of rotaviruses reveals common origin between human Wa-like and porcine rotavirus strains and human DS-1-like and bovine rotavirus strains. *Journal of Virology, Vol.*82, No.7, (April 2008), pp. 3204-3219, ISSN 0022-538X

Matthijnssens, J., Ciarlet, M., Rahman, M., Attoui, H., Bányai, K., Estes, M.K., Gentsch, J.R., Iturriza-Gómara, M., Kirkwood, C.D., Martella, V., Mertens, P.P., Nakagomi, O., Patton, J.T., Ruggeri, F.M., Saif, L.J., Santos, N., Steyer, A., Taniguchi, K., Desselberger, U., & Van Ranst, M. (2008b). Recommendations for the classification of group A rotaviruses using all 11 genomic RNA segments. *Archives of Virology,* Vol.153, No.8, (July 2008), pp. 1621-1629, ISSN 1432-8798

Maunula, L. & von Bonsdorff, C.H. (1998). Short sequences define genetic lineages: phylogenetic analysis of group A rotaviruses based on partial sequences of genome segments 4 and 9. *Journal of General Virology,* Vol.79, No.2, (February 1998), pp. 321-332, ISSN 1465-2099

Midthun, K. & Kapikian A.Z. (1996). Rotavirus vaccines: an overview. *Clinical Microbiology Reviews,* Vol.9, No.3, (July 1996), pp. 423-434, ISSN 0893-8512

Milich, D.R. (1990). Synthetic peptides: prospects for vaccine development. Seminars in Immunology, Vol.2, No.5, (September 1990), pp. 307-315, ISSN 1044-5323

Müller, G.M., Shapira, M., & Arnon, R. (1982). Anti-influenza response achieved by immunization with a synthetic conjugate. *Proceedings of the National Academy of Sciences USA,* Vol.79, No.2, (January 1982), pp. 569-573, ISSN 0027-8424

Nakagomi, T. & Nakagomi, O. (2009). A critical review on a globally-licensed, live, orally-administrable, monovalent human rotavirus vaccine: Rotarix. *Expert Opinion on Biological Therapy,* Vol.9, No.8, (August 2009), pp. 1073-1086, ISSN 1471-2598

Nishikawa, K., Hoshino, Y., Taniguchi, K., Green, K.Y., Greenberg, H.B., Kapikian, A.Z., Chanock, R.M., & Gorziglia, M. (1989). Rotavirus VP7 neutralization epitopes of serotype 3 strains. *Virology,* Vol.171, No.2, (August 1989), pp. 503-515, ISSN 0042-6822

Nokes, D.J., Peenze, I., Netshifhefhe, L., Abwao, J., De Beer, M.C., Seheri, M., Williams, T.N., Page, N., & Steele, D. (2010). Rotavirus genetic diversity, disease association and temporal change in hospitalized rural Kenyan children. *Journal of Infectious Diseases*, Vol.202, Suppl., (September 2010), pp. S180-S186, ISSN 0022-1899

Norrby, E. (2007). Yellow fever and Max Theiler: the only Nobel Prize for a virus vaccine. *Journal of Experimental Medicine*, Vol.204, No.12, (November 2007), pp. 2779-2784, ISSN 0022-1007

Ohshima, A., Takagi T., Nakagomi T., Matsuno S., & Nakagomi O. (1990). Molecular characterization by RNA-RNA hybridization of a serotype 8 human rotavirus with a super-short RNA electropherotype. *Journal of Medical Virology*, Vol.30, No.2, (February 1990), pp. 107-112, ISSN 1096-9071

Okada, J., Urasawa, T., Kobayashi, N., Taniguchi, K., Hasegawa, A., Mise, K., & Urasawa, S. (2000). New P serotype of group A human rotavirus closely related to that of a porcine rotavirus. *Journal of Medical Virology*, Vol.60, No.1, (January 2000), pp. 63-69, ISSN 1096-9071

Palombo, E.A. & Bishop, R.F. (1995). Genetic and antigenic characterization of a serotype G6 human rotavirus isolated in Melbourne, Australia. *Journal of Medical Virology*, Vol.47, No.4, (December 1995), pp. 348-354, ISSN 1096-9071

Palombo, E.A. (1999). Genetic and antigenic diversity of human rotaviruses: potential impact on the success of candidate vaccines. *FEMS Microbiology Letters*, Vol.181, No.1, (December 1999), pp. 1-8, ISSN 0378-1097

Palombo, E.A., Clark, R., & Bishop, R.F. (2000). Characterization of a "European-like" serotype G8 human rotavirus isolated in Australia. *Journal of Medical Virology*, Vol.60, No.1, (January 2000), pp. 56-62, ISSN 1096-9071

Panicali, D., Davis, S.W., Weinberg, R.L., & Paoletti, E. (1983). Construction of live vaccines by using genetically engineered poxviruses: biological activity of recombinant vaccinia virus expressing influenza virus haemagglutinin. *Proceedings of the National Academy of Sciences USA*, Vol.80, No.17, (September 1983), pp. 5364-5368, ISSN 0027-8424

Paoletti, E., Lipinskas, B.R., Samsanoff, C., Mercer, S., & Panicali, D. (1984). Construction of live vaccines using genetically engineered poxviruses: biological activity of vaccinia virus recombinants expressing the hepatitis B virus surface antigen and herpes simplex virus glycoprotein D. *Proceedings of the National Academy of Sciences USA*, Vol.81, No.1, (January 1984), pp. 193-197, ISSN 0027-8424

Park, S.I., Matthijnssens, J., Saif, L.J., Kim, H.J., Park, J.G., Alfajaro, M.M., Kim, D.S., Son, K.Y., Yang, D.K., Hyun, B.H., Kang, M.I., & Cho, K.O. (2011). Reassortment among bovine, porcine and human rotavirus strains results in G8P[7] and G6P[7] strains isolated from cattle in South Korea. *Veterinary Microbiology*, Vol.152, No.1-2, (August 2011), pp. 55-66, ISSN 0378-1135

Parra, G.I. & Espinola, E.E. (2006). Nucleotide mismatches between the VP7 gene and the primer are associated with genotyping failure of a specific lineage from G1 rotavirus strains. *Virology Journal*, Vol.3, (May 2006), pp. 35, ISSN 1743-422X

Parwani, A.V., Hussein, H.A., Rosen, B.I., Lucchelli, A., Navarro, L., & Saif, L.J. (1993). Characterization of field strains of group A bovine rotaviruses by using polymerase chain reaction-generated G and P type-specific cDNA probes. *Journal of Clinical Microbiology*, Vol.31, No.8, (August 1993), pp. 2010-2015, ISSN 0095-1137

Pattara, K., Aksara, T., Natthawan, C., Pattranuch, C., Shoko, O., Hiroshi, U., & Niwat, M. (2009). Evolutionary consequences of G9 rotaviruses circulating in Thailand. Infection, Genetics and Evolution, Vol.9, No.2, (December 2009), pp. 1394-1399, ISSN 1567-1348

Payne, D.C., Edwards, K.M., Bowen, M.D., Keckley, E., Peters, J., Esona, M.D., Teel, E.N., Kent, D., Parashar, U.D., & Gentsch, J.R. (2010). Sibling Transmission of Vaccine-Derived Rotavirus (RotaTeq) Associated With Rotavirus Gastroenteritis. *Pediatrics*, Vol.125, No.2, (February 1), pp. e438-e441, ISSN 0031-4005

Penelope, H.D. (2008). Rotavirus Vaccines: an Overview. *Clinical Microbiology Reviews*, Vol.21, No.1, (January 2008), pp. 198-208, ISSN 0893-8512

Perez-Schael, I., Guntinas, M.J., Perez, M., Pagone, V., Rojas, A.M., Gonzalez, R., Cunto, W., Hoshino, Y., & Kapikian, A.Z. (1997). Efficacy of the rhesus rotavirus-based quadrivalent vaccine in infants and young children in Venezuela. *New England Journal of Medicine*, Vol.337, (October 1997), pp. 1181-1187, ISSN 1533-4406

Perkus, M.E., Piccini, A., Lipinskas, B.R., & Paoletti, E. (1985). Recombinant vaccinia virus: immunisation against multiple pathogens. *Science*, Vol.229, No.4717, (September 1985), pp. 981-984, ISSN 0036-8075

Pongsuwanna, Y., Guntapong, R., Chiwakul, M., Tacharoenmuang, R., Onvimala, N., Wakuda, M., Kobayashi, N., & Taniguchi, K. (2002). Detection of a human rotavirus with G12 and P[9] specificity in Thailand. *Journal of Clinical Microbiology*, Vol.40, No.4, (April 2002), pp. 1390-1394, ISSN 0095-1137

Prevots, D.R., Sutter, R.W., Quick, L., Izurieta, H., & Strebel, P.M. (1996). Vaccine-associated paralytic poliomyelitis in the United States, 1980-1994: current risk and potential impact of a proposed sequential schedule of IPV followed by OPV [Abstract H90]. *Program and Abstracts of the 36th Interscience Conference on Antimicrobial Agents and Chemotherapy*, Washington, (September 1996)

Pringle, C.R. (1996). Temperature-sensitive mutant vaccines. *Methods in Molecular Medicine*, Vol.4, (n.d.), pp. 17-32, ISSN 1543-1894

Rahman, M., De Leener, K., Goegebuer, T., Wollants, E., Van der Donck, I., Van Hoovels, L., & Van Ranst, M. (2003). Genetic characterization of a novel, naturally occurring recombinant human G6P[6] rotavirus. *Journal of Clinical Microbiology*, Vol.41, No.5, (May 2003), pp. 2088-2095, ISSN 0095-1137

Rahman, M., Matthijnssens, J., Nahar, S., Podder, G., Sack, D.A., Azim, T., & Van Ranst, M. (2005a). Characterization of a novel P[25]G11 human group a rotavirus. *Journal of Clinical Microbiology*, Vol.43, No.7, (July 2005), pp. 3208-3212, ISSN 0095-1137

Rahman, M., Sultana, R., Podder, G., Faruque, A.S., Matthijnssens, J., Zaman, K., Breiman, R.F., Sack, D.A., Van Ranst, M., & Azim, T. (2005b). Typing of human rotaviruses: Nucleotide mismatches between the VP7 gene and primer are associated with genotyping failure. *Virology Journal*, Vol.2, (March 2005), pp. 24-28, ISSN 1743-422X

Rahman, M., Sultana, R., Ahmed, G., Nahar, S., Hassan, Z.M., Saiada, F., Podder, G., Faruque, A.S., Siddique, A.K., Sack, D.A., Matthijnssens, J., Van Ranst, M., & Azim, T. (2007). Prevalence of G2P[4] and G12P[6] rotavirus, Bangladesh. *Emerging Infectious Diseases*, Vol.13, No.1, (January 2007), pp. 18-24, ISSN 1080-6059

Rao, C.D., Gowda, K., & Reddy, B.S. (2000). Sequence analysis of VP4 and VP7 genes of nontypeable strains identifies a new pair of outer capsid proteins representing novel P and G genotypes in bovine rotaviruses. *Virology*, Vol.276, No.1, (October 2000), pp. 104-113, ISSN 0042-6822

Rennels, M.B., Glass, R.I., Dennehy, P.H., Bernstein, D.I., Pichichero, M.E., Zito, E.T., Mack, M.E., Davidson, B.L., & Kapikian, A.Z. (1996). Safety and efficacy of high-dose rhesus-human reassortant rotavirus vaccines—report of the National Multicenter Trial. *Pediatrics*, Vol.97, No.1, (January 1996), pp. 7-13, ISSN 0031-4005

Rice, C.M., Franke, C.A., Strauss, J.H., & Hruby, D.E. (1985). Expression of Sindbisvirus structural proteins via recombinant vaccinia virus: synthesis, proceeding and incorporation into mature Sindbis virions. *Journal of Virology*, Vol.56, No.1, (October 1985), pp. 227-239, ISSN 0022-538X

Ruiz, A.M., Lopez, I.V., Lopez, S., Espejo, R.T., & Arias, C.F. (1988). Molecular and antigenic characterization of porcine rotavirus YM, a possible new rotavirus serotype. *Journal of Virology*, Vol.62, No.11, (November 1988), pp. 4331-4336, ISSN 0022-538X

Ruiz-Palacios, G.M., Pérez-Schael, I., Velázquez, F.R., Abate, H., Breuer, T., Clemens, S.C., Cheuvart, B., Espinoza, F., Gillard, P., Innis, B.L., Cervantes, Y., Linhares, A.C., López, P., Macías-Parra, M., Ortega-Barría, E., Richardson, V., Rivera-Medina, D.M., Rivera, L., Salinas, B., Pavía-Ruz, N., Salmerón, J., Rüttimann, R., Tinoco, J.C., Rubio, P., Nuñez, E., Guerrero, M.L., Yarzábal, J.P., Damaso, S., Tornieporth, N., Sáez-Llorens, X., Vergara, R.F., Vesikari, T., Bouckenooghe, A., Clemens, R., De Vos, B., & O'Ryan, M. (2006). Safety and efficacy of an attenuated vaccine against severe gastroenteritis. *New England Journal of Medicine*, Vol.354, No.1, (January 2006), pp. 11-22, ISSN 1533-4406

Santos, N., Lima, R.C.C., Pereira, C.F.A., & Gouvea, V. (1998). Detection of rotavirus types G8 and G10 among Brazilian children with diarrhea. *Journal of Clinical Microbiology*, Vol.36, No.9, (September 1998), pp. 2727-2729, ISSN 0095-1137

Santos, N., Volotão, E.M., Soares, C.C., Albuquerque, M.C., da Silva, F.M., Chizhikov, V., & Hoshino, Y. (2002). VP7 gene polymorphism of serotype G9 rotavirus strains and its impact on G genotype determination by PCR. *Virus Research*, Vol.90, No.1-2, (December 2002), pp. 1-14, ISSN 0168-1702

Santos, N., Volotão, E.M., Soares, C.C., Albuquerque, M.C., da Silva, F.M., Chizhikov, V., & Hoshino, Y. (2003). VP7 gene polymorphism of serotype G9 rotavirus strains and its impact on G genotype determination by PCR. *Virus Research*, Vol.93, No.1, (May 2003), pp. 127-138, ISSN 0168-1702

Santos, N., & Hoshino, Y. (2005). Global distribution of rotavirus serotypes/genotypes and its implication for the development and implementation of an effective rotavirus vaccine. *Reviews in Medical Virology*, Vol.15, No.1, (January-February 2005), pp. 29-56, ISSN 1099-1654

Santosham, M., Moulton, L.H., Reid, R., Croll, J., Weatherholt, R., Ward, R., Forro, J., Zito, E., Mack, M., Brenneman, G., & Davidson, B.L. (1997). Efficacy and safety of high-dose rhesus-human reassortant rotavirus vaccine in Native American populations. *Journal of Pediatrics*, Vol.131, No.4, (October 1997), pp. 632-638, ISSN 0022-3476

Sereno, M.M., & Gorziglia, M.I. (1994). The outer capsid protein VP4 of murine rotavirus strain Eb represents a tentative new P type. *Virology*, Vol.199, No.2, (March 1994), pp. 500-504, ISSN 0042-6822

Shinozaki, K., Okada, M., Nagashima, S., Kaiho, I., & Taniguchi, K. (2004). Characterization of human rotavirus strains with G12 and P[9] detected in Japan. *Journal of Medical Virology*, Vol.73, No.4, (August 2004), pp. 612-616, ISSN 1096-9071

Smith, G. L., Mackett, M., & Moss, B. (1983). Infectious vaccinia virus recombinants that express hepatitis B surface antigen. *Nature*, Vol.302, (April 1983), pp. 490-495, ISSN 0028-0836

Steele, A.D., Parker, S.P., Peenze, I., Pager, C.T., Taylor, M.B., & Cubitt, W.D. (1999). Comparative studies of human rotavirus serotype G8 strains recovered in South Africa and the United Kingdom. *Journal of General Virology*, Vol.80, No.11, (November 1999), pp. 3029-3034, ISSN 1465-2099

Stefan, R. (2005). Edward Jenner and the history of smallpox and vaccination. *BUMC Proceedings*, Vol.18, No.1, (January 2005), pp. 21-25, ISSN 0899-8280

Tam, D-T., Salaheddin, M.M., Riccardo, P., & Eduardo, L.F. (2004). Polio vaccines, Simian Virus 40, and human cancer: the epidemiologic evidence for a causal association. *Oncogene*, Vol.23, (n.d.), pp. 6535-6540, ISSN 0950-9232

Taniguchi, K., Urasawa, T., Kobayashi, N., Gorziglia, M., & Urasawa, S. (1990). Nucleotide sequence of VP4 and VP7 genes of human rotaviruses with subgroup I specificity and long RNA pattern: implication for new serotype specificity. *Journal of Virology*, Vol.64, No.11, (November 1990), pp. 5640-5644, ISSN 0022-538X

Timenetsky Mdo, C., Gouvea, V., Santos, N., Carmona, R.C., & Hoshino, Y. (1997). A novel human rotavirus serotype with dual G5/G11 specificity. *Journal of General Virology*, Vol.78, No.6, (June 1997), pp. 1373-1378, ISSN 1465-2099

Trinh, Q.D., Pham, N.T., Nguyen, T.A., Phan, T.G., Khamrin, P., Yan, H., Hoang, P.L., Maneekarn, N., Li, Y., Kozlov, V., Kozlov, A., Okitsu, S., & Ushijima, H. (2007). Amino acid substitutions in the VP7 protein of human rotavirus G3 isolated in China, Russia, Thailand, and Vietnam during 2001–2004. *Journal of Medical Virology*, Vol.79, No.10, (October 2007), pp. 1611-1616, ISSN 1096-9071

Turner, G.S., Squires, E.J., & Murray, H.G.S. (1970). Inactivated smallpox vaccine. A comparison of inactivation methods. *Journal of Hygiene*, Vol.68, No.2, (June 1970), pp. 197-210, ISSN 0022-1724

Tung, G.P., Shoko, O., Niwat, M., & Hiroshi, U. (2007). Evidence of Intragenic Recombination in G1 Rotavirus VP7 Genes. *Journal of Virology*, Vol.81, No.18, (September 2007), pp. 10188-10194, ISSN 0022-538X

Uchida, R., Pandey, B.D., Sherchand, J.B., Ahmed, K., Yokoo, M., Nakagomi, T., Cuevas, L.E., Cunliffe, N.A., Hart, C.A., & Nakagomi, O. (2006). Molecular epidemiology of rotavirus diarrhea among children and adults in Nepal: detection of G12 strains with P[6] or P[8] and a G11P[25] strain. *Journal of Clinical Microbiology*, Vol. 44, No.10, (October 2006), pp. 3499-3505, ISSN 0095-1137

Ulmer, J.B., Donnelly, J.J., Parker, S.E., Rhodes, G.H., Felgner, P.L., Dwarki, V.J., Gromkowski, S.H., Deck, R.R., DeWitt, C.M., Friedman, D., Perry, H.C., Shiver, J.W., Montgomery, D.L., & Liu, M.A. (1993). Heterologous protection against influenza by injection of DNA encoding a viral protein. *Science*, Vol.259, No.5102, (March 1993), pp. 1745-1749, ISSN 0036-8075

Vesikari, T., Isolauri, E., D'Hondt, E., Delem, A., André, F.E., & Zissis, G. (1984). Protection of infants against rotavirus diarrhea by RIT 4237 attenuated bovine rotavirus strain vaccine. *Lancet*, Vol.5, No.1, (May 1984), pp. 977-981, ISSN 0140-6736

Vesikari, T., Matson, D.O., Dennehy, P., Van Damme, P., Santosham, M., Rodriguez, Z., Dallas, M.J., Heyse, J.F., Goveia, M.G., Black, S.B., Shinefield, H.R., Christie, C.D., Ylitalo, S., Itzler, R.F., Coia, M.L., Onorato, M.T., Adeyi, B.A., Marshall, G.S., Gothefors, L., Campens, D., Karvonen, A., Watt, J.P., O'Brien, K.L., DiNubile, M.J., Clark, H.F., Boslego, J.W., Offit, P.A., & Heaton, P.M. (2006). Safety and Efficacy of a pentavalent human-bovine (WC3) reassortant rotavirus vaccine. *New England Journal of Medicine*, Vol.354, No.1, (January 2006), pp. 23-33, ISSN 1533-4406

Vesikari, T., Karvonen, A., Allen, F.S., & Ciarlet, M. (2010). Efficacy of the pentavalent rotavirus vaccine, RotaTeq®, in Finnish infants up to 3 years of age: the Finnish Extension Study. *European Journal of Pediatrics*, Vol. 169, No.11, (November 2010), pp. 1379-1386, ISSN 1432-1076

Vyas, G.N. & Blum, H.E. (1984). Hepatitis B virus infection-Current concepts of chronicity and immunity. *West Journal of Medicine*, Vol.140, No.5, (May 1984), pp. 754-762, ISSN 0093-0415

Weil, A.J. & Gall, L.S. (1940). Studies on the immunization of rabbits with formalinized vaccine virus. *Journal of Immunology*, Vol.38, No.1, (January 1940), pp. 1-8, ISSN 0022-1767

Wen, L., Nakayama, M., Yamanishi, Y., Nishio, O., Fang, Z.-Y., Nakagomi, O., Araki, K., Nishimura, S., Hasegawa, A., Müller, W.E.G., & Ushijima, H. (1997). Genetic variation in the VP7 gene of human rotavirus serotype 3 (G3 type) isolated in China and Japan. *Archives of Virology*, Vol.142, No.7, (July 1997), pp. 1481-1489, ISSN 1432-8798

Wiktor, T.J., Macfarlan, R.I., Reagan, K.J., Dietzschold, B., Curtis, P.J., Wunner, W.H., Kieny, M.P., Lathe, R., Lecocq, J.P., Mackett, M., Moss, B., & Koprowski, H. (1984). Protection from rabies by a vaccinia virus recombinant containing the rabies virus glycoprotein gene. *Proceedings of the National Academy of Sciences USA*, Vol.81, No.22, (November 1984), pp. 7194-7198, ISSN 0027-8424

Wolff, J.A., Malone, R.W., Williams, P., Chong, W., Acsadi, G., Jani, A., & Felgner, P.L. (1990). Direct gene transfer into mouse muscle in vivo. *Science*, Vol.247, No.4949, (March 1990), pp. 1465-1468, ISSN 0036-8075

World Health Organization, 2000, Geneva, (February 2000), Available from: www.who.int/vaccines-documents/, Report of the meeting on the Future Directions for Rotavirus Vaccine Research in Developing Countries

Yap, I., Guan, R., & Chan, S.H. (1992). Recombinant DNA hepatitis B vaccine containing Pre-S components of the HBV coat protein-preliminary study on immunogenicity. *Vaccine*, Vol.10, No.7, (n.d.), pp. 439-442, ISSN 0264-410X

Zissis, G., Lambert, J.P., Marbehant, P., Marissens, D., Lobmann, M., Charlier, P., Delem, A., & Zygraich, N. (1983). Protection studies in colostrum-deprived piglets of a bovine rotavirus vaccine candidate using human rotavirus strains for challenge. *Journal of Infectious Diseases*, Vol.148, No.6, (December 1983), pp. 1061-1068, ISSN 0022-1899

7

Molecular Attenuation Process in Live Vaccine Generation for Arenaviruses

Sandra Elizabeth Goñi and Mario Enrique Lozano
Laboratorio de Ingeniería Genética y Biología Celular y Molecular, Área de Virosis Emergentes y Zoonóticas, Dept. of Sciences and Technology, National University of Quilmes, Argentina

1. Introduction

The arenaviruses are part of a growing viral family denominated *Arenaviridae*. Currently, there are 22 recognized members (Salvato *et al.*, 2005), listed in Table 1. Based on the geographic origin and distribution of their hosts, the arenaviruses can be classified in two groups: the New World Arenaviruses (NWA) and the Old World Arenaviruses (OWA). The first group comprised native American arenaviruses, while the Old World group is conformed by African viruses and the ubiquitous Lymphocytic Choriomeningitis virus (LCMV). This geographic distribution is determined by the species host range, with LCMV as the only one arenavirus with a worldwide distribution, mainly because *Mus musculus* is its rodent reservoir. Specific members of *Neotominae* and *Sigmodontinae* from the *Cricetidae* rodent's family are the principal hosts for the New World Arenaviruses (Cajimat *et al.*, 2007). From these 22 recognized species, only 6 were consistently detected in humans and were related to a set of clinical symptoms that allowed to establish the description of a disease: Lymphocytic Choriomeningitis (LCM, caused by LCMV), Lassa Fever (LF caused by LASV), Argentine Hemorrhagic Fever (AHF, caused by JUNV), Bolivian Hemorrhagic Fever (BHF, caused by MACV), Venezuelan Hemorrhagic Fever (VHF, caused by GTOV), and Brazilian Hemorrhagic Fever (BrHF, caused by SABV). The physiopathology of the hemorrhagic fevers produced by NWA is very similar. AHF and BHF were described in the middle of the twentieth century. GTOV was isolated from humans during an epidemic outbreak (at first mistaken for hemorrhagic dengue) that happened in Venezuela (Salas *et al.*, 1991). Because GTOV and PIRV share the same (geographic) area, different studies were made with the aim of predicting a re-emergence of a Venezuelan hemorrhagic fever variant (Cajimat & Fulhorst, 2004). The Brazilian hemorrhagic fever was established from a human fatal case, isolating the SABV (Lisieux *et al.*, 1994). Recently, a serological screening for arenavirus among the population of Nova Xavantina, State of Mato Grosso in Brazil, show that 1,4% of the serum samples presented antibody titers against arenavirus (Machado *et al.*, 2010).

In 2003 a hemorrhagic fever case was reported in Bolivia, and after an exhaustive analysis a new virus, denominated Chapare, was described (Delgado *et al.*, 2008). On the other side, in the year 2000, another three isolated cases were reported, one of them, related to WWAV, was a classical hemorrhagic fever (CDC, 2000), while the others, related to TCRV and FLEV, were mild feverish illness in laboratory workers (Charrel *et al.*, 2008).

Virus	Acronym	Evolutionary Lineage	Distribution	Reservoir	Human Disease
Flexal	FLEV	NWA-A	Brazil	*Oryzomys spp.*	LM
Pichindé	PICV	NWA-A	Colombia	*O. albigularis*	NR
Paraná	PARV	NWA-A	Paraguay	*O. buccinatus*	NR
Allpahuayo	ALLV	NWA-A	Perú	*Oecomys bicolor*	NR
Pirital	PIRV	NWA-A	Venezuela	*Sigmodon alstoni*	NR
Junín	JUNV	NWA-B	Argentina	*C. musculinus*	SD
Machupo	MACV	NWA-B	Bolivia	*C. callosus, C. laucha*	SD
Guanarito	GTOV	NWA-B	Venezuela	*Z. brevicauda*	SD
Sabia	SABV	NWA-B	Brazil	*Unknown*	LS
Chapare	-	NWA-B	Bolivia	*Unknown*	LS
Pinhal	-	NWA-B	Brazil	*Calomys tener*	NR
Tacaribe	TCRV	NWA-B	Trinidad	*Artibeus spp.*	LM
Cupixi	CPXV	NWA-B	Brazil	*O. capita*	NR
Amapari	AMAV	NWA-B	Brazil	*O. capita-N. guianae*	NR
Oiveros	OLVV	NWA-C	Argentina	*Bolomys obscurus*	NR
Pampa	-	NWA-C	Argentina	*Bolomys sp.*	NR
Latino	LATV	NWA-C	Bolivia	*Calomys callosus*	NR
Río Carcarañá	-	NWA	Argentina	*Bolomys obscurus*	NR
Catarina	-	NWA-RecA/B	USA, Texas	*Neotoma micropus*	NR
Skinner Tank	-	NWA-RecA/B	USA, Arizona	*Neotoma mexicana*	NR
North American	-	NWA-Rec A/B	USA	*Neotoma mexicana*	NR
Withewater Arroyo	WWAV	NWA-RecA/B	USA, Southwest	*N. albigula, N. mexicana*	LS
Tamiami	TAMV	NWA-RecA/B	USA, Florida	*Sigmodon hispidus*	NR
Bear Canyon	BCNV	NWA-RecA/B	USA, California	*Peromyscus sp.*	NR
Big Brushy Tank	-	NWA-Rec A/B	USA		
Tonto Creek	-	NWA-Rec A/B	USA		
LCM	LCMV	OWA	All world	*Mus musculus*	MD
Lassa	LASV	OWA	Nigeria, Ivory Coast, Guinea, Sierra Leone	*Mastomys sp.*	SD
Mopeia	MOPV	OWA	Mozambique	*Mastomys natalensis*	NR
Mobala	MOBV	OWA	Central African Republic	*Praomys sp.*	NR
Ippy	IPPYV	OWA	Central African Republic	*Arvicanthis sp.*	NR
Dandenong	-	OWA	Australia	*Unknown*	LM
Kodoko	-	OWA	Guinea	*Mus Nannomys minutoides*	NR
Morogoro	-	OWA	Tanzania	*Mastomys sp.*	NR
Lujo	-	OWA	South Africa	*Unknown*	LS

SD: Severe disease; MD: Mild disease; LS: Limited and severe disease; LM: Limited and mild disease; NR: not reported; OWA: Old World Arenavirus; NWA: New World Arenavirus; thereafter is indicated the lineage in which the New World members are classified: A, B, C and Rec A/B. The countries are listed based on viral isolation and not serology data. Table modified from Charrel & de Llambarie, 2003 and Charrel *et al.*, 2008.

Table 1. *Arenaviridae* family members list.

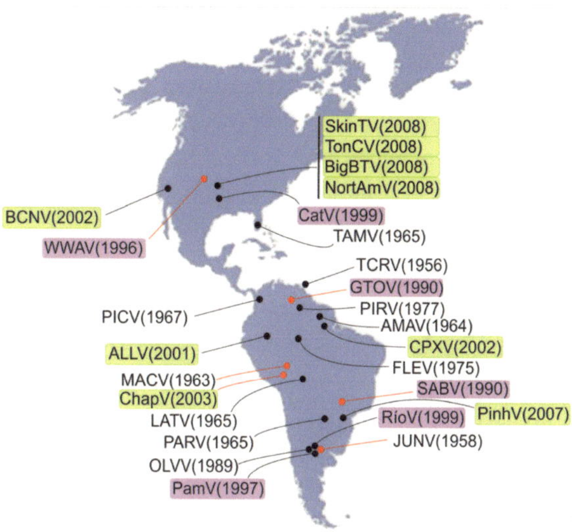

Fig. 1. Geographic distribution of New World Arenaviruses. The black points indicate those viruses not described as human pathogens, while the red points indicate the known pathogens that cause the different American hemorrhagic fevers. After each viral acronym, the year of isolation or description is added. The viruses identified after the year 2000 are shadowed in green, while those isolated in the past century's ´90s decade are in violet. The virus acronyms are indicated in Table 1, with the exception of the following: ChapV (Chapare), PamV (Pampa); RíoV (Río Carcarañá); PinhV (Pinhal); CatV (Catarina); NortAmV (North American); BigBTV (Big Brushy Tank); TontCV (Tonto Creek); and SkinTV (Skinner Tank), because they were not yet included as recognized arenavirus member.

In the course of the year 2008 the Dandenong virus was characterized, isolated from a transplanted patient, showing a high homology with LCMV (Palacios *et al.*, 2008). In that same year an outbreak of human nosocomial disease was reported in South Africa, with a high mortality rate (80%) and whose etiological agent was later characterized as an arenavirus. After 30 years, a new emerging member of the OWA group that caused a hemorrhagic fever (Briese *et al.*, 2009) was discovered. This virus was denominated Lujo virus, because the places where the first patients came from, the cities of Lusaka and Johannesburg. As can be seen in Figure 1, there is an evident increase in the information about arenavirus circulation in different places, with surprising findings in North America. Probably, their description is due to the active rodent capture program in different regions of USA and the search for arenaviral sequences by molecular techniques (with or without viral isolation). Most of these viruses still have to undergo taxonomic classification.

The LCM virus, detected in humans and rodents (Armostrong & Sweet, 1939; Lepine *et al.*, 1937; Rivers & Scott, 1935), is the causative agent of lymphocytic choriomeningitis and although it was associated to aseptic meningitis their infections in humans are unapparent in most cases. This virus has been a very important tool in the description of immunological mechanisms (Oldstone, 1987a, 1987b). The other arenaviruses, with the exception of LCMV, are found in restricted areas around the world. In fact, LCMV was also isolated in the AHF endemic region (Maiztegui *et al.*, 1972; Sabattini, 1977), where other arenavirus isolations were made, including OLVV and PamV which could be a variety of the same viral species. Another yet not completely characterized virus isolated in the AHF endemic area was denominated Río Carcarañá, and from the sequence data it could be a product of a recombination event between arenaviruses from lineages B and C. The arenavirus hemorrhagic fevers are characterized by a disease that develops in well-defined phases: prodromal, neurologic-hemorrhagic and convalescent (Enría *et al.*, 2004), with a short incubation period, high fever, headaches and a set of specific symptoms that depend on the arenavirus species related with the infection. The principal characteristics of the arenaviral hemorrhagic fevers are indicated in Table 2.

Agent (Virus)	Pathological Characteristics
Old World Lassa	Incubation: 3 to 21 days. Fever, headaches, myalgia, backaches, trembling and sickness. Generalized infection: hemorrhagic dissemination of the virus to several organs and systems via bloodstream, lymphatic system, respiratory and digestive tract. Black vomit, aqueous diarrhea (dehydration), decrease in quantity of lymphocyts and platelets, mild thrombocytopenia, abdominal, pleuritic and hepatic area pain. Extensive reticuloendothelial compromise: capillary injuries causing stomach, small intestine, kidneys, lungs and brain bleeding. Multifocal hepatocellular necrosis with Councilman-like bodies, hepatocites citoplasmatic degeneration and minimal inflammatory response. Adrenal focal necrosis and citoplasmatic inclusions. Respiratory system: interstitial pneumonia, cough, dyspnea, bronchitis, pneumonia and pleurisy. Cardiovascular system: pericarditis, tachycardia, bradycardia, hypertension, hypotension, thrombocytopenia, leukopenia and hiperuraemia, lymphadenopathy, elevated aminotransferases, decreased prothrombin levels, disorder of blood circulation and bleeding through the skin, lungs, gastrointestinal tract and other membranes mucosa. Nervous system: encephalitis, meningitis, uni- or bilateral hearing decrease, or convulsions.
New World Junín Machupo Guanarito Sabiá	Incubation: 6 to 14 days. First 4: decaying, fever, anorexia, nausea and vomiting, headaches and myalgia. Second stage: acute hemorrhagic syndrome (epistaxis and hematemesis, Melcom & Herskovits, 1981), or acute neurologic syndrome (Rugiero *et al.*, 1960). General: malaise, high fever, severe myalgia, anorexia, back pain, abdominal tenderness, conjunctivitis, retro-orbital pain, photophobia, and constipation. Acute phase of infection: lymphomonocytes periferic blood viral active replication (Ambrosio *et al.*, 1986). Oropharyngeal enanthem. Gums swollen, congested and bleeding (gingival border). Proteinuria high dehydration and hemoconcentration. In women, early menorrhagia. Multifocal hepatocellular necrosis with formation of Councilman-like bodies, nuclear pyknosis, cytoplasmic eosinophilia, cytolysis, inflammation and a mild cellular infiltration composed of mononuclear cells and neutrophils. Kidney damage: distal tubular cells and collecting ducts. Glomeruli or proximal tubules (Cossio *et al.*, 1975). In a few cases the presence of renal failure was described (Agrest *et al.*, 1969). Cardiovascular system: postural hypotension and relative bradycardia, arrhythmias are transient and benign. Different degrees of dehydration, uremia, proteinuria, hematuria and oliguria. Respiratory: dry cough, without sore throat. Pharyngeal enanthem broncho-pulmonary unchanged. Interstitial pneumonia or bronchial, pulmonary edema and hemorrhage.

Table 2. Arenaviral hemorrhagic fevers pathological characteristics. The principal pathological characteristics caused by Old World Arenaviruses (LASV, Lassa Fever), and New World Arenaviruses (JUNV, Argentinean Hemorrhagic Fever; MACV, Bolivian Hemorrhagic Fever; GTOV, Venezuelan Hemorrhagic Fever; SABV, Brazilian Hemorrhagic Fever) are listed.

As previously described, Argentine hemorrhagic fever (AHF) is a severe endemoepidemic disease characterized by vascular, renal, hematological, neurological, and immunological alterations with a mortality of 15 to 30% in untreated individuals. Since the disease was first recognized, annual outbreaks have occurred without interruption, principally in autumn and winter (Ambrosio *et al.*, 2006). In Figure 3 it is possible to see the number of notified and confirmed cases until 2008 (Enría *et al.*, 2008; Iserte *et al.*, 2010). In this figure, the black arrow indicates the start of vaccination of the population at risk at the endemic area, reflecting the decrease in the AHF annual case numbers. The vaccine efficacy for the 1992-2000 periods was estimated in a 98% (AHF National Control Program, 2007).

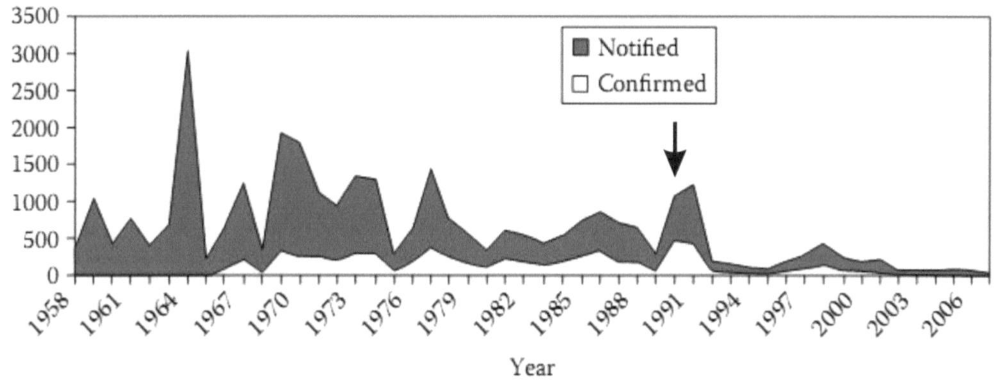

The arrow indicates the start of vaccination.

Fig. 3. AHF notified and confirmed cases (1958–2006).

The attempts to obtain a vaccine against AHF started in 1959. A collaborative effort conducted by the US and Argentine Governments led to the production of a live attenuated Junin virus vaccine. After rigorous biological testing in rhesus monkeys, the highly attenuated Junin virus variant, named Candid#1, was used in human volunteers, followed by an extensive clinical trial in the AHF endemic area. (Barrera Oro & Eddy, 1982, Maiztegui *et al.*, 1987). The vaccination consists in the administration of JUNV Candid#1 to generate the protective immune response. The diagram with the passage history in different systems until the attenuated strain was obtained can be observed in Figure 4. Records of the passage history of the XJ strain come from the Yale Arbovirus Research Unit, Connecticut, USA (J. Casals) and USAMRIID, Frederick, Maryland, USA (J. G. Barrera Oro). The phase I and II clinical studies were made between 1984 and 1988 in Argentine and USA. After these studies it was shown that Candid#1 is innocuous, because none of the inoculated volunteers presented alterations and the immunogenicity was demonstrated in 90% of the cases. Since 2005 the vaccine is being produced in the National Institute of Viral Human Diseases (INEVH) located in Pergamino city, Argentina.

For other arenaviruses, was not yet possible to obtain an effective vaccine to prevent the disease. This would be especially important for Lassa fever, which is endemic in West Africa with up to 500.000 reported cases (Ogbu *et al.*, 2007). In the effort to make an efficient vaccine to combat Lassa fever in Africa, several strategies were applied. One of them, is based upon generation of a reassortant virus that contains a genomic segment from Mopeia virus (non pathogenic) and the other segment from Lassa virus (Lukashevich *et al.*, 2005). The obtained results are promising, but still have to demonstrate coverage of all natural variants of Lassa virus to ensure the protective capacity of a vaccine.

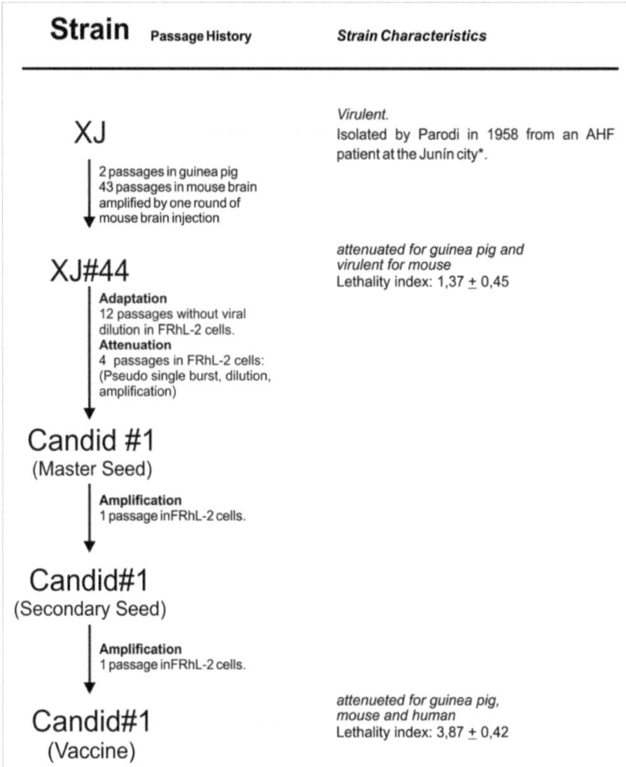

Fig. 4. Passage history of Junín virus, strain Candid#1. The genealogical relationships of the studied Junín virus strains are shown by arrows. The XJ strain was subjected to two passages in guinea-pigs (GP2) and 43 passages in mouse brain (MB43). Passage number 43 was amplified by one round of mouse brain injection (XJ#44). This brain homogenate was used to infect FRhL-2 cells. After 12 passages, one pseudo single burst growth was carried out, followed by cloning using two limiting dilution steps. After one amplification round, master and secondary seeds were obtained. The vaccine stock (Candid#1) was obtained by single amplification of the secondary seed. The lethality index was calculated as log10 p.f.u. that produce one LD50 (±1 SD) by intracerebral inoculation of mice (Parodi *et al.*, 1958).

2. Molecular features of arenaviruses

All arenaviruses shared morphological and biochemical properties. They are enveloped and their genome is composed of bipartite RNA (Martínez Segovia & Grazioli, 1969; Riviere *et al.*, 1985b). These RNAs are single-stranded and posses an approximate length of 7 kb (L RNA) and 3,5 kb (RNA S). The lipid envelope contains two viral glycoproteins, G1 and G2, inside of the virion there are three other arenavirus proteins, denominated N, Z and L. The majority of N protein is associated to the viral RNAs forming the nucleocapsids. The second, a protein of 11 kDa, is denominated Z because it has a Zinc finger structural motif and could be the counterpart of the matrix proteins of other RNA viruses (Pérez *et al.*, 2003). Furthermore, all virions contain a minimal proportion of a RNA dependent RNA polymerase, denominated L protein.

Each RNA segment directs the synthesis of two proteins; their open reading frames are arranged in opposite orientations (ambisense coding strategy) and are separated by a non-coding intergenic region that folds in a stable secondary structure (Auperin *et al.*, 1984). Furthermore, the ends of both genomic RNAs are complementary. The first 19 nucleotides at the 3' end base-pair with the complementary sequence at the 5' end forming a panhandle structure, which is conserved among the arenaviruses. The S RNA codes for the major structural proteins of the virion: the precursor of the envelope glycoproteins (GPC) and the viral nucleocapsid protein (N). Posttranslational cleavage of GPC renders a signal peptide (SP) and the two viral glycoproteins (G1 and G2). The L RNA segment codes for the viral RNA dependent RNA polymerase (L) and the small protein (Z). N and L proteins are translated from anti-genome-sense mRNAs, complementary to the 3′ portion of the viral S or L RNA, respectively. The GPC and Z proteins are translated from viral or genome-sense mRNAs corresponding to the 5′ region of the viral S or L RNA, respectively.

The secondary and tertiary structures present in the viral genomic RNAs play an essential regulatory role during the transcription, translation and assembly of new viral particles (Álvarez *et al.*, 2005). The intergenic region in both genomic fragments is arranged into a stable hairpin loop structure, which is crucial in the regulation between transcription and replication of the viral genome (Tortorici *et al.*, 2001b), while the panhandle structure at the ends of the genomic RNAs, could act as a promoter initiating replication, as occurs in Flavivirus (Álvarez *et al.*, 2005; Pérez & de la Torre, 2003; Salvato & Shimomaye, 1989).

In Figure 5, the morphological characteristics of the arenavirus particles are shown. They are pleomorphic with a diameter of 50 to 300 nm (Dalton *et al.*, 1968; Gschwender *et al.*, 1975; Murphy *et al.*, 1968, 1970; Murphy & Whitfield, 1975; Ofodile *et al.*, 1973; Speir *et al.*, 1970).

Once the virus enters the cell the ribonucleoproteins are released into the cytoplasm, and, transcription and replication are mediated by the L protein within the cytoplasm. The glycoproteins and Z are co-translated and processed in the ER and Golgi, while the N, and L proteins are translated on free ribosomes. Virus assembly initiates at the Golgi or plasma membrane. The N and L mRNAs are transcribed from the RNA S or L 3′ end, respectively. On the contrary, the GPC and Z mRNAs are transcribed from the 3′ end of the antigenomic S or L RNA. These processes and mechanisms are detailed in Figure 6.

The genomic S RNA is transcribed to only two antigenomic forms: the 1,8 kb N mRNA and the 3,4 kb full length antigenomic S RNA. This antigenomic S RNA serves as the replicative form of the virus and also as the template for GPC mRNA transcription. When translation is inhibited, transcription of Junín virus S RNA yields only the N mRNA. Apparently, the non-coding intergenic region form a secondary very stable hairpin loop acting as a transcription terminator (Franze Fernández *et al.*, 1987; Ghiringhelli *et al.*, 1991; Tortorici *et al.*, 2001a). This implies that the synthesis of a full length antigenomic copy of S RNA requires an antiterminator. This function is supplied by the N protein (Tortorici *et al.*, 2001a).

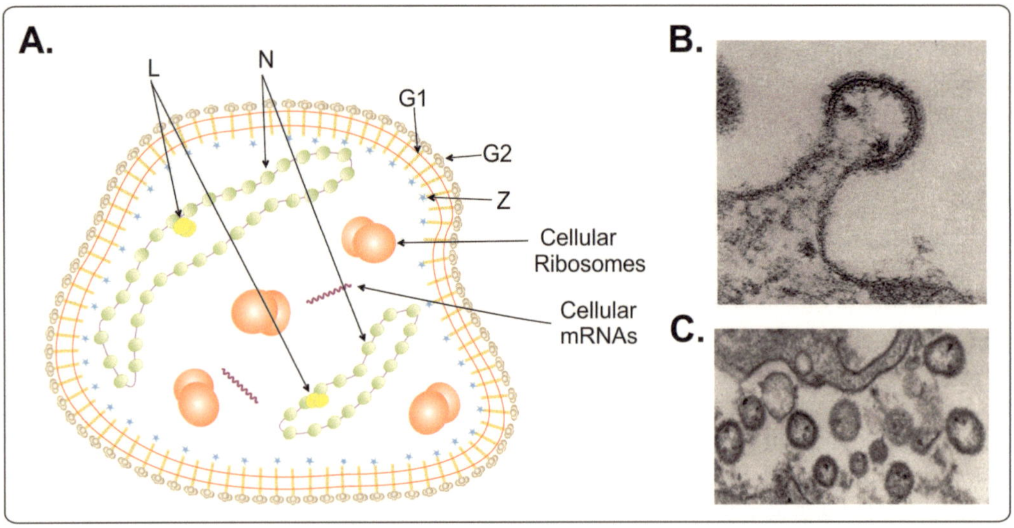

Fig. 5. Arenavirus viral particle.A. Virion structure diagram. The arenavirus particles have a lipid bilayer envelope (red lines), with envelope glycoprotein's (G1 and G2), and internal components that include two circular nucleocapsids with bead aspect, associated to the viral polymerase (L), cellular messengers and ribosomes. The nucleocapsids contain RNAs S and L and proteins (N, in several copies and L in few copies). The Z protein is found associated to the bilayer by the inner face. B. Electronic micrograph of a section showing a virion budding from an infected Vero cell. The viral envelope is more dense and different to the host cell membrane. The ribosomes are presents in the budding particle (173.000 X, Murphy *et al.*, 1968). C. Electronic micrograph of Junín virus particles in the extracellular space on the periphery of infected Vero cells (95.000 X). The particles are constituted by a heavy membrane envelope, containing several dense granules of 20 to 25 nm (Murphy *et al.*, 1970).

The glycoprotein precursor is processed into 3 peptides: the peripheral protein G1, the trans-membrane G2 and the signal peptide (Buchmeier & Oldstone, 1979; York *et al.*, 2004). Due to their characteristics, G1 is the protein that interacts with the cellular receptor. The Old World and C clade of New World arenaviruses share the same cellular receptor, the α-distroglycan (Cao *et al.*, 1998; Spiropoulou *et al.*, 2002). Later, it was found that for clade B of the New World arenaviruses, the receptor is a protein: the transferrin 1 receptor (TfR1, Radoshitzky *et al.*, 2007).

The arenavirus nucleoprotein has a weight of 63kDa and constitutes the principal component of the nucleocapsid, being the most abundant protein in the virion (near to 70%). This protein presents a dual function: structural and non-structural. On one side, it is involved in essential genome replication steps promoting the synthesis of the full length antigenomic segments, and on the other side it is associated to the viral genome to form the nucleocapsid. For that, the determinations of N-RNA interactions are very interesting study targets. Among the N described motifs, there is one RING finger domain whose folding requires zinc (Tortorici *et al.*, 2001b). There is one conserved region between amino acids 497 and 530 ($C_{497}X_2H_{500}X_{23}C_{525}X_4C_{530}$, Parisi *et al.*, 1996) and their function was experimentally studied (Tortorici *et al.*, 2001b). These results confirm the identity of the domain and also

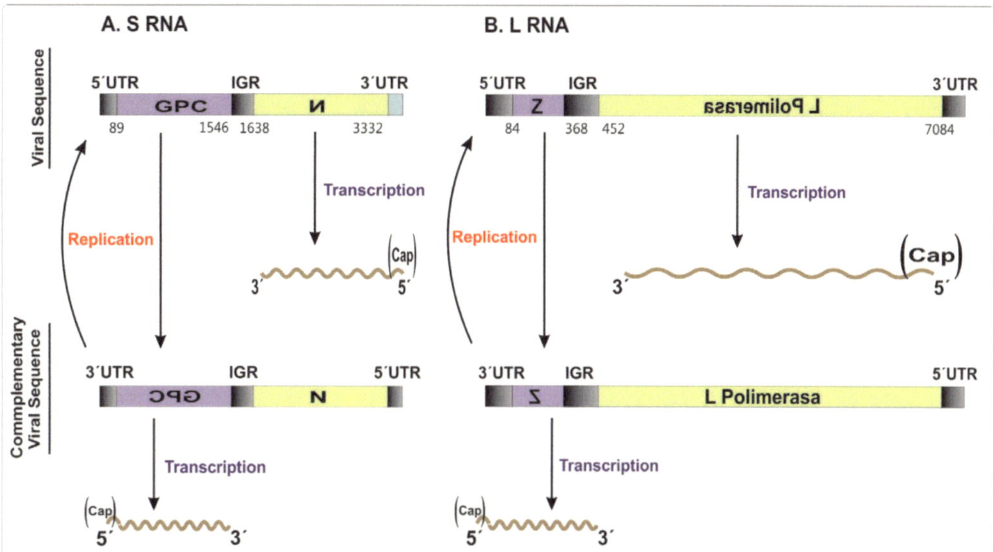

Fig. 6. Arenavirus replication/transcription strategy. The S and L genomic segments are schematized as horizontal rectangles. The ORFs that present a genomic or viral polarity (GPC and Z) are violet, while the antigenomic or viral complementary genes (N and L) are in green. The intergenic region (IGR) and untranslated terminal regions (UTR) are shown in gray. A. S RNA replication/transcription diagram. B. L RNA replication/transcription diagram.

showed the possibility of the presence of other motifs that enhance this activity. Another important functional aspect of the N protein is its capacity to avoid elimination by the adaptative immune response of the host. It was demonstrated that in LCMV infections, N inhibits the response by β-interpheron production interference (Martínez-Sobrido *et al.*, 2006).

The major ORF in the virus genome corresponds to the RNA dependent RNA polymerase denominated L protein. In the virion, this protein is associated to the viral nucleocapsid forming the ribonucleoprotein complex, and posseses the sequence motifs characteristically conserved between the RNA dependent RNA polymerases of the negative-stranded RNA viruses. The polymerase activity requires oligomerization through the formation of a L-L complex that is essential for the enzymatic function (Sánchez & de la Torre, 2005). Because of its size this protein is the target for different mutations that affect its capacity to different extents.

Finally, the smaller protein of this viral family is denominated Z protein. The role of Z in the virus life cycle is not completely elucidated, and homologues of Z are not found in other ambisense or negative-stranded RNA viruses. Z is a structural component of the virion (Salvato *et al.*, 1992), and by means of *in vivo* and *in vitro* experiments, the interaction of Z with several cellular factors has been reported, including the promyelocytic leukemia protein and the eukaryotic translation initiation factor 4E (Borden *et al.*, 1998a, b). Because of this latter interaction, it was proposed that Z inhibits Cap-mediated translation (Campbel *et al.*, 2000; Kentsis *et al.*, 2001). Other researchers suggested that Z could be a transcriptional regulator of the viral cycle (Garcín *et al.*, 1993) or even an inhibitor of viral replication (López *et al.*, 2001). Furthermore, Pérez and coworkers (Pérez *et al.*, 2003) proposed, for LCMV and

LASV, that Z is the functional counterpart of the matrix proteins found in other negative-stranded enveloped RNA viruses. Z protein have characteristic late domains (LDs), also found in matrix proteins from negative-stranded RNA viruses and in Gag protein from retroviruses. LDs, have an essential role in the viral budding process (Freed, 2002). Three types of motifs have been defined within viral LDs: P[TS]AP, PPxY, and YxxL (Pornillos *et al.*, 2002), where "x" is any amino acid. Later, Martín Serrano and coworkers (Martín Serrano *et al.*, 2004), redefined the last as: YPxL/LxxLF. LDs are highly conserved and have been shown to mediate interaction with host cell proteins, in particular with members of the vacuolar protein-sorting pathway (Bieniasz, 2006; Urata *et al.*, 2006). For instance, the PTAP motif from Ebola virus VP40 matrix protein and from HIV Gag protein interacts with Tsg101, a member of the vacuolar protein-sorting pathway.

3. Sequence analysis of the Junín virus vaccine related strains

To characterize the mutations associated with the attenuated phenotype in Junín virus, we obtained the complete nucleotide genomic sequence from the vaccine genealogy related strains and another field strains of Junin virus (Goñi *et al.*, 2006, 2010).

Sequence data was analyzed using a series of bioinformatics tools. When we compared the complete genomic sequence of Candid#1, XJ#44 and XJ13 strain, we found a set of differences that could be associated with the attenuated phenotype (Figure 7). Alignment of the coding sequences of the S RNA genes of Junín virus vaccine related strains showed twelve nucleotide changes implied in amino acid substitutions. As depicted in Figure 7.A.1, one of these changes is found in the signal peptide (I_{35}→V→V), four of them are at the middle portion of G1 (T_{168}→A→A; E_{186}→E→G; S_{206}→S→P and P_{208}→L→L), two are at the carboxyl terminus of G2 (F_{427}→F→I and T_{446}→T→S), and five more are at the amino half of N (V_{47}→V→E; K_{59}→R→R; I_{158}→V→V; E_{268}→D→D and T_{322}→I→I). An alignment of the coding sequences of the L genes of Junín virus strains showed only nine nucleotide changes between XJ13, XJ#44 and Candid#1 strains implicated in amino acid substitutions (Figure 7.B.1). Seven of these changes may be related with the attenuation process (H_{76}→Y→Y; V_{415}→V→A; D_{462}→N→N; L_{936}→L→P; R_{1156}→K→K; S_{1698}→S→F and I_{1883}→I→V) and two changes (R_{881}→G→R; S_{921}→G→S) could be considered reversions. All these changes are presented as XJ13 residue → XJ#44 residue → Candid#1 residue. On the contrary, no changes were found in the amino acid sequence as well as at the nucleotide level of the Z protein, among these three Junín virus strains.

3.1 Mutation analysis

Furthermore we compared the nucleotide sequences obtained from vaccine related strains with other reported Junín virus strains. There are only two other Junín virus strains whose genome was fully sequenced, Romero and MC2 strains. Romero strain, classified as a high virulence strain, was isolated from an AHF patient and was passed twice in fetal rhesus lung cells and once in Vero cells (McKee *et al.*, 1985; Yun *et al.*, 2008). This strain is named Rumero in Genebank, but this was derived from a typographical mistake. On the other hand, the MC2 strain was isolated from a rodent from the endemic area of AHF, and was classified as intermediate virulence strain (Berría *et al.*, 1967; Candurra *et al.*, 1989; Weissenbacher *et al.*, 1987). Moreover the complete S RNA and Z gene sequences were obtained for the Junín virus strain Cba-IV4454. This strain, classified as an intermediate virulence strain, was isolated from an AHF patient. Differences between deduced amino acid sequences from the six analyzed Junín virus strains are shown as vertical bars in Figure 7 and were classified into two types:

Type 1: Positions where the nucleotide or aminoacid sequence of one of the field strains of Junin virus (XJ13, Romero, IV4454 or MC2) was different from all other field strains, shown as vertical gray bars in Figure 7 located below each RNA scheme.

Type 2: Positions with mutations among the vaccine strains, shown as vertical red bars in Figure 7 located over each RNA scheme.

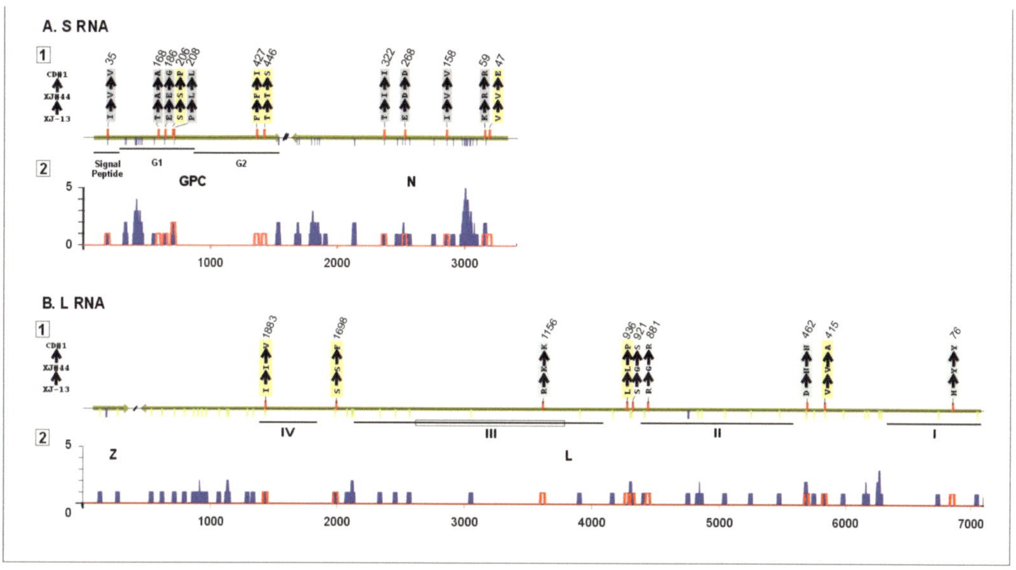

Fig. 7. Schematic of the changes detected in Junín virus proteins. Comparisons were done among all fully sequenced genomes from different Junín virus strains. A nucleotide rule is depicted below the diagram to facilitate the location of each position. **A.** S RNA, **1:** the open reading frames corresponding to the N and GPC genes are shown as open rectangles with arrowheads indicating the direction of translation. Non-coding sequences are shown as horizontal thin lines. The three cleavage products of GPC protein are shown by horizontal lines below the diagram. Amino acid changes detected between vaccine genealogy strains (XJ13, XJ#44, and Candid#1; type-2 mutation) are represented as vertical red lines over the genes. Above them, the detected changes and the position are indicated. Amino acid changes between field strains of Junín virus (XJ13, Romero, IV4454 and MC2; type-1 mutation) are indicated as vertical lines below the genes; **2:** plot of relative mutation frequency for type-1 mutations (blue areas) and for type-2 mutations (red line). **B.** L RNA, **1:** the open reading frames corresponding to the Z and L genes and the position of the changes in the amino acid sequence are shown as in (A.1.). The four conserved regions of the RNA polymerase of arenaviruses as described by Vieth *et al.* (Vieth *et al.*, 2004) are shown by horizontal lines below the diagram of the L RNA. Inside region III, the polymerase domain is signalized with an open box; **2:** plot of relative mutation frequency for type-1 mutations (blue areas) and for type-2 mutations (red line).

To identify those type 2 mutations that could be more confidently related with the attenuation process, we compare the homologous positions at the genomes obtained from field strains of Junín virus (XJ13, Romero, IV4454 and MC2). At positions GPC_{35}, N_{158}, N_{268} and N_{322} the same variations present between vaccine related strains was found among field strains. At positions L_{881} and L_{921}, there is a variation from XJ#44 to Candid#1. However, Candid#1 derived sequence is identical to the field strains (including XJ13) derived sequences. Thus, it is probable that these positions represent naturally generated mutations, non-related with the attenuation process. Furthermore, sequence variations among field strain are subject to natural selection pressure, whereas sequence variations among vaccine genealogy strains were subjected to an arbitrary selection pressure. We calculated a mutation frequency index defined as number of mutations per amino acid, and the graph was constructed with a program designed in our group by J.A. Iserte (unpublished results), using an overlapped windows-based strategy (11 residues) counting the number of mutations over each window and plotting the value at the middle of the window. This analysis was made along the Junín virus genome for both types of mutations (Figure 7.A.2 and 7.B.2). The regions of the S or L RNA with a high mutation frequency index for type 1 mutations are shown as closed blue areas while regions with a high mutation frequency index for type 2 mutations are shown as open, red outlined, areas. Mutations of type 2 found outside blue regions, identified at S RNA positions GPC_{168}, GPC_{427}, GPC_{446} and N_{47}, and L RNA positions L_{76}, L_{936}, L_{1156}, could be more confidently involved in the virulence attenuation process.

Furthermore, we searched for the presence of some of the type 2 mutations in a set of field samples. These Junín virus strains were isolated in the endemic area from human cases and captured rodents from the period of 1963-1991. Four genomic regions were selected for the analysis: i) G fragment: comprises the nucleotide positions 303 to 941 (in the glycoprotein precursor coding sequence), ii) N fragment, located between nucleotides 1632 and 2095 (in the nucleoprotein coding sequence), iii) L1 fragment, comprise between 1086 and 2005 nucleotide residues, covering the totality of RNA polymerase-RNA dependent IV motif, and iv) L2 fragment, covering the residues comprises between the 4234 and 4890 positions (C terminal of motif II). These regions include some of the type 2 mutations detected in previously. For 13 field JUNV strains, these regions were amplified and sequenced.

In the alignments of the different *in silico* translated proteins from sequenced fragments we search for the positions in which it was possible to identify variations between strains. However, for the positions included in this analysis, the variation observed between the attenuated JUNV strains was also present in some of the new field samples, taken from both rodents and human cases. As example, in Table 3 we showed some of the positions with type 2 mutations (potentially related to the virulence attenuation process) within the G fragment. The analyzed region spanned positions between residues 49 and 193 of glycoprotein 1 (G1), as well as the first 11 amino acids from glycoprotein 2 (G2), after the consensus sites for glycoprotein processing observed in other arenaviruses (York *et al.*, 2004). As a consequence, the relative importance of these variations in the attenuation process should be re-evaluated.

3.2 Non coding regions

It has been previously suggested that changes in the intergenic region could play a role in the attenuation processes of arenaviruses (Wilson & Clegg, 1991). However, our sequence analysis of the intergenic regions from XJ13, XJ#44 and Candid#1 revealed 100% conservation in both genomic RNAs. If nucleotide changes were not tolerated in this region, it could suggests that a major evolutive constraint is operating, perhaps related to the calculated secondary structure conformation and its proposed function in the transcription regulation process (Franze-Fernández *et al.*, 1993; Tortorici *et al.*, 2001a). Furthermore, the non-coding regions at the genomic ends are highly conserved among analyzed strains, varying between 93% and 97% of nucleotide sequence homology. The 3′ non-coding region, which in the virions shows a high degree of complementarity with the 5′ non-coding region, exhibits very few differences in independent clones of each strain and varies only slightly from one strain to another.

On the other hand, when infected cell-derived RNAs were sequenced, a high degree of sequence variability has been observed at the 5′ and 3′ non-coding regions among RNAs derived from the same strain. We did a RACE analysis to observe specifically the genomic or the antigenomic forms of Junín virus RNAs. For example, after RACE analysis, a series of non-template bases were found at the 5′end of Candid#1 L and S RNAs. In the comparison between the 5′end of genomic RNAs and the 3′end of antigenomic RNAs (which are used as a template for the former), at least one additional guanine is present in all 5′ end genomic clones comprising extra bases, similarly as detected for other arenavirus (Polyak *et al.*, 1995). The 3′ RACE analysis of genomic S and L RNA obtained from Candid#1 infected cells rendered several clones harboring short deletions. RNA secondary structure analysis from Candid#1 S and L RNA predicted a panhandle structure between 5′ and 3′ ends of both genomic RNAs. Deletions at the 3′ end were localized inside the panhandle (Figure 8).

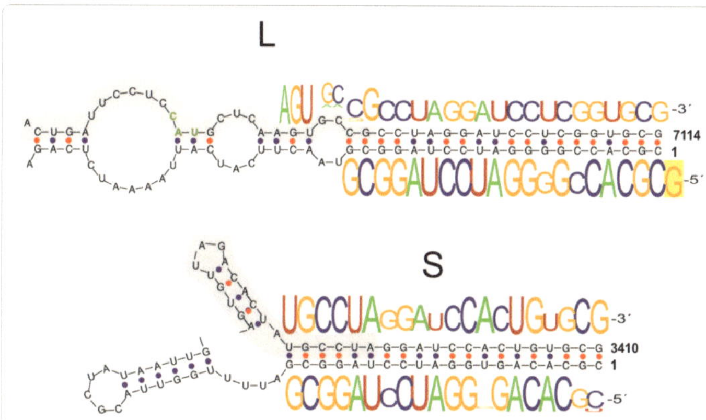

Fig. 8. End sequence determination of Junín virus, Candid#1 strain RNAs. Panhandle structures predicted for Candid#1, L and S RNAs. Shadowed with gray is the region present in all 3′-end clones. Sequence logos representing the distribution in the last nucleotides of 3′-end and 5′-end sequence of L and S RNA clones as determined by a genome specific RACE technique. Shadowed box corresponds to an additional extended G of the genomic sequence.

These results are consistent with a model that suggests the use of cellular RNAs to prime the viral RNA synthesis and the use of 5′ end sequences from viral RNA into a non-completed panhandle structure, as template for the 3′ end sequence completion. This heterogeneity could have arisen from different transcription-related editing of the subgenomic RNAs, reported previously for other arenaviruses (Garcin & Kolakofsky, 1992). However, the involvement of these regions in the attenuation process remains to be evaluated.

Interestingly, comparison between 5´ and 3´ ends sequences from both genomic RNAs (S and L segments), show highly conserved positions. These positions could be related with the minimal promoter sequence. The 5′ and 3′ non-coding sequences from Candid#1 S RNA have approximately 80 nucleotides in length, similarly to the 5′ end from L RNA non-coding sequences. However, 3′ non-coding sequences from L RNA have only 30 nucleotides in length. When comparing the 80 nucleotides from non-coding sequences, the homology between 5´ end sequences of the L and S RNAs was 60% while that from 3′ end sequences was only 50%. However, if we compare only 30 nucleotides from the 3′ end of both genomic RNAs the homology of this region ascends to 71%. Because both, genomic or antigenomic, non-coding regions must be recognized by the viral RNA polymerase to complete the viral replicative cycle, the promoter region should be present in the first 30 nucleotides of the antigenomic L RNA. Genomic ends of arenaviruses comprise a highly conserved region of 19 nucleotides, called arena region. Outside this region the 3′ end of Junín virus L RNA comprises only 11 nucleotides (GCTCAAGTGCC). These nucleotides show a high degree of homology with two regions of S RNA 3′ end sequences. Thus, two boxes at the S RNA appear to match with a unique box at the L RNA. The S RNA boxes (positions 1-12 and 35-45 in the alignment) could be related to translation or transcription processes. Other arenaviruses have similar characteristics at their genomic ends. For example, an extensive analysis using the genomic sequences from other New World arenaviruses belonging to B1 subclade (Machupo, Junín and Tacaribe viruses; Flanagan *et al.*, 2008), show that the 38-46 box (GCUCAAGUG for the Junín virus L RNA and GCUCAGUG for the Junin virus S RNA) was conserved in the group (Goñi *et al.*, 2010). Consequently, it is possible that a sequence motif could be present at the 3′ end of both genomic RNAs of arenaviruses. Furthermore, for Junín, Machupo and Tacaribe viruses, this motif, described by the sequence GSYC$(A)_{1-2}$GUR, shows a relative degree of conservation in position in the RNA secondary structure calculated by bioinformatic tools.

3.3 Phylogeny

An independent parsimony analysis was performed for each arenavirus gene (GPC, N, Z and L). An additive tree-file was constructed adding the obtained parsimony tree-files from each gene in order to obtain a consensus tree for the four genes. Clades and subclades of Old World and New World arenaviruses are in accord with Charrell *et al.* (2008). Phylogenetic analysis show that all Junín virus strains (Candid#1, XJ13, XJ#44, MC2 and Romero) grouped together with other hemorrhagic New World arenaviruses. Furthermore, the phylogeny correlates with the genealogy of the vaccine strain, Candid#1, and a small set of nucleotide changes seems to be central to define the phenotypic variation from virulence to attenuation. If this is confirmed in a more extensive study, any surveillance program designed to monitor the natural vaccine variations should search for possible point mutations at those positions related with attenuation.

4. Conclusions

Candid#1, the most attenuated Junín strain, has a set of putative attenuation markers into the GPC, N and L protein ORFs. Some of these changes could be associated more confidently with the attenuated phenotype. Initially, we focussed on changes detected into those genomic regions harboring a low wild type mutation frequency index (GPC_{168}, GPC_{427}, GPC_{446}, N_{47}, L_{76}, L_{936}, L_{1156}).

At present, we have made bioinformatic and phylogenetic analysis on the putative attenuation markers. For L proteins, the group of Vieth (Vieth *et al.*, 2004) describe four conserved regions among all arenaviruses. Inside of the region III, Lan and coworkers (Lan *et al.*, 2008), found the polymerase domain, and proposed the presence of four motifs: A, B, C and D. In this region we detect only one change (R→K→K), at the 1156 position. Although this change is classified as conservative, it could be related to the attenuation process because this region seems not to sustain mutations in nature. Other L changes are located between region II and III (L_{936}, L→L→P) or inside region I (L_{76}, H→Y→Y). Change L_{936}, in spite of being present in a region of high index for type 2 mutations, could only be associated with a structural change of the Candid#1 derived L protein based on the structural characteristics of the Proline residue. L_{76} change falls near the putative ATP/GTP binding site (P-loop) predicted using the Expasy web site (www.expasy.ch). Although our results, suggesting the involvement of the RNA polymerase in attenuation of virulence are preliminary, they are consistent with reports on other viruses (Endres *et al.*, 1991; Lan *et al.*, 2008; Riviere *et al.*, 1985a). Furthermore, some changes in the structural proteins, nucleoprotein and both mature glycoproteins, could be related with the attenuation of virulence. The carboxyl-terminus of N protein, which contains a zinc binding domain (Tortorici *et al.*, 2001b) is highly conserved, and the found N_{47} change (V→V→E) falls outside this region and would be associated with another characteristic of the protein, as the ability to oligomerize (N-N interactions, Levingston Macleod *et al.*, 2011). Therefore, N protein has a dual function during the virus life cycle. First, it is involved in essential steps of genome replication, promoting the synthesis of the full-length antigenomic copy of S RNA, and second, it associates with the genomic RNA to form the nucleocapsid. For the glycoprotein precursor, we found a mutation in the carboxyl-terminus of G1 (GPC_{168}, T→A→A). This change affects directly the conserved sequence ($N_{166}R_{167}T_{168}K_{169}$) for the principal N-glycosylation site predicted by NETNGLYC 1.0. G2 has three domains, the outer (caboxi-terminus) domain located outside the virion, the transmembrane domain and the inner (amino-terminus) domain, located inside the virion. The outer domain interacts with G1, the transmembrane domain interacts with the signal peptide, and the inner domain could interact with Z or the nucleocapsid (Capul *et al.*, 2007; York *et al.*, 2004). G2 changes fall inside the transmembrane domain (GPC_{427}, F→F→I) or at the cytoplasmic tail (GPC_{446}, T→T→S) and could affect such important interactions.

In terms of distribution of the potential attenuation markers, we find a lower level of nucleotide sequence conservation in the S RNA than in the L RNA, indicating a faster rate of evolution in the S polypeptides. Lan and colaborators (Lan *et al.*, 2008) showed the genome comparison of virulent and avirulent strains of the Pichinde arenavirus, and found a lower number of attenuation related mutations, but at comparable genomic regions. If we compared only the field strains of Junín virus (MC2, Romero, IV4454 and XJ13), the mutations distribute markedly differently among large and small segments. We considered specific changes for MC2, Romero or IV4454 when their sequences differed from XJ13 sequence, and specific changes for XJ13 when its sequence differed from all three Junín virus strains. Analyzing the protein sequences of the field strains, there were 45 divergence sites for the S RNA ORFs and 48 for the L RNA ORFs. Interestingly, 96% (46/48) of L RNA-derived divergence sites were XJ13-specific changes, and only 9% (4/45) of this type of changes were present when S RNA-derived divergence sites were analyzed.

The increasing sequence information from complete arenavirus genomes, especially of the JUNV species, contributed to the identification of putative markers of virulence attenuation. In this sense, Goñi *et al.* (2010) and the recent paper of Albariño *et al.* (2011a) publish sequence data involving seven members of the vaccine strain family (XJ13, XJ17, XJ34, XJ39, XJ44, XJ48 and Candid#1 strains). To investigate the role of different point mutations in the virulence attenuation process Albariño *et al.*, (2011a) used a reverse genetics system for JUNV they developed (Albariño *et al.*, 2011b). They show that point mutations located at the Candid#1 GPC ORF, conferred the attenuated phenotype.

Furthermore, with the objective of analyzing the mutation distribution in nature, Goñi *et al.* (2011) designed a molecular technique of RT-Nested-PCR and afterwards used with rodent and human samples from the endemic area. A previous study, performed on different genomic regions with another group of strains (García *et al.*, 2000), suggested a high degree of homology for the S RNA derived ORFs. The protein sequences we obtained by *in silico* translation of the four fragments were analyzed with different tools.

We compare the data collected for the GPC derived sequences (G fragment) after the results included in our studies and in the Albariño *et al.* (2011a) paper. In the Table 3 we show the positions with residue differences between G fragments encoded proteins from JUNV strains belonging to the vaccine family and JUNV strains collected from field samples. As noted above, the G fragment covered the sequence involved in the cleavage between G1 and G2 proteins. The possible recognition site is formed by the sequence QLPRRSLK_{251}↓AFF (Beyer *et al.*, 2003), or between the L_{250} and K_{251} (Lenz *et al.*, 2001), and cutting is done by the protease SKI-1/S1P. The sequenced samples reported here showed a high conservation degree in this zone. Only for isolate H_FHA5054, changes were observed at positions 244 and 245 (Q→H and L→F respectively), although it is possible that these modifications may not affect the recognition site. Some of the changes observed in the G fragment (63% of G1), could be related to the host jump process of a particular strain from rodents to humans (probably derived from the receptor affinity variation in the human isolates). These changes could be related to changes in the virulence (attenuation or increase) trough modification of the cellular tropism. Another important site in this fragment was determined by NETGLYC 1.0, comprising the target sequence $N_{166}R_{167}T_{168}K_{169}$ involved in the N-glycosylation of this protein. By observing the distribution of this target in the different isolates it can be seen that only 65% of the field strains have the target sequence, while the other 35% have an alanine residue (A_{168}).

The bioinformatics studies did not show important changes in the protein properties at this region (data not shown). On the other hand, a recent study resolved the importance of two positions strongly related to the N- glycosylation for JUNV and MACV (Bowden *et al.*, 2009). It was found that both residues and their environment are highly conserved. In any case, it was recently shown for LCMV, that each N-linked glycan in the arenavirus glycoprotein is involved in GPC expression, fusion with the host receptor and infectivity (Bonhomme *et al.*, 2011). Interestingly, all XJ13-derived attenuated strains have an A_{168} mutation.

Residue Position	XJ13	XJ17	XJ34	XJ39	XJ#44	XJ48	Candid#1	MC2	IV4454	Romero	AN_8640	AN_5185	AN_13365	AN_16501	AN_17058	AN_17246	AN_17116	AN_17064	H_Lye63	H_FHA5069	H_p1879	H_FHA5054	H_8027
107	S	S	S	S	S	S	S	S	**T**	S	S	S	S	S	S	S	S	S	S	**T**	**T**	**T**	S
109	Q	Q	Q	Q	Q	Q	Q	**K**	**M**	**M**	Q	Q	Q	**M**	Q	Q	**M**	**M**	Q	**M**	**M**	**M**	Q
111	S	S	S	S	S	S	S	S	**T**	S	S	S	S	S	T	S	S	S	S	**T**	**T**	**T**	S
116	A	A	A	A	A	A	A	A	A	E	A	A	A	A	A	A	A	A	A	A	A	A	A
121	Q	Q	Q	Q	Q	Q	Q	E	Q	Q	Q	Q	E	Q	Q	Q	Q	Q	Q	Q	Q	Q	Q
125	I	I	I	I	I	I	I	I	**V**	I	I	I	I	I	**V**	I	I	I	I	**V**	**V**	**V**	I
133	S	S	S	S	S	S	S	S	S	S	S	S	S	**N**	S	S	**N**	**N**	S	S	S	S	S
143	W	W	W	W	W	W	W	W	W	W	W	W	W	W	W	W	W	W	W	**R**	**R**	**R**	W
151	A	A	A	A	A	A	A	A	A	A	A	A	A	A	A	A	A	A	A	**V**	**V**	**V**	A
157	H	H	H	H	H	H	H	**Y**	**Y**	H	H	H	H	H	H	H	H	H	H	H	H	H	H
168	T	**A**	**A**	**A**	**A**	**A**	**A**	T	T	T	**A**	**A**	T	T	**A**	**A**	T	T	**A**	T	T	T	**A**
184	V	V	V	V	V	V	V	**I**	V	V	V	V	V	V	V	V	V	V	V	V	V	V	V
186	E	E	E	E	E	E	**G**	E	E	E	**G**	**G**	E	E	**G**	**G**	E	E	**G**	E	E	E	**G**
206	S	S	S	S	S	S	P	S	S	S	P	P	S	S	P	P	S	S	P	S	S	S	P
208	P	**L**	**L**	**L**	**L**	**L**	**L**	**L**	**L**	**L**	**L**	**L**	**L**	**L**	**L**	**L**	**L**	**L**	**L**	**L**	**L**	**L**	**L**
209	N	N	N	N	N	N	N	D	S	N	N	N	N	N	N	N	N	N	N	**S**	**S**	**S**	N
244	Q	Q	Q	Q	Q	Q	Q	Q	Q	Q	Q	Q	Q	Q	Q	Q	Q	Q	Q	Q	Q	**H**	Q
245	L	L	L	L	L	L	L	L	L	L	L	L	L	L	L	L	L	L	L	L	L	**F**	L

Letters in bold indicate the residues that are different from the residue present in the reference XJ13 strain. The amino acids are shown in the one letter code. The type 2 mutations between vaccine family strains are shadowed in grey.

Table 3. Positions with residue differences between G fragment encoded proteins.

We hypothesized that those mutations found among field strains are of minor importance in the phenomenon of virulence attenuation. None of the type 2 mutations here analyzed, were absent in natural samples. In this context, the data presented in Table 3, could indicate that none of the mutations found in G1 is important to define the attenuated phenotype. This result is in accordance with those published by Albariño *et al.*, (2011a), who located the most important mutations for attenuation in G2.

In summary, the present work shows a set of mutations that could be related to the virulence attenuation phenomenon. Furthermore, most of both described types of mutations (type 1 and type 2) could be grouped into a few regions (Figure 7). In order to analyze genomic variability in Junín virus and to search for the presence of mutations of type 1 or type 2 among field strains, we designed a set of primers that are used in a rapid method, based on RT-PCR and nucleotide sequencing. This method could be useful in order to observe the biodiversity in nature or to develop an epidemiologic surveillance program of vaccinated people. The information accumulated by sequence analysis of viral genomes with different degrees of virulence will certainly serve as a starting point to study this biological phenomenon. Our results contribute to the generation of the sequence data of field isolates that should prove highly useful in the selection of residues potentially involved in different viral survival mechanisms and are a potential target for mutagenesis studies.

5. Acknowledgment

We are very grateful to Dr. Antonio Tenorio Matanzo from Carlos III Health Institute (ISCIII, Madrid, Spain) and Dr. Marta S. Contigiani from Virology Institute "Dr. J. M. Vanella" (Fac. de Medicina, Córdoba National University, Argentina), and the students Javier A. Iserte, Betina I. Stephan and Cristina S. Borio, who contributed to the development of this work. We also thank Dr. J. G Barrera Oro from USAMRJID (Frederick, Maryland, USA) who provided us with an XJ#44 seed, and to Dr. Ana María Ambrosio and Dr. María del Carmen Saavedra from National Institute of Viral Human Diseases (INEVH, Pergamino, Argentina), who prepared Candid#1 virions. This work was supported by the National University of Quilmes (UNQ) and by PICT 38138 from ANPCYT and PIP5813 from CONICET (Argentina). S.E.G. has a research fellowship from CONICET. M.E.L. is member of the research career of CONICET. SEG and MEL are Professors at UNQ.

6. References

Agrest, A., Avalos, J.C.S. & Slepoy, M.A. (1969). Fiebre hemorrágica argentina y coagulopatía por consumo. *Medicina (Buenos Aires)*. 29, 194-201.

AHF National Control Program. (2007) Recopilation and Edition: Instituto Nacional de Enfermedades Virales Humanas "Dr. Julio I. Maiztegui"- Pergamino, Editors: Dra Ana M. Briggiler, Lic. María Rosa Feuillade. Ministerio de Salud de la Nación, Ministerio de Salud de las Pcias. de Buenos Aires, de Santa Fe, de Córdoba y de La Pampa. *Edition Forth.*

Albariño, C.G.; Bird, B.H.; Chakrabarti, A.K.; Dodd, K.A.; Flint, M.; Bergeron, E.; White, D.M. & Nichol, S.T. (2011a) The major determinant of attenuation in mice of the Candid1 vaccine for argentine hemorrhagic Fever is located in the g2 glycoprotein transmembrane domain. *J Virol.* 85(19):10404-8.

Albariño, C.G.; Bird, B.H.; Chakrabarti, A.K.; Dodd, K.A.; White, D.M.; Bergeron, E.; Shrivastava-Ranjan, P. & Nichol, S.T. (2011b). Reverse genetics generation of chimeric infectious Junin/Lassa virus is dependent on interaction of homologous glycoprotein stable signal peptide and G2 cytoplasmic domains. *J. Virol.* 85(1), 112-122.

Álvarez, D.E.; Lodeiro, M.F.; Ludueña, S.J.; Pietrasanta, L.I. & Gamarnik, A.V. (2005) Long-Range RNA-RNA Interactions Circularize the Dengue Virus Genome. *J Virol.*; 79(11): 6631-6643.

Ambrosio, A.M., Enría, D. & Maiztegui, J.I. (1986). Junín virus isolation from lympho-mononuclear cells of patients with Argentine hemorrhagic fever. *Intervirology*. 25, 97-102.

Ambrosio, A.M.; Saavedra, M.C.; Riera, L.M.; Fassio, R.M. (2006) La producción nacional de vacuna a virus Junín vivo atenuado (Candid#1) anti-fiebre hemorrágica argentina. *Acta Bioquím Clín Latinoam;* 40 (1): 5-17.

Armstrong, C. & Sweet, L.K. Lymphocytic choriomeningitis. (1939) Report of two cases, with recovery of the virus from gray mice (Mus musculus) trapped in the two infected households. *Public Health Report*. 54, 673-684.

Auperin, D.D.; Romanowski, V.; Galinski, M.S. and Bishop, D.H.L. (1984) Sequencing studies of Pichinde arenavirus S RNA indicate a novel coding strategy, an ambisense viral S RNA. *Journal of Virology*. 52, 987-904.

Barrera Oro, J.G. & Eddy, G.A. (1982) Characteristics of candidate live attenuated Junín virus vaccine. *Fourth International Conference on Comparative Virology*, Banff, Alberta, Canadá. October 17-22.

Berría, M.I.; Gutman Frugone, L.F.; Girda, R. & Barrera Oro, J.G. (1967) Estudios inmunológicos con virus Junín. I. Formación de anticuerpos en cobayos inoculados con virus vivos. *Medicina* (Buenos Aires). 27, 93-98.

Beyer, W.R.; Pöpplau, D.; Garten, W.; von Laer, D. & Lenz, O. (2003) Endoproteolytic processing of the lymphocytic choriomeningitis virus glycoprotein by the subtilase SKI-1/S1P. *J Virol.*; 77(5):2866-72. 2003.

Bieniasz, P.D. (2006) Late budding domains and host proteins in enveloped virus release. *J Virol.* Vol. 344. pp. 55-63.

Bonhomme, C.J.; Capul, A.A.; Lauron, E.J.; Bederka, L.H.; Knopp, K.A. & Buchmeier, M.J. (2011). Glycosylation modulates arenavirus glycoprotein expression and function. *Virology* 409 (2), 223–233.

Borden, K.L.; Campbell-Dwyer, E.J.; Carlile, G.W.; Djavani, M. & Salvato, M.S. (1998a) Two RING finger proteins, the oncoprotein PML and the arenavirus Z protein, colocalize with the nuclear fraction of the ribosomal P proteins. *J. Virol.* Vol. 72. pp. 3819–3826.

Borden, K.L; Campbell-Dwyer, E.J. & Salvato, M.S. (1998b) An arenavirus RING (zinc-binding) protein binds the oncoprotein promyelocyte leukemia protein (PML) and relocates PML nuclear bodies to the cytoplasm. *J. Virol.* Vol. 72. pp. 758–766.

Bowden, T.A.; Crispin, M.;Graham, S.C.; Harvey, D.J.;Grimes, J.M.; Jones, E.Y. & Stuart, D.I. (2009) Unusual Molecular Architecture of the Machupo Virus Attachment Glycoprotein. *Journal of Virology*, p. 8259-8265, Vol. 83, No. 16.

Briese, T.; Paweska, J.T.; McMullan, L.K.; Hutchison, S.K.; Street, C.; Palacios, G.; Khristova, M.L.; Weyer, J.; Swanepoel, R.; Egholm, M.; Nichol, S.T. & Lipkin, W.I. (2009) Genetic Detection and Characterization of Lujo Virus, a New Hemorrhagic Fever-Associated Arenavirus from Southern Africa. *PLoS Pathog.* Volume 4, Issue 5, 1-8.

Buchmeier, M.J. & Oldstone, M.B.A. (1979) Protein structure of lymphocytic choriomeningitis virus: evidence for a cell-associated precursor of the virion glycopeptides. *Virology*. 99, 111-120.

Cajimat, M.N.B. & Fulhorst, C.F. (2004) Phylogeny of the Venezuelan arenaviruses. *Virus Research* 102: 199–206.

Cajimat, M.N.B; Milazzo, M.L.; Hess, B.D.; Rood, M.P. & Fulhorst, C.F. (2007) Principal host relationships and evolutionary history of the North American arenaviruses. *Virology*. 367(2): 235–243.

Campbell Dwyer, E.J.; Lai, H.; MacDonald, R.C.; Salvato, M.S. & Borden, K.L. (2000) The lymphocytic choriomeningitis virus RING protein Zassociates with eukaryotic initiation factor 4E and selectively represses translation in a RING-dependent manner. *J. Virol.* Vol. 74. pp. 3293–3300.

Candurra, N.A.; Damonte, E.B. & Coto, C.E. (1989) Antigenic relationships among attenuated and pathogenic strains of virus Junín. *Journal of Medical Virology*. 27, 145.

Cao, W.; Henry, M.D.; Borrow, P.; Yamada, H.; Elder, J.H.; Ravkov, E.V.; Nichol, S.T.; Compans, R.W.; Campbel, K.P. & Oldstone, M.B. (1998) Identification of alpha-dystroglycan as a receptor for lymphocytic choriomeningitis virus and Lassa fever virus. *Science*. 282, 2079-2081.

Capul, A.A.; Pérez, M.; Burke, E.; Kunz, S.; Buchmeier, M.J. & de la Torre, J.C. Arenavirus Z-glycoprotein association requires Z myristoylation but not functional RING or late domains. *J Virol.*; 81(17):9451-60. 2007.

CDC. Center for Disease Control and Prevention. (2000). Fatal illnesses associated with a New World Arenavirus - California, 1999-2000. *MMWR Morb. Mortal. Wkly. Rep.* 49, 709-711

Charrel, R.N. & de Lamballerie, X. (2003) Arenaviruses other than Lassa virus. *Antiviral Res.*; 57 (1-2): 89-100.

Charrel, R.N.; de Lamballerie X. & Emonet, S. (2008) Phylogeny of the genus Arenavirus. *Curr Opin Microbiol.* 11 (4):362-8.

Cossio, P.M.; Laguens, R.P.; Arana, R.M.; Segal, A. & Maiztegui, J.I. (1975). Ultrastructural and immunohistochemical study of the human kidney in Argentine hemorrhagic fever. *Virchows Archives*. 368, 1.

Dalton, A.J.; Rowe, W.P.; Smith, G.H.; Wilsnack, R.E. & Pugh, W.E. (1968) Morphological and cytochemical studies on lymphocytic choriomeningitis virus. *Journal of Virology*. 2, 1465-1478.

Delgado, S.; Erickson, B.R.; Agudo, R.; Blair, P.J.; Vallejo, E.; Albariño, C.J.; Vargas, J.; Comer, J.A.; Rollin, P.E.; Ksiazek, T.G.; Olson, J.G. & Nichol, S.T. (2008) Chapare Virus, a Newly Discovered Arenavirus Isolatedfrom a Fatal Hemorrhagic Fever Case in Bolivia. *PLOS Pathogens*. 4(4): e1000047.

Endres, M.J.; Griot, C.; Gonzalez-Scarano, F. & Nathanson, N. (1991) Neuroattenuation of an avirulent bunyavirus variant maps to the L RNA segment. *Journal of Virology*, 65: 5465-5470.

Enría, D.A.; Bowen, M.D.; Mills, J.N.; Shieh,W.J.; Bausch, D. & Peters, C.J. (2004) Arenavirus infections. In: Guerrant, R.L.,Walker, D. H.,Weller, P.F., Saunders, W.B. (Eds.), *Tropical Infectious Diseases: Principles, Pathogens, and Practice,* vol. 2, pp. 1191–1212 (Chapter 111).

Enría, D.A.; Briggiler, A.M. & Sánchez, Z. (2008) Treatment of Argentine hemorrhagic fever. *Antiviral Res.*;78(1):132-9.

Flanagan, M.L.; Oldenburg, J.; Reignier, T.; Holt, N.; Hamilton, G.A.; Martin, V.K.; Cannon, P.M. (2008). New world clade B arenaviruses can use transferrin receptor 1 (TfR1)-dependent and -independent entry pathways, and glycoproteins from human pathogenic strains are associated with the use of TfR1. *J Virol*; 82(2):938-48.

Franze Fernández, M.T.; Zetina, C.; Iapalucci, S.; Lucero, M.A.; Boissou, C.; López, R.; Rey, O.; Daheli, M.; Cohen, G. & Zalein, M. (1987) Molecular structure and early events in the replication of Tacaribe Arenavirus S RNA. *Virus Research*. 7, 309-324.

Franze-Fernandez, M.T.; Iapalucci, S.; Lopez, N. & Rossi, C. (1993) Subgenomic RNAs of Tacaribe virus. In *The Arenaviridae*, pp. 113-132. Edited by M. S. Salvato. New York: Plenum Press.

Freed, E.O. (2002) Viral late domains. *J. Virol.* Vol. 76. pp. 4679–4687.

García, J.B.; Morzunov, S.P.; Levis, S.; Rowe, J.; Calderón, G.; Enría, D.; Sabattini, M.; Buchmeier, M.J.; Bowen, M.D. & St. Jeort, S.C. (2000). Genetic diversity of the Junín virus in Argentina: geographic and temporal patterns. *Virology* 272, 127–136.

Garcin, D. & Kolakofsky, D. Tacaribe arenavirus RNA synthesis in vitro is primer dependent and suggests an unusual model for the initiation of genome replication. *J. Virol.* 66:1370–1376. 1992.

Garcin, D.; Rochat, S. & Kolakofsky, D. (1993) The Tacaribe arenavirus small zinc finger protein is required for both mRNA synthesis and genome replication. *J. Virol. Vol.* 67. pp 807–812.

Ghiringhelli, P.D.; Rivera Pomar, R.V.; Lozano, M.E.; Grau, O. & Romanowski, V. (1991) Molecular organization of Junín virus S RNA: complete nucleotide sequence, relationship with the other members of Arenaviridae and unusual secondary structures. *Journal of General Virology.* 72, 2129-2141.

Goñi, S.E.; Iserte, J.A.; Ambrosio, A.M.; Romanowski, V.; Ghiringhelli, P.D. & Lozano, M.E. (2006) Genomic features of attenuated Junín virus vaccine strain candidate. *Virus Genes*, 32:37-41.

Goñi, S.E.; Iserte, J.A.; Stephan, B.I.; Borio, C.S.; Ghiringhelli, P.D. & Lozano, M.E. (2010) Molecular analysis of the virulence attenuation process in Junín virus vaccine genealogy. *Virus Genes.* 40(3):320-8.

Gschwender, H.H.; Brummund, M. & Lehmann-Grube, F. (1975) Lymphocytic choriomeningitis virus. I. Concentration and purification of the infectious virus. *Journal of Virology.* 15, 1317-1322.

Iserte, J.A.; Enría, D.A.; Levis, S.C. & Lozano, M.E. (2010) Junín virus (Argentine hemorrhagic fever). In: Chapter 65. Molecular Detection of Human Viral Pathogens. Edited by Dongyou Liu. *Taylor & Francis CRC Press.* In Press.

Kentsis, A.; Dwyer, E.C; Perez, J.M.; Sharma, M.; Chen, A.; Pan, Z.Q. & Borden, K.L. (2001) The RING domains of the promyelocytic leukemia protein PML and the arenaviral protein Z repress translation by directly inhibiting translation initiation factor eIF4E. *J. Mol. Biol.* Vol. 312. pp. 609–623.

Lan, S.; McLay, L.; Aronson, J.; Ly, H. & Liang; Y. (2008) Genome comparison of virulent and avirulent strains of the Pichinde arenavirus. *Archives of Virology*, 153 (7):1241-1250.

Lenz, O.; ter Meulen, J.; Klenk, H.D.; Seidah, N.G.; Garten, W. (2001). The Lassa virus glycoprotein precursor GP-C is proteolytically processed by subtilase SKI-1/S1P. *Proc Natl Acad Sci* ; 98(22):12701-5.

Levingston Macleod, J.M.; D'Antuono, A.; Loureiro, M.E.; Casabona, J.C.; Gomez, G.A. & Lopez, N. (2011) Identification of Two Functional Domains within the Arenavirus Nucleoprotein. *J Virol.* 85(5): 2012–2023.

Lepine, P.; Mollaret, P. & Kreis, B. (1937) Receptivite de l'homme au virus murin de la choriomeningite lymphocytaire. Reproduction experimentale de la meningite lymphocytaire benigne. *C.R. Academy of Science Paris.* 204, 1846-1848.

Lisieux, T.; Coimbra, M.; Nassar, E.S.; Burattini, M.N.; de Souza, L.T.; Ferreira, I.; Rocco, I.M.; da Rosa, A.P.; Vasconcelos, P.F.; Pinheiro, F.P. (1994) New arenavirus isolated in Brazil. *Lancet.* ; 343 (8894): 391-2.

López, N.; Jácamo, R. & Franze-Fernández, M.T. (2001) Transcription and RNA replication of Tacaribe virus genome and antigenome analogs require N and L proteins: Z protein is an inhibitor of these processes. *J Virol.* Vol. 75. pp. 12241-12251.

Lukashevich, I.S.; Patterson, J.; Carrion, R.; Moshkoff, D.; Ticer, A.; Zapata, J.; Brasky, K.; Geiger, R.; Hubbard, G.B.; Bryant, J. & Salvato, M.S. (2005) A Live Attenuated Vaccine for Lassa Fever Made by Reassortment of Lassa and Mopeia Viruses. *Journal of Virology*, p. 13934–13942 Vol. 79, No. 22.

Machado, Alex Martins, Figueiredo GG, Campos GM, Lozano ME, Machado AR, Figueiredo LT. (2010). Standardization of an ELISA test using a recombinant nucleoprotein from the Junin virus as the antigen and serological screening for arenavirus among the population of Nova Xavantina, State of Mato Grosso. *Rev. Soc. Bras. Med. Trop.*, 43, 229-233.

Maiztegui, J.I.; Sabattini, M.S. & Barrera Oro, J.G. (1972) Actividad del virus de la coriomeningitis linfocitaria (LCM) en el área endémica de Fiebre Hemorrágica Argentina (FHA). 1. Estudios serológicos en roedores capturados en la ciudad de Pergamino. *Medicina* (Buenos Aires). 32, 131-137.

Maiztegui, J.I.; Feinsod, F.; Briggiler, A.M.; Peters, C.J.; Enría, D.A.; Lupton, H.W.; Ambrosio, A.M.; Tiano, E.; Feuillade, M.R.; Gamboa, G.; Conti, O.; Vallejos, D.; Mac Donald, C. & Barrera Oro, J.G. (1987). Inoculation of Argentine volunteers with a live-attenuated Junín virus vaccine. *VII International Congress of Virology*, Edmonton, Canada (Abstract book, p. 69, R.3.49).

Martín Serrano, J.; Pérez Caballero, D. & Bieniasz, P.D. (2004) Context-Dependent effects of L domains and ubiquitination on viral budding. J.Virol. Vol. 78. pp. 5554-5563.

Martínez Segovia, Z.M. & Grazioli, F. (1969) The nucleic acid of Junín virus. *Acta Virologica*. 13, 264-268.

Martínez-Sobrido, L.; Zúñiga, E.I.; Rosario, D.; García-Sastre, A. & de la Torre, J.C. (2006) Inhibition of the Type I Interferon Response by the Nucleoprotein of the Prototypic Arenavirus Lymphocytic Choriomeningitis Virus. *J Virol.* 80(18): 9192–9199.

McKee, K.T. Jr, Mahlandt, B.G.; Maiztegui, J.I.; Eddy, G.A. & Peters, C.J. (1985) Experimental Argentine hemorrhagic fever in rhesus macaques: viral strain-dependent clinical response. *J Infect Dis.* 152(1):218-21.

Melcon, M.O. & Herskovits, E. (1981) Complicaciones neurológicas tardías de la fiebre hemorrágica argentina. *Medicina (Buenos Aires)* 41: 137.

Murphy, F.A. & Whitfield, S.G. (1975) Morphology and morphogenesis of arenaviruses. *Bulletin WHO.* 52, 409-419.

Murphy, F.A.; Webb, P.A.; Johnson, K.M. & Whitfield, S.G. (1968) Morphological comparison of Machupo with lymphocytic choriomeningitis virus: basis for a new taxonomic group. *Journal of Virology.* 4, 535-541.

Murphy, F.A.; Webb, P.A.; Johnson, K.M.; Whitfield, S.G. & Chappel, W.A. (1970) Arenaviruses in Vero cells: ultrastructural studies. *Journal of Virology.* 6, 507-518.

Ofodile, A.; Padnos, M.; Molomut, N. & Duffy, J.L. (1973) Morphological and biological characteristics of the M-P strain of lymphocytic choriomeningitis virus. *Infect. Immun.* 7, 309-315.

Ogbu, O.; Ajuluchukwu, E. & Uneke C.J. (2007) Lassa fever in West African sub-region: an overview. *J Vector Borne Dis.* 44(1):1-11.

Oldstone, M.B.A. (1987a). Arenaviruses: biology and immunotherapy (edit). Current Topics in Microbiology and Immunology. 134, 1.

Oldstone, M.B.A. (1987b). Immunotherapy for virus infection. Current Topics in Microbiology and Immunology. 134, 211-229.

Palacios, G.; Druce, J.; Du, L.; Tran, T.; Birch, C.; Briese, T.; Conlan, S.; Quan, P.L.; Hui, J.; Marshall, J.; Simons, J.F.; Egholm, M.; Paddock, C.D.; Shieh, W.J.; Goldsmith, C.S.; Zaki, S.R.; Catton, M. & Lipkin, W.I. (2008) A New Arenavirus in a Cluster of Fatal Transplant-Associated Diseases. *N Engl J Med.* 6;358(10):991-8.

Parisi, G.; Echave, J.; Ghiringhelli, P. D. & Romanowski, V. (1996) Computational characterization of potential RNA-binding sites in arenavirus nucleocapsid proteins. *Virus Genes* 13, 249-256.

Parodi, A.S.; Greenway, D.J.; Rugiero, H.R.; Rivero, E.; Frigerio, M.J.; Mettler, N.E.; Garzon, F.; Boxaca, M.; Guerrero, L.B. de & Nota, N.R. (1958) Sobre la etiología del brote epidémico en Junín. *Día Médico.* 30, 2300-2302.

Pérez, M. & de la Torre, J.C. (2003) Characterization of the Genomic Promoter of the Prototypic Arenavirus Lymphocytic Choriomeningitis Virus. *Journal of Virology.* p. 1184–1194 Vol. 77, No. 2.

Pérez, M.; Craven, R.C. & de la Torre, J.C. (2003) The small RING finger protein Z drives arenavirus budding: implications for antiviral strategies. *Proc. Natl. Acad. Sci.;* 100:12978–12983.

Polyak, S.J.; Zheng, S. & Harnish, D.G. (1995). 5′ Termini of Pichinde arenavirus S RNAs and mRNAs contain nontemplated nucleotides. *J. Virol.* 69:3211–3215.

Pornillos, O.; Garrus, J.E. & Sundquist, W.I. (2002) Mechanisms of enveloped RNA virus budding. *Trends Cell Biol.* Vol. 12. pp. 569–579.

Radoshitzky, S.R.; Abraham, J.; Spiropoulou, C.F.; Kuhn, J.H.; Nguyen, D.; Li, W.; Ángel, J.; Schmidt, P.J.; Nunberg, J.H.; Andrews, N.C.; Farzan, M. & Choe, H. (2007) Transferrin receptor 1 is a cellular receptor for New World haemorrhagic fever arenaviruses. *Nature.* 446(7131):92-6.

Rivers, T.M. & Scott, T.F.M. (1935) Meningitis in man caused by a filterable virus. *Science.* 81, 439-440.

Riviere, Y.; Ahmed, R.; Southern, P.J.; Buchmeier, M.J. & Oldstone, M.B.A. (1985a) Genetic mapping of lymphocytic choriomeningitis virus pathogenicity: virulence in guinea pigs is associated with the L RNA segment. *Journal of Virology.* 55, 704-709.

Riviere, Y.; Ahmed, R.; Southern, P.J.; Buchmeier, M.J.; Dutko, F.J. & Oldstone, M.B.A. (1985b) The S RNA segment of lymphocytic choriomeningitis virus codes for the nucleoprotein and the glycoproteins 1 and 2. *Journal of Virology.* 53, 966-968.

Rugiero, H.R.; Címtora, F.; Libonatti, E.; Magnoni, C.; Castiglioni, E. & Locisero, R. (1960) Formas nerviosas de la Fiebre Hemorrágica Epidémica. *Pren. Méd. Argent.* 47: 1845

Sabattini, M.S.; Gonzalez de Ríos, L.E.; Díaz, G. & Vega, V.R. (1977) Infección natural y experimental de roedores con virus Junín. *Medicina* (Buenos Aires). 37 Supl. 3, 149-161.

Salas, R.; Manzione, N.; Tesh, R.B.; Rico-Hesse, R.; Shope, R.; Betancourt, A.; Godoy, O.; Bruzual, R.; Pacheco, M.; Ramos, B.; Taibo, M.E.; García Tamayo, J.; Jaimes, E.; Vasquez, C.; Araoz, F. & Quarales, J. (1991) Venezuelan hemorrhagic fever. *Lancet.* 338, 1033-1036.

Salvato, M.S. & Shimomaye, E.M. (1989) The completed sequence of lymphocytic choriomeningitis virus reveals a unique RNA structure and a gene for a zinc finger protein. *Virology*. 173 (1), 1-10.

Salvato, M.S.; Clegg, J.C.S.; Buchmeier, M.J.; Charrel, R.N.; Gonzalez, J.P.; Lukashevich, I.S.; Peters, C.J.; Rico-Hesse, R. and Romanowski, V. Family Arenaviridae. In: Van Regenmortel, M.H.V., Fauquet, C.M., Mayo, M.A., Maniloff, J., Desselberger, U. & Ball, L.A. (Eds.) (2005). *Virus Taxonomy, Eighth report of the International Committee on Taxonomy of Viruses*. Academic Press.

Salvato, M.S.; Schweighofer, K.J.; Burns, J. & Shimomaye, E.M. (1992) Biochemical and immunological evidence that the 11 kDa zinc-binding protein of lymphocytic choriomeningitis virus is a structural component of the virus. *Virus Res.* Vol. 22. pp. 185–198.

Sánchez, A.B. & de la Torre, J.C. (2005) Genetic and Biochemical Evidence for an Oligomeric Structure of the Functional L Polymerase of the Prototypic Arenavirus Lymphocytic Choriomeningitis Virus. *J Virol.*; 79(11): 7262–7268.

Speir, R.W.; Wood, O.; Liebhaber, H. & Buckley, S.M. (1970) Lassa fever, a new virus disease of man from west Africa. IV. Electron microscopy of Vero cell cultures infected with Lassa virus. *American Journal of Tropical Medicine and Hygene*. 19, 692-694.

Spiropoulou, C.F.; Kunz, S.; Rollin, P.E.; Campbell, K.P. & Oldstone, M.B. (2002) New World arenavirus clade C, but not clade A and B viruses, utilizes alpha-dystroglycan as its major receptor. *J. Virol.* 76 (10), 5140-5146.

Tortorici, M.A.; Ghiringhelli, P.D. Lozano, M.E.; Albariño, C.G. & Romanowski, V. (2001a) Zinc-binding properties of Junín virus nucleocapsid protein. *Journal of General Virology*, 82: 121–128.

Tortorici, M.A.; Albariño, C.G.; Posik, D.M.; Ghiringhelli, P.D.; Lozano, M.E.; Rivera Pomar, R.V. & Romanowski, V. (2001b) Arenavirus nucleocapsid protein displays a transcriptional antitermination activity *in vivo*. *Virus Research* 73, 41–55.

Urata, S.; Noda, T.; Kawaoka, Y.; Yokosawa, H. & Yasuda, J. (2006) Cellular factors required for Lassa virus budding. *J Virol.* Vol. 80. pp. 4191-5.

Vieth, S.; Torda, A.E.; Asper, M.; Schmitz, H. & Günter, S. (2004) Sequence analysis of L RNA of Lassa virus. *Virology*, 318: 153-168.

Weissenbacher, M.C.; Laguens, R.P. & Coto, C.E. (1987) Argentine hemorrhagic fever. *Curr Top Microbiol Immunol.*; 134:79-116.

Wilson, S.M. & Clegg, J.C.S. (1991). Sequence analysis of the S RNA of the African arenavirus Mopeia: an unusual secondary structure feature in the intergenic region. *Virology* 180: 543-552.

York, J.; Romanowski, V.; Lu, M. & Nunberg, J.H. (2004) The Signal Peptide of the Junín Arenavirus Envelope Glycoprotein Is Myristoylated and Forms an Essential Subunit of the Mature G1-G2 Complex. *Journal of Virology*, 78 (19): 10783-10792.

Yun, N.E.; Linde, N.S.; Dziuba, N.; Zacks, M.A.; Smith, J.N.; Smith, J.K.; Aronson, J.F.; Chumakova, O.V.; Lander, H.M.; Peters, C.J. & Paessler, S. (2008) Pathogenesis of XJ and Romero Strains of Junin Virus in Two Strains of Guinea Pigs. *Am. J. Trop. Med. Hyg.*, 79(2), pp. 275–282.

Part 3

Point Mutation in Bacteria: Human Activity-Driven Evolution

8

Mutational Polymorphism in the Bacterial Topoisomerase Genes Driven by Treatment with Quinolones

Maja Velhner and Dragica Stojanović
Scientific Veterinary Institute Novi Sad, Serbia

1. Introduction

Overuse of antimicrobial agents in human and veterinary medicine is a serious problem worldwide. Bacteria have developed resistance mechanisms decades ago, even before wide application of antibiotics had started. Naturally they had learned to cope with an unfavourable environment well before man changed it. Bacteria can develop resistance utilizing different mechanisms. Through mobile genetic elements bacteria transfer resistance to progeny, raising concerns about not being able to control the infection (Velhner et al., 2011). An understanding of resistance mechanisms is essential for developing new therapeutics and overcoming current problems in therapy.

Single point mutations in target genes is sufficient to develop resistance (Giraud et al., 1999).

Quinolones are directed to the complex of DNA and the enzyme Gyrase A and/or topoisomerase IV. They disturb replication of bacteria by changing the topology of DNA. Mutations in genes coding these important enzymes enable bacteria to develop resistance, creating a favourable environment for their survival. Gyrase A consists of two subunits encoded by genes *gyrA* and *gyrB*. In the *gyrA* gene, there is a quinolone resistance-determining region (QRDR) where mutations occur, if bacteria are exposed to antimicrobials (rev. by Velhner et al., 2010). The QRDR extends from codon 67 to 106, but upon quinolone treatment, mutations mostly occur on codons 83 and 87 (Yoshida et al., 1990). In the *gyrB* gene, the QRDR region extends from codons 426 to 447 in *E. coli* and also in *Salmonella* (Yoshida et al., 1991). Gyrase A is a target enzyme in gram negative bacteria. Topoisomerase IV is a target enzyme for gram positive and a secondary target in gram negative bacteria. Topoisomerase IV is encoded by two genes termed *parC* and *parE*. In environments where antimicrobials are persistently in use, multiple resistances develop and genes for both enzymes can be mutated. To monitor the level of resistance it is important to estimate minimal inhibitory concentration (MIC) for certain antibiotics since this would tell us what the risk of antimicrobial use is and whether to expect mutations on target genes.

The focus of the present review will be on resistance development in bacteria that cause food-borne illness and are most often found in livestock industry. Three genera have been selected because of their significance in both human and veterinary medicine: *Salmonella* spp., *Escherichia coli* and *Campylobacter* spp. These bacteria are transferred to humans through the food chain and tend to persist in farms, alimentary and medical settings. Salmonellae are very invasive and spread very quickly from animal to animal. The rate of *Salmonella* Enteritidis isolation in groups of chickens infected orally with 10^2 cfu/0.1 ml (group A), the sentinels (group C) and group of chickens infected orally with 10^4 cfu/0.1ml and sentinels (group D) is presented in Fig 1. The low infective doses did not prevent horizontal spread of SE to contact chickens during 14 days post infection. *Salmonella* Enteritidis could be isolated in highest percent (group C and D) from birds exposed by contact (Velhner et al., 2005). If chickens are infected during the growth *Salmonella* will be transmitted in slaughterhouses, contaminating food. E*scherichia coli* are widely distributed among farm animals. Pathogenic isolates but also commensals, tend to harbour different resistance mechanisms. Genetic polymorphism in target genes is noted in quinolone resistant strains. However, just recently identical extended-spectrum β-lactamase genes were found among *E. coli* isolates from humans and retail chicken meat in The Netherlands. This implicates spread of *E. coli* to people through the food chain, raising concern about prudent use of antimicrobial agents in farm animals. To minimize health problems in humans caused by infection with food borne bacteria, it is also important to develop strict measures to prevent contamination during food processing and handling (Overdevest et al., 2011). *Campylobacter* species gain resistance to quinolones easily and as such present a risk for consumer's safety. Usually they are not pathogenic for animals, but if humans are infected through food this can cause gastrointestinal diseases. Resistance to quinolones is of special concern because proper medical treatment could be difficult if patients are infected with multiple resistant microorganism. Children, elderly people and immunocompromised patients are at highest risk in such situation. Monitoring of antimicrobial resistance is therefore necessary and in most countries is introduced as a part of the national programs in human and veterinary medicine.

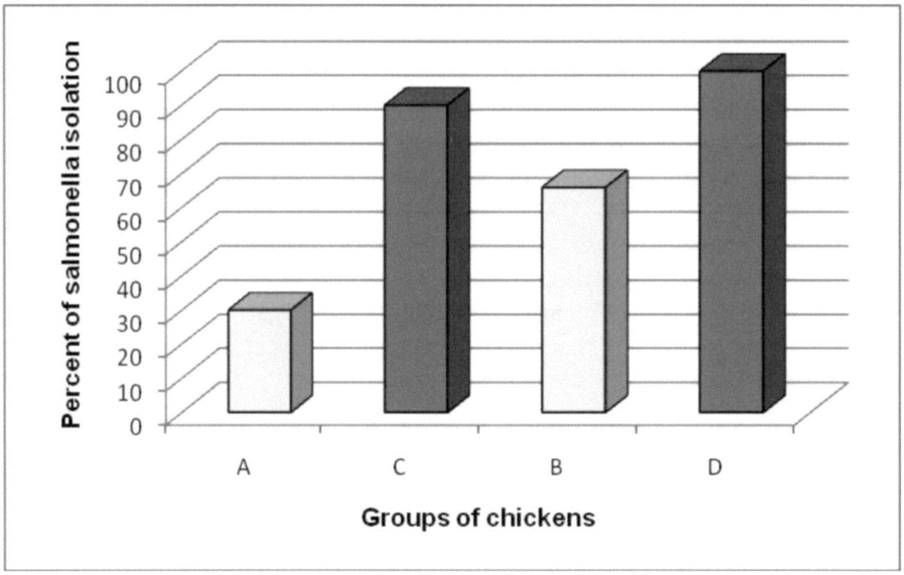

Fig. 1. Incidence of salmonella isolation from cloacal swabs during the experiment. Groups C and D are sentinel chickens.

2. Point mutations in topoisomerase genes of *Salmonella*

There are over 2000 serotypes of the genus *Salmonella* and most of them are pathogens for humans. They are usually transmitted by food of animal origin and animal products. *Salmonellae* are invasive, tend to spread clonally and also gain multiple resistance phenotypes. There is a number of papers dealing with the resistance mechanisms to quinolones in *Salmonella*. Every decade is marked with the predominance of certain serotypes and distinctive resistance patterns. Most frequently quinolones will induce the apparition of point mutations in the *gyrA* gene but there are reports on mutations in other topoisomerase genes. If bacteria are highly resistant to fluoroquinolones (FQ) and MIC exceeds the clinical breakpoint, a double mutant can be expected. Nevertheless in quinolone resistant *Salmonella*, the most frequent mutations are on the *gyrA* gene, while mutations in multiple loci are reported occasionally. We will summarize recent reports concerning mutations in topoisomerase genes and present our current opinion about resistance mechanisms.

Giraud et al. (1999) proposed that in veterinary isolates the most common amino acid substitution in *gyrA* gene is Ser83→Phe, because of wide application in animal husbandry of enrofloxacin, a fluorinated quinolone derivate. A similar result was obtained by spontaneous mutant selection with nalidixic acid (NAL), ciprofloxacin (CIP) and enrofloxacin (ENR). Enrofloxacin selects mutants with Ser83→Phe substitution on *gyrA*, while NAL and CIP favour substitutions on codon 87 (Levy et al., 2004). Therefore mutations on topoisomerase genes depend on antimicrobial agents to which *Salmonella* are exposed (Giraud et al., 2006). In a collection of isolates from farm animals in England and Wales, mutation at codon Ser83 induced higher MIC to ciprofloxacin compared to mutations at Asp87 (Liebana et al., 2002). Mutational polymorphism is prominent in topoisomerase genes in Salmonella and sometimes depends on serotype, country of origin or continent (Escribano et al., 2004; Hopkins et al., 2005; Lindstedt et al., 2004; Piddock et al., 1998; San Martin et al., 2005). The most frequent are mutations on *gyrA*, Ser83→Tyr, Phe or Ala and on codon Asp87→Asn, Gly, Tyr or Lys, (Giraud et al., 2006; Hopkins et al., 2005; Lee et al., 2004). In one clinical isolate of *Salmonella* Enteritidis described in the research work of Lindstedt et al. (2004), a novel mutation was found on *gyrA* at Gly81→His. This mutation coupled with Ser83→Tyr exchange, increased the MIC to CIP to 8 μg/ml (doubled in comparison to single mutant). Mutations on Gly81→Ser do not cause resistance to quinolone and FQ in *Salmonella* Typhimurium when spontaneous mutants are induced *in vitro*. The substitution to serine is too weak to induce resistance to FQ (Reyna et al., 1995). In another experiment Gly81→Cys *in vitro* mutants induced significant increase in MIC to NAL and CIP compared to the parent strain (Giraud et al., 2003). Novel mutants were found in clinical *Salmonella* isolates from patients that were hospitalized because of enteric infection in Tehran, Iran. These novel mutations on *gyrA* are: Ala118→Thr, Ser111→Thr, Arg47→Ser, Leu41→Pro, Asp147→Gly and Gly133→Glu coupled with mutations either on 83 or 87. The significance of these novel substitutions is not known (Hamidian et al., 2011). *Sallmonella* gain resistance to FQ during the therapy. In two immunocompromised patients, *Salmonella* Enteritidis and *Salmonella* Typhimuirum susceptible to FQ were isolated. After the therapy with norfloxacin (patient 1) and cefotaxime (patient 2), the resistant mutants (Ser83→Tyr, Ser83→Phe) were found when the treatment was completed. *In vivo* mutant and pre-therapy isolates were of the same clone, supporting the opinion that quinolone selection can occur *in vivo* during antibiotic treatment (Ouabdesselam et al., 1996). The role of mutation of *gyrB* to yield quinolone resistance was studied by Gensberg et al. (1995). The authors found a novel mutation on *gyrB* at codon Ser463→Tyr, located outside the QRDR. Complementation experiment with the *E. coli* carrying plasmid pBP548, having the wild type GyraseB, have shown that one isolate, termed L18, regains a susceptible phenotype to quinolones. The mutated region in L18 did not change the hydrophobicity of the enzyme but possibly introduced a conformational change in the molecule. Heisig (1993) and Heisig et al. (1995) reported that in the early 1990's, a *Salmonella* Thyphimuirum var. Copenhagen multiple resistant clonally spread from cattle to humans. These isolates had two point mutations on *gyrA* Ser83→Ala and Asp87→Asn or Tyr. Complementation experiments have provided the evidence that target gene *gyrA*, if mutated, plays a role in resistance to fluoroquinolones and that also *gyrB* is implicated in resistance development. Guerra et al. (2003) found three point mutations in two *Salmonella* Typhimurium var. Copenhagen from the early 1990 that were sent to National Salmonella Reference Laboratory in Germany. The mutations were found on codon Ser83 →Ala and on codon Asp87→Asn in *gyrA*. A novel mutation was found on *gyrB* at codon Ser464→Phe and one additional mutation was found on QRDR of *parC* (Ser80→Ile). Casin et al. (2003) reported that high level resistance to ciprofloxacin was found in two patients (74 year old man, isolate STmA and 3 years old boy, isolate STmB) and that 5 strains had the same point mutations on *gyrA* (Ser83→Phe and Asp87→Asn), while on *gyrB* mutation was found at Ser464→Phe. In STmA, a mutation was found on *parC* (Glu84→Lys) while in an isolate from a 3 year old boy, the mutation was Ser80→Arg. The two isolates were not clonally related. The isolate STmA could acquire resistance during treatment with ciprofloxacin, although it is still hard to explain why the isolate STmB from the boy was floroquinolone resistant and yet the patient had never been exposed to ciprofloxacin. It is possible that both Salmonellas appeared independently from the environment, suggesting the presence of multiple resistant ST in communities in France. A comprehensive research on mutational polymorphism in *Salmonella enterica* in the United Kingdom is provided by Eaves et al., 2004. In this strain collection among 182 isolates, five had a novel substitution on *gyrB*. In *Salmonella enterica* serovar Seftenberg Tyr420 is mutated to Cys and in serovar Newport Arg at 437 was mutated to Leu. These mutations were also found in *Salmonella* Enteritidis and serovar Mbandaka. The authors stated that the mutations occur in close proximity to the quinolone binding pocket, most likely contributing to decreased binding of quinolones. The first report on *parC* mutations in Salmonella was provided by Ling et al. (2003). They discovered that a single point mutation in *parC* confers resistance to quinolones and the highest resistance level was obtained if double mutation occurs in Ser83 and Asp87 on *gyrA* gene. Double mutants were common in clinical isolates reported in the research by Ling et al., 2003. Another interesting observation about *parC* mutations comes from Eaves et al. (2004) who found out that the *parC* mutations, single or coupled with *gyrA* mutation, in *Salmonella* induce lower geometric mean (GMM) and MIC_{50} comparing to single *gyrA* mutant, suggesting compensatory mechanism of *parC* point mutation at 57. This observation was not found by other authors or in *E. coli*, but there is evidence that Thr57→Ser substitution in *parC* (C→G transversion) does not induce quinolone resistance *per se* (Baucheron et al., 2005; Kim et al., 2011).

High fluoroquinolone resistance in *Salmonella* is not very common and sometimes depends on serovar and the rate of exposition to antimicrobial agents. Heisig et al. (1995) stated that clinical resistance to fluoroquinolones is rare due to the high antibacterial activity against *Salmonella*, because of the lack of enzymatic inactivation of the drug and because it is hard to transfer such resistance. Fluoroquinolone resistant *Salmonella* Typhimurium mutants selected *in vitro* and *in vivo* have shown a low fitness cost indicated by an impaired growth rate comparing to susceptible strains. However, if a compensatory mutation occurs, bacteria have more chance to survive in the presence of antibiotics. In survivors, the role of overexpressed multidrug pumps is also evident (Giraud et al., 2003). Indeed, most often high resistance to fluoroquinolone is coupled with multiple resistance phenotypes. If bacteria harbor resistance to ampicillin, chloramphenicol, sulfa drugs and fluoroquinolones the therapy of ill individuals that require treatment could be difficult. There is an opinion that in such cases different resistance mechanisms are involved in selecting mutants that are capable of surviving in the environment. Three major mechanisms are: mutation in topoisomerase II and IV, overexpression of efflux pump and decreased outer membrane permeability (Cloeckaert & Chaslus-Dancla, 2001; Giraud et al., 2006; Hopkins et al., 2005).

In Spain, the rate of NAL resistant *Salmonella* isolated from humans increased during the year 1994 and peaked at 2001 to 46.2%. In 2003 NAL resistance was found in 38.5% isolates. Out of 164 non-typhoid *Salmonella* from food collected from 1999 to 2003, 124 isolates were NAL resistant. Point mutations were found dominantly at codon 87 and also codon 83. The first *Salmonella* isolate from humans resistant to CIP was reported in March 2003. Subsequently in the same year, 2 more CIP resistant isolates were found. Three *Salmonella* were isolated from children and two from patients aged 49 and 47. These strains possessed three point mutation in QRDR of the *gyrA* gene (aa substitution were at Ser83→Phe and Asp87→Asn) and additional mutation was found on *parC* at Ser80→Arg (Marimon et al., 2004). Similar increase in number of NAL resistant clinical isolates of *Salmonella enterica* was recorded in Korea. In 1996 NAL resistance was found in 1.8% isolates and by 2000-2002 it increased to 21.8%. Single mutation were at codon 87 (39 strains) and at codon 83 in 4 strains (Choi et al., 2005). An increase from 0.4% in 1996 to 2.3% in 2003 was also recorded for NAL resistant *Salmonella enterica* in the USA. In 14 CIP resistant isolates, double mutations were found at *gyrA* at 83 (Ser83→Tyr or Ser83→Phe) and on 87 (Asp87→Gly or Asp87→Asn). Mutations on *gyrB*, *parC* and *parE* were not detected (Stevenson et al., 2007). *Salmonella* Seftenberg isolated during a nosocomial outbreak in Florida were included in the study of Whichard et al. (2007). In these isolates point mutations were found on *gyrA* at Ser83→Tyr and Asp87→Gly and on *parC* (Ser80→Ile and/or Thr57→Ser) while MIC to CIP was >4μg/ml. Most of the *Salmonella* Seftenberg isolates from their collection also contained mechanism of extended-spectrum cephalosporin resistance. Such co-resistance in *Salmonella* Seftenberg maybe plays a role in the epidemiology of *Salmonella*.

If a high resistance to fluoroquinolone occurs, several point mutations are usually detected in target genes. In *Salmonella* collected in Hong Kong in the period from 1990 to 2001, highly resistant strains to fluoroquinolone were recorded. Two isolates harbour mutations at *gyrA* (Ser83→Phe, Asp87→Asn) and on *parC* at Ser80→Arg. MIC to ciprofloxacine was 8-16 μg/ml for these isolates. In 4 additional isolates, point mutations were found on *gyrA* (Ser83→Phe, Asp87→Gly), in *parC* (Ser80→Arg) and in *parE*, with a new substitution at Ser458→Pro. In these *Salmonella* MIC for ciprofloxacin was even higher (16-32 μg/ml). For the first time a mutation, Thr57→Ser in *parC*, alone or coupled with *gyrA* mutation, was reported. Single *parC* mutant were less susceptible to CIP (MIC < 0.12 μg/ml) suggesting that such mutation is a marker of low level resistance to FQ (Ling et al., 2003). A first report of infection with fluoroquinolon resistant *Salmonella* in the USA was published by Olsen et al. in 2001. The infection occurred in nursing homes, where *Salmonella enterica* serotype Schwarzenground spread among residents in two distant facilities. The patient, who returned from the Philippines and was hospitalized in New York and afterwards resided in a nursery home, was most likely a vehicle for the transmission. In fact, after comprehensive epidemiological survey *Salmonella* Schwarzenground was found in two environmental samples taken from the mattress and door handle in the room of the ill resident. Twenty nine months *Salmonella* Schwarzenground was present in the environment and this infection lead to the death of 3 people in the nursing home. PFGE pattern was similar for all the strains and the same *gyrA* mutations were found during survey (Ser83→Phe and Asp87→Gly). MIC to ciprofloxacin was 4μg/ml. The first report on clinical *Salmonella* Typhimurium DT12 highly resistant to fluoroquinolones in Japan comes from Nakaya et al. (2003). The STDT12 was isolated from a stool of an infant with diarrhoea. The isolate was resistant to ampicillin, streptomycin, gentamycin, tetracycline, chloramphenicol, sulfamethoxazole/trimetoprim, nalidixic acid and fluoroquinolones. It exhibited resistance also to levofloxacin (MIC 8 μg/ml), ciprofloxacin (MIC 8 μg/ml) and norfloxacin (MIC 16 μg/ml). Three point mutations were distributed on *gyrA* Ser83→Phe and Asp87→Asn and on *parC*, Ser80→Arg. Therapy was successful with fosfomycin, a drug prescribed for babies and children. *Salmonella* isolated from cattle in Japan did not posses such resistance phenotype and could not be linked to this outbreak at the time being. However, in 2005, the spread of multiple resistant *Salmonella enterica* serovar Typhimurium DT104 was found in Japan (Izumiya et al., 2005). The isolates harboured mutations on *gyrA* gene Ser83→Phe and Asp87→Asn and on *parC* Ser80→Arg was found. Besides the same point mutations, similar resistotypes were detected in human and nonhuman isolates in their study. Genetically related ciprofloxacin resistant *Salmonella* Typhimurium and *Salmonella* Choleraesuis were found in Taiwan in people and pigs. In human isolates MIC for ciprofloxacin was 8-64 μg/ml while in pig isolates MIC range from $\geq$ 0.125 to 64 μg/ml. In *Salmonella* Typhimurium from patients, mutations were found in *gyrA* (Ser83→Phe and Asp87→Gly) and additional mutations were found on *parC* at Ser80→Arg or Glu84→Lys. In *Salmonella* Choleraesuis from patients, *gyrA* mutations were found on codons Ser83→Phe and Asp87→Asn while mutation on *parC* was at Ser80→Ile. The same mutations were found in *Salmonella* Typhimuirum from pigs. In serovar Choleraesuis from pigs the mutations were at Ser83→Phe, Asp87→Asn, or Asp87→Gly coupled with *parC* mutations on Ser80→Ile. Interestingly in both human and pig *Salmonella* Choleraesuis isolates resistant to CIP, the same point mutation was also found on *acrR* (efflux repressor gene) at Gln78→Stp. The molecular typing survey has shown that *Salmonella* Typhimurium and *Salmonella* Choleraesuis spread from animals to humans in Taiwan (Chiu et al., 2004; Hsueh et al., 2004). Other research supports the finding that double and triple mutant of *Salmonella enterica* serovar Choleraesusis circulates in several pig farms and that multiple mutations on topoisomerase genes confer resistance to fluoroqionolones in Taiwan (Huang et al., 2004). Clinical report on ciprofloxacin/ceftriaxone resistant *Salmonella* Choleraesuis infection in three patients admitted to Medical Centre in Southern Taiwan, reveals the same PFGE profile and point mutations on *gyrA* Ser83→Phe, Asp87→Asn and on parC Ser80→Ile. All five isolates from patients also possess the bla_{CMY-2} gene. It was postulated that NAL resistant

Salmonella tend to cause higher death rate comparing to susceptible strains (Ko et al., 2005). Recently, one *Salmonella* Typhi isolate from a patient who returned from India was reported to have high MIC to ciprofloxacin (32μg/ml) and subsequently two point mutations were discovered in *gyrA* Ser83→Phe and Asp87→Gly (Hassing et al., 2011). Recurrent infection with *Salmonella enterica* serovar Typhimurium DT104 occurred in a patient admitted to the hospital in Denmark. Initially the bacteria were susceptible to fluoroquinolones. The patient received low doses of ciprofloxacin and during the next year STDT104 emerged as quinolone resistant (MIC to CIP 0.190 μg/ml), due to the single point mutation, on *gyrA* Ser83→Phe (Kristiansen et al., 2003). In *Salmonella* one single point mutation on *gyrA* gene is sufficient to induce high level resistance to quinolones. Double mutations in *gyrA* or *gyrA* and other target genes for quinolones are not so common as in *E. coli*. However, if double mutations occur it usually leads to elevated or high resistance to FQ. High resistance to quinolones due to double and triple mutations is sometimes reported in patients who returned from Asia and/or Mediterranean countries. It is evident that Salmonella differs from continent to continent and depends on the medical treatment prescribed and overuse of antimicrobials in both human and veterinary medicine. In China it is also possible that stool specimens were sometimes collected after the onset of the disease and after the therapy had already been applied. This is due to easy access to the medication that is not under appropriate control of a physician (Cui et al., 2008). *Salmonella* is also the most frequent cause of traveller's diarrhoea. Clinical isolates obtained in a five year study from the patients who returned from different countries (India, Mexico, Egypt, Peru, Kenya, Ivory Coast, Gambia, Senegal, Mali and Bolivia) were tested for antimicrobial resistance. In quinolone resistant strains a single amino acid substitution was found on Asp87→Tyr and in one isolate a Ser83→Tyr substitution was found. Amino acid substitution was not found on *parC* in this strain collection (Cabrera et al., 2004). *Salmonella enterica* serovar Typhi was found in the year 2006 and 2007, in two patients from Kuwait who returned from Bangladesh. In these isolates four point mutations were detected on QRDR, namely: **Leu55→Trp**, Ser83→Phe, **Asp87→Ala, Gln106→Arg** in gyrA gene. On *parC* gene mutations were found on Glu84→Lys, Trp106→Gly and **Tyr128→Asp** (in bold are mutations reported for the first time in *gyrA* and *parC* genes) (Dimitrov et al., 2009). Reduced susceptibility in *Salmonella enterica* isolates from Finland was most frequent in patients who acquired infection abroad. Following mutations were reported on *gyrA* gene: Ser83→Phe, Ser83→Tyr, Asp87→Asn, Gly or Tyr. Mutations on *parC* were not recorded in this survey (Hakanen et al., 1999; Hakanen et al., 2001).

A research work from veterinary field is shortly presented here and clonal spread of *Salmonella* is described. Treatment of pigs infected with quinolone resistant *Salmonella* Typhimuirum DT104 with enrofloxacin cause higher shedding of resistant microorganism comparing to untreated control. This means that antibiotic treatment of pigs before slaughter will induce increased shedding and impose higher risk concerning food safety (Delsol et al., 2004). In chicken experiments it was shown that enrofloxacin treatment cause elevated MIC to ciprofloxacin (MIC 0.12-0.5 μg/ml) if birds are infected with a susceptible strain of *Salmonella enterica* serovar Typhimurium DT104. In the same experiment a multidrug-resistant (MDR) derivate of the same strain appeared in the presence of enrofloxacin, exhibiting higher MIC to CIP (0.25-1μg/ml). This isolate was cyclohexane tolerant, implicating the role of efflux pump in MDR strains (Randall et al., 2005).

```
                                83          87
1. gyrA/ST nctc atccccacggcgattccgcagtgtatgacaccatcgttcgtatggcgcagccattctcgc
2. gyrA/EC ATCC atccccacggcgattccgcagtgtatgacaccatcgttcgtatggcgcagccattctcgc
3. gyrA/9568    ..........................aac...............................
4. gyrA/501     ..........................aac...............................
5. gyrA/75      ..........................aac...............................
6. gyrA/7938    ..............ttc...........................................
7. gyrA/74      ..........................aac...............................
8. gyrA/33641   ..........................aac...............................
9. gyrA/317526  ............................................................
10. gyrA/1898   ..........................ggc...............................
11. gyrA/228020 ..........................aac...............................

1. gyrA/ST nctc tgcgttacatgctggtggatggtcagggtaacttcggttctattgacggcgactccgcgg
2. gyrA/EC ATCC tgcgttacatgctggtggatggtcagggtaacttcggttctattgacggcgactccgcgg
3. gyrA/9568    ............................................................
4. gyrA/501     ............................................................
5. gyrA/75      ............................................................
6. gyrA/7938    ............................................................
7. gyrA/74      ............................................................
8. gyrA/33641   ............................................................
9. gyrA/317526  ............................................................
10. gyrA/1898   ............................................................
11. gyrA/228020 ............................................................
```

Fig. 2. Multiple alignment of quinolone resistant *Salmonella Enteritidis*, isolated from stool, food and poultry in Serbia. Point mutations are presented in bold. This region encompasses codons 83 and 87. The reference strain is number 2 (*Escherichia coli*, ATCC 25922), in strain 317526 the mutation was not found, implying another mechanism of resistance to quinolones

Intercontinental spread of *Salmonella* Typhimurium definitive phage type 104 (STDT104) is well documented. Clonal spread of *Salmonella* Enteritidis PT1, resistant to quinolones (MIC for nalidixic acid >128 μg/ml) also harbouring one unique point mutation on *gyrA* (Asp87→Tyr) is reported in Ireland by Kilmartin et al. (2005). *Salmonella* Virchow has for many years been a common serotype in Israel. It is resistant to nalidixic acid and possesses the point mutation Asp87→Tyr on *gyrA* gene (Solnik-Isaac, 2007). Since the year 2000, in the Netherlands and Germany *Salmonella* Java clonally spreads and is more prevalent compared to other serovars. This strain is resistant to chloramphenicol, sulphonamide, tetracycline, trimetoprim and often to kanamycin, neomycin and nalidixic acid. It is postulated that S. Java has emerged in the poultry industry due to the frequent use of antibiotics and because vaccination was implemented to eradicate *Salmonella* Enteritidis (van Pelt et al., 2003). Clonal spread of multiple resistant *Salmonella* Infantis (nalidixic acid, streptomycin, sulphonamide and tetracycline) is reported in Hungary where poultry isolates were linked to human's (Nógrády et al., 2007). *Salmonella enterica* serovar Haardt resistant to quinolones with elevated MIC to ciprofloxacin (MIC 0.25-2 μg/ml) was found on chicken meat collected in various stores. Point mutation was detected on *gyrA* (Ser83→Tyr). PFGE analysis implies clonal spread of NAL resistant S. Haardt in Korea (Lee et al., 2008). In Serbia S. Enteritidis isolated from humans, food and poultry was typed by Random Amplified Polymorphic DNA analysis (RAPD). In a collection of 60 strains, 9 were resistant to nalidixic acid. In these strains 3 different single point mutations were found on *gyrA*, namely Asp87→Asn in 6 strains, Asp87→Gly in 1 strain and Ser83→Phe in one strain (Fig 2). For these isolates, MIC for NAL was 128-512 μg/ml and MIC for CIP was 0.256-0,512 μg/ml. In this strain collection multiple resistances was found in three isolates. *Salmonella* Enteritidis from one day old chicken was resistant to ampicillin (AMP), cephalothin (CFT), nalidixic acid (NAL) and tetracycline (TET). One isolate from stool was resistant to AMP, TET, trimetoprim-sulfamethoxasole (SXT) and another isolate from stool exhibited resistance to AMP, TET, SXT and neomycin (NEO) (Kozoderović et al., 2011). There was an increase of *Salmonella* Enteritidis isolates in Serbia in 2005 and clonal spread was suspected. However, from 2005 to 2008, the percentage of quinolone resistant *Salmonella* Enteritidis appeared to decrease from 9% to 1% in the Northern part of the country (Kozoderović et al., 2009).

3. Point mutations in topoisomerase genes of *E. coli*

Resistance to fluoroquinolones in *E. coli* has been extensively studied. Mutational polymorphism on topoisomerase genes in *E. coli* is frequent in clinical settings but also in commensal. First step mutations occur on *gyrA* gene, most frequently at codon 83, where substitution of Leucine for Serine is found (Chen et al., 2001; Conrad et al., 1996; Everett et al., 1996; Gales et al., 2000; Heisig and Tschorny, 1994; del Mar Tavio et al., 1999). The first report of double mutation in *gyrA* was provided by Heisig et al. (1993). The mutations in *E. coli* isolate 205096, highly resistant to FQ, were located on Ser83→Leu and on Asp87→Gly. Complete sequencing of the gene revealed additional mutation in less conserved region of the *gyrA*, at Asp678→Glu. This mutation is not implicated in FQ resistance. Throughout the coding region, 52 silent mutations were also found. The authors stated that mutations at 83 and 87 encompass part of the enzyme responsible for cleavage and sealing of the DNA. This is necessary to obtain negative supercoiling prior to strand separation. The quinolones prevent contact between DNA and enzyme thus aborting bacterial replication (Drlica & Zhao, 1997). In clinical *E. coli* isolated from urine samples of outpatients who did not receive FQ therapy, a novel mutation was found: Asp87→Tyr. Concomitant mutation of Ser83→Leu and Asp87→Asn or Tyr, induced clinical resistance to CIP (MIC $\geq$ 8 μg/ml). The significance of the double mutant for high fluoroquinolone resistance is warranted (Vila et al., 1994). In clinical isolates of *E. coli* (MIC to CIP > 1 μg/ml) mutations were found on *gyrA* and *parC* gene. Mutational polymorphism in this strain collection is briefly presented here. Mutant with MIC to CIP of < 1 μg/ml have only one mutation at Ser83→Leu. If MIC to CIP is from 8-128 μg/ml, 3-4 mutations were found on gyrA (Ser83→Leu or Asp87→Tyr or Asn) and parC genes (Ser80→Arg or Ile) and /or Glu84→Lys or Val). In two isolates (1319 and 1383) four mutations were found. The MIC to ciprofloxacin was 64 μg/ml and 128 μg/ml and mutations were arranged as follows: Ser83→Leu, Asp87→Asn, Ser80→Ile and Glu84→Val in isolate marked 1319, while a mutation's on Ser83→Leu, Asp87→Tyr, Ser80→Ile and Glu84→Lys were found in isolate marked 1318. This was the first report of *parC* mutation in *E. coli* (Vila et al., 1996). The role of *parC* mutations in highly quinolone resistant *E. coli* was studied by Kumagai et al., 1996. In the QRDR of the *parC* gene three missense mutations on codons Gly78, Ser80 and Glu84 were described corresponding to the *gyrA* mutations on codons Ser83, Gly81 and Ap87. In this research the importance of mutations in topoisomerase IV, in building resistance to FQ in *E. coli* was emphasized. The role of mutations on FQ resistance was also studied by Heisig (1996). In *parC* mutant a reduction in MIC to CIP was recorded after introduction of the wild type gene to mutants. If $parC^{1-80}$ allele (a single mutant) is introduced into isolates that have two point mutations on *parC,* an increase of susceptibility is noted, while introduction of resistant *parC* allele to *gyrA* mutants will induce an increase of MIC to CIP. Mutation of *parC* in *E. coli* having two point mutations on *gyrA* is a prerequisite for high FQ resistance phenotype. The mutations induced by FQ occur in stepwise manner and the primary target for CIP is Gyrase (Bagel et al., 1999). The level of quinolone/fluoroquinolone resistance correlates well with the type and number of mutations on topoisomerase genes. The CLSI breakpoint for FQ is obtained if double mutations on *gyrA* are combined with single or double *parC* mutant (Morgan-Linnell and Zechiedrich 2007; Sáenz et al., 2001). If a mutation on *parC* occurs in a single *gyrA* mutant, second mutation on *gyrA* is selected (Morgan-Linnell and Zechiedrich 2007). Therefore *gyrA* mutation is indispensable for clinical resistance to quinolones and it mostly occurs before *parC* mutations, especially in clinical isolates. Single *parC* mutation does not induce resistance to FQ (Bagel et al., 1999). If *E. coli* is exposed to quinolones, a stepwise mutagenesis may lead to development of a new feature that is beneficial for these bacteria. Usually selection pressure is imposed by application of various quinolones or fluroquinolones in agriculture. In such scenario a single step mutant can become predominate in the population. This will contribute to developing multiple mutations and high resistance to fluoroquinolones in clinical isolates after therapy has been introduced (Piddock et al., 1996). Infection with Fluoroquinolone resistant *E. coli* acquired in hospitals is of special concern. The resistant strains usually evolve independently and the therapy may be difficult to introduce. In the mid 1990, the percent of fluoroquinolone resistant *E. coli* increased in many countries. Lehn et al. (1996) described resistotype and mutations on *gyrA* in a collection of 19 *E. coli* resistant to CIP in hospital settings in Munich, Germany. The majority of isolates were multiple resistant to the following antibiotics: nalidixic acid, ciprofloxacin, norfloxacin, aminoglycosides, co-trimoxazole, ampicillin, ampicillin and sulbactam and piperacillin. Most isolates obtained for the study were from Urology Department, from Gynecology, Surgery and Internal Medicine. PFGE typing implicates diversity of the strains but resistotype was quite similar. Also, the mutations on topisomerase were documented on Ser83→Leu, Asp87→Asn in 16 strains. In two strains Asp was mutated to Gly. Resistance of *E. coli* to FQ is equally reported in developed and developing countries. At highest risk are patients that are hospitalized and treated with antibiotic. Several studies have dealt with various aspects of infection with *E. coli* in hospitals and outpatient clinics. In a study from Taiwan, a total of 1203 isolates of *E. coli* from 44 hospitals were tested on antimicrobial susceptibility and it was found that 11.3% isolates were resistant to FQ. Decreased susceptibility to CIP was found in 21.7% isolates. A single point mutation was found on *gyrA* among FQ resistant and isolates with reduced susceptibility. The authors postulated that such single mutation is a prerequisite for resistance development. In FQ highly resistant strains (MIC >32µg/ml) three or four point mutations were found in QRDR of the *gyrA,* and *parC.* These included substitution at Ser83→Leu, Asp87→Asn, coupled also with Ser80→Ile (9 isolates) or Ser80→Arg (one isolate), Ala81→Pro (one isolate) and Glu84→Gly or Lys (one isolate). The survey in Taiwan reveals high risk on FQ resistance in clinical *E. coli* isolates. It was noted that patients diagnosed with cancer were predisposed to infection with resistant *E. coli.* Nalidixic acid and pipemidic acid are still in medical practice and these practices pose a risk for higher FQ resistance in Taiwan (McDonald et al., 2001). Two or more mutation on topisomerase II and

IV were found in a hospital strain collection in South Korea. In fact, the number of acquired mutations was proportional to MIC for ciprofloxacin. The CIP resistant isolates were divided into 4 groups depending of the number of mutations in topoisomerase genes. It was concluded that second step mutant will induce double mutation on *parC* and that double *parC* mutant are highly resistant to fluoroquinolones. All of the *parE* mutations were outside the QRDR. Three novel *parE* mutations were reported on Leu445→Ile, Ser458→Pro and Ser458→Trp. These single mutations on *parE* significantly increased MIC to CIP, norfloxacin and gatifloxacin. In this strain collection three to four mutations on topisomerase II and IV were common. Mutations on *gyrB* were not found. Combination of double mutations on *parC* or single *parC* and *parE* mutation increases MIC of ciprofloxacin (Chan Moon et al., 2010). Mutational polymorphism was found in clinical isolates of *E. coli* in New Delhi, India, revealing that a number of isolates possess several mutation on topisomerase genes and that mutation on *parE* was prominent since 44.4% of isolates are mutated on *parE*, outside of QRDR. The substitutions found on *parE* were Ser458→Ala and Glu460→Asp. Mutations on both genes (*parC* and *parE*) being the secondary target for FQ contributed to higher MIC >0.25 µg/ml for ciprofloxacin (Bansal and Tandon, 2011). Asian Network for Surveillance of Resistant Pathogens provided 68 *E. coli* isolates resistant to FQ, to carry out a research on geographic distribution of mutational polymorphism. Clonal spread was not evident. Continentally distributed isolates possessed a variety of mutation in topoisomerase genes but those with three or more mutations were increasingly resistant to CIP. This high increase was attributed also to the mutation of the *parE* gene (Uchida et al., 2010). *E. coli* isolates from healthy patients in Teaching Hospital and Microbiology Department at the University in Ghana were studied with respect to FQ resistance. About 50 to 90% of faecal isolates from healthy individuals were multiple resistant to the following antimicrobial agents: ampicillin, streptomycin, tetracycline, sulphonamides and trimethoprim. The obtained results revealed that in the year 2008, 18.2% of isolates were resistant to NAL and 9.9% were resistant to FQ. In resistant isolates the most frequent substitution was Ser80→Leu often combined with Asp87→Asn in *gyrA* and on *parC* the most frequent substitution was at Ser80→Ile. The mutation in topoisomerase that was found was attributed to old and recently introduced drugs in clinical practice in Ghana. Presence of multiple resistances in commensal microflora in patients is noted and the prudent use of fluoroquinolones is warranted (Namboodiri et al., 2011). Bacteria change phenotype, depending on the selection pressure. This has been shown in research on resistance mechanisms in laboratory mutants and clinical isolates. We have learned that careful use of antibiotics is essential and must be under control or it will be impossible to cope with the infections acquired in hospitals and the environments from which subsequent transfer of resistant bacteria is common. Topoisomerase mutators can have prohibitive fitness cost or might have selection advantage.

E. coli with single point mutation on *gyrA* was found in veterinary isolates and it was suggested that the digestive tract of animals can be a reservoir of low level resistance to quinolones. If such bacteria find their way to humans through the food chain, clinical resistance will occur in patients that needs therapy (Everett et al., 1996). A heterogenic population of quinolone resistant *E. coli* collected from poultry, poultry farmers and poultry slaughterers was described by van den Bogaard et al. (2001). Only in few isolates a link between poultry and poultry farmers was noted, implying that *E. coli* from animals could also infect people. Mutations on topoisomerase genes in *E. coli* isolated from faeces of healthy chickens in six broiler and 4 breeder farms in Korea was described by Lee et al. (2005). All isolates resistant to ciprofloxacin and enrofloxacin exhibited mutations on Ser83→Leu. Many isolates also harbour second mutation on Asp87→Asn, Ala, Gly, His or Tyr. In this strain collection, mutations were also found on *parC*, the most prevalent being Ser80→Arg, Ile, Phe and Gly and in some isolates, mutation were found on Glu84→Lys, Ile and Tyr. The MIC breakpoint to CIP and ENR was >3 µg/ml and 2 µg/ml respectfully. The isolates with two mutations distributed on *gyrA* and *parC* had elevated MIC to ciprofloxacin (0.5-3 µg/ml) while MIC to ENR was 1 to 32 µg/ml. Isolates presented by greater MIC than clinical breakpoint had two mutations on *gyrA* (at codons 83 and 87) with or without substitution on *parC* . Khan et al. (2005) found out that the poultry litter collected from poultry and turkey farms in the Arkansas, USA becomes an important source of quinolone resistant *E. coli*. In isolates resistant to CIP (> 2 µg/ml) two point mutations were found at Ser83→Leu and Asp87→Asn. Single point mutation in MIC < 2 µg/ml was found on Ser83→Leu. Beef, pork and poultry are considered as the main reservoir of quinolone resistant *E. coli*, *Salmonella* and *Campylobacter* (Mayrhofer et al., 2004). Nine *E. coli* isolates from wild birds that died from septicemia were tested on quinolone resistance. It was found that all the strains had one mutation on *gyrA* gene at Ser80→Leu. Mutations on other target genes (*gyrB*, *parC* and *parE*) were not found (Jiménez Gómez et al., 2004). The high incidence of quinolone resistant *E .coli* from nosocomial and community acquired infections is linked to a high incidence of FQ resistant *E. coli* in poultry and pigs. The clear connection between human and poultry isolates was not, however, found in Spain but it was postulated that the infection of humans occurs via contaminated food of animal origin Garau et al. (1999). Indeed, it is difficult to explicitly claim that the link exists between poultry related food and humans but the similarities are present in resistant isolates, compared to susceptible strains. The general statement is that the misuse of quinolones largely contributes to the spread of resistant bacteria through the food chain (Johnson et al., 2006).

It is difficult to explain how FQ resistance evolves in *E. coli* and how it spreads in clinical settings. It seems that *E. coli* mutates to a higher extent compared to *Salmonellae* and is capable of accumulating several point mutations at the same time or in a stepwise manner. Since the FQ resistant phenotype arises exclusively after *de novo* mutations (Mooij et al., 2005) it seems that microorganisms harbouring one single amino acid substitution are prone to mutate and more easily survive in the environment. High mutation rates could also lead to the development of deleterious mutations. Strong mutators therefore do not always have an evolutionary advantage. If the high mutation rate of *E. coli* will not favour its survival, then the only way to explain the presence of resistant population in a certain zone is exposure of bacteria to antimicrobials. *E. coli* tends not to spread clonally in hospital settings (Lautenbach et al., 2006) and also in the environment (Khan et al., 2005). It is not clear whether isolates with multiple mutations on target genes have some evolutionary advantage so it appears that multiple mutations have low fitness cost. If such mutations are accumulated, compensatory mutations will support growth. On the contrary there are examples where multiple mutations have actually increased bacterial fitness. This also takes place in the absence of antibiotics. Mutations on regulatory genes have the highest influence on bacteria fitness, since those genes regulate transcription and also efflux mechanisms (Marcusson et al., 2009).

4. Point mutations in topoisomerase genes in *Campylobacter* spp

Infections caused by *Campylobacter* usually have a very silent course in animals (Stojanov et al., 2004). However, Campylobacteriosis is the most frequent reason for gastroenteritis in humans. If food producing animals (pigs and poultry) are treated with enrofloxacin (a fluoroquinolone antibiotic) *Campylobacter* develops resistance that lasts well beyond withdrawal of the therapy (Delsol et al., 2004; Griggs et al., 2005; Luo et al., 2005). Subsequently food can be contaminated during processing, increasing the possibility of transmission to humans. Ciprofloxacin resistant Campylobacter emerged on the European continent in the early 1990 and this coincides with the agricultural practice to treat animals with enrofloxacin. At that time in the United Kingdom human *Campylobacter* infections were reported most frequently in travellers returned from abroad, while ciprofloxacin resistant *Campylobacter* was found in poultry carcasses imported from Europe (Gaunt and Piddock, 1996). In Northern Ireland, ciprofloxacin resistance of *Campylobacter* rose in 1998. This was attributed to dietary habits of the consumers in the UK. Chicken and pork meat consumption increased because of Bovine spongioform encephalopathy. Subsequently the import of poultry meat from the European countries might have contributed to the spread of fluoroquinolone resistance (Moore et al., 2001). The National Antimicrobial Resistance Monitoring Program (NARMS) was conducted from 1997 to 2001 to identify susceptibility of *Campylobacter* for the following antimicrobials: chloramphenicol, ciprofloxacin, clindamycin, erythromycin, nalidixic acid, tetracycline, azithromycin and gentamycin. Isolates were collected based on a questionnaire that included: history of recent illness, exposure to animals, food consumption or travelling. Retail chicken meat products from domestic brand were also included in the study. An increase of ciprofloxacin resistant *Campylobact*er from 13% in 1997 to 21% in 2001 was found. Foreign travel was identified as a risk of FQ resistant *Campylobacter* infection in humans but also consumption of chicken meat. The increase of CIP resistant *Campylobacter* coincides with the increasing use of fluoroquinolones in human medicine and livestock industry in the USA (Gupta et al., 2004). Infection with CIP resistant *Campylobacter* in a Minnesota community was related to travels abroad and seasonal peaks were identified. Overall increase in *Campylobacter* isolates resistant to CIP from the year 1996 to 1998 was attributed also to domestically acquired infections. Poultry meat and products were identified as a source of infection and a genetic correlation between human and poultry isolates was determined (Smith et al., 1999). However, *Campylobacter* is genetically quite diverse and clear links between food of animal origin and humans is not easily confirmed. In fact, diverse *Campylobacter* isolates were noted on a single swine farms and slaughter plant in the USA (Thakur and Gebreyes, 2005). Similar results were obtained in Senegal in a two-year period, applying multilocus sequence approach in *Campylobacter* isolated on chicken carcasses. Allelic profiles in *Campylobacter* jejuni (Kinana et al., 2006) and *Campylobacter* coli (Kinana et al., 2007a) imply genetic differences in this strain collection. The link between genotype and quinolone resistance was not found with certainty in their research. Even for the isolates of the same sequence type, different silent mutations were found on *gyrA* gene. In the research conducted in France an increase in FQ resistant *Campylobacter* was recorded for the period 1986 to 2004. The FQ resistance pattern was similar between human, pig and poultry isolates. In *C. coli* the overall resistance rate was higher comparing to C. jejuni. In pigs, C. coli predominated over C. jejuni and it was more frequently resistant to CIP. The higher rate of C. coli isolation in pigs and chickens is not explained. The FQ resistance pattern was similar in C. jejuni isolates found in humans and broilers. Resistance decreased to lesser extend in human C. jejuni comparing to chicken. This is explained in part by restrictive use of antimicrobials as food additives in livestock industry and may also be related to various routes of infection in humans and therapeutic practice in human medicine (Gallay et al., 2007). Overall, it has been shown that people are infected from food of animal origin and that intensive use of quinolones and fluoroquinolones in livestock industry undoubtedly contributes to the development of resistance. Molecular typing of the *Campylobacter* species revealed quite diverse genetic backgrounds and apparent clonal distribution was not identified. The prudent use of FQ antibiotics is necessary to build up safe environment and safe food production.

The ability of *Campylobacter* to acquire resistance to quinolones/fluoroquinolones is rather impressive. The most frequent missense mutation in *gyrA* gene is Thr86→Ile. The codon 86 in *Campylobacter* corresponds to *gyrA* codon 83 in *E. coli* and Salmonella (Beckmann et al., 2004; Griggs et al., 2005; Hakanen et al., 2002; Sonnevend et al., 2006; Wang et al., 1993, Zirnstein et al., 2000). This single point mutation confers resistance to ciprofloxacin and MIC is $\geq$ 32μg/ml. Less frequent mutation in QRDR of the *gyrA* in *Campylobacter* are Asp90→Asn, Thr86→Lys, Thr86→Ala, Thr86→Val and Asp90→Tyr. Double mutant are found on Thr86→Ile-Pro104→Ser and Thr86→Ile-Asp90→Asn (rev by Payot et al., 2006). *Campylobacter* isolates originating from broilers, turkeys and humans resistant and sensitive to NAL were examined for mutations within QRDR. In 135 resistant strains the most frequent mutation was Thr86→Ile and thereafter mutations were found on Thr86→Ala, Asp90→Asn and Pro104→Ser. It is not known whether mutation on Pro104→Ser influence the resistance to FQ. In susceptible isolates as well as in resistant strains, silent mutations were on codons Gly78, His 81, Gly110 and Ser119. Genetic variation is therefore common in C. jejuni isolated from chickens, turkeys and humans (Beckman et al., 2004). Mutations on *gyrB* gene are rare in *Campylobacter* resistant to NAL and CIP. Piddock et al. (2003) reported silent mutation on *gyrB* in few isolates of *Campylobacter* species. In clinical isolates of C. coli, C. jejuni, C. lari and C. fetus obtained from UK, Germany and the Netherlands, from the period 1990 to 1995, the most frequent mutation on *gyrA* was Thr86→Ile. In one isolate mutation on Asp90→Asn was found and one isolate was double mutant (Thr86→Ile-Pro104→Ser). Silent mutations were found on *gyrA* in *C. jejuni* suggesting genetic and epidemiological differences between the isolates. In Senegal silent mutation of *gyrB* was found in a collection of isolates from chicken carcasses. These silent mutations were identified from codons 371-540. Besides silent mutations the dominant transition on *gyrA* was Thr86→Ile and six isolates mutated on Thr86→Ala. The amino acid substitution Thr86→Ala was found also in two chicken isolates susceptible to CIP and MIC to NAL was 16 μg/ml. In 17 isolates mutations were found at Asn203→Ser, downstream *gyrA* and in 3 isolates mutations were found also at Ala206→Thr. The *parC* gene could not be amplified (Kinana et al., 2007b). In a strain collection of CIP resistant *C. coli*, isolated from humans, food and animals in Italy, a novel mutation at codon 86 was described. This was a double nucleotide substitution at ACT → GTT changing Thr86→Val in three C. coli isolates. This type of transition did not induce additional increase of MIC to CIP. In C. coli different *gyrA* alleles were found, but the mutations were silent, pointing only to the genetic diversity of the unrelated isolates from Italy. Mutation Thr86→Ile on *gyrA* was associated with high MIC to ciprofloxacin (MIC $\geq$32 μg/ml) (Carattoli et al., 2002). In six clinical isolates from the research of McIver et al. (2004) mutation was identified on Thr86→Ile, but in laboratory derived mutants three non-synonymous substitution were identified at Asp90→Asn, Asp85→Tyr and Thr86→Ala. This was a first report of double mutation Asp85→Tyr-Thr86→Ile in *Campylobacter* after *in vitro* exposition to sub-inhibitory concentration of ciprofloxacin. Silent mutations apparently do not improve *in vivo* fitness cost of the resistant *Campylobacter* nor its colonization ability, which is preserved even in the absence of antibiotics. Its viability is solely due to single point mutation in *gyrA* gene. This is probably the reason why FQ resistant *Campylobacter* persist in farm animals over a long period and because once contaminated with such bacteria the farm presents a hazard in food production (Luo et al., 2005). Double *gyrA* mutant is reported from Thailand in C. coli isolated from pigs. Mutations were found in *gyrA* at Thr86→Ile and Gly119→Ser and in three isolates also amino acid substitution on *gyrB* were Lys382→Gln or Arg. These additional mutations did not increase MIC to CIP or NAL, so its possible role in resistance mechanism needs to be determined in the future (Ekkapobyotin et al., 2008). Double mutations on *gyrA* (Thr86→Ile) and *parC* (Arg139→Gln) were found in clinical isolates of C. jejuni in patient that were treated with fluoroquinolones because of profound diarrhea. The mutation on *parC* gene is rare and is coupled with amino acid transition on *gyrA*. The influence of *parC* mutation on MIC for CIP is not clear (Gibreel et al., 1998).

Implications of gene mutations to NAL resistance phenotype was studied by Jesse et al. (2006) and an observation was made that single point mutation on Thr86→Ala confers the resistance to NAL but not to CIP. Most isolates from their strain collection, obtained from chicken carcasses and cattle faeces, also possessed one or more silent mutations in the *gyrA* gene. Silent mutations, double mutant in *gyrA* gene and also mutations outside of the QRDR/gyrA, usually do not change the MIC significantly but contribute in allelic diversity and in that respect can be used as a typing tool or in research on correlation between strains found in humans and animals. Multilocus sequence *fla* typing successfully discriminated C. jejuni and C. coli in the strain collection from the Institute of Veterinary Bacteriology at the University of Bern, Switzerland. This method can be used in epidemiology research and in studying phylogenetic relation and divergence in large collection of isolates over a longer period of time (Korezak et al., 2009). The *fla* Restriction Fragment Length Polymorphism (RFLP) is a good alternative in research on genetic diversity of *Campylobacter* spp. (Keller & Perreten, 2006, Sonnevend et al., 2006). *Campylobacter fetus* subsp. fetus (wild type isolate and laboratory obtained mutants) is intrinsically resistant to NAL and resistance to CIP is obtained from the single transition of Asp91→Tyr. The MIC to CIP does not exceed 8μg/ml for laboratory mutants. For clinical isolates the obtained MIC was 16 μg/ml (Taylor & Chau, 1997). *Campylobacter fetus* was isolated in two immunodeficient patients. The clinical symptoms of gastrointestinal disorder relapsed after therapy with fluoroquinolones. In re-isolated *Campylobacter* a mutation on *gyrA* gene was found at Asp87→Thr. The authors stated that in immunodeficient patients it is very important to control resistance status before, during and after the treatment to enable successful therapy and prevent a failure (Meier et al., 1998). *Campylobacter hyointestinalis* subsp. hyointestinalis, isolated from reindeer and bovine fecal samples from the northern Finland were tested on antimicrobial resistance and *gyrA* mutations obtained *in vitro*. *C. hyointsetinalis* is intrinsically resistant to NAL and susceptible to CIP. In isolate naturally resistant to NAL an amino acid substitution Thr86→Ile was found. The same transition (Thr86→Ile) was recorded from *in vitro* obtained mutants (grown in a gradually increasing concentration of ciprofloxacin) with MIC of ≥64 μg/ml. In the strains that exhibit

MIC to CIP ≤32 μg/ml, *gyrA* was not mutated implicating other mechanism of inherent resistance, was not mutated implicating other mechanism of inherent resistance (Laatu et al., 2005).

Mutational polymorphism in QRDR region of the *gyrA* gene in *Campylobacter* species is not exclusively driven by antimicrobial therapy in livestock industry but also occurs after therapy of patients. To decrease spreading of resistant bacteria in agriculture, since 2005 fluoroquinolones have been banned in poultry and swine industry in the USA. Other antimicrobial agents must be used to treat *E. coli* infections in pigs and poultry in North America. The most important approach to combat resistance in bacteria is therefore good management, food safety and good cooking practice. It is hard to expect that the problems of antibiotic resistance will be entirely resolved since bacteria find ways to survive under selective pressure created by man but also in their own environment and communities. Permanent monitoring of antimicrobial resistance and resistance mechanism is essential and must be carried out in each country under national programs and preferable supported by international projects. Point mutations in a single gene of topoisomerase enzymes are a good example of the smart game that bacteria play to survive and spread in nature.

5. Conclusion

Antibiotic resistance monitoring is compulsory in developed countries but is also conducted at similar level in developing countries. Since resistance development is attributed to the use of antimicrobial agents in clinical therapy and livestock industry, medical and veterinary sector is equally involved in resistance monitoring. We have learned that resistance to "old" antibiotics can lead to bacteria that inherit more than one mechanism of resistance, that could develop MDR phenotype and that the new feature is sometimes fitness cost effective. Mutations on target genes selected *in vitro* do not necessarily resemble the nature of mutational frequency *in vivo,* but with certainty enable scientist to understand how resistance develops and what the risk is of antibiotic use. Epidemiologists have put much effort to explain the spread of resistant bacteria and to find their origin. They have tried to explain their intercontinental appearance. Vehicles for the transmission are numerous and it is usually impossible to find the exact path of their spread in humans and also animals. By utilizing molecular biology methods, clones and links that are attributed to their transfer from one setting to another can be identified. Mutations on topoisomerase genes determine the genetic background of the bacteria and in some instances increase the success of their survival in nature.

6. Acknowledgment

This paper is dedicated to late Dr Slavko Đurišić, who was our mentor, dear colleague and friend. We thank Mrs Lidija Orčić for English editing. This work is supported by a grant from the Ministry of Education and Science, Republic of Serbia, Project number TR 31071

7. References

Bagel S,; Hüllen V, Wiedemann B. & Haisig P. (1999). Imapct of *gyrA* and *parC* mutations on quinolone resistance, doubling time and supercoiling degree of *Escherichia coli*. Antimicrobial Agents and Chemotherapy, Vol.43, No.4, pp. 868-875, ISSN 0066-4804

Bansal S. & Tandon V. (2011). Contribution of mutations in DNA gyrase and topisomerase IV genes to ciprofloxacin resistance *in Escherichia coli* clinical isolates. International Journal of Antimicrobial Agents, Vol.37, pp. 253-255, ISSN 0924-8579

Baucheron S,; Chiu CH. & Butaye P. (2005). High-level resistance to fluoroquinolones linked to mutations in *gyrA* and *parC* and *parE* in *Salmonella enterica* serovar Schwarzengrund isolates from humans in Taiwan. Antimicrobial Agents and Chemotherapy, Vol.49, No.2, pp. 862-863, ISSN 0066-4804

Beckman L.; Müller M, Luber P., Schrader C., Bartelt E. & Klein G. (2004). Analysis of *gyrA* mutations in quinolone-resistant and susceptible *Campylobacter jejuni* isolates from retail poultry and human clinical isolates by non-radioactive single-strand conformation polymorphism analysis and DNA sequencing. Journal of Applied Microbiology, Vol. 96. pp. 1040-1047, ISSN 1364-5072

Cabrera R,; Ruiz J, Marco F, Oliveira I, Arroyo M, Aladueña A, Usera MA, Teresa Jiménez De Anita MT, Gascón J. & Vila J. (2004). Mechanism of resistance to several antimicrobial agents in *Salmonella* clinical isolates causing traveler's diarrhea. Antimicrobial Agents and Chemotherapy, Vol.48, No.10, pp 3934-3939, ISSN 0066-4804

Carattoli A,; Dionisi AM. & Luzzi I. (2002). Use of a LightCycler *gyrA* mutation assay for identification of ciprofloxacin-resistant *Campylobacter coli*. FEMS Microbiology Letters, Vol.214, pp. 87-93, ISSN 0378-1097

Casin I.; Breuil J., Jean Pierre D., Guelpa C. & Collatz E.(2003). Fluoroquinolone resistance linked to GyrA, GyrB and ParC mutations in *Salmonella enterica* Typhimurium isolates in humans. Emerging Infectious Diseases, Vol.9, No.11, pp. 1455-1457 ISSN 1080-6040

Chan Moon D,; Yong Seol S, Gurung M, Sook Jin J, Hee Choi C, Kim J, Chul Lee Y, Taek Cho D. & Chul Lee JC. (2010). Emergence of a new mutation and its accumulation in the topoisomerase IV gene confers high levels of resistance to fluoroquinolones in *Escherichia coli* isolates. International Journal of Antimicrobial Agents, Vol.35, pp. 76-79, ISSN 0924-8579

Chen JY,; Siu LK, Chen YH, Lu PL, HoM. & Peng CF. (2001). Molecular epidemiology and mutations at *gyrA* and *parC* genes of ciprofloxacin resistant *Escherichia coli* isolates from a Taiwan medical centre. Microbial Drug Resistance, Vol.7, No.1, pp. 47-53, ISSN 1076-6294

Chiu CH,; Wu TL, Su LH, Liu JW. & Chu C. (2004). Fluoroquinolone resistance in *Salmonella enterica* serotype Choleraesuis Taiwan, 2000-2003. Emerging Infectious Diseases, Vol.10, No.9, pp. 1674-1676, ISSN 1080-6040

Chiu CH.; Su LH, Chu C, Chia JH, Wu TL, Lin TY, Lee YS. & Ou JT. (2004). Isolation of *Salmoenella eneterica* serotype Choleraesuis resistant to ceftriaxone and ciprofloxacin. Lancet, Vol.363 (April 17), Issue 9417, pp. 1285-1286, ISSN 0140-6736

Choi SH,; Woo JH, Lee JE, Park SJ, Choo EJ, Kwak YG, Kim MN, Choi MS, Lee NY, Lee BK, Kim NJ, Jeong JY, Ryu J. & Kimm YS. (2005). Increasing incidence of quinolone resistance in human non-typhoid *Salmonella enterica* isolates in Korea and mechanisms involved in quinolone resistance. Journal of Antimicrobial Chemotherapy, Vol.56, pp. 1111-1114, ISSN 0305-7453

Cloeckaert A. & Chaslus-Dancla E. (2001). Mechanisms of quinolone resistance in *Salmonella*. Veterinary Record, Vol. 32, pp. 291-300, ISSN 0042-4900

Conrad S, Oethinger M, Kaifel K, Klotz G, Marre R. & Kern WV. (1996). *gyrA* mutations in high-level fluoroquinolone-resistant clinical isolates of *Escherichia coli.* Journal of Antimicrobial Chemotherapy, Vol.38, pp. 443-455, ISSN 0305-7453

Cui S, Li J, Sun Z, Hu C, Jin S, Guo Y, Ran L. & Ma Y. (2008). Ciprofloxacin-resistant Salmonella enterica serotype Typhimuirum, China. Emerging Infectious Diseases, Vol.14, No.3, pp. 493-495, ISSN 1080-6040

del Mar Tavio M,; Vila J, Ruiz J, Martin-Sánchez AM. & Jiménez de Anta MT. (1999). Mechanisms involved in the development of resistance to fluoroquinolones in *Escherichia coli* isolates. Journal of Antimicrobial Chemotherapy, Vol.44, pp. 735-742, ISSN 0305-7453

Delsol A.; Woodward MJ. & Roe JM (2004). Effect of 5 day enrofloxacin treatment on *Salmonella enterica* serotype Typhimurium DT104 in the pig. Journal of Antimicrobial Chemotherapy, Vol.53, pp. 396-398 ISSN 0305-7453

Delsol AA, Sunderland J, Woodward MJ, Pumbwe L, Piddock LJV. & Roe JM. (2004). Emergence of fluoroquinolone resistance in the native *Campylobacter coli* population of pigs exposed to enrofloxacin. Journal of Antimicrobial Chemotherapy, Vol.53, pp. 872-874, ISSN 0305-7453

Dimitrov T, Dashti AA, Albaksami O, Udo EE, Jadaon MM. & Albert MJ. (2009). Ciprofloxacin-resistant *Salmonella enterica* serovar Typhi from Kuwait with novel mutations in *gyA* and *parC* genes. Journal of Clinical Microbiology, Vol.47, No.1, pp 208-211, ISSN 0095-1137

Drlica K. & Zhao X. (1997). DNA gyrase, topoisomerase IV and the 4-Quinolones. Microbiology and Molecular Biology Reviews, Vol.61, No.3, pp. 377-392, ISSN 1092-2172

Eaves DJ.; Randall L., Gray DT, Buckley A., Woodward MJ., White AP. & Piddock LJV. (2004). Prevalence of mutations within the quinolone resistance-determining region of *gyrA*, *gyrB*, *parC* and *parE* and association with antibiotic resistance in quinolone-resistant *Salmonella enterica*. Antimicrobial Agents and Chemotherapy, Vol.48, No.10, pp. 4012-4015, ISSN 0066-4804

Ekkapobyotin C,; Padungtod P. & Chuanchuen R. (2008). Antimicrobial resistance of *Campylobacter coli* isolates from swine. International Journal of Food Microbiology, Vol.128, pp. 325-328, ISSN 0168-1605

Escribano I,; Rodríguez JC. & Royo G. (2004). Mutations in the *gyrA* in *Salmonella enterica* clinical isolates with decreased ciprofloxacin susceptibility. International Journal of Antimicrobial Agents, Vol.24, pp. 102-105, ISSN 0924-8579

Everett MJ, Jin YF, Ricci V. & Piddock LJV. (1996). Contributions of individual mechanisms to fluoroquionolone resistance in 36 *Escherichia coli* strains isolated from humans and animals. Antimicrobial Agents and Chemotherapy, Vol.40, No.10, pp. 2380-2386, ISSN 0066-4804

Gales AC, Gordon KA, Wilke WW, Pfaller MA. & Jones RN. (2000). Occurrence of single point *gyrA* mutations among ciprofloxacin-susceptible *Escherichia coli* isolates causing urinary tract infections in Latin America. Diagnostic Microbiology and Infectious Disease, Vol.36, pp. 61-64, ISSN 0732-8893

Gallay A.; Prouzet-Mauléon V., Kempf I., Lehours P., Labadi L., Camou C., Denis M., de Valk H., Desenclos JC. & Mégraud F. (2007). *Campylobacter* antimicrobial drug resistance among humans, broiler chickens, and pigs, France. Emerging Infectious Diseases, Vol.13, No.2, pp .259-266, ISSN 1080-6040

Garau J.; Xercavins M., Rodríiguez-Caraballeira M., Ramón Gómez-Vera J., Coll I., Vidal D., Llovet T. & Ruíz-Bremón A.(1999). Emergence and dissemination of quinolone-resistant *Escherichia coli* in the community. Antimicrobial Agents and Chemotherapy, Vol.43, No.11, pp. 736-2741, ISSN 0066-1137

Gaunt PN. & Piddock LJV. (1996). Ciprofloxacin resistant *Campylobacter* spp. in humans: an epidemiological and laboratory study. Journal of Antimicrobial Chemotherapy, Vol.37, pp. 747-757, ISSN 0305-7453

Gensberg K,; Jin YF. & Piddock LJV (1995). A novel *gyrB* mutation in a fluoroquinolone-resistant clinical isolate of *Salmonella* typhimurium. FEMS Microbiology Letters, Vol.132, pp. 57-60, ISSN 0378-1097

Gibreel A,; Sjögren E, Kaijser B, Wretlind B. & Sköld O. (1998). Rapid emergence of high-level resistance to quinolones in *Campylobacter jejuni* associated with mutational change in *gyrA* and *parC*. Antimicrobial Agents and Chemotherapy, Vol.42, No.12, pp. 3276-3278, ISSN 0066-4804

Giraud E,; Cloeckaert A, Baucheron S, Mouline C. & Chaslus-Dancla E. (2003). Fitness cost of fluoroquinolone resistance in *Salmonella enterica* serovar Typhimurium. Journal of Medical Microbiology, Vol.52, pp 697-703, ISSN 0022-2615

Giraud E.; Baucheron S. & Cloeckaert A.(2006). Resistance to fluoroquinolones in Salmonella: emerging mechanisms and resistance prevention strategies. Microbes and Infection, Vol.8, pp. 1937-1944, ISSN 1286-4579

Giraud E.; Brisabois A., Martel JL. & Chaslus-Dancla E. (1999). Comparative studies of mutations in animal isolates and experimental in vitro and in vivo-selected mutants of *Salmonella* spp., suggest a counterselection of highly fluoroquinolone-resistant strains in the field. Antimicrobial Agents and Chemotherapy, Vol. 43, No.9, pp. 2131-2137, ISSN 0066-4804

Grrigs DJ; Johnson MM, Frost JA, Humphrey T, Jørgensen F. & Piddock LJV. (2005). Incidence and mechanism of ciprofloxacin resistance in *Campylobacter* spp., isolated from commercial poultry flocks in the United Kingdom before, during and after fluoroquinolone treatment. Antimicrobial Agents and Chemotherapy, Vol.49, No.2, pp. 699-707, ISSN 0066-4804

Guerra B.; Malorny B., Schroeter A. & Helmuth R. (2003). Multiple resistance mechanisms in fluoroquinolone-resistant *Salmonella* isolates from Germany. Antimicrobial Agents and Chemotherapy, Vol.47, No.6, pp. 2059, ISSN 0066-4804

Gupta A,; Nelson JM, Barrett TJ, Tauxe RV, Rossiter SP, Frideman CR, Joyce KW, Smith KE, Jones TF, Hawkins MA, Shiferaw B, Beebe JL, Vugia DJ, Rabatsky-Ehr T, Benson JA, Root TP. & Angulo FJ. (2004). Antimicrobial resistance among *Campylobacter* strains, United States, 1997-2001. Emerging Infectious Diseases, Vol.10, No.6, pp. 1102-1109, ISSN 1080-6040

Hakanen A,; Jalava J, Kotilainen P, Jousimies-Somer H, Siitonen A. & Huovinen P. (2002). *gyrA* polymorphism in *Campylobacter jejuni*: Detection of *gyrA* mutations in 162 C. jejuni isolates by single-strand conformation polymorphism and DNA sequencing. Antimicrobial Agents and Chemotherapy, Vol.46, No.8, pp. 2644-2647, ISSN 0066-4804

Hamidian M,; Tajbakhsh M, Tohidopour A, Rahbar M, Reza Zali M. & Walther-Rasmussen J. (2011). Detection of novel *gyrA* mutation in nalidixic acid-resistance isolates of Salmonella enterica from patients with diarrhea. International Journal of Antimicrobial Agents, vol.37, pp. 360-364, ISSN 0924-8579

Hassing RJ,; Menezes GA, van Pelt W, Petit PL, van Genderen PJ. & Goessens WHF. (2011). Analysis of mechanisms involved in reduced susceptibility to ciprofloxacin in *Salmonella enterica* serotype Typhi and Paratyphi A isolates from travellers to Southeast Asia. International Journal of Antimicrobial Agents, Vol.37, pp. 240-243, ISSN 0924-8579

Heisig P, Schedletzky H. & Falkenstein-Paul H. (1993). Mutations in the *gyrA* gene of a highly fluoroquinolone-resistant clinical isolate of *Escherichia coli*. Antimicrobial Agents and Chemotherapy, Vol 37, No.4, pp. 696-701, ISSN 0066-4804

Heisig P,; (1996). Genetic evidence for a role of *parC* mutations in development of high-level fluoroquinolone resistance in *Eschericihia coli*. Antimicrobial Agents and Chemotherapy, Vol.40, No.4, pp. 879-885, ISSN 0066-4804

Heisig P. & Tschorny R. (1994). Characterization of fluoroquinolone-resistant mutants of *Escherichia coli* selected in vitro. Antimicrobial Agents and Chemotherapy, Vol.38, No.6, pp. 1284-1291, ISSN 0066-4804

Heisig P.; Kratz B, Halle E, Gräser Y, Altwegg M, Rabsch W. & Faber JP (1995). Identification of DNA Gyrase A mutations in ciprofloxacin-resistant isolates of *Salmonella typhimurium* from men and cattle in Germany. Microbial Drug Resistance, Vol.1, No3, pp. 211-218, ISSN 1076-6254

Hopkins KL.; Davies RH. & Threlfall EJ.(2005). Mechanisms of quinolone resistance in *Escherichia coli* and *Salmonella*: Recent developments. International Journal of Antimicrobial Agents, Vol.25, pp. 358-373, ISSN 0924-8579

Hsueh PR,; Teng LJ, Tseng SP, Chang CF, Wan JH, Yan JJ, Lee CM, Chuang YC, Huang WK, Yang D, Shyr JM, Yu KW, Wang LS, Lu JJ, Ko WC, Wu JJ, Chang FY, Yang YC, Lau YJ, Liu YC, Liu CY, Ho SW. & Luh KT (2004). Ciprofloxacin-resistant *Salmonella enterica* typhimurium and Choleraesuis from pigs to humans, Taiwan. Emerging Infectious Diseases, Vol.10, No.1, pp. 60-68, ISSN 1080-6040 http://www.eurosurveillance.org/ViewArticle.aspx?Articled=398

Huang TM,; Chang YF. & Chang CF. (2004). Detection of mutations in the *gyrA* gene and class I integron from quinolone-resistant *Salmonella enterica* serovar Choleresuis isolated in Taiwan. Veterinary Microbiology, Vol.100, pp. 247-254, ISSN 0378-1135

Izumiya H,; Mori K, Kurazono T, Yamaguchi M, Higashide M, Konishi N, Kai A, Morita K, Terajima J. & Watanabe H. (2005). Characterization of isolates of *Salmonella enterica* serovar Typhimurium displaying high level fluoroquinolone resistance in Japan. Journal of Clinical Microbiology, Vol.43, No.10, pp. 5074-5079, ISSN 0095-1137

Jesse TW,; Englen MD, Pittenger-Alley LG. & Fedorka-Cray PJ. (2006). Two distinct mutations in *gyrA* to ciprofloxacin and nalidixic acid resistance in *Campylobacter coli* and *Campylobacter jejuni* isolated from chickens and beef cattle. Journal of Applied Microbiology, Vol.100, pp. 682-688, ISSN 1364-5072

Jiménez Gómez PA,; García de los Ríos JE, Mendoza Rojas A, de Pedro Ramonet P, Garcia Albiach R. & Reche Sainz MP. (2004). Molecular basis of quinolone resistance in *Escherichia coli* from wild birds. The Canadian Journal of Veterinary Research, Vol.68, pp. 229-231, ISSN 0830-9000

Johnson JR.; Kuskowski MA., Menard M., Gajewski A., Xercavins M. & Garau J.(2006). Similarity between human and chicken *Escherichia coli* isolates in relation to ciprofloxacin resistance status. The Journal of Infectious Diseases, Vol.194, pp. 71-78, ISSN 0022-1899

Keller J. & Perreten V. (2006). Genetic diversity in fluoroquinolone and macrolide-resistant *Campylobacter coli* from pigs. Veterinary Microbiology, Vol.113, pp. 103-108, ISSN 0378-1135

Khan AA.; Nawaz M.S., West S, Khan SA. & Lin J. (2005). Isolation and molecular characterization of fluoroquinolone-resistant *Escherichia coli* from poultry litter. Poultry Science , Vol. 84, pp. 61-66, ISSN 0032-5791

Kilmartin D.; Morris D., O'Hare C., Corbett-Feeney G. & Cormican M. (2005). Clonal expansion may account for high levels of quinolone resistance in *Salmonella enterica* serovar Enteritidis. Applied and Environmental Microbiology, Vol.71, No.5, pp. 2587-2591, ISSN 0099-2240

Kim KY,; Park JH, Kwak HS. & Woo GJ. (2011). Characterization of the quinolone resistance mechanism in foodborne *Salmonella* isolates with high nalidixic acid resistance. International Journal of Food Microbiology, Vol.146, pp. 52-56, ISSN 0168-1605

Kinana AD,; Cardinale E, Bahsoun I, Tall F, Sire JM, Breurec S, Garin B, Saad-Bouh Boye C. & Perrier-Gros-Claude JD. (2007a). *Campylobacter coli* isolates derived from chickens in Senegal: Diversity, genetic exchange with *Campylobacter jejuni* and quinolone resistance. Research in Microbiology, Vol.158, pp. 138-142, ISSN 0923-2508

Kinana AD,; Cardinale E, Bahsoun I, Tall F, Sire JM, Garin B, Saad-Bouh Boye C, Dromigny JA. & Perrier-Gros-Claude JD. (2007b). Analysis of topoisomerase mutations in fluoroquinolone-resistant and susceptible *Campylobacter jejuni* strains isolated in Senegal. International Journal of Antimicrobial Agents, Vol.29, pp.397-401, ISSN 0924-8579

Kinana AD,; Cardinale E, Tall F, Bahsoun I, Sire JM, Garin B, Breurec S, Saad-Bouh Boye C. & Perrier-Gros-Claude JD. (2006). Genetic diversity and quinolone resistance in *Campylobacter jejuni* isolates from poultry in Senegal. Applied and Environmental Microbiology, Vol72, No.5, pp. 3309-3313, ISSN 0099-2240

Ko WC,; Yan JJ, Yu WL, Lee HC, Lee NY, Wang LR. & Chuang YC. (2005). A new therapeutic challenge for old pathogens: Community-acquired invasive infections caused by ceftriaxone and ciprofloxacin resistant *Salmonella enterica* serotype Choleraesuis. Clinical Infectious Diseases, Vol.40, pp. 315-8, ISSN 1058-4838

Korezak BM,; Zurfluh M, Emler S, Kuhn-Oertli J. & Kuhnert P. (2009). Multiplex strategy for multilocus sequence typing *fla* typing and genetic determination of antimicrobial resistance of *Campylobacter jejuni* and *Campylobacter coli* isolates collected in Switzerland. Journal of Clinical Microbiology, Vol.47, No.7, pp. 1996-2007, ISSN 0095-1137

Kozoderović G., Jelesić Z. & Velhner M.: Resistance to quinolones among *Salmonella* Enteritidis isolates in Vojvodina. Microbiologia Balkanica 2009, Book of abstracts and Programme, 6th Balkan Congress of Microbiology, Ohrid, 28-31. Oktober, Macedonia, Skopje, Macedonian Medical Association, 2009, p. 120, ISSN 0025-1097

Kozoderović G.; Velhner M., Jelesić Z., Stojanov I., Petrović T., Stojanović D. & Golić N. (2011). Molecular typing and antimicrobial resistance of *Salmonella* Enteritidis isolated from poultry, food and humans in Serbia. Folia Microbiologica, Vol. 56, pp. 66-71, ISSN 0015-5632

Kristiansen MAM,; Sandvang D. & Rasmussen TB. (2003). In vivo development of quinolone resistance in *Salmonella enterica* serotype Typhimuirum DT104. Journal of Clinical Microbiology, Vol.41, No.9, pp. 4462-4464, ISSN 0095-1137

Kumagai Y,; Kato JI, Hoshino K, Akasaka T, Sato K. & Ikeda H. (1996). Quinolone-resistant mutants of *Escherichia coli* DNA topoisomerase IV *parC* gene. Antimicrobial Agents and Chemothreapy, Vol.40, No.3, pp. 710-714, ISSN 0066-1137

Laatu M,; Rautelin H. & Hänninen ML. (2005). Susceptibility of *Campylobacter hyointestinalis* subsp. *hyointestinalis* to antimicrobial agents and characterization of quionolone-resistant strains. Journal of Antimicrobial Chemotherapy, Vol.55, pp. 182-187, ISSN 0305-7453

Lautenbach E,; Fishman NO, Metlay JP, Mao X., Bilker WB, Tolomeo P. & Nachamkin I. (2006). Phenotypic and genotypic characterization of fecal *Escherichia coli* isolates with decreased susceptibility to fluoroquinolones: Results from a large hospital-based surveillance initiative. The Journal of Infectious Diseases, Vol.194, pp. 79-85, ISSN 0022-1899

Lee K,; Lee M, Lim J, Jung J, Park Y. & Lee Y. (2008). Contamination of chicken meat with *Salmonella enterica* serovar Haardt with nalidixic acid resistance and reduced fluoroquinolone susceptibility. Journal of Microbiology Biotechnology, Vol.18, No.11, pp. 1853.-1857, ISSN 1017-7825

Lee YJ,; Kim KS, Kim JH. & Tak RB. (2004). *Salmonella gallinarum gyrA* mutations associated with fluoroquinolone resistance. Avian Pathology, Vol.33, No.2, pp 251-257, ISSN 0307-9457

Lee YJ.; Cho JK., Kim KS., Tak RB., Kim AR., Kim JW., Im SK. & Kim BH.(2005). Fluoroquinolone resistance and *gyrA* and *parC* mutations of *Escherichia coli* isolated from chickens. The Journal of Microbiology, Vol.43, No.5, pp. 391-397, ISSN 1225-8873

Lehn N,; Stöwer-Hoffmann J, Kott T, Strassner C, Wagner H, Krönke M. & Schneider-Brachert W. (1996). Characterization of clinical isolates of *Escherichia coli* showing high levels of fluoroquinolone resistance. Journal of Clinical Microbiology, Vol.34, No.3, pp. 597-602, ISSN 0095-1137

Levy DD.; Sharma B. & Cebula TA.(2004). Single-nucleotide polymorphism mutation spectra and resistance to quinolones in Salmonella enterica Serovar Enteritidis with a mutator phenotype. Antimicrobial Agents and Chemotherapy, Vol.48, No.7, pp. 2355-2363, ISSN 0066-4804

Liebana E.; Clouting C, Cassar CA, Randall LP, Walker RA, Threlfall EJ, Clifton-Hadley FA, Ridley AM. & Davies RH. (2002). Comparison of *gyrA* mutations, cyclohexane resistance, and the presence of Class I integrons in *Salmonella enterica* from farm animals in England and Wales. Journal of Clinical Microbiology, Vol.40, No.4, pp. 1481-1486, ISSN 0095-1137

Lindstedt BA,; Aas L. & Kapperud G. (2004). Geographically dependent distribution of *gyrA* gene mutations at codons 83 and 87 in *Salmonella* Hadar, and a novel codon 81 Gly to His mutation in *Salmonella* Enteritidis. APMIS, Vol.112, No. 3, pp. 165-71, ISSN 0963-4641

Ling JM.; Chan EW., Lam AW. & Cheng AF. (2003). Mutations in topoisomerase genes of fluoroquinolone-resistant Salmonellae in Hong Kong. Antimicrobial Agents and Chemotherapy, Vol.47, No.11, pp. 3567-3573, ISSN 0066-4804

Luo N,; Pereira S, Sahin O, Lin J, Huang S, Michel L. & Zhang Q. (2005). Enhanced *in vivo* fitness of floroquinolone-resistant *Campylobacter jejuni* in the absence of antibiotic selection pressure. PNAS, Vol.102, No.3, pp. 541-546, ISSN 0027-8424

Luo N,; Sahin O, Lin J, Michel LO. & Zhang Q. (2003). In vivo selection of *Campylobacter* isolates with high levels of fluoroquinolne resistance associated with *gyrA* mutations and the function of the CmeABC efflux pump. Antimicrobial Agents and Chemotherapy, Vol47, No.1, pp. 390-394, ISSN 0066-4804

Marcusson LL,; Frimodt-Moller N. & Hughes D. (2009). Interplay in the selection of fluoroquinolone resistance and bacterial fitness. PLOSPathogens, Vol.5, No.8, pp. 1-7, ISSN 1553-7366

Marimon JM, Gomariz M, Zigorraga, Cilla G. & Pérez-Trallero E. (2004). Increasing prevalence of quinolone resistance in human nontyphoid *Salmonella enterica* isolates obtained in Spain from 1981 to 2003. Antimicrobial Agents and Chemotherapy, Vol.48, No.10, pp. 3789-3793, ISSN 0066-4804

Mayrhofer S.; Paulsen P., Smulders FJM. & Hilbert F. (2004). Antimicrobial resistance profile of five major food-borne pathogens isolated from beef, pork and poultry. International Journal of Food Microbiology, Vol.97, pp. 23-29, ISSN 0168-1605

Mc Donald CL,; Chen FJ, Lo HJ, Yin HC, Lu PL, Huang CH, Chen P, Lauderdale TL & Ho M. (2001). Emergence of reduced susceptibility and resistance to fluoroquinolones in *Escherichia coli* in Taiwan and contributions of distinct selective pressures. Antimicrobial Agents and Chemotherapy, Vol.45, No.11, pp. 3084-3091, ISSN 0066-4804

McIver CJ,; Hogan TR, White PA. & Tapsall JW. (2004). Patterns of quinolone susceptibility in *Campylobacter jejuni* associated with different *gyrA* mutations. Pathology, Vol.36, No.2, pp. 166-169, ISSN 0031-3025

Meier PA,; Dooley DP, Jorgensen JH, Sanders CC, Huang WM. & Patterson JE. (1998). Development of quinolone-resistant *Campylobacter fetus* bacteriemia in human immunodeficiency virus/infected patients. Tha Journal of Infectious Diseases, Vol.177, pp. 951-954, ISSN 0022-1899

Mooij MJ, Schouten I, Vos G, van Belkum A, Vandenbroucke-Grauls CMJE, Savelkoul PHM. & Schultsz C. (2005). Class 1 integrons in ciprofloxacin-resistant *Escherichia coli* strains from two Dutch hospitals. Clinical Microbiology and Infection, Vol.11, pp. 898-902, ISSN 1198-743X

Moore JE,; Crowe M, Heaney N. & Crothers E. (2001). Antibiotic resistance in *Campylobacter* spp. isolated from human faeces (1980-2000) and foods (1887-2000) in Northern Ireland: an update. Journal of Antimicrobial Chemotherapy, Vol.48, pp. 455-457, ISSN 0305-7453

Morgan-Linnell SK. & Zechiedrich L. (2007). Contributions of the combined effect of topoisomerase mutations toward fluoroquinolone resistance in *Escherichia coli*. Antimicrobial Agents and Chemotherapy, Vol.51, No.11, pp. 4205-4208, ISSN 0066-4804

Nakaya H.; Yasuhara A, Yoshimura K, Oshihoi Y, Izumiya H. & Watanabe H (2003). Life threatening infantile diarrhea from fluoroquinolone-resistant *Salmonella enterica*

Typhimurium with mutations in both *gyrA* and *parC*. Emerging Infectious Diseases, Vol.9, No.2, pp. 255-257, ISSN 1080-6040

Namboodiri SS,; Opintan JA, Lijek RS, Newman MJ. & Okeke IN. (2011). Quinolone resistance in *Escherichia coli* from Accra, Ghana. BMC Microbiology, Vol.11:44, ISSN 1471-2180

Nógrády N.; Tóth Á, Kostyák Á, Pászti J. & Nagy B. (2007). Emergence of multidrug-resistant clones of *Salmonella* infantis in broiler chickens and humans in Hungary. Journal of Antimicrobial Chemotherapy, Vol.60, pp. 645-648, ISSN 0305-7453

Olsen SJ.; De Bess EE, McGivern TE, Marano N, Eby T, Mauvais S., Balan VK, Zirnstein G., Cieslak PR. & Angulo FJ (2001). A nosocomial outbreak of fluoroquinolone-resistant salmonella infection. New England Journal of Medicine, Vol.344, No.21, (May 24), pp. 1572-1578, ISSN 0028-4793

Ouabdesselam S,; Tankovic J. & Soussy CJ, (1996). Quinolone resistance mutations in the *gyrA* gene in clinical isolates of Salmonella. Microbial Drug Resistance, Vol. 2, No.3, pp. 299-302, ISSN 1076-6254

Overdevest I,; Willemsen I, Rijnsburger M, Eustace A, Xu L, Hawkey P, Heck M, Savelkoul P, Vandenbroucke-Grauls C, van der Zwaluw K, Huijsdens X. & Kluytmans J. (2011). Extended-spectrum β-lactamase genes of *Escherichia coli* in chicken meat and humans, the Netherlands. Emerging Infectious Diseases, Vol. 17, No. 7 pp. 1216-1222, ISSN 1080-6040

Payot S.; Bolla JM., Corcoran D., Fanning S., Mégraud F. & Zhang Q.(2006). Mechanisms of fluoroquinolone and macrolide resistance in *Campylobacter* spp. Microbes and Infection, Vol.8, pp. 1967-1971, ISSN 1286-4579

Piddock LJV (1996). Does the use of antimicrobial agents in veterinary medicine and animal husbandry select antibiotic-resistant bacteria that infect man and compromise antimicrobial chemotherapy. Journal of Antimicrobial Chemotherapy, Vol. 38, pp. 1-3, ISSN 0924-8579

Piddock LJV, Ricci V, Pumbwe L, Everett MJ. & Griggs DJ. (2003). Fluoroquinolone resistance in *Campylobacter* species from man and animals: detection of mutations in topoisomerase genes. Journal of Antimicrobial Chemotherapy, Vol.51, pp. 19-26, ISSN 0305-7453

Piddock LJV.; Ricci V., McLaren I. & Griggs DJ. (1998). Role of mutation in the *gyrA* and *parC* genes of nalidixic-acid-resistant salmonella serotypes isolated from animals in the United Kingdom. Journal of Antimicrobial Chemotherapy, Vol.41, pp. 635-641, ISSN 0305-7453

Randall LP.; Eaves DJ, Cooles SW, Ricci V, Buckley A, Woodward MJ. & Piddock LJV (2005). Fluoroquinolone treatment of experimental *Salmonella enterica* serovar Typhimuirum DT104 infections in chickens select for both *gyrA* mutations and changes in efflux pump gene expression. Journal of Antimicrobial Chemotherapy, Vol.56, pp. 297-306, ISSN 0305-7453

Reyna F,; Huesca M, González V. & Fuchs LY. (1995). *Salmonella typhimurium gyrA* mutations associated with fluoroquinolone resistance. Antimicrobial Agents and Chemotherapy, Vol.39, No.7, pp. 1621-1623, ISSN 0066-4804

Sáenz Y,; Zarazaga Z, Briñas L, Ruiz-Larrea F. & Torres C. (2001). Mutations in *gyrA* and *parC* genes in nalidixic acid-resistant *Escherichia coli* strains from food products, humans and animals. Journal of Antimicrobial Chemotherapy, Vol51, pp. 1001-1005, ISSN 0305-7453

San Martin B,.; Lapierre L., Toro C., Bravo V., Cornejo J., Hormazabal JC. & Borie C. (2005). Isolation and molecular characterization of quinolone resistant *Salmonella* spp from poultry farms. Veterinary Microbiology, Vol.110, pp. 239-244, ISSN 0378-1135

Smith KE,; Besser JM, Hedberg CW, Leano FT, Bender JF, Wicklund JH, Johnson BP, Moore KA. & Osterholm MT.(1999). Quinolone-resistant Campylobacter jejuni infections in Minnesota, 1992-1998. New England Journal of Medicine, Vol.340,m (May 20), pp.1525-1532, ISSN 0028-4793

Solnik-Isaac H.; Weinberger M, Tabak M, Ben-David A, Shachar D. & Yaron S. (2007). Quinolone resistance of *Salmonella enterica* serovar Virchow isolates from human and poultry in Israel: Evidence for clonal expansion. Journal of Clinical Microbiology, Vol. 45, No.8, pp. 2575-2579, ISSN 0095-1137

Sonnevend A,; Rotimi VO, Kolodziejek J, Usmani A, Nowotny N. & Pál T. (2006). High level of ciprofloxacin resistance and its molecular background among *Campylobacter jejuni* strains isolated in the United Arab Emirates. Journal of Medical Microbiology, Vol.55, pp. 1533-1538, ISSN 0022-2615

Stevenson JE, Gay K, Barrett TJ, Medalla F., Chiller TM. & Angulo FJ. (2007). Increase in nalidixic acid resistance among non-typhi *Salmonella enterica* isolates in the United States from 1996 to 2003. Antimicrobial Agents and Chemotherapy, Vol.51, No.1, pp. 195-197, ISSN 0066-4809

Stojanov IM,; Velhner M. & Orlić DB. (2004). Presence of Campylobacter spp. in nature. Zbornik Matice Srpske, No.107, pp. 75-83, ISSN 0352-4906

Taylor DE. & Chau ASS. (1997). Cloning and nucleotide sequence of the *gyrA* gene from *Campylobacter fetus* subsp fetus ATCC 27374 and characterization of ciprofloxacin-resistant laboratory and clinical isolates. Antimicrobial Agents and Chemotherapy, Vol.41, No.3, pp. 665-671, ISSN 0066-4804

Thakur S. & Gebreyes WA. (2005). *Campylobacter coli* in swine production: Antimicrobial resistance mechanisms and molecular epidemiology. Journal of Clinical Microbiology, Vol.43, No.11, pp. 5705-5714, ISSN 0095-1137

Uchida Y,; Mochimaru T, Morokuma Y, Kiyosuke M, Fujise M, Eto F, Harada Y, Kadowaki M, Shimono N. & Kang D. (2010). Geographic distribution of fluoroquinolone-resistant *Escherichia coli*. International Journal of Antimicrobial Agents, Vol. 35, pp. 387-391, ISSN 0924-8579

van den Bogaard AE,; London N, Driessen C. & Stobberingh EE. (2001). Antibiotic resistance of faecal *Escherichia coli* in poultry, poultry farmers and poultry slaughterers. Journal of Antimicrobial Chemotherapy, Vol.47, pp. 763-771 ISSN 0305-7453

van Pelt W.; van der Zee H, Wannet WJB, van de Giessen AW, Mevius DJ, Bolder NM, Komijn RE. & van Duynhoven YTHP (2003). Explosive increase of Salmonella Java in poultry in the Netherlands: Consequences for public health. Eurosurveillance, Vol.8, No.2, pii=398. Available online:

Velhner M.; Petrović J, Stojanov I., Ratajac R. & Stojanović D. (2011). Mehanizmi prenošenja rezistencije kod bakterija, Arhiv Veterinarske Medicine, Vol.3, pp. -92, ISSN 1820-9955.

Velhner M.; Stojanov I, Potkonjak D, Kapetanov M., Orlić D. & Rašić Z. (2005). Salmonella Enteritidis isolation from broiler chickens infected with low doses. Acta Veterinaria, Vol. 55, pp. 183-191, ISSN 0567-8315.

Velhner Maja,; Kozoderović Gordana, Jelesić Zora, Stojanov I, Ratajac R. & Stojanović Dragica. (2010). Rezistencija bakterija na hinolone i njen uticaj na zdravlje ljudi i životinja. Veterinarski glasnik, Vol.64, No.3-4, pp. 277-285, ISSN 0350-2457

Vila J, Ruiz J, Goñi P. & Jimeneze de Anta MT.(1996). Detection of mutations in *parC* in quinolone-resistant clinical isolates of *Escherichia coli.* Antimicrobial Agents and Chemotherapy, Vol 40, No.2, pp. 491-493, ISSN 0066-4804

Vila J, Ruiz J, Marco F, Barcelo A, Goñi P, Giralt E. & Jimeneze de Anta T. (1994). Association between double mutation in *gyrA* gene of ciprofloxacin-resistant clinical isolates of *Eschericihia coli* and MICs. Antimicrobial Agents and Chemotherapy, Vol. 38, No10, pp. 2477-2479, ISSN

Wang Y,; Huang WM. & Taylor DE. (1993). Cloning and nucleotide sequence of the *Campylobacter jejuni gyrA* gene and characterization of quinolone resistance mutations. Antimicrobial Agents and Chemotherapy, Vol.37, No.3, pp. 457-463, ISSN 00664804

Whichard JM, Gay K, Stevenson JE, Joyce KJ, Cooper KL, Omondi M, Medalla F, Jacoby GA. & Barrett TJ. (2007). Human *Salmonella* and concurrent decreased susceptibility to quinolones and extended-spectrum cephalosporins. Emerging Infectious Diseases, Vol.13, No.11, pp. 1681-1687, ISSN 1080-6040

Yoshida H,; Nakamura M, Bogaki M, Ito H, Kojima T, Hattori H. & Nakamura S. (1993). Mechanism of action of quinolones against *Escherichia coli* DNA gyrase. Antimicrobial Agents and Chemotherapy, Vol.37, No.4, pp. 839-845, ISSN 0066-4804

Yoshida H.; Bogaki M., Nakamura M. & Nakamura S. (1990). Quinolone resistance-determining region in the DNA Gyrase *gyrA* gene of *Escherichia coli.* Antimicrobial Agents and Chemotherapy, Vol. 34, No.6, pp. 1271-1272, ISSN 0066-4804

Zirnstein G, Helsel L, Li Y, Swaminathan B. & Besser J. (2000). Characterization of *gyrA* mutations associated with fluoroquinolone resistance in *Campylobacter coli* by DNA sequence analysis and MAMA PCR. FEMS Microbiology Letters, Vol. 190, pp. 1-7, ISSN 0378-1097

Part 4

Point Mutation in Eukaryote: From Pathogens to Cigarette Smoke

9

Point Mutation in Surveillance of Drug-Resistant Malaria

Sungano Mharakurwa[1,2]
[1]*Johns Hopkins Bloomberg School of Public Health, Baltimore,*
[2]*Malaria Institute at Macha,*
[1]*USA*
[2]*Zambia*

1. Introduction

Simple point mutations can confer profound phenotypes on pathogens and parasites of major public health importance, such as malaria. In particular, single nucleotide polymporphisms (SNPs) are known to easily arise, where one base changes occur in the parasite genomic sequence. These SNPs may confer resistance to malaria therapeutic or preventive drugs, or even render other as yet uncharacterized phenotypes of public health concern, such as virulence. Modern advances in parasite molecular biology and genomics allow the typing of parasites with a range of levels of detail. Particular SNPs or combinations of these are identified which are associated with resistance, followed by confirmation through genetic cross experiments. Using simple polymerase chain reaction (PCR) techniques, the point mutations are now increasingly applied as molecular markers for tracking and containment of resistant malaria. These marker point mutations are particularly instrumental surveillance tools as they enable efficient detection of drug-resistant parasites or pathogens before escalation to a public health toll.

1.1 Drug resistance and malaria control

Malaria persists as a major global public health problem, affecting more than 100 countries in Africa, Asia, the South Pacific region, Latin America and the Indian sub-continent, as well as a vast assemblage of non-immune travellers continually visiting such areas. Notwithstanding substantial technological advances, the old scourge currently claims a global toll of 225 million cases and 781,000 deaths every year, mostly children in Africa [1,2]. This has been a relative improvement from 500 million cases and at least 2.3 million annual deaths that were occurring as recently as early-mid 2000s [3,4], with an escalating trend in overall burden of the disease. Thanks to the Roll Back Malaria programme, the President's Malaria Initiative and other public-private sector initiatives, and notably the Bill and Melinda Gates Foundation, endemic countries have scaled up vector control and artemisinin-based combination therapy (ACT) interventions against malaria[5,6], resulting in widespread reduction of burden[7,8]. A number of countries have presently been earmarked for possible local or regional malaria elimination[9,10], including those in southern Africa, which are located towards the natural fringes of transmission. However, the resilient scourge prevails in significant segments of resident communities as asymptomatic[11] and often low-grade, sub-microscopic[12] infections.

Recent epidemiological studies have shown a striking link between availability of effective treatment drugs and historical successes in major reduction of the burden of malaria throughout the world[13,14]. Correspondingly, the emergence of antimalarial drug resistance, especially in *Plasmodium falciparum*, has proved a major obstacle for malaria control and elimination efforts since the eradication campaigns of the 1950s[15,16,17,18,19]. Drug resistance in *P. ovale* and *P. malariae* has not been documented, while in *P. vivax* the phenomenon, has been recently increasing[20,21,22].

The potential of the malaria parasite to generate genetic diversity through its complex genome and a proliferative life cycle involving sexual and asexual stages, means that drug resistance will remain a problem to contend with, escalating in the wake of wider introduction of each antimalarial. *P. falciparum* has repeatedly demonstrated this adaptation against virtually all antimalarial drugs[23,24,25], including the new regimens with or without artemisinin[26,27,28,29]. To minimize suffering and mortality due to use of drug regimens which are no longer effective, the epidemiology of drug resistance in malaria endemic regions needs continual monitoring[6].

1.2 Definition of drug resistance

Because of the immense amount of work that has gone into the subject, a number of related terms have evolved around "drug resistance", with distinguishable applications, depending on the objectives of the characterization and methods used. These are summarized as follows, for clarity.

1.2.1 Classical definition of drug resistance

Antimalarial drug resistance has been defined as "the ability of a parasite strain to survive and (or) multiply despite administration and absorption of the usually recommended, or slightly higher doses of a drug, within limits of tolerance of the host"[30,31]. This original definition generally holds for most drugs, but in the light of the pharmacokinetic characteristics of some antimalarials, a qualification was subsequently added, that "the form of the active drug against the parasite must gain access to the parasite, or the infected erythrocyte, for the duration of time necessary for its normal action"[32]. The qualification was added to cater for drug bioavailability and narrow down the reason of drug failure to parasite resistance. This definition of drug resistance therefore, in the strict sense, attempts to centre on the response of a parasite to an antimalarial, excluding host factors. Resistance has been assayed by *in vitro* methods, primarily based on the system developed by Rieckman *et al*[33]. *In vivo* methods[19,31] have also been used, but discrepancies with *in vitro* findings have been common because host factors, especially immunity, cannot be entirely precluded *in vivo*.

1.2.2 Therapeutic failure concept

For public health purposes, the importance and relevance of *in vivo* resistance has been increasingly recognized in drug policy decisions[34,35] since it is net parasite response to antimalarial medication in the human host that is paramount. However, *in vivo* resistance can, and indeed has, still occurred without much clinical relevance in the human population of interest, which may harbour resistant parasitaemias asymptomatically, especially in endemic areas[36,37]. Over time *in vivo* approaches have therefore been progressively modified to assess the parasitological and clinical response to antimalarial drugs[38,39,40]. These approaches measure the therapeutic efficacy of antimalarials and the corresponding parasitological and clinical resistance, which is termed therapeutic failure. Drug resistance *per se* may or may not lead to therapeutic failure, depending on malaria endemicity and concomitant level of immunity in the resident populations.

1.2.3 Treatment failure

Under routine operational conditions in primary health care, resistance parasitologically and (or) clinically is frequently encountered. It is usually not feasible in these situations to completely supervise drug administration and confirm bioabsorption. The apparent resistance is termed treatment failure, and may be caused by true drug resistance, malabsorption or incomplete dose compliance by outpatients.

1.2.4 Summary

Albeit often confused and interchangeably used, the foregoing terms have distinct applications. In this chapter drug resistance refers to the original sense, based on parasite response as ascertained *in vivo* or *in vitro*. Where reference to the other conditions is made the appropriate terms shall be used.

2. Armamentarium of current antimalarials and mode of action

Despite a seemingly extensive list of potent compounds, the net armamentarium of effective, safe and usable antimalarials is limited, relative to the epidemiological magnitude and evolutionary potential of malaria parasites. Owing to the advent of drug resistance, there is a need to develop more antimalarials. The antimalarial drugs in current use can in effect be grouped into blood schizontocides and antimetabolites of the folate pathway.

2.1 Blood schizontocides

Blood schizontocides act directly on intraerythrocytic stages responsible for symptoms and tend to be fast acting compounds usually preferred for treatment of acute disease. They include: aryl amino alcohols; 4-aminopyridine analogues; and the more recently widely introduced artemisinin and derivatives. Compounds in the first two groups are often referred to as quinoline-containing drugs (QCD's).

The aryl amino alcohols include the old cinchona alkaloid drug, quinine; the quinolinemethanol, mefloquine; and the phenanthrenemethanol drug, halofantrine. Quinine has been used for treatment and, in some cases prophylaxis, since the 17th century, as crude cinchona (Peruvian) bark, and from the 19th century as the pure drug. In contrast, halofantrine is a relatively new compound, which was first registered in France and francophone African countries in 1988. The 4-aminopyridine analogues include amopyraquine, mepacrine and the 4-aminoquinolines: chloroquine and amodiaquine. The 4-

aminoquinolines were introduced among the first generation of synthetic antimalarials in the late 1940's, following the search for safer compounds, for use both as treatment and prophylaxis. Artemisinin and derivatives include the parent compound artemisinin, a sesquiterpene lactone which constitutes the active principle of the Chinese herb *quingaosu*, and its derivatives. The Chinese herb was used for hundreds of years to cure malarial fevers, but only recently purified and introduced on a wider scale for treatment of multidrug-resistant malaria. Water and oil-soluble derivatives of artemisinin were subsequently developed which include the salt, sodium (or potassium) artesunate; the methyl ether derivative, artemether; and the ethyl ether derivative, arteether.

Blood schizontocides are believed to target the haemoglobin digestion and excretion process in the parasite food vacuole. Chloroquine, one of the 4-aminoquinolines most extensively studied, is thought to act by inhibiting polymerization of the parasite's haemoglobin digestion by-product, haem (ferriprotoporphyrin IX), which is toxic to the parasite if allowed to accumulate[41]. The non-toxic polymer that the parasite generates in the absence of inhibiting drug is haemozoin, or malaria pigment. Artemisinin and its derivatives have a unique endoperoxide bridge that is thought to undergo reactive cleavage by ferriprotoporphyrin IX. This generates free carbon-centred radicals that alkylate biomolecules and kill the parasite cells.

2.2 Antimetabolites of the folate pathway

Antimetabolites of the folate pathway (often referred to as antifolates) tend to attack all growing stages of the malaria parasites, including the early growing stages in the liver (causal prophylactic effect) and developing infective stages in the mosquito (antisporogonic effect). Like 4-aminoquinolines, the antimetabolites were also introduced in the late 1940's. They include the dihydrofolate reductase (DHFR) inhibitors (pyrimethamine, trimethoprim, cycloguanil and chlorcycloguanil) and dihydropteroate synthetase (DHPS) inhibitors or sulfa drugs (sulfadoxine, sulfalene, dapsone, sulfamethoxazole). Antifolates are usually used as combinations, e.g. sulfadoxine/pyrimethamine, sulfalene/pyrimethamine, or dapsone/pyrimethamine (prophylaxis).

The mode of action of antifolate drugs is among the most well understood. Malaria parasites synthesize folates during biosynthesis of pyrimidines which they cannot scavenge from the host. Antifolate drugs block two sequential steps within the folate synthesis pathway, eventually leading to (i) decreased pyrimidine synthesis and arrest of DNA replication; (ii) decreased methionine and serine production; and (iii) ultimate cell cycle arrest and death of the parasites. Dihydrofolate reductase inhibitors act by competing with substrate for the enzyme dihydrofolate reductase, while sulfa drugs are paraminobenzoic acid (PABA) analogues which competitively inhibit dihydropteroate synthetase in the preceding reaction.

3. Mechanisms of drug resistance

3.1 Quinoline-containing drugs

3.1.1 Group I blood schizontocides

Group I blood schizontocides are the dibasic QCD's, mainly the 4-aminoquinolines.

The mechanism of resistance to these drugs is due not to altered drug target, but to reduced drug accumulation in the parasite food vacuole[42]. Resistant parasites survive by accumulation of less drug than their sensitive counterparts. How the low drug levels are accumulated in resistant parasites is still not fully understood. A drug efflux mechanism has been proposed [43,44], and so has reduced drug uptake[45,46].

Enhanced Drug Efflux

Chloroquine-resistant isolates are known to expel intracellular chloroquine 40-50 times as rapidly as chloroquine-sensitive strains[44]. This process is energy-dependent and susceptible to ATP blockage[43]. Compelling evidence for a drug efflux mechanism has been the demonstration of reversal of chloroquine resistance by calcium channel blockers such as verapamil as well as some tricyclic compounds such as desipramine, *in vitro* and *in vivo*[47,48,49]. Reversal of chloroquine resistance by verapamil is independent of the weak base effect and is specific to resistant strains[50]. Although there were conflicting findings among earlier *in vivo* studies[51], subsequent work has abundantly illustrated chloroquine resistance reversal in malaria patients, with the antihistaminic agent chlopheniramine[52,53], and with promethazine[54]. The observations on reversal of chloroquine resistance by calcium channel blockers have led to the theory that a similar system to the multidrug resistance (*mdr*) phenomenon in mammalian cancer cells[55] is responsible. The *mdr* phenomenon in mammalian cancer cells is mediated by an ATP-dependent transporter, P-glycoprotein, which resides on the surface of the cell and has affinity for a wide range of compounds, including anti-cancer drugs which it actively expels. The mammalian *mdr* phenotype is reversed by a broad range of compounds that compete for affinity for the P-glycoprotein, including calcium channel blockers like verapamil, calmodulin antagonists and other compounds. P-glycoprotein homologues were subsequently isolated in *Plasmodium falciparum*, pfPgh1 and pfPgh2[56] encoded by the genes *Pfmdr1* and *Pfmdr2*.

These genes have shown partial association with chloroquine resistance controversy, with some workers reporting no association between *Pfmdr1* and chloroquine resistance[57], although the chloroquine efflux trait genetically segregated as a single locus[58]. Others have reported amino acid changes in *Pfmdr1* linked with chloroquine resistance[59], including the single substitution N86Y (the K1 allele), and four substitutions Y184P, N1032D, S1034C and D1246Y (7G8 allele). However, the most convincing demonstration for the role of *Pfmdr1* has come from recent allelic exchange studies which show that replacement of the wild type allele in chloroquine-sensitive strains with resistant alleles resulted in decreased drug sensitivity[60]. There is evidence that more than one gene is involved in coding for the chloroquine resistance phenotype.

The P. falciparum Chloroquine Resistance Transporter Gene (Pfcrt)

Through transfection and allelic exchange experiments between resistant and sensitive parasites a chloroquine resistance transporter (*Pfcrt*) gene was identified, which exhibited polymorphisms that matched the chloroquine resistance phenotype without exception. An *in vivo* study in Mali demonstrated close association between *Pfcrt* and chloroquine therapeutic failure[61].

3.1.2 Group II blood schizontocides

These are monobasic quinoline containing drugs (QCD's), which include quinine, mefloquine and halofantrine. Although their mode of action is thought to be essentially similar to that of the chloroquine group in interfering with haemoglobin digestion[62], the mechanism of resistance to these antimalarials is not clearly understood.

Increased drug efflux as seen with chloroquine-resistant *P. falciparum*, has not been demonstrated with the group II blood schizontocides. Moreover, it is believed unlikely that group II schizontocides, which are monobasic, can accumulate sufficiently in food vacuoles to reach levels required to inhibit haem polymerization[42], yet at least some of these drugs are more potent inhibitors of parasite growth than chloroquine. In addition, resistance to mefloquine has been associated with *Pfmdr1* amplification and cross-resistance to quinine and halofantrine, but decreased resistance to chloroquine[63].

3.2 Resistance to antifolate drugs

Antifolates include dihydrofolate reductase (DHFR) inhibitors (pyrimethamine, trimethoprim, cycloguanil, chlorcycloguanil) and dihydropteroate synthetase (DHPS) inhibitors (sulfones and sulfonamides, e.g. sulfadoxine, sulfamethoxazole, dapsone). These drugs were also among the first generation of synthetic antimalarials introduced in late 1940's [64]. Combinations of pyrimethamine and sulfonamides have been used as second line medication to treat chloroquine-resistant *P. falciparum* infections since the mid-1960's. Prophylactic usage was terminated owing to high risk of adverse reactions, except with pyrimethamine alone or dapsone/pyrimethamine which remains an alternative prophylactic used in a few countries.

Resistance to pyrimethamine became widespread in large areas soon after introduction of the drug, but the potentiating combination with sulfonamides retained effectiveness for longer. Resistance to the antifolate combinations initially became a problem in Indochina and South America in early 1980's. Pyrimethamine/sulfonamide combinations lost therapeutic adequacy in wide areas of South East Asia, western Oceania and South America and although they are still relatively effective in Africa, resistance is on the increase. Like chloroquine, antifolates have remained useful for relatively longer in Africa compared to Asia owing to substantial host immunity reducing the levels of *in vivo* therapeutic failure.

3.2.1 Mechanism of resistance to antifolate drugs

Unlike resistance to chloroquine and other quinoline containing drugs, the mechanism of antifolate drug resistance is directly related to the mode of drug action. The mechanism is also relatively well understood. Resistance to antifolates is known to be due to alterations in target enzymes which reduce drug binding affinity[65,66]. These structural alterations are caused by point mutations in the dihydrofolate/thymidylate synthetase (DHFR-TS) gene, for DHFR inhibitors[67,68] or in the dihydro-6-hydroxymethylpterin pyrophosphokinase-dihydropteroate synthetase (PPPK-DHPS) gene, for DHPS inhibitors[69,70].

Antifolate Resistance Point Mutations in the DHFR-TS gene

Point mutations conferring resistance to DHFR inhibitors have been well described for pyrimethamine and cycloguanil. A single point mutation (from wild type serine to asparagine) at amino acid position 108 in the DHFR domain of the DHFR-TS gene is associated with resistance to pyrimethamine, and only marginal decrease in susceptibility to cycloguanil. Additional mutations N51I and C59R have been associated with high levels of pyrimethamine resistance when they occur in combination with the S108N mutation. A mutation S108T, coupled with the mutation A16V, confers resistance to cycloguanil, with marginal effect on pyrimethamine sensitivity[71,72]. Cross-resistance to pyrimethamine and cycloguanil is conferred by a combination of mutations S108N and I164L, and is even heightened when the C59R mutation is also present.

Polymerase chain reaction (PCR) based assays have been developed, to detect pyrimethamine and cycloguanil resistant parasites and their correlation with standard *in vitro* or *in vivo* drug response profiles have been explored[73,74,75].

Antifolate Resistance Mutations in the PPPK-DHPS gene

Mutations conferring resistance to DHPS inhibitors have been also characterized, especially for sulfadoxine and sulfamethoxazole, frequently used in synergistic combinations with DHFR inhibitors. Point mutations at positions 436, 437, 540, 581 and 613 of the DHPS domain of the PPPK-DHPS gene have been implicated[69], with those at positions 436, 437, and 581 being reportedly the most common. As with the DHFR inhibitors, a corresponding PCR-based assay for detecting PPPK-DHPS mutations conferring resistance to sulfa drugs (sulfadoxine and sulfamethoxazole) has been developed.

4. Point mutations as molecular markers for drug-resistance

The gold standard approach for monitoring drug resistance is by performing *in vivo* antimalarial drug therapeutic efficacy assessments[35,40]. A complex protocol is implemented, where a sentinel group of malaria patients, mostly aged 5 years or less, is subjected to supervised drug treatment and followed up for periods usually lasting 28 days. Parasitological and clinical response to treatment is monitored during follow-up to ascertain whether clearance takes place within the stipulated time consistent with adequate drug efficacy. To distinguish persistent or recrudescent parasitaemia from reinfections, pre- and post-treatment samples must be subjected to genotyping using polymorphic markers, usually *P. falciparum* MSP1, MSP2 and GLURP genes. This approach is labour-intensive and costly, often with losses to follow-up, while some of the patients do not meet eligibility criteria at recruitment. Accrual of significant sample sizes on which to base incisive policy conclusions is therefore sometimes constrained, especially as malaria cases decrease.

Needless to say, the molecular detection of point mutations that confer drug resistance has proved a highly efficient approach for tracking and containment of drug resistant malaria. To date these molecular markers for drug resistance are best characterized for chloroquine and antifolate drugs (Table 1). Furthermore, the nature and combination of mutations that correlate most closely with clinical failure are characterized by standardizing against the *in vivo* assessment gold standard, making for highly instrumental surveillance tools. In antifolate resistance, combinations point mutations (double, triple, quadruple quintuple mutants) in the parasite DHFR and DHPS genes confer increasing levels of resistance. Research is under way to characterize markers for the other major antimalarials in use.

Gene	Molecular Marker (Point Mutation)	Antimalarial Drug
PfCRT	K76T	Chloroquine
DHFR-TS	S108N, S108T, N51I, C59R, A16V, I164L	DHFR inhibitors pyrimethamine, cycloguanil
PPK-DHPS	S436A(F/C), A437G, L540E, A581G, A613S(T)	DHPS inhibitors Sulfadoxine

Table 1. Point mutations widely used to track drug-resistant malaria

With molecular markers, resistant parasites can now be monitored both in the human and vector hosts, enabling containment long before escalation to a public health toll (Figure 1).

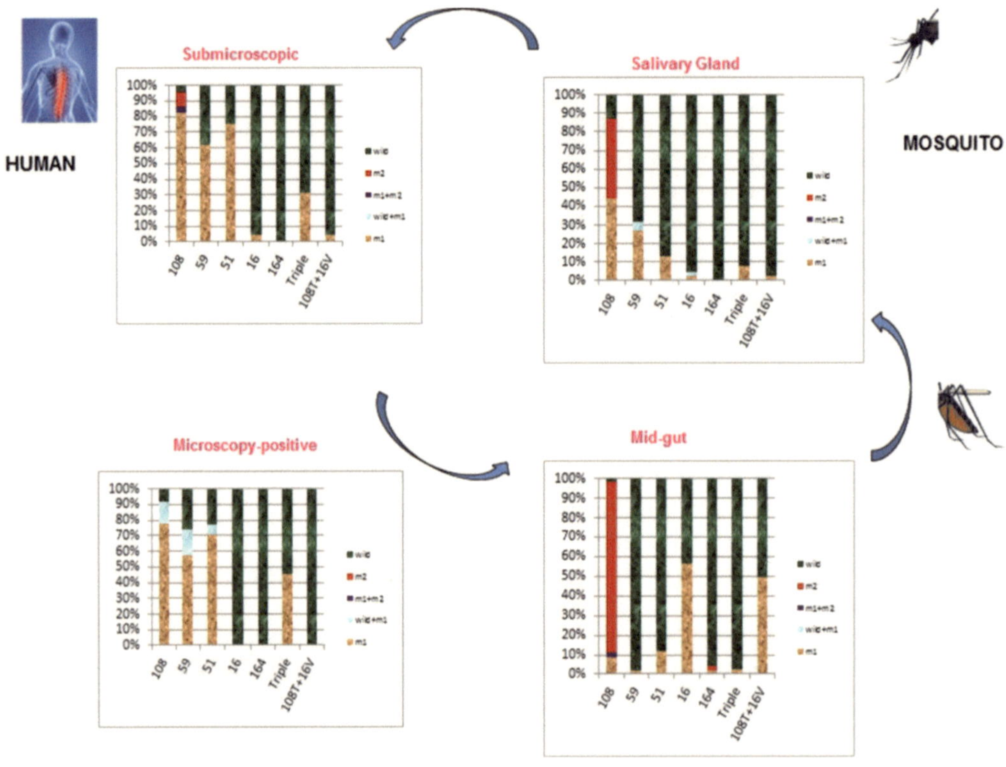

Fig. 1. Distribution of *P. falciparum* antifolate drug resistance alleles in human and mosquito hosts. Note major differences reflecting drug and immune selection. Using point mutations as molecular markers, drug resistance can be tracked in any phase of the parasite, enabling pre-emptive interventions before patient clinical failures set in.

4.1 Parasite bar-coding

Recently, SNPs located in numerous sections across the parasite genome have been applied as a potent tool to finger-print or bar-code malaria infections. This enables sensitive detection of changes in population structure or epidemiology of malaria in a given area in relation to interventions or re-invasion.

A typical bar-code[76] comprises 20-24 SNPs from across all the chromosomes of the malaria parasite, enabling medium-high resolution typing of malarial infections.

5. Conclusion

P. falciparum drug resistance persists as a key strategy by which malaria frustrates control and elimination efforts. The complex genomic blueprint of *P. falciparum* has repeatedly proven its ability to overcome any widely introduced antimalarial with relative ease. It is therefore imperative to develop and implement not only new antimalarial drugs, but also effective strategies for the surveillance and containment of drug resistance. Combination therapy is now stipulated as standard treatment for malaria by WHO, where constituent drugs protect each other from resistance development and the chances of resistance to both are less likely to occur. Artemisinin-based combination therapy (ACT) is preferred, containing artemisinin or its derivative as one of the partner drugs, since it is fast-acting and shows signs of relatively slow resistance development.

Simple point mutations can confer resistance to most antimalarial drugs. In the diverse and dynamic epidemiology of malaria, point mutations are increasingly adopted as efficient molecular markers for surveillance of drug resistant malaria in endemic countries. These molecular markers are readily standardizable and independent of host immune status, drug history or other confounding factors incorporated in the strict eligibility criteria for gold standard *in vivo* drug efficacy assessments. They are also less laborious and require much less time to perform once standardized against the gold standard *in vivo* assessments. Well characterized molecular markers for resistance to chloroquine and antifolate drugs have become standard surveillance tools, with global data being fed into world resistance monitoring programmes such as the World-wide Antimalarial Resistance Network (WWARN).

In recent times point mutations are also being utilized to identify malaria strains and detect changes in population structure during interventions or resurgences by bar-coding.

Furthermore, molecular markers for resistance to other major antimalarial drugs are being actively sought, placing the simple point mutation in good stead to be the future of surveillance in malaria and other diseases.

6. References

[1] WHO (2010) World Malaria Report. World Health Organization, Geneva.
[2] Kitua A, Ogundahunsi O, Lines J, Mgone C (2011) Conquering malaria: enhancing the impact of effective interventions towards elimination in the diverse and changing epidemiology. J Glob Infect Dis 3: 161-165.
[3] Greenwood B, Mutabingwa T (2002) Malaria in 2002. Nature 415: 670-672.
[4] Sachs J, Malaney P (2002) The economic and social burden of malaria. Nature 415: 680-685.
[5] Nabarro D (1999) Roll Back Malaria. Parassitologia 41: 501-504.
[6] Bosman A, Mendis KN (2007) A major transition in malaria treatment: the adoption and deployment of artemisinin-based combination therapies. Am J Trop Med Hyg 77: 193-197.

[7] Chanda E, Masaninga F, Coleman M, Sikaala C, Katebe C, et al. (2008) Integrated vector management: the Zambian experience. Malar J 7: 164.
[8] Nabarro D, Mendis K (2000) Roll back malaria is unarguably both necessary and possible. Bull World Health Organ 78: 1454-1455.
[9] Greenwood B (2009) Can malaria be eliminated? Trans R Soc Trop Med Hyg 103 Suppl 1: S2-5.
[10] Mendis K, Rietveld A, Warsame M, Bosman A, Greenwood B, et al. (2009) From malaria control to eradication: The WHO perspective. Trop Med Int Health 14: 802-809.
[11] Nwagha UI, Ugwu VO, Nwagha TU, Anyaehie BU (2009) Asymptomatic Plasmodium parasitaemia in pregnant Nigerian women: almost a decade after Roll Back Malaria. Trans R Soc Trop Med Hyg 103: 16-20.
[12] Babiker HA (1998) Unstable malaria in Sudan: the influence of the dry season. Plasmodium falciparum population in the unstable malaria area of eastern Sudan is stable and genetically complex. Trans R Soc Trop Med Hyg 92: 585-589.
[13] Trape JF, Pison G, Spiegel A, Enel C, Rogier C (2002) Combating malaria in Africa. Trends Parasitol 18: 224-230.
[14] Trape JF (2001) The public health impact of chloroquine resistance in Africa. Am J Trop Med Hyg 64: 12-17.
[15] Bjorkman A, Bhattarai A (2005) Public health impact of drug resistant Plasmodium falciparum malaria. Acta Trop 94: 163-169.
[16] Bjorkman A, Phillips-Howard PA (1990) The epidemiology of drug-resistant malaria. Trans R Soc Trop Med Hyg 84: 177-180.
[17] Bloland PB, Ettling M (1999) Making malaria-treatment policy in the face of drug resistance. Ann Trop Med Parasitol 93: 5-23.
[18] Trape JF, Pison G, Preziosi MP, Enel C, Desgrees du Lou A, et al. (1998) Impact of chloroquine resistance on malaria mortality. C R Acad Sci III 321: 689-697.
[19] WHO (1984) Advances in malaria chemotherapy. Report of a WHO Scientific Group. Geneva: World Health Organization.
[20] Wernsdorfer WH (1994) Epidemiology of drug resistance in malaria. Acta Trop 56: 143-156.
[21] Ketema T, Getahun K, Bacha K (2011) Therapeutic efficacy of chloroquine for treatment of Plasmodium vivax malaria cases in Halaba district, South Ethiopia. Parasit Vectors 4: 46.
[22] Rieckmann KH, Davis DR, Hutton DC (1989) Plasmodium vivax resistance to chloroquine 2 1183-1184. . Lancet 2: 1183-1184.
[23] Brockman A, Price RN, van Vugt M, Heppner DG, Walsh D, et al. (2000) *Plasmodium falciparum* antimalarial drug susceptibility on the north-western border of Thailand during five years of extensive use of artesunate-mefloquine. *Transactions of the Royal Society of Tropical Medicine and Hygiene* 94 537-544.
[24] Noranate N, Durand R, Tall A, Marrama L, Spiegel A, et al. (2007) Rapid dissemination of Plasmodium falciparum drug resistance despite strictly controlled antimalarial use. PLoS ONE 2: e139.
[25] Foote SJ, Cowman AF (1994) The mode of action and the mechanism of resistance to antimalarial drugs. Acta Trop 56: 157-171.

[26] Crabb C (2003) Plasmodium falciparum outwits Malarone, protector of travellers. Bull World Health Organ 81: 382-383.
[27] Fivelman Q, Butcher G, Adagu I, Warhurst D, Pasvol G (2002) Malarone treatment failure and in vitro confirmation of resistance of Plasmodium falciparum isolate from Lagos, Nigeria. Malaria Journal 1: 1.
[28] Dondorp AM, Yeung S, White L, Nguon C, Day NP, et al. Artemisinin resistance: current status and scenarios for containment. Nat Rev Microbiol 8: 272-280.
[29] Noedl H, Se Y, Schaecher K, Smith BL, Socheat D, et al. (2008) Evidence of artemisinin-resistant malaria in western Cambodia. N Engl J Med 359: 2619-2620.
[30] WHO (1965) Resistance of malaria parasites to drugs. Geneva: World Health Organization.
[31] WHO (1973) Chemotherapy of malaria and resistance to antimalarials. . Geneva: World Health Organization.
[32] Bruce-Chwatt LJ, Black RH, Canfield CJ, Clyde DF, Peters W, et al. (1986) Chemotherapy of Malaria, 2nd revised Edition. WHO Monograph Series
[33] Rieckmann KH, Campbell GH, Sax LJ, Mrema JA (1978) Drug sensitivity of Plasmodium falciparum: an in vitro micro technique. *Lancet* 1: 22-23
[34] WHO (1990) Practical chemotherapy of malaria. Geneva: World Health Organization.
[35] WHO (2005) Susceptibility of *Plasmodium falciparum* to Antimalarial Drugs. Geneva: World Health Organization.
[36] Mutabingwa TK, Malle LN, Mtui SN (1991) Chloroquine therapy still useful in the management of malaria during pregnancy in Muheza, Tanzania. Trop Geogr Med 43: 131-135.
[37] Henry MC, Docters van Leeuwen W, Watson P, Jansen A, Jacobs K, et al. (1994) In vivo sensitivity of Plasmodium falciparum to chloroquine in rural areas of Cote d'Ivoire. Acta Tropica 58: 275-281.
[38] WHO (1994) Antimalaria drug policies: data requirements, treatment of uncomplicated malaria and management of malaria in pregnancy. Report of an informal consultation, Geneva 14-18 March 1994. Geneva: World Health Organization.
[39] WHO (1996) Assessment of the Therapeutic Efficacy of Antimalarial Drugs for the Treatment of Uncomplicated Malaria in Africa in Areas with Intense Transmission. Geneva: World Health Organization.
[40] WHO (2003) Assessment and Monitoring of Antimalarial Drug Efficacy for the Treatment of Uncomplicated Falciparum Malaria . . Geneva: World Health Organization.
[41] Slater AF, Cerami A (1992) Inhibition by chloroquine of a novel haem polymerase enzyme activity in malaria trophozoites. Nature 355: 167-169.
[42] Slater AF (1993) Chloroquine: mechanism of drug action and resistance in Plasmodium falciparum. Pharmacol Ther 57: 203-235.
[43] Krogstad DJ, Gluzman IY, Herwaldt BL, Schlesinger PH, Wellems TE (1992) Energy dependence of chloroquine accumulation and chloroquine efflux in Plasmodium falciparum. Biochem Pharmacol 43: 57-62.
[44] Krogstad DJ, Gluzman IY, Kyle DE, Oduola AM, Martin SK, et al. (1987) Efflux of chloroquine from Plasmodium falciparum: mechanism of chloroquine resistance. Science 238: 1283-1285.

[45] Geary TG, Divo AD, Jensen JB, Zangwill M, Ginsburg H (1990) Kinetic modelling of the response of Plasmodium falciparum to chloroquine and its experimental testing in vitro. Implications for mechanism of action of and resistance to the drug. Biochem Pharmacol 40: 685-691.

[46] Geary TG, Jensen JB, Ginsburg H (1986) Uptake of [3H]chloroquine by drug-sensitive and -resistant strains of the human malaria parasite Plasmodium falciparum. Biochem Pharmacol 35: 3805-3812.

[47] Martin SK, Oduola AM, Milhous WK (1987) Reversal of chloroquine resistance in Plasmodium falciparum by verapamil. Science 235: 899-901.

[48] Bitonti AJ, McCann PP (1989) Desipramine and cyproheptadine for reversal of chloroquine resistance in Plasmodium falciparum. Lancet 2: 1282-1283.

[49] Bitonti AJ, Sjoerdsma A, McCann PP, Kyle DE, Oduola AM, et al. (1988) Reversal of chloroquine resistance in malaria parasite Plasmodium falciparum by desipramine. Science 242: 1301-1303.

[50] Martiney JA, Cerami A, Slater AF (1995) Verapamil reversal of chloroquine resistance in the malaria parasite Plasmodium falciparum is specific for resistant parasites and independent of the weak base effect. J Biol Chem 270: 22393-22398.

[51] Warsame M, Wernsdorfer WH, Bjorkman A (1992) Lack of effect of desipramine on the response to chloroquine of patients with chloroquine-resistant falciparum malaria. Trans R Soc Trop Med Hyg 86: 235-236.

[52] Sowunmi A, Fehintola FA, Ogundahunsi OA, Arowojolu AO, Oduola AM (1998) Efficacy of chloroquine plus chlorpheniramine in chloroquine-resistant falciparum malaria during pregnancy in Nigerian women: a preliminary study. J Obstet Gynaecol 18: 524-527.

[53] Sowunmi A, Oduola AM (1997) Comparative efficacy of chloroquine/chlorpheniramine combination and mefloquine for the treatment of chloroquine-resistant Plasmodium falciparum malaria in Nigerian children. Trans R Soc Trop Med Hyg 91: 689-693.

[54] Oduola AM, Sowunmi A, Milhous WK, Brewer TG, Kyle DE, et al. (1998) In vitro and in vivo reversal of chloroquine resistance in Plasmodium falciparum with promethazine. Am J Trop Med Hyg 58: 625-629.

[55] Endicott JA, Ling V (1989) The biochemistry of P-glycoprotein-mediated multidrug resistance. Annu Rev Biochem 58: 137-171.

[56] Cowman AF, Karcz S, Galatis D, Culvenor JG (1991) A P-glycoprotein homologue of Plasmodium falciparum is localized on the digestive vacuole. J Cell Biol 113: 1033-1042.

[57] Wellems TE, Panton LJ, Gluzman IY, do Rosario VE, Gwadz RW, et al. (1990) Chloroquine resistance not linked to mdr-like genes in a Plasmodium falciparum cross. Nature 345: 253-255.

[58] Wellems TE (1991) Molecular genetics of drug resistance in Plasmodium falciparum malaria. Parasitol Today 7: 110-112.

[59] Foote SJ, Kyle DE, Martin RK, Oduola AM, Forsyth K, et al. (1990) Several alleles of the multidrug-resistance gene are closely linked to chloroquine resistance in Plasmodium falciparum. Nature 345: 255-258.

[60] Reed MB, Saliba KJ, Caruana SR, Kirk K, Cowman AF (2000) Pgh1 modulates sensitivity and resistance to multiple antimalarials in Plasmodium falciparum. Nature 403: 906-909.

[61] Djimde A, Doumbo OK, Cortese JF, Kayentao K, Doumbo S, et al. (2001) A molecular marker for chloroquine-resistant falciparum malaria. N Engl J Med 344: 257-263.

[62] Peters W, Howells RE, Portus J, Robinson BL, Thomas S, et al. (1977) The chemotherapy of rodent malaria, XXVII. Studies on mefloquine (WR 142,490). Ann Trop Med Parasitol 71: 407-418.

[63] Wilson CM, Volkman SK, Thaithong S, Martin RK, Kyle DE, et al. (1993) Amplification of pfmdr 1 associated with mefloquine and halofantrine resistance in Plasmodium falciparum from Thailand. Mol Biochem Parasitol 57: 151-160.

[64] Wernsdorfer WH, Payne D (1991) The dynamics of drug resistance in Plasmodium falciparum. Pharmacol Ther 50: 95-121.

[65] McCutchan TF, Welsh JA, Dame JB, Quakyi IA, Graves PM, et al. (1984) Mechanism of pyrimethamine resistance in recent isolates of Plasmodium falciparum. Antimicrob Agents Chemother 26: 656-659.

[66] Chen GX, Mueller C, Wendlinger M, Zolg JW (1987) Kinetic and molecular properties of the dihydrofolate reductase from pyrimethamine-sensitive and pyrimethamine-resistant clones of the human malaria parasite Plasmodium falciparum. Mol Pharmacol 31: 430-437.

[67] Cowman AF, Morry MJ, Biggs BA, Cross GA, Foote SJ (1988) Amino acid changes linked to pyrimethamine resistance in the dihydrofolate reductase-thymidylate synthase gene of Plasmodium falciparum. Proc Natl Acad Sci U S A 85: 9109-9113.

[68] Peterson DS, Walliker D, Wellems TE (1988) Evidence that a point mutation in dihydrofolate reductase-thymidylate synthase confers resistance to pyrimethamine in falciparum malaria. Proc Natl Acad Sci U S A 85: 9114-9118.

[69] Brooks DR, Wang P, Read M, Watkins WM, Sims PF, et al. (1994) Sequence variation of the hydroxymethylpterin pyrophosphokinase-dihydropteroate synthase gene in lines of the human malaria parasite, *Plasmodium falciparum*, with differing resistance to sulfadoxine. European Journal of Biochemistry 224: 397-405.

[70] Triglia T, Cowman AF (1994) Primary structure and expression of the dihydropteroate synthetase gene of *Plasmodium falciparum*. Proc Natl Acad Sci U S A 91: 7149-7153.

[71] Peterson DS, Milhous WK, Wellems TE (1990) Molecular basis of differential resistance to cycloguanil and pyrimethamine in Plasmodium falciparum malaria. Proc Natl Acad Sci U S A 87: 3018-3022.

[72] Foote SJ, Galatis D, Cowman AF (1990) Amino acids in the dihydrofolate reductase-thymidylate synthase gene of Plasmodium falciparum involved in cycloguanil resistance differ from those involved in pyrimethamine resistance. Proc Natl Acad Sci U S A 87: 3014-3017.

[73] Peterson DS, Di Santi SM, Povoa M, Calvosa VS, Do Rosario VE, et al. (1991) Prevalence of the dihydrofolate reductase Asn-108 mutation as the basis for pyrimethamine-resistant falciparum malaria in the Brazilian Amazon. Am J Trop Med Hyg 45: 492-497.

[74] Gyang FN, Peterson DS, Wellems TE (1992) Plasmodium falciparum: rapid detection of dihydrofolate reductase mutations that confer resistance to cycloguanil and pyrimethamine. Exp Parasitol 74: 470-472.
[75] Plowe CV, Djimde A, Bouare M, Doumbo O, Wellems TE (1995) Pyrimethamine and proguanil resistance-conferring mutations in Plasmodium falciparum dihydrofolate reductase: polymerase chain reaction methods for surveillance in Africa. Am J Trop Med Hyg 52: 565-568.
[76] Daniels R, Volkman SK, Milner DA, Mahesh N, Neafsey DE, et al. (2008) A general SNP-based molecular barcode for Plasmodium falciparum identification and tracking. Malar J 7: 223.

10

Correlations with Point Mutations and Severity of Hemolitic Anemias: The Example of Hereditary Persistence of Fetal Hemoglobin with Sickle Cell Anemia and Beta Thalassemia

Anderson Ferreira da Cunha[1], Iran Malavazi[1],
Karen Simone Romanello[1] and Cintia do Couto Mascarenhas[2]
[1]*Departamento de Genética e Evolução,*
Centro de Ciências Biológicas e da Saúde,
Universidade Federal de São Carlos,
[2]*Centro de Hematologia e Hemoterapia,*
Universidade Estadual de Campinas,
Brazil

1. Introduction

Hemolytic anemias are a group of diseases characterized by a reduction in red blood cells (RBC) life span mainly caused by a deregulation in the hemoglobin formation. Among these diseases, Sickle Cell Disease (SCD) and Beta Thalassemia (βThal) are the most common disorders involved in the premature destruction of RBC. Understanding the molecular mechanisms involved in the outcome of these diseases as well as the metabolic pathways surrounding its onset constitutes a very useful approach to target treatment strategies for such diseases. In this chapter we will discuss the state-of-the-art aspects about this theme highlighting the importance of several point mutations in hemolytic anemia using β thalassemia and sickle cell disease as examples. In addition, the molecular aspects involved in the Hereditary Persistence of Fetal Hemoglobin (HPFH), also an important disorder caused by point mutations and deletions, and its association with the severity of βThal and SCD will be also discussed. In this context lies the manifestation of better prognostic to patients having an increase in fetal hemoglobin and SCD or βThal concomitantly. Therefore a parallel discussion towards the advances currently described in the literature and associations of gene expression and different drugs that increase the production of fetal hemoglobin (HbF) are pointed out as a mechanism to improve the quality of life of SCD and βThal patients.

2. The erythroid cell

Erythroid proliferation is a precisely regulated process, in which hematopoietic stem cells (HSCs) differentiate into lineage-restricted erythroid progenitors through a process called erythropoiesis. While in adult humans the process occurs basically in the bone marrow (BM), the primitive hematopoiesis occurs initially in the yolk sac (YS). (Fig. 01) The regulation of cellular proliferation, survival and differentiation is a strictly regulated process in all the producing cells and are stimulated by extracellular signaling molecules, particularly erythropoietin (EPO), a hormone synthesized by the kidney. This hormone functionally activates its receptor called EPOR on the surface of red blood cells (RBCs) precursor cells in the BM. The first cell line formed after this stimulus is known as Burst Forming Unit-Erythroid (BFU-E) (Hoffman et al. 2008).

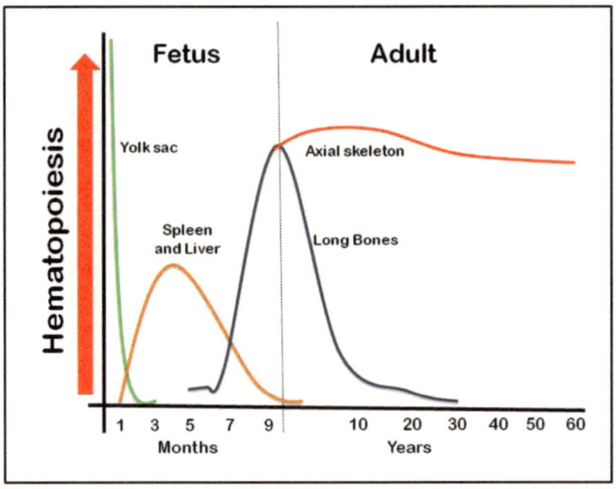

Fig. 1. Sites of hematopoesis during the human development. During the very first weeks of human development the hematopoiesis occurs in the yolk sac. After the first month, the hematopoietic site is switched to spleen and liver and after the seventh month all the hematopoiesis occurs in long bones. Following the birth and during the adult life the hematopoesis site is in the axial skeleton.

After the EPO stimulus, cells undergo several modifications that lead to the formation of RBCs. The first step occurs when the Burst forming unit erythroid cells (BFU-E) originates the colony-forming units erythroid (CFU-E), which differentiates to the first morphologically identifiable stage of the erythroid cells, the proerythroblasts. Successive modifications lead the cell to several transforming processes generating the basophilics erythroblasts, polychromatophilics erythroblasts, orthochromics erythroblasts. At this stage, the nucleus becomes picnotic and is extruded of the cell forming the reticulocyte. This cell presents a biconcave shape and contains residual remaining RNA. Reticulocytes are released into the blood and develop into mature erythrocytes within about two days (Fig. 02) (Hoffman et al. 2008; Tsiftsoglou et al. 2009).

Under normal conditions, erythrocytes life span is about 120 days. After this time, the erythrocytes undergo several morphological changes, specially caused by reduction in its metabolic activity and the hemoglobin content oxidation (Ghaffari 2008). These cell alterations are ultimately recognized by mononuclear phagocyte system (MPS). The cells are then removed from bloodstream in that the majority of the cell components are recycled and used in the production of new cells. The MPS consists of phagocytic cells (macrophages and monocytes) residents in the liver and spleen which are the major organs responsible for

RBCs removal. An increase in RBCs destruction independent from the etiology results in a clinical disorder generally called anemia. This unbalanced destruction of the RBC population is the most important feature found in several hemolytic diseases like sickle cell disease and βThal that will be further discussed in detail later on in this chapter (Telen et al. 1999; Hoffman et al. 2008).

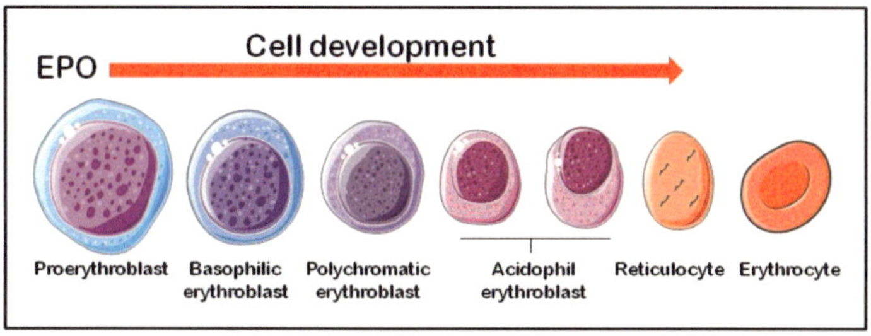

Fig. 2. Morphological changes during erythropoiesis in humans - After EPO stimulus the erythroid cell undergo several morphological changes that lead to the formation of mature erythrocytes. For details see the text. Figure was produced using Servier Medical Art, http://www.servier.co.uk/medical-art-gallery/SlideKit.asp?kit=18.

3. The hemoglobin

The main function of erythrocytes is the transport of oxygen from lung to peripheral tissues and carbon dioxide from them to the lung. This function is performed by the hemoglobin (Hb) molecule, a protein tetramer which comprises 95% of the whole protein content in RBC.

Hemoglobin synthesis requires the coordinated production of different globin proteins combined with a non-protein heme group as a prosthetic group. Heme molecule consists of an iron (Fe) ion held in a heterocyclic ring, known as a porphyrin. The protoporphyrin present in erithrocytes is the protoporphyrin IX which is a complex structure of a tetrapyrole structure. This molecule comprises four pyrole rings having eight sites for side chain groups substituents at its periphery. The protoporphyrin IX can then be described as 1,3,5,8 methyl; 2,4 vinyl; 6,7 propionic acid-porphiryn. The designation of protoporphiryn IX refers to the fact that from the 15 possible isomers of protoporphyrin, the ninith one that Hans Fischer (the pioneer in the chemical foundations of proptoprphyrin molecules) synthetized was exactly the same naturally occurring in the heme molecule. Therefore, the IX isomer is the only one found in nature (Greer et al. 2008).

Iron is the site of oxygen binding when it is in the ferrous (Fe^{2+}) oxidation state. The hemoglobin can be saturated with oxygen molecules (oxyhemoglobin), or desaturated without oxygen (deoxyhemoglobin). Two distinct globin chains are combined to form hemoglobin, the alpha and non-alpha (Fig. 3a).

The alpha cluster located at chromosome 16 is responsible for the production of ζ and α globin. On the other hand, the production of non-alpha chains occurs in the β cluster located at chromosome 11. In this latter cluster the ε, γ, δ and β globin are produced. (Fig. 3b) (Tang et al. 2008).

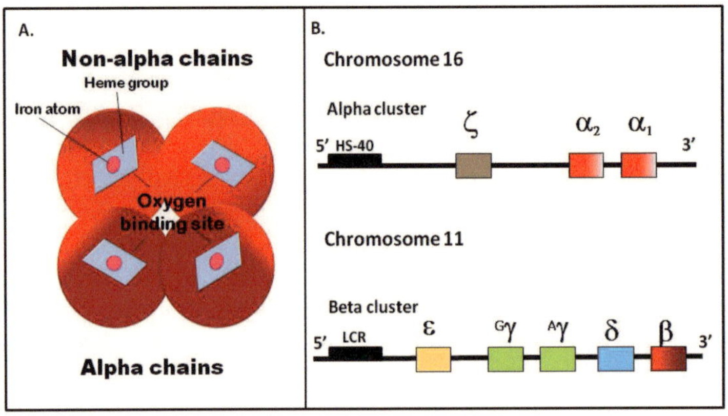

Fig. 3. Formation of hemoglobin during the human development - (A) Schematic representation of hemoglobin showing its molecules. (B) The hemoglobin is composed by the combination of two alpha and two non-alpha chains. The proteins are produced by the expression of several genes located in the α and β cluster at Chromosome 16 and 11 respectively.

The ontogeny of globin synthesis during development is complex and dynamic having different proteins being produced by different clusters. During the first weeks of embryogenesis the predominant globin chain synthetized by α cluster is the ζ globin. After this time, the globin chain produced by the α cluster is always represented by the α globin. However, the β cluster can produce several different globin proteins as shown in Fig. 3. During the fetal period, the non-alpha globins produced are the ε (2 - 6 weeks) and γ (after the 6th week). After the birth, the γ gene is silenced and the transcription of the β and δ gene starts indefinitely. The most abundant globin occurring after the birth expressed by β cluster is the β globin that represents about 98% of non-alpha chains found in the mature erythrocyte The control mechanisms of the transcription modulation of globin genes are not completely understood. Some studies showed that the Locus Control Region (LCR) present in β cluster and the HS40 (Hypersensitive site 40) region in α cluster bend on the promoter of each gene enhancing its transcription. When these regions fold up in the subsequent promoter, the silencing of the preceding gene occurs with the consequent activation of transcription in the subsequent gene. The transcription factors involved in LCR and HS40 movements remains unclear but some relevant aspects of this regulation module will be discussed later in this section. The combination of two α chains and two non-α chains produces a complete hemoglobin molecule (Palstra et al. 2003; Hoffman et al. 2008).

In humans, as for the expression of globin genes, the production of Hb is also ontogenetically regulated. Therefore, different types of hemoglobin are produced according to the developmental cell stage (i. e. embryonic, fetal and adult). Embryonic Hbs are produced early during hematopoiesis when erythropoiesis is predominantly in the yolk sac. The first hemoglobin produced in embryo is the gower 1 formed by the combination of two ζ globins and two ε globins ($\zeta_2\varepsilon_2$). The hemoglobin Gower 2 is then formed by the combination of two α and two ε globin ($\alpha_2\varepsilon_2$). The Portland hemoglobin is the third class of globins produced in embryos as a result of the association of two ζ and two γ globin ($\zeta_2\gamma_2$). During the fetal period the first hemoglobin switching takes place when the α globin is combined with γ globin ($\alpha_2\gamma_2$), producing the fetal hemoglobin (HbF). In this period, the hemoglobin is synthesized in the liver. During the first six weeks after the birth, occurs the second hemoglobin switching. At this stage the γ globin synthesis is drastically decreased and the production of β globin starts. The combination of α and the newly β globin produced results in the major hemoglobin counterpart found during the adult life which is called HbA1 ($\alpha_2\beta_2$). There is also another adult normal hemoglobin formed by the combination of α and δ globins the HbA2 ($\alpha_2\delta_2$), that represents 1.5-3.5%. The Fig. 4 shows the ontogenetic production of hemoglobin depicting the sites of production and the time of development where the different globin chains peaks in concentration (Fig. 04) (Stamatoyannopoulos 2005).

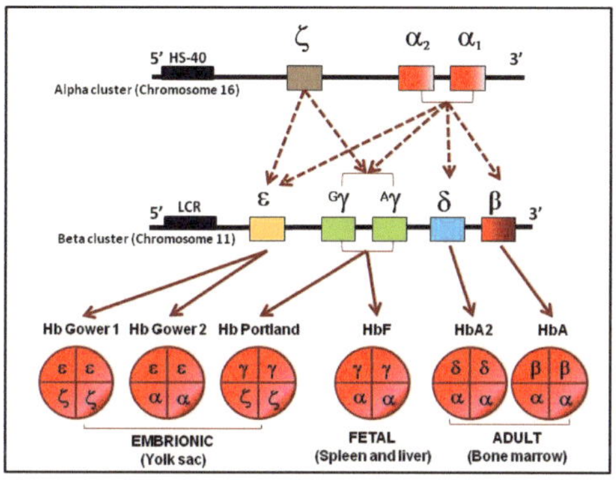

Fig. 4. The production of different types of hemoglobins during human development - During human development different types of hemoglobin are produced. In the embryonic phase de Hb Gower 1 and 2 and also Hb Portland are produced. In the fetal phase the combination of γ and α proteins produced the HbF. After the birth, two hemoglobins are produced, the HbA2 that represents about 1.5- 3.5% of total hemoglobin in adult blood and the HbA that represents 95 - 98% of hemoglobin.

3.1 The genetic regulation of globin genes

As discussed earlier, the genetic control of hemoglobin production is not completely understood, however several studies showed that globin genes can be expressed and repressed upon the regulation of several transcription factor that can interact with the globin gene promoters. As mentioned before, in the β globin cluster, the LCR can interact with the different globin genes in this cluster forming the different types of hemoglobin. This region is comprised of hypersensitive sites, which are DNA stretches with marked sensitivity to *in vitro* DNAse treatment. The precise function of LCR is not still completely clear. Several studies have shown that it acts as a "super-enhancer" DNA sequence that is thought to interact with each globin gene in the cluster by the interactions with several transcription factors. There are some other important regions surrounding the globin genes that are probably involved in its own transcription. One of these regions is a sequence spanning -80 and -120 bp upstream the start codon called the TATA and CAT box, respectively. These regulatory regions bind to and interacts with RNA polymerase in the beginning of globin gene transcription. Also of seminal importance is the region located at 3' region of the transcription start site, called as the GATA binding sequence. In such region, a transcription factors called GATA, a zinc-finger family of transcription factors (GATA 1-6), interacts with DNA and can both activate and repress target genes involved in erythroid development (Strauss et al. 1992; Strauss et al. 1992; Cao et al. 2011).

Specially in α- and β-globin loci, several binding sites for this family are found, suggesting an important role of these proteins in the regulation of these genes. The same motif is also found in the promoters of several genes that are also regulated during the erythroid development. GATA1 is the main member of these family involved in erythroid cell maturation *in vivo*. Its expression is essential for the formation of erythroid definitive lineage and several studies showed that erythroid Gata1-null cells can not mature beyond the proerythroblast stage. GATA1 seems to be also involved in the switching of the fetal to adult hemoglobin. Mutation in GATA1 gene has been described as involved in congenital erythropoietic porphyria and elevated levels of HbF. However the exact mechanism that links this gene to the elevation of γ globin is still not completely clear (Weiss et al. 1994; Blobel et al. 1995; Weiss et al. 1995; Blobel et al. 1996; Weiss et al. 1997; Blobel et al. 1998).

As mentioned before, these DNA sequences are well recognized as sites of bona fide globin gene expression regulation. The presence of mutations in such regions leads to a deregulation in the expression of globin genes causing either interruption or a decreased expression of such genes.

Besides this, regulation involving the gene transcription licensing, several other genetic factors have been described up to now as involved in the globin gene regulation. The *BCL11A* gene, as the GATA family is a zinc-finger protein, firstly identified as a potentially important factor in globin regulation and as a master regulator in the switch of the fetal to adult hemoglobin in humans. This gene is under the transcriptional regulation of a transcription factor known as KLF1 (Kruppel-like factor). KLF1 binds to a CACCC motif and this association is also strictly correlated to γ to β-globin gene switching. Mutation in this binding motif is associated with human βThal and Hereditary Persistence of Fetal Hemoglobin that will be discussed later on (Sankaran et al. 2008; Xu et al. 2010).

Another important set of genes involved in the erythroid terminal differentiation is SOX6 and *ALAS2*. *SOX6* is a transcription factor expressed in several human tissues. Specifically in erythroid cells, it has been reported that *SOX6* expression is crucial to promote erythroid final maturation, since an increased number of nucleated and immature red cells are observed in blood stream when this gene is deleted in mouse. ALAS2 is the enzyme catalysing the first and regulatory step of heme synthesis. Its expression is restricted to erythroid precursor cells. Therefore, reported mutations in ALAS2 have been linked to ineffective erythropoiesis and associated to X-linked sideroblastic anaemia (Ducamp et al. 2010; Wilber et al. 2011).

3.2 Hemolytic anemia

Despite many studies focusing on the understanding of the complete regulation of hemoglobin formation highlighted in the previous section, many aspects of this regulation are still to be addressed. Deregulation of hemoglobin formation is involved in the reduction of red blood cells leading to a important disorder called hemolytic anemia After the normal life span of about 120 days, the red blood cells need to be removed from the circulation.

Spleen and liver are the most important tissues responsible for the destruction and recycling of red blood cells components. In normal conditions, the destruction of these cells is balanced with their production in the bone marrow and the number of circulating red blood cells is physiologically maintained (Hoffman et al. 2008).

An unbalanced rate of destruction and production of RBC can increase or reduce the population of circulating cells. The increase of these cells is denominated policytemia and this clinical condition is present in several proliferative disorders. On the other hand, the reduction of RBC number consists of anemia and can be developed by several reasons, including some erythroid diseases including sickle cell disease and βThal. In these cases, the anemia is called hemolytic because the established condition is caused by an increase in hemolysis of the RBC.

The anemia is most often diagnosed through hematological tests in which a decrease in hemoglobin concentration and in RBC cell count are detected. Despite the laboratory diagnosis, the clinical history and physical examination can provide important clues about the presence of hemolysis and its underlying cause. The patient may complain of dyspnea or fatigue (caused by anemia). Dark urine and, occasionally, back pain may be reported by patients with intravascular hemolysis. The skin may appear jaundiced or pale. A resting tachycardia with a flow murmur may be present if the anemia is pronounced. Leg ulcers occur in some chronic hemolytic states, such as sickle cell anemia. Hepatosplenomegaly suggest an abnormal RBC destruction caused by accentuated hemolysis (Hoffman et al. 2008).

Besides the anemia, another important laboratory feature that indicates an accelerated hemolysis is reticulocytosis which is characterized by an increase in reticulocytes in peripheral blood (see Fig. 02). This increased prevalence of reticulocytes is the physiological bone marrow response attempting to the restoration (in number) of the cells loosen. In the absence of concomitant bone marrow disease, a brisk reticulocytosis should be observed within three to five days after a decline in hemoglobin. After this period, in a normal condition the RBCs production is compensated, leading to a normal and stable hemoglobin concentration.

In contrast, in the hemolytic anemia, although a marked reticulocytosis is observed after the RBCs destruction, the bone marrow is not able in compensate the formation of normal RBCs. The main cause for this fail is the fact that the primary event affecting RBCs involves an absence, reduction or malformation of hemoglobin. In the next sections we will discuss two important erythroid diseases that culminate to chronic hemolytic anemias whose main genetic alteration is accounted by a point mutation: the sickle cell disease and βThal. We will also discuss another important disorder generated by a point mutation that importantly has beneficial effects on the described diseases: the Hereditary Persistence of Fetal Hemoglobin.

4. Sickle Cell Disease

Sickle cell disease (SCD) is a worldwide health problem and one of the most common inherited disorders firstly reported in America by James Herrick in 1910. In 1949, Linus Pauling and colleagues demonstrated that sickle hemoglobin had a different migration compared to the normal hemoglobin in an electrophoretic field and recognized that this disease must be associated with a variant hemoglobin molecule (Pauling et al. 1949) The genetic alteration that leads to this autosomal recessive inherited disorder was described in 1957 by Ingram and colleagues, as a missense mutation (A - T) that introduces a substitution of a glutamic acid, a polar negatively charged aminoacid (in hemoglobin A) to valine, non polar aminoacid (in hemoglobin S) at position 6 of the globin β-chain causing an impairment in hemoglobin structure and function (Ingram 1957).

Since SCD has a Mendelian segregation, individuals can be homozygous or heterozygous. The genetic diagnostic of the disease can identify an important prognostic in the homozygous for the sickle gene (SS) once their erythrocytes contain at least 90% hemoglobin S. Those who are heterozygous (AS) have sickle cell trait and their erythrocytes contain both hemoglobin A (about 50-60%) and hemoglobin S (about 30-40%). Sickle cell trait is a clinical state that is clinically benign except under conditions of severe acidosis or low partial oxygen pressure (Pace 2007).

An important piece of information about the prognostic of patients carrying SCD was described by several studies that identified single nucleotide polymorphism (SNPs) in the β globin locus. These haplotypes were firstly defined in African population and identified in different regions that could be linked to different gene mutations. These regions are Benin, Senegal, Central African Republic (Bantu) and Cameroon. Another important haplotype was described in Saudi Arabia and India. The identification of these haplotypes was possible by digesting the β globin locus with several restriction enzymes. The pattern of each haplotype can be seen in Fig. 05. The occurrence of these is very broad worldwide but mainly in America, what is a direct consequence of the forced migration of Africans to America as slavers. The identification of these haplotypes is a very important tool for evaluating the prognostic of the disease, since several studies showed that different haplotypes accounts for different clinical evolution of the disease. For example, the Bantu haplotype is associated with a worse prognostic than others in the majority of cases (Pagnier et al. 1984; Nagel et al. 1985; Pace 2007).

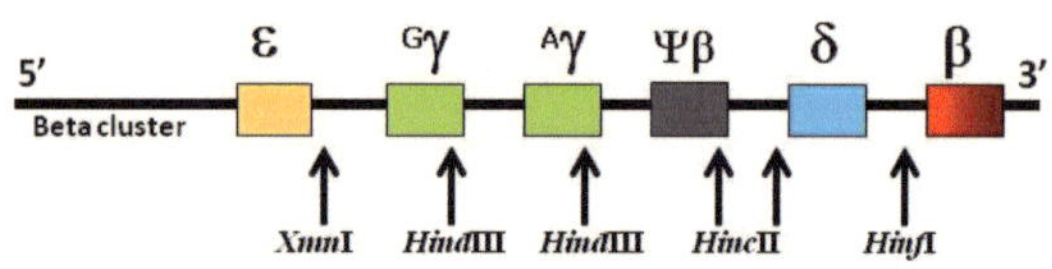

Haplotypes	Digestion (+) / Undigestion (-)					
Senegal	+	+	-	+	+	+
Benin	-	-	-	-	+	-
CAR (Bantu)	-	+	-	-	-	-
Saudi	+	+	-	+	+	-
Cameron	-	+	+	-	+	+

Fig. 5. Different haplotypes found in association with Sickle Cell Disease (SCD). Using different restriction enzymes, several haplotypes could be found and associated with the better or worse prognostic in SCD.

A significant association between endemic regions of malaria infestation and spontaneous β globin mutation were described by Carlson et al based on natural selection, since people with sickle cell trait are more resistant to malaria than people with two normal β globin genes. This is a very elegant example of a point mutation as a factor eliciting a direct consequence in the adaptation of a pathogen to the host (Carlson et al. 1994).

Under oxygenated conditions both hemoglobin S and hemoglobin A have similar function. However, when hemoglobin is in the deoxygenated state, cells carrying hemoglobin S become deformed and acquire sickle shape. The alterations observed in the HbS cell morphology is due the appearance of a new hydrophobic site in hemoglobin S that interact with another HbS protein leading to a formation of a long and multi-stranded fibers. This leads to several alterations such as red cell membrane damage, chronic hemolysis, altered interactions between sickle red blood cells and vascular endothelial cells, and inflammatory responses from such interactions (Fig. 6) (Pace 2007; Hoffman et al. 2008).

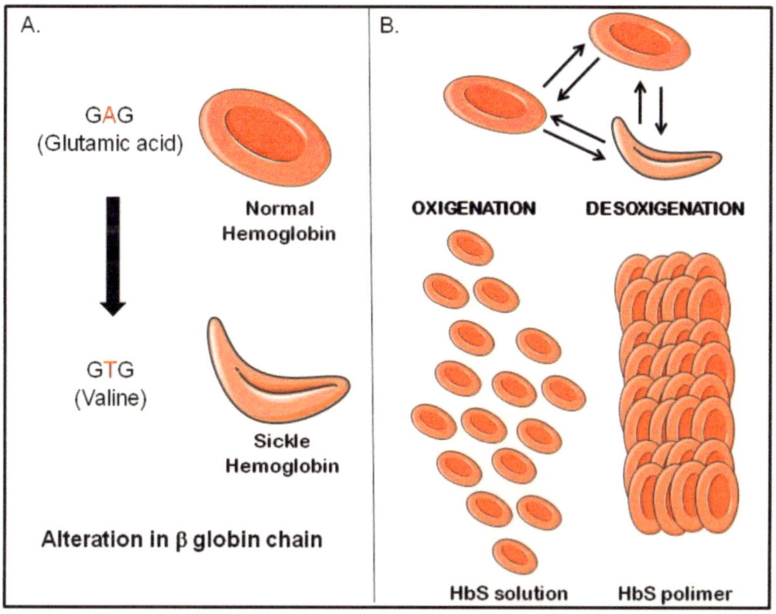

Fig. 6. Pathophysiology of sickle cell disease - The single point mutation (GAG - GTG) at β globin gene leads to a formation of sickle hemoglobin(HbS). This alteration is caused by a change of a Glutamic acid by a Valine at position six of the protein (A). Under oxygenation state the HbS have the same function than a normal Hb, however at absence of oxygen these cells interact with other HbS cells forming a HbS polimer that adhere to blood vessels leading to several alterations observed in this disease (B). Figure was produced using Servier Medical Art, http://www.servier.co.uk/medical-art-gallery/SlideKit.asp?kit=18.

Another hallmark event caused by the alteration in red blood cells shape is the sequestration of blood cells in the spleen and liver, resulting in a preeminent hepatosplenomegaly typically observed in SCD patients. In a first moment, the bone marrow increases the production of reticulocytes. As a consequence, the level of these cells that normally represents about 1% can be as high as 10% under these conditions. With the continued destruction of red blood cells associated to the hemolysis in the bloodstream, a great decrease in the number of circulating red blood cells can be observed culminating with an anemic condition (Pace 2007).

The primary event involved in the pathophysiology of SCD is the vaso-occlusion outcome that can promote strokes, resulting in tissues infarctation, painful episodes, acute chest syndromes and thrombosis of cerebral vessels (Shapiro et al. 1995).

Several studies support the idea that exists a genetic predisposition to stroke associated with the different β globin haplotypes (Powars et al. 1994). The increase of sequenced data from Human Genome Project, associated with the improvement of bioinformatics tools and high-throughput genotyping platforms and sequencing, called as the "genomic revolution", accelerated the identification and association of SNPs with several diseases, including SCD. The association of this information is a powerful tool in the discovery of new associations between novel haplotypes and SCD prognostic (Pace 2007).

Red cell transfusion and therapy with the use of Hydroxyurea (HU) are methods used to prevent the complications of SCD. The use of HU, a chemotherapy agent largely used in the treatment of mieloproliferative disease, in the SCD treatment was first demonstrated by the Multicenter Study of Hydroxyurea in Sickle Cell Anemia (MSH). This study showed that by the use of this pharmacological agent, the rate of painful episodes and the need for transfusions were decreased. Another important finding is the correlation of HU treatment and the increase of HbF. This point will be discussed later on in this chapter (Steinberg et al. 2003).

The only curative therapy for SCD is the hematopoietic stem cell transplantation, but this therapy has some important complications such as acute and late toxicities that need to be considered before its use. The evolution of the transplantation method with the possibility of alternate use of stem cell source such as cord blood could be improve the cure of this disease for a large number of individuals (Pace 2007).

5. Thalassemia

The thalassemia term was first used for anemia often found in Italian people and the Greek shores and nearby islands. Today the term is used to refer to inherited defects in the biosynthesis of globin chains (Hoffman et al. 2008; Cao et al. 2010).

The thalassemias are a group of inherited disorders characterized by alterations in the synthesis of one or more globin chain subunits in the hemoglobin tetramer. The clinical features associated with thalassemia arise due to an imbalanced production of globin, which leads to ineffective erythropoiesis and consequently hemolytic anemia. Thalassemic individuals may be asymptomatic or the clinical manifestations can vary from a hypochromic and microcytic anemia to changes that become incompatible with life.

These differences in clinical manifestations arise from defects of varying severity in primary biosynthesis and modulation inherited factors, such as increased synthesis of fetal globin subunits. In more severe forms of disease, iron overload can occurs as a consequence of either blood transfusions (which is used as palliative treatment) or alloimmunization and blood-borne infections (Thein 1998).

Thalassemias represent one of the most common group of genetic disorders known, thus constituting a public health problem. Molecular analysis of these disorders, mainly the study of molecular changes underlying the thalassemia syndromes, has led to fundamental advances in understanding the structure and function of eukaryotic genes. The classification, pathophysiology and genetic basis of this disease were used as a model to understand the production and the formation of hemoglobin and their main function as carriers of oxygen molecules bounded to heme group.

The thalassemia syndromes are named according to the globin chain whose synthesis is affected. Therefore, the α-globin chains are absent or reduced in patients with α-thalassemia, and β-globin chain production is altered in patients with βThal, the δ and β chains globin production are altered in patients with δβ-thalassemia among others. This nomenclature is also important to subdivide the patients depending on the level of production of each globin chain, which can be reduced (eg α or β^{+}- thalassemia) or absent (eg α or β^{0}- thalassemia). In this topic we will focus on βThal (Hoffman et al. 2008).

Heterozygote individuals for β thalassemia, called thalassemia trait, may develop anemia, yet can have a normal life. Whereas individuals who are homozygous can be classified into different groups: (i) thalassemia intermedia - in which individuals has moderate anemia due to reduced production of β-globin, and (ii) thalassemia major or Cooley's anemia - characterized by severe reduction or absence of production of β-globin. These patients with βThal major are dependent on periodic blood transfusions and as a consequence of this procedure, they may have a significant accumulation of iron in multiple organs and tissues. Thus, the treatment with iron chelating drugs, such as deferoxamine is mandatory, and can also cause death. Currently the only curative treatment available for these patients is bone marrow transplantation (Wheatherall et al. 2001).

5.1 Beta talassemia

Strikingly, more than two hundred mutations have been described to date as associated with this disease. Total gene deletion which could account for the total absence of β chain synthesis is rarely observed in βThal. The majority of the mutations found so far are mainly either single nucleotide substitutions and deletions or insertions of nucleotides on frameshift leading. Although there are several mutations described, only about nine of them usually represent more than 90% of cases of βThal in a particular ethnic group or region. Mutations can be divided into those that affect the transcription of mRNA (mutation on the promoter region and termination codon), those affecting mRNA processing (splicing junctions mutations, new signs of splicing, cleavage and recombination deficient) and those affecting the translation (Cao et al. 2011).

As we discussed before, different types and amounts of human hemoglobin are determined by the selective expression of specific genes encoding each globin chain. Also encoded within the genes are the signals that permit the enzymatic machinery within the nucleus to excise precisely the introns from the mRNA precursor and bring together the exons to form a mature mRNA. Many mutations are related to transcription of the β globin genes. These mutations alter the promoter region upstream of the β-globin mRNA coding sequence. In addition, other mutations can alter the sequence used for signaling the addition of the tail poly (A) of mRNA upstream of the β globin mRNA coding sequence. These events ultimately affects the mRNA synthesis resulting in abnormal division and polyadenylation of mRNA precursor leading to reduction of mature mRNA (Table 1 and fig. 7) (Hoffman et al. 2008).

DEFECT	TYPE OF THALASSEMIA
mRNA non-functional	
1. Premature Finish Codon a. CD 15 G→A, b. CD 17 A→T, c. CD 35 C→A, d. CD 39 C→T, e. CD 43 G→T, f. CD 121 A→T	β^0
2. Short Deletion Shift Base (*frameshift*) a. CD 5 -CT, b. CD 6 -C, c. CD 8/9 +G, d. CD 16 -C , e. CD 35 -C, f. CD 41/42 -TTCT, g. CD 76 -C, h. CD 109/110 1nt del	β^0
3. Mutation of the Start Codon ATG a. ATG→AGG, b. ATG→ACG	β^0
Abnormal Processing RNA	
1. Mutations Inside Introns a. IVS-1 nt 110 G→A, b. IVS-2 nt 705 T→G, c. IVS-2 745 C→G d. IVS-1 nt 116 T→G, e. IVS-2 nt 654 C→T	β^+
2. Activation of Cryptic Sites of *Splicing* a. CD 19 A→G, b. CD 26 G→A, c. CD 27 C→T	β^{+*}
3. Mutations in exon-intron limits a. IVS-1 nt 1 G→A, b. IVS-1 nt 1 G→T, c. IVS-1 nt 2 T→G, d. IVS-2 nt 849 A→G, e. IVS-2 nt 849 A→C	β^0
f. IVS-1 nt 5 C→G, g. IVS-1 nt 5 G→T, h. IVS-1 nt 128 T→G, i. IVS-2 nt 843 T→G	β^+

DEFECT	TYPE OF THALASSEMIA
Mutations in the promoter region	
4. Reduction in the mRNA transcription	
a. -101 C→T,	
b. -92 C→T,	β^+
c. -88 C→T,	
d. -31 A→G,	
e. -30 T→A,	
f. -28 A→C	
Mutations in polyadenylation site mRNA (AATAAA)	
a. AACAAA,	
b. AATAAG,	β^+
c. AATGAA,	
d. AATAGA,	
e. A (del AATAA)	
Structural Mutations (elongated chains or hyperunstable)	β^+
a. CD 49 +TG (Hb Agnana),	
b. CD 110 TC (Hb Showa- Yakushiji),	
c. CD 114 -CT +G (Hb Genebra)	

Table 1. Frequent examples of point mutations causing thalassemias in humam population, according to their location in the molecule, the functional defect associated and the consequence on globin synthesis.

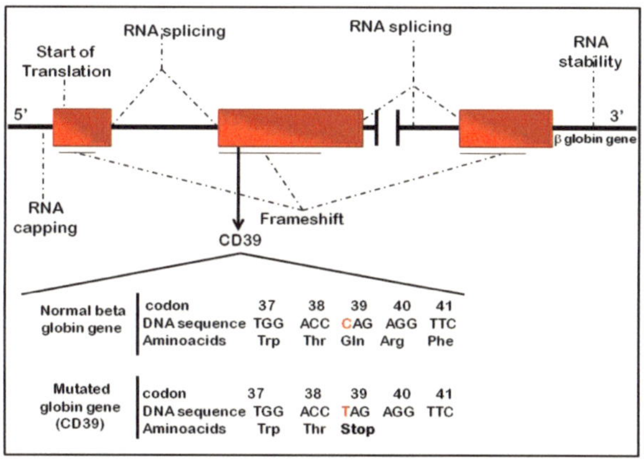

Fig. 7. Different types of point mutation involved in the development of βThal - Point mutations can alter the start of translation, RNA capping, the frameshift of protein translation and the RNA stability. The creation of a stop codon, as in the CD39 type of βThal, is responsible by a formation of a non-functional protein that is degraded causing β^0 thalassemia.

Specifically in the splicing process, which is necessary the recognition of specific sequences by the spliceosome in the intronic region, point mutations are responsible by the impaired globin production. In fact, various forms of βThal are caused by mutations that either damage the process of splicing of the mRNA precursor to mature mRNA in the nucleus or block translation of mRNA in the cytoplasm.

Some point mutations change the dinucleotide (GT) or (AG), which are extremely important in the exon-intron junctions on the conventional processing, completely block the production of mature RNA. Therefore, the β-globin molecules are not produced, leading to the appearance of a β^0 thalassemia.

Other mutations can change the consensus sequences surrounding the invariant dinucleotide AG and GT. This consequently decreases the efficiency of conventional splicing which shall occur at a level between 70% and 95%, resulting in β + talassemia. Another mechanism of change is the result of splicing mutations that do not occur close to any normal splice site. Such changes could occur in a region located in intron region which is crucial for regular splicing of the gene, called crypt splice sites. They resemble the consensus sequences of local splice, but usually do not support splicing . The mutations are able to activate these sites through the alteration to GT or AG site, generating a consensus sequence that stimulate the splicing machinery (Fig. 8) (Hoffman et al. 2008).

There may be mutations that suppres the translation in several regions along the mRNA, and it is a common cause of β^0 thalassemia. The most common form of β^0 thalassemia in people of the region of Sardinia (Italy) is the result of a base substitution, which changes the codon encoding the amino acid 39 of the β globin gene (CAG-TAG), whose sequence equivalent (UAG) characterizes the termination of translation of the mRNA, forming a premature stop codon that prevents the ability of mRNA to be translated into normal β-globin. This phenomenon can also result in frameshift mutations causing small deletions or insertions of a few bases, or multiples of 3, which alter the sequence of nucleotides that is read during translation (see Fig. 7).

Two groups of partial deletions of the β gene are known: (i) loss of 600 bases before the start of the gene, including the exon 1, intron 1 and part of exon 2, and (ii) loss of 619 nucleotides at the end of β gene. In both cases, the synthesis of β chain does not occur. This type of βThal is common in northwestern India and on Pakistan (Khan et al. 1998; Madan et al. 1998).

A study in Turkey aiming to determine the origin of some of the mutations related to βThal identified twelve haplotypes, demonstrating a remarkable level of heterogeneity. From 22 analyzed mutations in the β-globin gene, 18 were related to a single sequence haplotype. This simple association encouraged an attempt to determine the origin of these mutations by comparing their frequencies in Turkey with other countries and / or the worldwide distribution of haplotype carrying them. However, the presence of several exceptions to "one haplotype / one mutation" cluster showed that the β-globin gene is not static. Each of the mutations - IVS-I-10 (G -> A), Cd 39 (C -> T), IVS-I-6 (T -> C) and -30 (T -> A) - in the β globin was associated with a minimum of two sequences of haplotypes. This fact can be explained by the potential existence of recombination mechanisms which are continuously activated (Bilgen et al. 2011).

Some genetic factors may reduce phenotypic effects of some cases of βThal. A mechanism that exerts positive effects on βThal phenotypic traits is the decrease of the unbalanced production of the globin chains making the precipitation of these chains lower.

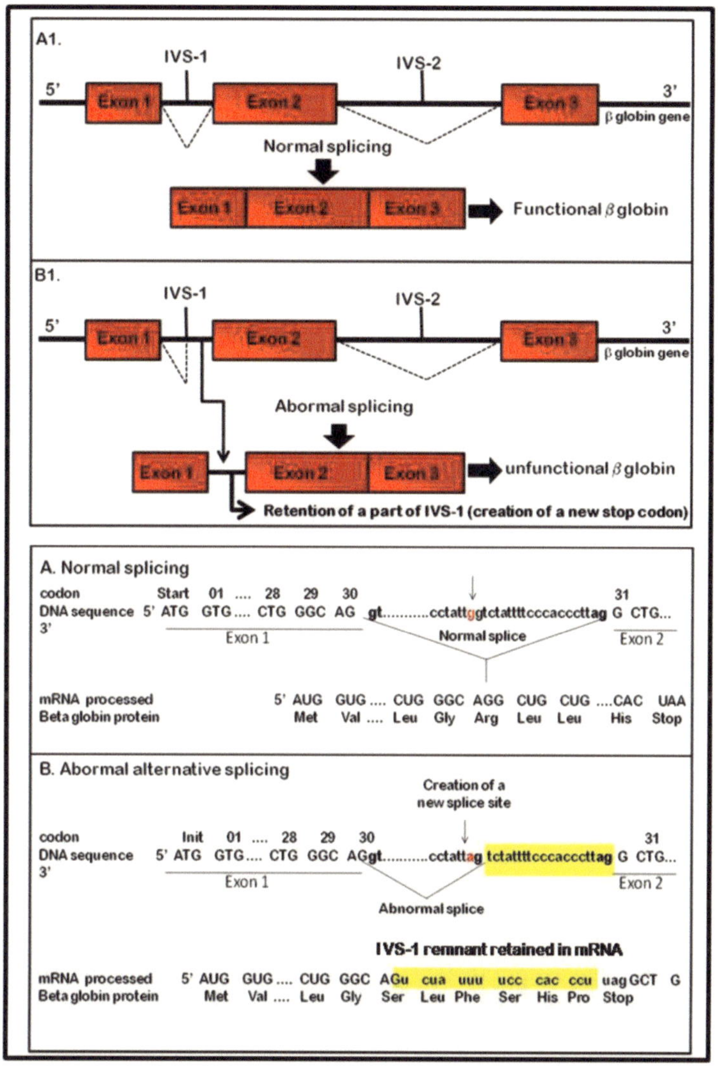

Fig. 8. Point mutations in the splicing sites are responsible for the formation of a non-functional hemoglobin - The introduction of point mutations in the splicing sites at intronic regions can create a new splicing site (highlighted in black) that can alter the structure of the β globin through the retention of a portion of intron forming an non-functional globin polypeptide.

This feature leads to reduced production of α chains thus reducing the overall imbalance of α and β chains. The persistence in the production of γ globin also acts reducing the imbalance between the globin chains. This persistence of HbF production relies on the transmission co-genetic factors. Hereditary persistence of fetal hemoglobin (HPFH) in adults can be present in two forms according to the distribution of HbF within red blood cells, i. e. homogeneous or heterogeneous distribution. The aspects of this disorder will be discussed in the next section below.

6. Hereditary persistence of fetal hemoglobin

The hereditary persistence of fetal hemoglobin (HPFH) is a group of genetic disorders characterized by continued expression of fetal hemoglobin (HbF) in adulthood. HPFH could be divided in (i) pancellular with homogeneus distribution of HbF among all red cells and (ii) heterocellular with an increase in HbF in some cells called F cells (Pace 2007).

On a molecular point of view, pancellular HPFH is in the most of cases caused by extensive deletions in the group β, called deletional HPFH (dHPFH). Point mutations in the promoter region of both γ globin genes, called non-deletional HPFH (ndHPFH) are found in the most of cases diagnosed as heterocellular HPFH (Hoffman et al. 2008).

6.1 Deletional HPFH

The increase in HbF caused by dHPFH is associated with deletions in DNA sequences in the β globin cluster, with the preservation of the γA and γG globin gene. Heterozygous individuals for delecional HPFH have an increase in the HbF up to 20% to 30% of total hemoglobin in the erythrocytes with homogeneous distribution (pancellular).

The mechanism responsible for the increase in HbF in dHPFH has not been completely elucidated. Some hypotheses have been proposed to explain these mechanisms and the more accepted one is that the deletion removes competitive regions of γ globin gene like the δ and β globin genes that under normal conditions would interact with the LCR, silencing the γ globin expression and starting the HbA production. Together with the deletion of these genes, the removal of the silencer elements located in the region between genes γ^A and δ globin helps in the increment of HbF observed in this hematological disorder (Pace 2007; Ngo et al. 2011).

To date, six different types of dHPFHs have been characterized: The HPFH-1 and HPFH-2 is characterized as a large deletion of approximately 105 kb in DNA sequence of the δ and β globin gene region; in the HPFH-3 and HPFH-4 the deletions are shorter with approximately 50 kb of DNA sequence from Ψβ to β globin removed; HPFH-5 is the smaller deletion characterized by the removal of approximately 3 kb upstream to δ globin until 0.7 kb downstream from the β globin gene. Finally HPFH-6 had similar deletions profiles observed in type 1 and 2 with the involvement of γ^A globin gene deletion (Fig. 9)

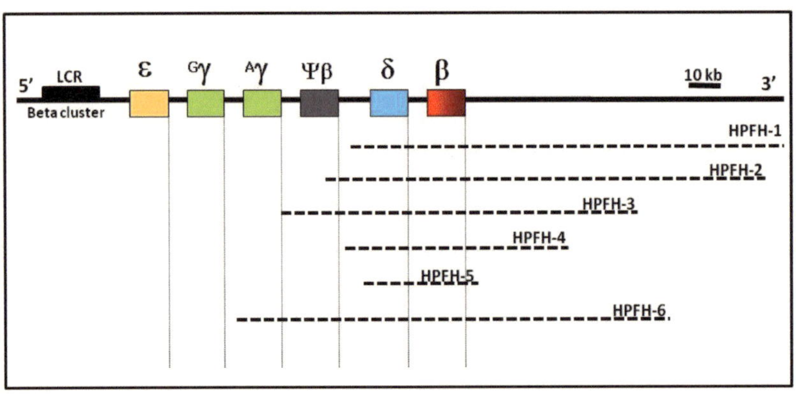

Fig. 9. The deletional form of HPFH – Position of deletions involved in the increase of fetal hemoglobin after the birth are shown in the β globin gene cluster.

6.2 Non delecional HPFH

The non deletional HPFH is characterized by a point mutation in the promoter region of the γ^G globin gene or the γ^A globin gene. In contrast to dHPFH there are several mutations involved in the increment of fetal globin in the ndHPFH that are clustered in three regions of the γ gene promoters centered around positions -200, -175, and -115 of both γ^A and γ^G, relative to the transcriptional start site Some examples of ndHPFHs described in the literature are: Georgiana type (γ^A -114 C-T), Greek type (γ^A -117 G-A); African type (γ^A -175 T-C), Brazilian type (γ^A -195 C-G), Italian type (γ^A -196 C-T), English type (γ^A –198 T-C), African type (γ^A –202 C-T), Switzerland type (γ^G –110 A-C), Algeria type (γ^G –114 C-A), Japanese type (γ^G –114 C-T), Australian type (γ^G –114 C-G) Sardinian type (γ^G –175 T-C) and African type (γ^G - 202 C-G) (as summarized in (Pace 2007).

The mechanisms involved in the reactivation of γ globin were not completely understood for the most mutations described. It is suggested that these mutations interfere with the specific binding of some elements, mainly transcription factors, restricting or facilitating the connection of elements, suppressing the binding of transcription activators.

Some studies support this hypothesis, since several authors identified many transcription factors that could interact with these regions which are able to activate the γ globin promoter. In the ndHPFH English type, –198 T-C, the creation of a new site of interaction, CACCC box occurs which has high affinity for the transcription factor SP1 therefore increasing the strength of the γ^A globin gene promoter (Ronchi et al. 1989; Fischer et al. 1990; Gumucio et al. 1991). This event allows the CACCC box interaction with the LCR, increasing the production of mRNA for γ globin production. Besides SP1, Olave and colleagues identified in the same mutation (-198 T-C) another activator protein complex formed by DNMT1, CDC5-like protein, RAP74, SNEV and P52, that can bind to the promoter region of the γ^A globin gene, also reactivating the expression of this gene (Olave et al. 2007).

In the Greek type ndHPFH, the –117 G-A mutation deletes the repressor binding site of the transcription factor NF-E3, reducing its interaction with the globin gene promoter γ^A allowing the interaction of CP-1, an activator of transcription (Mantovani et al. 1989).

Mutations –175 T-C and –173 T-C prevents the formation of the protein complex containing GATA-1, OCT-1 and other transcriptional factors. It is suggested that this protein complex contributes to the formation of a repressive chromatin structure in the region -170 to -191 of the globin γ^A promoter, leading to the silencing of this gene in erythrocytes. In addition, Magis and Martin hypothesized in 1995 that the transcription factor HMG1 binds in the region -175 of the γ^A gene promoter and interacts with the GATA-1 (Magis et al. 1995).

The -195 mutation, that characterize the ndHPFH Brazilian type, was identified by Costa and colleagues in 1990, through the study of a Caucasian patient bearer of hereditary spherocytosis and splenectomized, with HbF levels of 7% (13.9% of chains γ^G and 86.1% of chains γ^A). Two brothers of these individuals also had elevated HbF (4.5% and 4.7%) with predominance of the γ^A chains, however, they were not suffering from spherocytosis (Costa et al. 1990). Analysis of DNA-protein interaction demonstrated that the increased synthesis of HbF, due to the –195 C-G mutation is not mediated by the protein and SP1 or a new site CACCC box creation (Takahashi et al. 2003). Thus, the mechanism of increased levels of HbF in patients with ndHPFH Brazilian type is different from the -198 mutation that occurs in the ndHPFH English type. In order to evaluate if the -195 mutation is able to increase the HbF *in vivo,* Cunha and colleagues in 2009 developed an *in vivo* study in which the -195 mutation was inserted into the γ globin gene promoter at a β globin cluster cloned in a cosmid. This construction was inserted in a transgenic mouse and through RT-PCR and RNAse Protection Assay (RPA) the authors demonstrated that the -195 mutation, together with all the β globin cluster is enough to raise levels of HbF in all phases of development of transgenic mice. This observation was supported by an increase in γ globin gene expression in yolk sac, fetal liver and other organs of these mice compared to expression in mice carrying the wild β globin cluster. The results showed that the presence of the mutation -195 together with the entire β globin cluster is sufficient to develop the phenotype of ndHPFH-B in mice (da Cunha et al. 2009). Even with these detailed studies, the complete mechanism involved in the reactivation of the globin gene in the Brazilian type γ^A ndHPFH is not elucidated.

Understanding the mechanisms involved in these mutations may be important for the development of new therapies based on reactivation of γ globin gene which can assist in the treatment of hemoglobinopathies.

7. Expression of gamma globin and the regulation of severity of sickle cell disease and beta thalassemia

As we discussed above, in SCD a point mutation leads to a structural alteration in β globin protein, that in absence of oxygen acquires the ability of forming long and multi-stranded fibers that alters the red blood cell shape increasing the destruction of these cells in spleen and liver and finally causing an important hemolytic anemia. In βThal, the point mutations or deletions observed in β globin gene are responsible for altering the production of β globin protein. In the most severe form of βThal, the β thalassemia major, there is no production of this protein. As a result, the α globin normally produces precipitates inside the red blood cells leading to an increased destruction of these cells causing hemolytic anemia, as also observed in SCD patients. In both cases, when a high expression of γ globin is observed, the patient has a very mild clinical disorder when compared to patients with a low expression of this protein. This better condition is due to the increment of production of fetal hemoglobin (HbF), as we have presented before as caused by the assembly of two α chains with 2 γ chains ($\alpha 2\gamma 2$). The clinical benefit induced by the increase of HbF in SCD patients has been repeatedly demonstrated by several authors. In this disease, the beneficial effects of HbF is due to its interaction with the HbS polypeptide, that form an asymmetric hybrid hemoglobin, referred to as HbF/S ($\alpha 2\gamma\beta^S$). This molecul directly affects the stability of the sickle hemoglobin polymer, preventing its deleterious alteration in cell morphology. Moreover, the premature destruction of sickle erythrocytes increases the number of cells where HbF concentration is high (Pace 2007).

Several studies over the last 20 years attempted to identify pharmacological agents able to increase the HbF in these patients. Several compounds that broadly influence epigenetic modifications, including DNA methylation and histone deacetylation were tested.

In the beginning of 1990, the use of Hydroxyurea (HU) was proposed for the treatment of SCD patients. This compound was firstly synthesized in 1869 and is widely used as an antineoplastic drug mainly employed to traet myeloproliferative disorders. During the 90's several experiments were conducted mainly by the Multicenter Study of Hydroxyurea in Sickle Cell Anemia (MSH) and the results showed that HU were able to decrease the morbidity of SCA in adults, reducing the incidence of painful episodes and acute chest syndrome. These studies also revealed that this compound could be used to increase fetal hemoglobin (HbF) concentration therefore reducing the vaso-occlusive complications and diminishing hemolysis (Steinberg et al. 2003). The ability of HU in the generation of Nitric Oxide (NO) is reported as the main property which can partially explain the augment of γ globin production. In this sense, NO could act as a second messenger in a signaling cascade leading to the activation of several important genes. The results found in these first studies triggered other trials that used HU in βThal. Although the results were considered very promising, the augment of HbF in βThal was not observed in all patients (Lou et al. 2009).

To date, HU is the most widely used drug for adult SCD patients and is also highly used in β thalassemia patients. Despite of several studies addressing this issue, the metabolic pathways and the set of genes expressed upon induction by HU are not completely known. Recently, some studies have evaluated patients and cultured cells before and after HU treatment in order to identify metabolic pathways and genes that could shed some light in the mechanism of action of this drug. In one of these studies conducted in 2006 by Costa et al, the mechanisms surrounding the in vivo action of HU were evaluated using a global gene expression analysis in cells obtained from the bone marrow of a SCD patient before and after HU treatment. The results suggested that HU induced significant changes in the gene expression pattern of SCD patient, mainly in global signal transduction pathways. This gene expression alteration may have a direct effect in the induction of globin genes and in genes associated with channel or pore class transporter. These pore transporter genes are thought to interfere in the hydratation status of cells, interfering with the rheological properties of them, what is very important in SCD (Costa et al. 2007). Having the same objectives and similar experimental design, another important study was conducted by Moreira et al (2007) using suppression subtractive hybridization (SSH) in HU-treated and -untreated reticulocytes of patients with SCD . In this report, similar pathways initially described by Costa were also identified after HU treatment. Additionally were also found some genes involved in chromatin modifications like *SUDS3*, *FZD5* and *PHC3*. Although these studies have contributed to elucidate the transcriptional response influenced by HU, the molecular mechanisms involved in HU treatment remain unclear (Moreira et al. 2008).

After the demonstration that some chemical agents are able to increase HbF concentration many efforts have been developed in order to find other inducers or a combination of agents able in ameliorate the symptoms of SCD and βThal. Several potential therapeutic agents and its combination have been investigated to use in these hemoglobinopathies. Table 2 shows some clinical trials used in βThal patients and their hematologic responses.

Despite the clear beneficial effects observed after HU treatment, the use of this pharmacological agent is limited since long-term treatment has been associated with several deleterious effects. In order to diminish the HU treatment effects many efforts are made to find new therapeutic alternatives to treat SCD symptoms without side effects. Recently, dos Santos et al designed a new molecule by molecular hybridization combining portions of thalidomide and HU and tested as potential use in the oral treatment of sickle cell disease symptoms. The results showed that this molecule was able to increase the levels of NO donor, as observed in HU treatment, and also demonstrated that different from what is observed in HU treatment, this new molecule had analgesic and anti-inflamatory properties, reducing the levels of tumor necrosis factor α (TNFα) thus representing an alternative approach to HU treatment (dos Santos et al. 2011).

Terapeutic Agent	Action	Thalassemia Syndromes	Increase in Total Hb (g/dl) (range)	Responses
5- Azacytidine	Hypomethylation +/- cytotoxicity	Thalassemia Intermedia	2.5 [1.5 - 4]	1/1 1/1 3/3
Hydroxyurea (HU)	Cytotoxicity and erythroid regeration →high- F BFU- E	HbE/β-talassemia Thalassemia Intermedia HbE/β-talassemia	20 [1-3.3] 27 [2.2 - 3.2] 0.6 [0 - 1.7] 1.0 0.9	3/3 2/2 (β globin) 11/13 3/8 7/19
Sodium Phenybutyrate (SPB)	? HDACi effect	Thalassemia Intermedia and Major	2.1 [1.2 - 2.8]	4/8 untransfused
Arginine Butyrate and AB+ Erithropoietin (EPO)	Activates γ globin gene promoter, (SSP binding), (? HDACi effect)	Thalassemia Intermedia and Major	2.7 [0 .6 - 5]	7/10 (AB +/- EPO)
Isobutyramide	Activates γ globin gene promoter	Thalassemia Intermedia and Major	Increase in HbF, Reduced Transfusion Requeriments	6/10 2/4
EPO	Stimulates Erythroid Proliferation, promotes erythroid cell survival	Thalassemia Intermedia and Major	2 [1 - 3] 2.5 2 Reduced Transfusion Requeriments	5 - 7/10 4/4 8/10 3/26 5/10
Darbepoietin	Stimulates Erythropoiesis	Thalassemia Intermedia	1.6 [0.7 - 3.8]	4/6
HU+EPO	As Above	Thalassemia Intermedia HbE/β-talassemia	1.7 [0.5 - 4] 1.2	 1/5
HU+SPB	As Above	β Lepore	3 [2 - 4]	2/2

Table 2. Hematologic Responses to Fetal Globin Gene Inducers or Erithropoietin (EPO) in βThal Patients (Perrine 2005).

8. Molecular biology and the identification of targets to treat SCD and beta thalassemia diseases

It has been a very well established concept the benefits in the increment of γ-globin levels in the treatment of patients SCD or βThal (Cao et al. 2011; Ngo et al. 2011).

Therefore the development of new therapies targeting the increment of γ globin production can become possible through the identification of the molecular mechanisms involved in fetal globin gene silencing and its reactivation which needs to be known in depth. An excellent model to study these mechanisms is the HPFH, a disorder in which the γ globin production is not silenced, as described above. The mechanisms involved in the reactivation of γ globin have been scrutinized in several studies. Olave et al. studied the proteins able to bind at the γ globin promoter in the presence of a point mutation that leads to an English form of HPFH (-198T→C). The results showed that a protein complex binds to this region and is able to increase the HbF production. The authors suggested that DNMT1 protein, one member of this putative complex, acts as a chromatin remodeling protein opening the chromatin and triggering the γ globin expression (Olave et al. 2007). In another interesting study developed by Andrade et al., the pattern of gene expression was evaluated in reticulocytes of an individual with the deletional form of PHHF. In this study the authors also identified the up-regulation of chromatin remodeling proteins (ARID1B and TSPYL1) as also involved in the reactivation of γ globin (de Andrade et al. 2006).

Despite the studies with HPFH, several authors have described the interaction of genes with the activation or silencing of γ globin promoter. Among these genes *EKLF* has been pointed out in numerous reports as the main responsible for the regulation of β globin expression. The increase in the expression of this gene occurs in accordance with the increase of β globin producing and γ globin silencing. The main function of this protein seems to be in the activation of another gene called *BCL11A* whose gene product is able to bind at γ globin genes promoter repressing its transcription (Figure 10). The control of EKLF and BCL11A production could be further explored as a therapeutical strategy to increase the production of HbF and ameliorate hemoglobin disorders such as βThal and sickle cell disease (Sankaran et al. 2008; Xu et al. 2010; Jawaid et al. 2011; Wilber et al. 2011).

Another important contribution aiming to clarify the understanding of γ-globin genes silencing is the results found in the analysis of the hematopoietic transcription factor GATA-1. This gene, as we discussed before is a zinc finger protein that binds to WGATAR elements located mainly in the regulatory regions of erythroid genes, including the α and β globin genes (Weiss et al. 1995; Weiss et al. 1997).

A direct interaction between GATA1 and γ-globin silencing was highlighted in two different studies. In the first one, the authors showed the importance of a 352-bp region harboring a conserved GATA element at position -566 5'of the *HBG1* is required for γ-globin silencing in transgenic mice. In the second report, the authors correlated a mutation found in GATA site in the *HBG2* gene with the increase in γ globin expression in a family with HPFH. These results showed that GATA-1 can act as a repressor of γ globin gene despite its widely described role in the literature as an activator of α and β globin genes. The mechanism whereby GATA-1 exerts these distinct functions remains unresolved. Some evidences

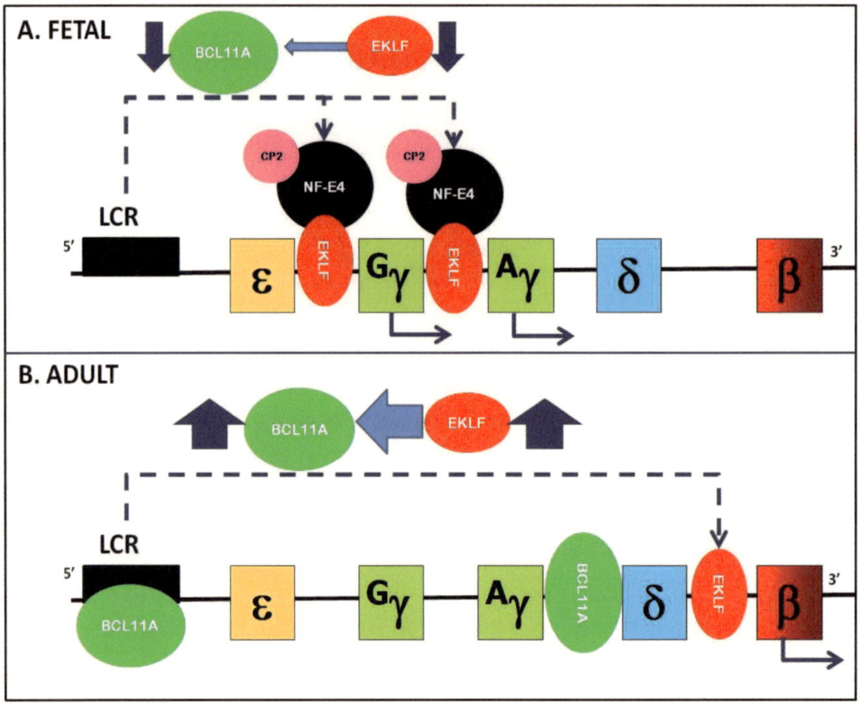

Fig. 10. EKLF levels coordinate the hemoglobin switching. The activation of globin genes is dependent of the production of EKLF protein. A low level of EKLF is observed during the fetal stage. Since EKLF is essential for the activation of BCL11A, low levels of this gene is also reduced. The lowly expressed BCL11A is unable to repress γ-globin genes and EKLF with the recruitment of the NFE4 and CP2, preferentially interacts with the γ-globin promoters. This interaction stimulates the assembly of LCR elements activating the production of γ-globin protein and consequently the HbF formation. In the adult stage, high levels of EKLF is observed. The increase of this protein promotes an overexpression of BCL11A ultimately repressing the γ-globin genes under these circunstances. In this situation the EKLF binds preferentially to the β-globin promoter activating the β-globin gene with the recruitment of the LCR. This figure was adapted from (Wilber et al. 2011).

showed that this repression mechanisms could occurs via two other genes: *FOG-1* and *NuRD*. FOG-1 is also a zinc finger protein that binds to GATA-1 acting as an important player in both activation and repression of genes modulated by GATA-1. FOG-1 interacts with several protein complexes, including NuRD (nucleosome remodeling and histone deacetylase), that is a co-repressor complex that interacts with several N-terminal motifs found in other transcriptional repressors, for instance, the BCL11A gene. In an experiment using transgenic mice bearing three different mutations that completely abrogate the binding between NuRD and FOG-1, the authors showed that animals homozygous for these mutations were anemic and displayed defects in platelet formation. These results indicate that this interaction is essential for normal erythroid and megakaryocyte development. The same authors concluded that the FOG-1/NuRD interaction is indispensable for the expression of β-globin gene and this interaction was not required for the repression of human γ-globin *in vivo* (Miccio et al. 2010; Xu et al. 2010).

Despite several attempts, the complete molecular mechanism involved in the switching of globins and the reactivation of γ globin remains to be elucidated. Is clear that chromatin remodeling in the γ globin region is the main process whereby HbF reactivation occurs, once the expression of genes involved in this process are found in most of gene expression profiling studies using HPFH as a model. However, additional studies are necessary in order to identify a complete overview of metabolic pathways able to increase the HbF production and raise the possibility for the identification of new targets that could be used as therapeutical agents to treat SCD and βThal.

9. Conclusion

The mechanisms underlying the hemolytic anemia are very complex and the prognosis of this group of diseases is greatly influenced by the gain or loss-of function in key genes involved in the regulation of synthesis and destruction of globin proteins. Several molecular events can be linked to the alteration in gene function. In this chapter, we focused on point mutations interfering in the nature and the severity of SCD and βThal. The comprehension of the molecular basis and the identification of proteins involved in the onset and development of a disease can enable the development of drugs specially designed to targeted therapy. There are some well succeeded examples of the use of molecular biology to design drugs to treat a specific disease. One of the most classical examples comes from the study of another hematological disease: the Chronic Myeloid Leukemia (CML). The development of this CML is characterized by the expression of a BCR-ABL protein produced by a genetic translocation event. Using molecular biology approaches, the BCR-ABL inhibitor imatinib was the first molecular targeted cancer therapy designed to bind inactive the translocated product of BCR-ABL protein. The employment of such molecular approach in the field of hemolytic anemias can open up new avenues of investigation taking advantage of the large scale studies to found new point mutation in genes involved in these diseases and correlate with the prognosis of each patient. Although many decades of efforts have been devoted to the mechanism elucidation of these diseases, much more remains to be done concerning to the identification of new point mutations conferring function on the disease progression,. In this context, the current scenery worldwide seen to be very prolific due to the recent large investments in the genomic revolution of next generation sequencing approaches. These approachs can be easely exploited through the large scale transcriptome (RNAseq) dissecation of hemolytic anemias. It may provide interesting links between the expressed genes by a specific disease, such as SCD and βthal, and help in better understanding the association between the mutations and the metabolic pathways activated in each case. Thus the dissection of the involved metabolic pathways can identify key genes responsible for the disease development and progression. In addition, although important studies using molecular biology techniques highlighted the function of several genes involved in the hemolytic anemias, several questions are currently partially understood. For example, what are the transcriptome and proteome difference between patients that have the same mutations causing βThal but that have different phenotypes (major and intermedia)? The answer for this question is a promising strategy to identify new genes involved in the severity of these disease. Also, which are the genes that are modulated in each type of HPFH? The identification of these genes could help in the elaboration of new therapies to increase the fetal hemoglobin in SCD and βThal. Once the modulation and severity of these diseases is strictly correlated with mutations and haplotypes, this feature make them a very interesting and fruitful model for study of point mutation and genome plasticity using molecular biology approach seeking for further improvements for patients built on the field regenerative medicine and genetic therapy.

10. Acknowledgment

The authors would like to thank fundings from the Brazilian agencies FAPESP (Fundação de Amparo à Pesquisa do Estado de São Paulo) and CAPES (Coordenação de Aperfeiçoamento de Pessoal de Nível Superior)

11. References

Bilgen, T., Y. Arikan, D. Canatan, A. Yesilipek and I. Keser (2011). "The association between intragenic SNP haplotypes and mutations of the beta globin gene in a Turkish population." *Blood Cells Mol Dis* 46(3): 226-9.

Blobel, G. A., T. Nakajima, R. Eckner, M. Montminy and S. H. Orkin (1998). "CREB-binding protein cooperates with transcription factor GATA-1 and is required for erythroid differentiation." *Proc Natl Acad Sci U S A* 95(5): 2061-6.

Blobel, G. A. and S. H. Orkin (1996). "Estrogen-induced apoptosis by inhibition of the erythroid transcription factor GATA-1." *Mol Cell Biol* 16(4): 1687-94.

Blobel, G. A., C. A. Sieff and S. H. Orkin (1995). "Ligand-dependent repression of the erythroid transcription factor GATA-1 by the estrogen receptor." *Mol Cell Biol* 15(6): 3147-53.

Cao, A. and R. Galanello (2010). "Beta-thalassemia." *Genet Med* 12(2): 61-76.

Cao, A., P. Moi and R. Galanello (2011). "Recent advances in beta-thalassemias." *Pediatr Rep* 3(2): e17.

Carlson, J., G. B. Nash, V. Gabutti, F. al-Yaman and M. Wahlgren (1994). "Natural protection against severe Plasmodium falciparum malaria due to impaired rosette formation." *Blood* 84(11): 3909-14.

Costa, F. C., A. F. da Cunha, A. Fattori, T. de Sousa Peres, G. G. Costa, T. F. Machado, D. M. de Albuquerque, S. Gambero, C. Lanaro, S. T. Saad and F. F. Costa (2007). "Gene expression profiles of erythroid precursors characterise several mechanisms of the action of hydroxycarbamide in sickle cell anaemia." *Br J Haematol* 136(2): 333-42.

Costa, F. F., M. A. Zago, G. Cheng, J. F. Nechtman, T. A. Stoming and T. H. Huisman (1990). "The Brazilian type of nondeletional A gamma-fetal hemoglobin has a C----G substitution at nucleotide -195 of the A gamma-globin gene." *Blood* 76(9): 1896-7.

da Cunha, A. F., A. F. Brugnerotto, M. A. Corat, E. E. Devlin, A. P. Gimenes, M. B. de Melo, L. A. Passos, D. Bodine, S. T. Saad and F. F. Costa (2009). "High levels of human gamma-globin are expressed in adult mice carrying a transgene of the Brazilian type of hereditary persistence of fetal hemoglobin ((A)gamma -195)." *Hemoglobin* 33(6): 439-47.

de Andrade, T. G., K. R. Peterson, A. F. Cunha, L. S. Moreira, A. Fattori, S. T. Saad and F. F. Costa (2006). "Identification of novel candidate genes for globin regulation in erythroid cells containing large deletions of the human beta-globin gene cluster." *Blood Cells Mol Dis* 37(2): 82-90.

dos Santos, J. L., C. Lanaro and C. M. Chin (2011). "Advances in sickle cell disease treatment: from drug discovery until the patient monitoring." *Cardiovasc Hematol Agents Med Chem* 9(2): 113-27.

Ducamp, S., C. Kannengiesser, M. Touati, L. Garcon, A. Guerci-Bresler, J. F. Guichard, C. Vermylen, J. Dochir, H. A. Poirel, F. Fouyssac, L. Mansuy, G. Leroux, G. Tertian, R. Girot, H. Heimpel, T. Matthes, N. Talbi, J. C. Deybach, C. Beaumont, H. Puy and B. Grandchamp (2010). "Sideroblastic anemia: molecular analysis of the ALAS2 gene in a series of 29 probands and functional studies of 10 missense mutations." *Hum Mutat* 32(6): 590-7.

Fischer, K. D. and J. Nowock (1990). "The T----C substitution at -198 of the A gamma-globin gene associated with the British form of HPFH generates overlapping recognition sites for two DNA-binding proteins." *Nucleic Acids Res* 18(19): 5685-93.

Ghaffari, S. (2008). "Oxidative stress in the regulation of normal and neoplastic hematopoiesis." *Antioxid Redox Signal* 10(11): 1923-40.

Greer, J. P., J. Foerrster, G. Rodgers, F. Paraskevas, B. Glader, D. A. Arber and J. Means, R. T. (2008). *Wintrobe's clinical hematology*, Lippincott Williams & Wilkins

Gumucio, D. L., K. L. Rood, K. L. Blanchard-McQuate, T. A. Gray, A. Saulino and F. S. Collins (1991). "Interaction of Sp1 with the human gamma globin promoter: binding and transactivation of normal and mutant promoters." *Blood* 78(7): 1853-63.

Hoffman, R., B. Furie, P. McGlave, P. E. Silberstein, S. J. Shattil, E. J. Benz Jr. and H. Heslop (2008). *Hematology: Basic Principles and Practice*. New York, Churchil Livingstone - ELSEVIER.

Ingram, V. M. (1957). "Gene mutations in human haemoglobin: the chemical difference between normal and sickle cell haemoglobin." *Nature* 180(4581): 326-8.

Jawaid, K., K. Wahlberg, S. L. Thein and S. Best (2011). "Binding patterns of BCL11A in the globin and GATA1 loci and characterization of the BCL11A fetal hemoglobin locus." *Blood Cells Mol Dis* 45(2): 140-6.

Khan, S. N. and S. Riazuddin (1998). "Molecular characterization of beta-thalassemia in Pakistan." *Hemoglobin* 22(4): 333-45.

Lou, T. F., M. Singh, A. Mackie, W. Li and B. S. Pace (2009). "Hydroxyurea generates nitric oxide in human erythroid cells: mechanisms for gamma-globin gene activation." *Exp Biol Med (Maywood)* 234(11): 1374-82.

Madan, N., S. Sharma, U. Rusia, S. Sen and S. K. Sood (1998). "Beta-thalassaemia mutations in northern India (Delhi)." *Indian J Med Res* 107: 134-41.

Magis, W. and D. I. Martin (1995). "HMG-I binds to GATA motifs: implications for an HPFH syndrome." *Biochem Biophys Res Commun* 214(3): 927-33.

Mantovani, R., G. Superti-Furga, J. Gilman and S. Ottolenghi (1989). "The deletion of the distal CCAAT box region of the A gamma-globin gene in black HPFH abolishes the binding of the erythroid specific protein NFE3 and of the CCAAT displacement protein." *Nucleic Acids Res* 17(16): 6681-91.

Miccio, A. and G. A. Blobel (2010). "Role of the GATA-1/FOG-1/NuRD pathway in the expression of human beta-like globin genes." *Mol Cell Biol* 30(14): 3460-70.

Moreira, L. S., T. G. de Andrade, D. M. Albuquerque, A. F. Cunha, A. Fattori, S. T. Saad and F. F. Costa (2008). "Identification of differentially expressed genes induced by hydroxyurea in reticulocytes from sickle cell anaemia patients." *Clin Exp Pharmacol Physiol* 35(5-6): 651-5.

Nagel, R. L., M. E. Fabry, J. Pagnier, I. Zohoun, H. Wajcman, V. Baudin and D. Labie (1985). "Hematologically and genetically distinct forms of sickle cell anemia in Africa. The Senegal type and the Benin type." *N Engl J Med* 312(14): 880-4.

Ngo, D. A., B. Aygun, I. Akinsheye, J. S. Hankins, I. Bhan, H. Y. Luo, M. H. Steinberg and D. H. Chui (2011). "Fetal haemoglobin levels and haematological characteristics of compound heterozygotes for haemoglobin S and deletional hereditary persistence of fetal haemoglobin." *Br J Haematol.*

Olave, I. A., C. Doneanu, X. Fang, G. Stamatoyannopoulos and Q. Li (2007). "Purification and identification of proteins that bind to the hereditary persistence of fetal hemoglobin -198 mutation in the gamma-globin gene promoter." *J Biol Chem* 282(2): 853-62.

Pace, B. (2007). *Renaissance of Sickle Cell Disease research in the genome era.* London, Imperial College Press.

Pagnier, J., J. G. Mears, O. Dunda-Belkhodja, K. E. Schaefer-Rego, C. Beldjord, R. L. Nagel and D. Labie (1984). "Evidence for the multicentric origin of the sickle cell hemoglobin gene in Africa." *Proc Natl Acad Sci U S A* 81(6): 1771-3.

Palstra, R. J., B. Tolhuis, E. Splinter, R. Nijmeijer, F. Grosveld and W. de Laat (2003). "The beta-globin nuclear compartment in development and erythroid differentiation." *Nat Genet* 35(2): 190-4.

Pauling, L., H. A. Itano and et al. (1949). "Sickle cell anemia a molecular disease." *Science* 110(2865): 543-8.

Perrine, S. P. (2005). "Fetal globin induction--can it cure beta thalassemia?" *Hematology Am Soc Hematol Educ Program*: 38-44.

Powars, D. R., H. J. Meiselman, T. C. Fisher, A. Hiti and C. Johnson (1994). "Beta-S gene cluster haplotypes modulate hematologic and hemorheologic expression in sickle cell anemia. Use in predicting clinical severity." *Am J Pediatr Hematol Oncol* 16(1): 55-61.

Ronchi, A., S. Nicolis, C. Santoro and S. Ottolenghi (1989). "Increased Sp1 binding mediates erythroid-specific overexpression of a mutated (HPFH) gamma-globulin promoter." *Nucleic Acids Res* 17(24): 10231-41.

Sankaran, V. G., T. F. Menne, J. Xu, T. E. Akie, G. Lettre, B. Van Handel, H. K. Mikkola, J. N. Hirschhorn, A. B. Cantor and S. H. Orkin (2008). "Human fetal hemoglobin expression is regulated by the developmental stage-specific repressor BCL11A." *Science* 322(5909): 1839-42.

Shapiro, B. S., D. F. Dinges, E. C. Orne, N. Bauer, L. B. Reilly, W. G. Whitehouse, K. Ohene-Frempong and M. T. Orne (1995). "Home management of sickle cell-related pain in children and adolescents: natural history and impact on school attendance." *Pain* 61(1): 139-44.

Stamatoyannopoulos, G. (2005). "Control of globin gene expression during development and erythroid differentiation." *Exp Hematol* 33(3): 259-71.

Steinberg, M. H., F. Barton, O. Castro, C. H. Pegelow, S. K. Ballas, A. Kutlar, E. Orringer, R. Bellevue, N. Olivieri, J. Eckman, M. Varma, G. Ramirez, B. Adler, W. Smith, T. Carlos, K. Ataga, L. DeCastro, C. Bigelow, Y. Saunthararajah, M. Telfer, E. Vichinsky, S. Claster, S. Shurin, K. Bridges, M. Waclawiw, D. Bonds and M. Terrin (2003). "Effect of hydroxyurea on mortality and morbidity in adult sickle cell anemia: risks and benefits up to 9 years of treatment." *Jama* 289(13): 1645-51.

Strauss, E. C., N. C. Andrews, D. R. Higgs and S. H. Orkin (1992). "In vivo footprinting of the human alpha-globin locus upstream regulatory element by guanine and adenine ligation-mediated polymerase chain reaction." *Mol Cell Biol* 12(5): 2135-42.

Strauss, E. C. and S. H. Orkin (1992). "In vivo protein-DNA interactions at hypersensitive site 3 of the human beta-globin locus control region." *Proc Natl Acad Sci U S A* 89(13): 5809-13.

Takahashi, T., R. Schreiber, J. E. Krieger, S. T. Saad and F. F. Costa (2003). "Analysis of the mechanism of action of the Brazilian type (Agamma-195 C --> G) of hereditary persistence of fetal hemoglobin." *Eur J Haematol* 71(6): 418-24.

Tang, Y., Y. Huang, W. Shen, G. Liu, Z. Wang, X. B. Tang, D. X. Feng, D. P. Liu and C. C. Liang (2008). "Cluster specific regulation pattern of upstream regulatory elements in human alpha- and beta-globin gene clusters." *Exp Cell Res* 314(1): 115-22.

Telen, M. and R. Kaufman (1999). The mature erythrocyte. *Wintrobe's Clinical Hematology*. J. Greer and F. J. Philadelphia, Lippincott Williams & Wilkins: 217–47.

Thein, S. L. (1998). "Beta-thalassaemia." *Baillieres Clin Haematol* 11(1): 91-126.

Tsiftsoglou, A. S., I. S. Vizirianakis and J. Strouboulis (2009). "Erythropoiesis: model systems, molecular regulators, and developmental programs." *IUBMB Life* 61(8): 800-30.

Weiss, M. J., G. Keller and S. H. Orkin (1994). "Novel insights into erythroid development revealed through *in vitro* differentiation of GATA-1 embryonic stem cells." *Genes Dev* 8(10): 1184-97.

Weiss, M. J. and S. H. Orkin (1995). "Transcription factor GATA-1 permits survival and maturation of erythroid precursors by preventing apoptosis." *Proc Natl Acad Sci U S A* 92(21): 9623-7.

Weiss, M. J., C. Yu and S. H. Orkin (1997). "Erythroid-cell-specific properties of transcription factor GATA-1 revealed by phenotypic rescue of a gene-targeted cell line." *Mol Cell Biol* 17(3): 1642-51.

Wheatherall, D. J. and J. B. Clegg (2001). *The Thalassemia Syndromes*, Blackwell Science Ltd.

Wilber, A., A. W. Nienhuis and D. A. Persons (2011). "Transcriptional regulation of fetal to adult hemoglobin switching: new therapeutic opportunities." *Blood* 117(15): 3945-53.

Xu, J., V. G. Sankaran, M. Ni, T. F. Menne, R. V. Puram, W. Kim and S. H. Orkin (2010). "Transcriptional silencing of {gamma}-globin by BCL11A involves long-range interactions and cooperation with SOX6." *Genes Dev* 24(8): 783-98.

11

Point Mutations That Reduce Erythrocyte Resistance to Oxidative Stress

Dmitriy Volosnikov and Elena Serebryakova
The Chelyabinsk State Medical Academy, Russia

1. Introduction

Oxygen transport is a primary goal of erythrocytes. The high maintenance of oxygen in erythrocytes defines high speed of formation of active forms of oxygen - superoxide ($O2^-$), a hydrogen peroxide (H2O2) and a hydroxyl radical (·OH). A constant source of active forms of oxygen in erythrocytes is hemoglobin oxidation in a methemoglobin with formation of superoxide ($O2^-$). Therefore erythrocytes should have a powerful antioxidant system, which prevents the toxic action of active forms of oxygen on hemoglobin and erythrocyte membrane. Mature erythrocytes have neither cytoplasmic organelles nor a nucleus and consequently are not capable to synthesize proteins and lipids, to carry out oxidative phosphorylation or to maintain tricarboxylic acid cycle reactions. The energy of erythrocytes comes for the most part from anaerobic glycolysis - via the Embden-Meyerhof-Parnas pathway (EMP pathway). Thus, glucose catabolism provides preservation of structure and function of hemoglobin, integrity of an erythrocyte membrane and formation of energy for the work of ionic pumps. Anaerobic glycolysis in itself is a power-consuming process. Glucose arrives in erythrocytes by the facilitated diffusion by glucose transporter type 1. Hexokinase is the first enzyme of EMP pathway, it provides glucose phosphorylation. Further during consecutive reactions with participation of glucose-6-phosphate isomerase, phosphofructokinase, aldolase, glyceraldehydes 3-phosphate dehydrogenase, phosphoglycerate kinase, phosphoglycerate mutase, enolase, pyruvate kinase one molecule of glucose gives 4 molecules of adenosine triphosphate (ATP) and 2 molecules of restored nicotinamide adenine dinucleotide (NADH), and at the same time, 2 ATP molecules are spent at the initial stage of EMP pathway. A certain quantity of glucose with formation of restored compounds - glutathione (GSH) and nicotinamide adenine dinucleotide phosphate (NADPH) is taken away through pentose phosphate pathway (aerobic glycolysis). Glucose-6-phosphate dehydrogenase and 6-phosphogluconate dehydrogenase provide the stages of pentose phosphate pathway. The hydroxyl radical, the most active component of oxidative stress, is neutralized by GSH. Methemoglobin reductase restores a methemoglobin into hemoglobin, NADPH being the donor of hydrogen, which is formed in EMP pathway and NADPH is in its turn formed in pentose phosphate pathway. Superoxide dismutase 1 enzyme contributes superoxide ($O2^-$) to turn into hydrogen peroxide. The hydrogen peroxide is destroyed by catalase and glutathione peroxidase, GSH being the donor of hydrogen. Peroxiredoxin 2 is an antioxidant enzyme that uses cystein residues to decompose peroxides. Peroxiredoxin 2 is the third most abundant protein in erythrocytes, and competes effectively with catalase and glutathione peroxidase to scavenge low levels of hydrogen peroxide, including that derived from hemoglobin autoxidation. GSH reductase restores oxidized GSH at the expense of NADPH energy. The final step in GSH synthesis is catalysed by the glutathione synthetase. Thus, resistance of erythrocytes to oxidative stress will depend on the activity of glucose transporter type 1, glycolysis enzymes, glutathione synthetase, glutathione reductase, glutathione peroxidase, peroxiredoxin 2, superoxide dismutase 1, catalase and nucleotide metabolism. Activation of oxidative stress occurs in case of infection, hypoxic ischemia, acidosis, effect of some medications and toxins. Low resistance of erythrocytes to oxidative stress leads to hemoglobin precipitation and erythrocytes hemolysis. Thus, erythrocytes become sources of active forms of oxygen. Oxidative stress has been implicated in many human diseases. Activity of erythrocyte antioxidant enzymes is closely studied to reveal oxidative stress status in various pathological conditions.

Herein we describe the recent updates regarding point mutations, which contribute to the decrease of antioxidant protection of erythrocytes.

2. Point mutations in proteins and enzymes providing a metabolism of erythrocytes

2.1 Point mutation in glucose transporter GLUT 1

GLUT1 was the first glucose transporter isoform to be identified, and is one of 13 proteins that comprise the human equilibrative glucose transporter family. GLUT1 is a membrane-spanning glycoprotein of 492 amino acids, containing 12 transmembrane domains with both *N*- and *C*-termini located in cytosol, and its gene being located on chromosome 1 (1p35-31.3) is composed of ten exons and nine introns. GLUT1 is expressed at the highest levels in the plasma membranes of proliferating cells forming the early developing embryo, in cells forming the blood-tissue barriers, in human erythrocytes and astrocytes, and in cardiac muscle (Carruthers et al., 2009). Heterozygous mutations in the GLUT1 gene have been reported in sporadic patients and results in autosomal dominant pedigrees. Expression of mutant transporters resulted in a significant decrease in transport activity of GLUT1. Impaired glucose transport across brain tissue barriers is reflected by hypoglycorrhachia and results in epilepsy, mental retardation and motor disorders. The first autosomal dominant missense mutation (G272A) has been reported within the human GLUT1 gene and wos shared by three affected family members. Substitution of glycine-91 by site-directed mutagenesis with either aspartate or alanine was studied in oocytes. The data agree with 3-O-methyl-glucose uptake into patient erythrocytes and indicate that the loss of glycine rather than a hydrophilic side chain (Gly91→Asp) defines the functional consequences of this mutation. (Klepper et al., 2001). Recently, mutations in GLUT1 gene have been identified as a cause in some patients with autosomal dominant paroxysmal exercise-induced dyskinesias (PED). PED are involuntary intermittent movements triggered by prolonged physical exertion. Some patients had a predating history of childhood absence epilepsy and a current history of hemiplegic migraine as well as a family history of migraine (Schneider et al., 2009). In certain cases PED was accompanied by hemolytic anemia with echinocytosis, and altered erythrocyte ion concentrations. Using a candidate gene approach, a causative deletion of 4 highly conserved amino acids (Q282_S285del) in the pore region of GLUT1 was identified. Functional studies in Xenopus oocytes and human erythrocytes revealed that this mutation decreased glucose transport and caused a cation leak that alters intracellular concentrations of sodium, potassium, and calcium. In families where PED is combined with epilepsy, developmental delay, or migraine, but not with hemolysis or echinocytosis 2 GLUT1 mutations were identified (A275T, G314S) that decreased glucose transport but did not affect cation permeability (Weber et al., 2008). The causative mutations for some forms of hereditary stomatocytosis have been found to result from mutations in SLC2A1, encoding GLUT1. Stomatocytosis was associated with a cold-induced cation leak, hemolytic anemia and hepatosplenomegaly but also with cataracts, seizures, mental retardation and movement disorder (Flatt et al., 2011).

2.2 Point mutation in glycolysis enzymes

2.2.1 Point mutation in hexokinase

Hexokinase (HK) catalyses the phosphorylation of glucose to glucose-6-phosphate using adenosine triphosphate as a phosphoryl donor. The four isozymes of the HK family (HK1, HK2, HK3, and glucokinase) contribute to commit glucose to the glycolytic pathway, each of which is encoded by a separate gene. The predominant HK1 isozyme is expressed in the vast majority of cells and tissues, including cells that are strictly dependent on glucose uptake for their metabolic needs. While most tissues express more than one HK isozyme, erythrocytes glucose metabolism only depends on HK1 activity. HK1 is one of the rate-limiting enzymes in erythrocytes glycolysis. Gene structure and exon-intron organization of the HK1 gene have been elucidated from a sequence of three contiguous genomic clones localized at human chromosome 10. The sequence spans about 131 kb, and consists of 25 exons, which include 6 testis- and 1 erythroid-specific exons. The HK1 and erythroid-specific HK-R transcripts being produced by using two distinct promoters. Thus, the first and second exons are specifically utilized for the erythroid-specific HK-R and ubiquitously expressed HK1 isozymes respectively (Kanno 2000; Murakami et al., 2002; van Wijk at al., 2003; Bonnefond et al., 2009). In humans, mutations including nonsynonymous substitutions in the active site of HK1 and intragenic deletions have been shown to cause HK1 enzymatic deficiency associated with autosomal recessive severe nonspherocytic hemolytic anemia (Bonnefond et al., 2009). Mutation affecting the substrate affinites of the enzyme, regulatory properties, heat stability have been described (Rijksen et al., 1983; Magnani et al., 1985). HK deficiency is a very rare disease with a clinical phenotype of hemolysis. PCR amplification and sequence of the cDNA in patients with HK deficiency revealed the presence of a deletion and of a single nucleotide substitution, both in heterozygous form. In particular, the deletion, 96 bp long, concerns nucleotides 577 to 672 in the HK cDNA sequence and was not found in the cDNAs of 14 unrelated normal subjects. The sequence of the HK allele without deletion showed a single nucleotide substitution from T to C at position 1667 which causes the amino acid change from Leu529 to Ser (Bianchi et al., 1995). The T1667→C substitution, causing the amino acid change Leu529→Ser, is responsible for the complete loss of the hexokinase catalytic activity, while the 96 bp deletion causes a drastic reduction of the hexokinase activity (Bianchi et al., 1997). A homozygous missense mutation in exon 15 (2039C→G, HK Utrecht) of HK1, the gene that encodes red blood cell-specific hexokinase-R, in a patient previously diagnosed with hexokinase deficiency has been reported. The Thr680→Ser substitution predicted by this mutation affects a highly conserved residue in the enzyme's active site that interacts with phosphate moieties of adenosine diphosphate, adenosine triphosphate, and glucose-6-phosphate inhibitor (van Wijk et al. 2003). On the paternal allele in a patient with chronic hemolysis two mutations in the erythroid-specific promoter of HKI: 373A→C and 193A→G were identified. Transfection of promoter reporter constructs showed that the 193A→G mutation reduced promoter activity to 8%. Hence, 193A→G is the first mutation reported to affect red blood cell-specific hexokinase specific transcription. On the maternal allele there was a missense mutation in exon 3: 278G→A, encoding an arginine to glutamine substitution at residue 93 (Arg93→Glu), affecting both hexokinase-1 and erytrocytes specific-hexokinase. This missense mutation was shown to compromise normal pre-mRNA processing. Reduced erythroid transcription of HK1 together with aberrant splicing of both hexokinase-1 and erytrocytes specific-hexokinase results in HK deficiency and mild chronic hemolysis (de Vooght et al. 2009).

2.2.2 Point mutation in glucose-6-phosphate isomerase

Glucose-6-phosphate isomerase (GPI) catalyzes interconversion of glucose-6-phosphate and fructose 6-phosphate in the Embden-Meyerhof glycolytic pathway. GPI is an essential enzyme for carbohydrate metabolism in all tissues. In humans, the GPI gene locus is located on chromosome 19, and the gene spans more than 40 kb, including 18 exons and 17 introns. The cDNA sequence encodes 558 amino acid residues. The enzyme consists of two identical subunits. In mammals, GPI can also act as an autocrine motility factor, neuroleukin, and maturation factor. GPI deficiency is a well-known congenital autosomal recessive disorder with the typical manifestation of nonspherocytic hemolytic anemia of variable severity in humans. GPI deficiency is one of the most common cause of congenital nonspherocytic hemolytic anemia caused by deficiency of glycolytic enzymes, the commonest being deficiency of glucose-6-phosphate dehydrogenase and pyruvate kinase. Patients with inherited GPI deficiency present with nonspherocytic anemia of variable severity and with neuromuscular dysfunction. Mutations in the GPI gene usually have negative influences on catalytic parameters, particularly k(cat), as well as structure stability. Mutations at or close to the active site, including R273H, H389R, and S278L, cause great damage to the catalytic function, yet those at distance can still reduce the magnitude of k(cat). At the nucleotide level, 29 mutations have been reported. Mutations decrease the enzyme tolerance to heat by mechanisms of decreasing packing efficiency (V101M, T195I, S278L, L487F, L339P, T375R, I525T), weakening network bonding (R75G, R347C, R347H, R472H, E495K), increasing water-accessible hydrophobic surface (R83W), and destabilizing the ternary structure (T195I, R347C, R347H, and I525T). A300P, L339P, and E495K mutations may also negatively affect the protein folding efficiency (Merkle S. at al., 1993; Kanno H. at al., , 1996; Kugler W. at al., 2000; Haller J.F. et al., 2009; Haller J.F., et al., 2010). The neurologically affected patient (GPI Homburg) is compound heterozygous for a 59 A→C (H20P) and a 1016 T→C (L339P) exchange. Owing to the insertion of proline, the H20P and L339P mutations are likely to affect the folding and activity of the enzyme. Point mutations identified at 1166 A→G (H389R) and 1549 C→G (L517V), which are located at the subunit interface showed no neurological symptoms. Thus mutations that lead to incorrect folding destroy both catalytic

(GPI) and neurotrophic activities, thereby leading to the observed clinical symptoms (GPI Homburg). Those alterations at the active site, however, that allow correct folding retain the neurotrophic properties of the molecule (GPI Calden) (Kugler, 1998). The similarity of the mutant enzymes to the allozymes found in human GPI deficiencies indicates the GPI deficient mouse mutants to be excellent models for the human disease (Padua et al., 1978; Pretsch et al., 1990). A heterozygous mouse mutant exhibiting approximately 50% of wild-type GPI activity. Biochemical and immunological studies revealed no differences in physicochemical, kinetic and immunological properties between the erythrocytic enzyme of heterozygous and wild-type mouse. The genetic and physiological analyses provided no indications for further altered traits in heterozygous animals including fertility, viability and several other traits. Homozygous null mutants died at an early post-implantation stage of embryogenesis (West et al., 1990; Merkle et al., 1992). Homozygous GPI deficiency in humans are responsible for chronic nonspherocytic hemolytic anemia. The homozygous missense A346H mutation replacement in cDNA position 1040G→A, which causes a loss of GPI capacity to dimerize, which renders the enzyme more susceptible to thermolability and produces significant changes in erythrocyte metabolism was described in patient with chronic nonspherocytic hemolytic anemia (Repiso et al., 2005). Biochemical and molecular genetic studies performed with the enzyme variants of GPI Zwickau and GPI Nordhorn showed that in both cases the simultaneous occurrence of a single amino acid substitution affecting the active site, together with a nonsense mutation leading to the loss of major parts of the enzyme probably explains the severe clinical course of the disease (Huppke et al., 1997). Molecular characteristics of erythrocytes GPI deficiency were described in Spanish patients with chronic nonspherocytic hemolytic anemia. Residual GPI activity in erythrocytes of around 7% (GPI-Catalonia), in an individual is homozygous for the missense mutation 1648A→G (Lys550→Glu) in exon 18 was described and residual activity in erythrocytes of around 20% (GPI-Barcelona), was found in a compound heterozygote for two different missense mutations: 341A→T (Asp113→Val) in exon 4 and 663T→G (Asn220→Lys) in exon 7. Molecular modeling using the human crystal structure of GPI as a model was performed to determine how these mutations could affect enzyme structure and function (Repiso et al., 2006). Chinese hamster (CHO) cell lines with ethylmethane sulfonate induced mutations in GPI and consequent loss of GPI activity have been reported. GPI activity was reduced by 87% in GroD1 isolated from this population. Expression cloning and sequencing of the cDNA obtained from GroD1 revealed a point mutation Gly189→ Glu. This resulted in a temperature sensitivity and severe reduction in the synthesis of glycerolipids due to a reduction in phosphatidate phosphatase (PAP). Overexpression of lipin 1 in the GPI-deficient cell line, GroD1 resulted in increased PAP activity, however it failed to restore glycerolipid biosynthesis. Fluorescent microscopy showed a failure of GPI-deficient cells to localize lipin 1α to the nucleus. Glucose-6-phosphate levels in GroD1 cells were 10-fold over normal. Lowering glucose levels in the growth medium partially restored glycerolipid biosynthesis and nuclear localization of lipin 1α. Thus, GPI deficiency results in an accumulation of glucose-6-phosphate, and possibly other glucose-derived metabolites, leading to activation of mTOR and sequestration of lipin 1 to the cytosol, preventing its proper functioning. These results may also help to explain neuromuscular symptoms associated with inherited GPI deficiency (Haller et al., 2010; 2011). GPI deficiency was found to be the cause of recurrent haemolytic crises that has required frequent blood transfusion.

Hemolysis is often ameliorated by splenectomy (Neubauer et al., 1990; Shalev et al., 1994; Alfinito et al., 1994). GPI deficiency can become a clinically relevant consequence of the administration of drugs. GPI deficiency can lead to impairment of the system that removes free radicals generated by amoxicillin, thereby resulting in oxidation of hemoglobin and destabilization of erythrocytes membranes, with acute hemolysis and severe hemoglobinuria (Rossi et al., 2010).

2.2.3 Point mutation in phosphofructokinase

Phosphofructo-1-kinase (PFK) is a tetrameric enzyme that phosphorylates fructose-6-phosphate to fructose-1,6-bisphosphate, committing glucose to glycolysis. Three PFK isoenzymes, encoded by separate genes, have been identified in mammals: muscle-type (PFKM), liver-type (PFKL), and platelet-type (PFKP), all of which are expressed in a tissue specific manner. Skeletal muscle expresses only PFKM homotetramers, liver mainly PFKL homotetramers, while erythrocytes contain PFKM and PFKL heterotetramers (Vora et al., 1983). Inherited deficiency of muscle PFK is known to occur in man and dog (Vora et al., 1983; Skibild et al., 2001). PFK deficiency was the first recognized disorder that directly affects glycolysis. Ever since the discovery of the disease in 1965, a wide range of biochemical, physiological and molecular studies of the disorder have been carried out (Nakajima et al., 2002). Several mutations in PFKM cause type VII glycogen storage disease (GSDVII), which is a rare disease described by Tarui (Tarui's disease). GSDVII is characterized by the coexistence of a muscle disease and a hemolytic process. Clinical manifestations of the disease range from the severe infantile form, leading to death during childhood, to the classical form, which presents mainly with exercise intolerance. Typically, the disease begins in early childhood and consists of easy fatigability, transient weakness and muscle cramps and myoglobinuria after vigorous exercises (Vora et al., 1987; García et al., 2009). A G-to-A transition at codon 209-in exon 8 of the PFK-M gene, changing an encoded Gly to Asp, is responsible for the GSDVII in a homozygous French Canadian patient. The Swiss patient is a genetic compound, carrying a G-to-A transition at codon 100 in exon 6 (Arg to Gln) and a G-to-A transition at codon 696 in exon 22 (Arg to His) (Raben et al., 1995). PFK deficiency include isolated hemolytic anemia, compensated hemolysis or asymptomatic state (Etiemble et al., 1983; Fogelfeld et al., 1990). The concomitant haemolysis in patients with inherited PFK deficiency of the muscle isoenzyme may be explained by a diminished erythrocyte deformability due to Ca2+ overload (Ronquist et al., 2001). PFK deficiency include early-onset neonatal seizures (Al-Hassnan et al., 2007). Portal and mesenteric vein thrombosis in patient with a known case of PFK deficiency has been described (Madhoun et al., 2011).

2.2.4 Point mutation in aldolase

Aldolase, a homotetrameric protein encoded by the ALDOA gene, converts fructose-1,6-bisphosphate to dihydroxyacetone phosphate and glyceraldehyde-3-phosphate. Three isozymes are encoded by distinct genes. The sole aldolase present in erythrocytes and skeletal muscle is the A isozyme. Aldolase B is mainly expressed in the liver, kidney and small intestine, where it plays a role in exogenous fructose utilization. Aldolase C is expressed predominantly in the brain. Aldolase B deficiency has been widely described in humans, because it causes hereditary fructose intolerance, which is an autosomal recessive disease that may induce severe liver damage, leading, in extreme cases, to death if fructose is not eliminated from the diet. To date, nearly 25 HFI-related aldolase B mutants have been identified. In contrast, cases of aldolase A deficiency, which has been associated with nonspherocytic haemolytic anemia, are much rarer (Esposito et al., 2004). Human aldolase A is composed of four identical subunits encoded by a single gene located on chromosome 16 (16q22-q24). Aldolase A deficiency has been reported as a rare, autosomal recessive disorder (Kreuder et al., 1996; Yao et al., 2004). Alterations in the aldolase A gene leading to amino acid substitutions: Asp128→Gly (Kishi et al., 1987), Glu206→Lys (Kreuder et al., 1996), Gly346→Ser (Esposito et al., 2004) have been described. The Glu206→Lys mutation destabilizes the aldolase A tetramer at the subunit interface, the Gly346→Ser mutation limits the flexibility of the C-terminal region. Biochemical and thermodynamic data are available for the Asn128→Gly mutant have never been characterized. Yao D.C. et al. described the case of a girl of Sicilian descent with aldolase A deficiency. Clinical manifestations included transfusion-dependent anemia until splenectomy at age 3 and increasing muscle weakness, with death at age 4 associated with rhabdomyolysis and hyperkalemia. Sequence analysis of the ALDOA coding regions revealed 2 novel heterozygous ALDOA mutations in conserved regions of the protein. The paternal allele encoded a nonsense mutation, Arg303X, in the enzyme-active site. The maternal allele encoded a missense mutation, Cys338→Tyr, predicted to cause enzyme instability as reported (Yao et al., 2004). Hemolytic crisis in patients with aldolase A deficiency can be provoked by fever (Kiriyama et al., 1993) and upper respiratory infections (Miwa et al., 1981).

2.2.5 Housekeeping genes in glyceraldehyde 3-phosphate dehydrogenase

Glyceraldehyde-3-phosphate dehydrogenase (GAPDH) specifically catalyzes the simultaneous phosphorylation and oxidation of glyceraldehyde-3-phosphate to 1,3-biphosphoglycerate. GAPDH comprises a polypeptide chain of 335 amino acids. Structural studies identified two regions, namely the glyceraldehyde-3-phosphate catalytic site and the nicotinamide adenine dinucleotide binding site. The glycolytic function mainly relies on critical amino acids that include Cys152 and His179, and on its tetrameric structure composed of four identical 37-kDa subunits (Colell et al., 2009). GAPDH was considered a classical glycolytic protein involved exclusively in cytosolic energy production. However, recent evidence suggests that it is a multifunctional protein displaying diverse activities distinct from its conventional metabolic role. New investigations establish a primary role for GAPDH in a variety of critical nuclear pathways apart from its already recognized role in apoptosis. These new roles include its requirement for transcriptional control of histone gene expression, its essential function in nuclear membrane fusion, its necessity for the recognition of fraudulently incorporated nucleotides in DNA, and its mandatory participation in the maintenance of telomere structure. Other investigations relate a substantial role for nuclear GAPDH in hyperglycemic stress and the development of metabolic syndrome. GAPDH is a highly conserved gene and protein, with a single mRNA transcribed from a unique gene (Sirover 1997, 2005, 2011). GAPDH has been referred to as a "housekeeping" protein and based on the view that GAPDH gene expression remains constant under changing cellular conditions, the levels of GAPDH mRNA have frequently been used to normalize northern blots (Tatton, 2000). Evidence of an impairment of GAPDH glycolytic function in Alzheimer's and Huntington's disease subcellular fractions despite unchanged gene expression has been reported (Mazzola & Sirover, 2001).

2.2.6 Point mutation in phosphoglycerate kinase

Phosphoglycerate kinase (PGK) plays a key role for ATP generation in the glycolytic pathway. The PGK, which exists universally in various tissues of various organisms, is encoded by a single structural gene on the X-chromosome q13 in humans. The PGK consists of 417 amino acid residues with acetylserine at the NH2-terminal and isoleucine at the COOH-terminal and is a monomeric enzyme that is expressed in all tissues (Huang et al. 1980; Maeda et al. 1991). PGK deficiency is generally associated with chronic hemolytic anemia, although it can be accompanied by either mental retardation or muscular disease (Cohen-Solal et al. 1994). The structure of some PGK mutants has been described. PGK Matsue variant is a point mutation, a T/A→C/G transition in exon 3, that cause Leu88→Pro substitution associated with severe enzyme deficiency, congenital nonspherocytic hemolytic anemia, and mental disorders (Maeda et al. 1991). PGK Shizuoka variant is a single nucleotide substitution from guanine to thymine at position 473 of PGK messenger RNA, associated with chronic hemolysis and myoglobinuria. This nucleotide change causes a single amino acid substitution from Gly157→Val (Fujii et al. 1992). PGK Créteil variant arises from a G→A nucleotide interchange at position 1022 in cDNA (exon 9), resulting in amino acid substitution Asp314→Asn associated with rhabdomyolysis crises but not with hemolysis or mental retardation. PGK Amiens/New York variant, which is associated with chronic hemolytic anemia and mental retardation is a point mutation, an A→T nucleotide interchange at position 571 in cDNA (exon 5); this leads to amino acid substitution Asp163→Val (Cohen-Solal et al., 1994; Flanagan et al., 2006). Variants of PGK Barcelona and PGK Murcia are described in Spain. PGK Barcelona variant, which causes chronic hemolytic anemia associated with progressive neurological impairment is a point mutation, 140 T→A substitution that produces an Ile46→Asn change. The increase of 2,3-bisphosphoglycerate and the decrease of adenosine triphosphate levels in erythrocytes are the detected metabolic changes that could cause hemolytic anemia. PGK Murcia variant is a point mutation, 958 G→A transition that cause a Ser319→Asn substitution. The crystal structure of porcine PGK was used as a molecular model to investigate how these mutations may affect enzyme structure and function. In both cases – the mutations did not modify any of the PGK binding sites for ATP or 3PG, so their effect is probably related to a loss of enzyme stability rather than a decrease of enzyme catalytic function (Noel N. et al., 2006; Ramírez-Bajo M.J. et al., 2011). Mutants PGK München (Krietsch et al., 1980), PGK Herlev (Valentin et al., 1998), PGK Uppsala (Hjelm et al., 1980), PGK San Francisco (Guis et al., 1987), PGK II (Huang et al., 1980), PGK Michigan, PGK Tokyo (Cohen-Solal et al., 1994) are also described.

2.2.7 Point mutation in phosphoglycerate mutase

Phosphoglycerate mutase (PGAM) is a glycolytic enzyme that catalyses the interconversion of 2-phosphoglycerate and 3-phosphoglycerate, with 2,3-bisphosphoglycerate being required, in mammals, as a co-factor. In mammals, PGAM is present in three isozymes which result from the homodimeric and heterodimeric combinations of two different subunits, M and B, coded by two different genes, although the gene coding subunit B is unknown. Only the homodimer BB is present in erythrocytes. Only one PGAM BB deficiency has been reported. In a patient with clinical diagnosis of Hereditary Spherocytosis and partial deficiency (50%) of erythrocytes PGAM activity, a homozygous point mutation with cDNA 690G→A substitution that produces a Met230→Ile change has recently been reported. The mutated PGAM shows an abnormal behaviour on ion-exchange chromatography and is more thermo-labile that the native enzyme. The increased instability of the mutated enzyme can account for the decreased erythrocytes PGAM activity (Repiso et al., 2005; de Atauri et al., 2005).

2.2.8 Point mutation in enolase

Enolase, an essential enzyme of glycolysis and gluconeogenesis, catalyses the interconversion of 2-hosphoglyceric acid and phosphoenolpyruvate. Enolases from most species are dimeric, with subunit molecular masses of 40000–50000 Da. Mammals have three genes for enolase, coding for the α, β and γ subunits; the subunits associate to form both homo- and heterodimers. The α gene is expressed in many tissues, γ primarily in neurones and β in muscle (Zhao et al., 2008). Erytrocytes enolase deficiency is rare, and its pathogenesis, inheritance and clinical manifestation have not been firmly established. Enolase deficiency is known to be associated with chromosome 1p locus mutations (1 pter-p36.13) and to cause chronic nonspecific hemolytic anemia (Boulard-Heitzmann et al., 1984). Lachant et al. (1986) described four generations of a Caucasian family with hereditary erytrocytes enolase deficiency. Stefanini (1972) described chronic hemolytic anemia associated with erythrocyte enolase deficiency exacerbated by ingestion of nitrofurantoin.

2.2.9 Point mutation in pyruvate kinase

Pyruvate kinase (PK) catalyses the last step of the Embden–Meyerhof metabolic pathway, in which an ATP molecule is produced. Among the four PK isozymes present in humans (M1, M2, L and R), both PK-L (found in the liver, kidney and gut) and PK-R present in erythrocytes are encoded by the same gene, which is localised on hromosome 1q21. The respective expression of these two isozymes is under the control of specific promoters leading to structural differences in the N-terminal part of the protein. PK-R is a 574 amino acid-long protein, which associates into tetramers according to a double dyad symmetry pattern, resulting in allosteric enzymatic kinetics. PK deficiency is the most frequent red cell enzymatic defect responsible for hereditary nonspherocytic hemolytic anemia and is transmitted according to a recessive autosomal mode. Based on the gene frequency of the 1529A mutation in the white population and on its relative abundance in patients with hemolytic anemia caused by PK deficiency, the prevalence of PK deficiency is estimated at 51 cases per million white population (Beutler et al., 2000). The degree of haemolysis varies widely, ranging from very mild or fully compensated forms, to life-threatening neonatal anemia and jaundice necessitating exchange transfusions. Heterozygous carriers usually display very mild symptoms. Therefore, the defect is frequently ignored and its prevalence is difficult to establish. Severe disorders are described in homozygous or compound heterozygous patients (Zanella et al., 2005). According to the most recent database, more than 180 mutations have been reported on the PK-LR gene. Two mutations, both located in exon 11, are recurrent (Arg510 → Gln, Arg486 → Trp). Arg510→ Gln is the most frequent mutation found in northern Europe, central Europe and the USA (Pissard S. at al., 2006, as citated Wang et al., 2001) and Arg486 → Trp in southern Europe (Spain, Portugal and Italy) and in France (Pissard et al., 2006, as citited Zanella et al, 1997; Zarza et al, 1998; Pissard et al., 2006). The most frequent mutations of PKLR gene in the Indian population appear to be 1436G→A (19.44%), followed by 1456C→T (16.66%) and 992A→G (16.66%) (Kedar et al.,

2009). Erythrocyte PK plays an important role as an antioxidant during erythroid differentiation. Glycolytic inhibition by erythrocyte PK gene mutation augmented oxidative stress, leading to activation of hypoxia-inducible factor-1 as well as downstream proapoptotic gene expression (Aisaki et al., 2007). Extended molecular analysis is useful for studying how several interacting gene mutations contribute to the clinical variability of pyruvate kinase deficiency (Perseu et al., 2010).

2.2.10 Point mutation in glucose-6-phosphate dehydrogenase

Glucose 6-phosphate dehydrogenase (G6PD) is a ubiquitous enzyme, which is critical in the redox metabolism of all aerobic cells. It catalyzes the first, rate-limiting step of the pentose phosphate pathway, coupled to NADPH synthesis and to ribose availability which is essential for the production of nucleotide coenzymes and replication of nucleic acids (Sodiende O., 1992). The pentose phosphate pathway is the unique source of NADPH, which enables erytrocytes to counterbalance the oxidative stress triggered by several oxidant agents preserving the reduced form of glutathione. GSH protects the sulfhydryl groups in hemoglobin and in the red cell membrane from oxidation (Mason et al., 2007). G6PD is a dimer and each subunit contains a single active site. G6PD-enzyme is encoded by a human X-linked gene (Xq2.8) consisting of 13 exons and 12 introns, spanning nearly 20 kb in total. G6PD gene is probably the most polymorphic locus in humans, with over 400 allelic variants known (Minucci et al., 2009). G6PD, the most common enzyme deficiency worldwide, causes a spectrum of disease including neonatal hyperbilirubinemia, acute hemolysis, and chronic hemolysis. Persons with this condition also may be asymptomatic. Approximately 400 million people are affected worldwide. Homozygotes and heterozygotes can be symptomatic, although the disease typically is more severe in persons who are homozygous for the deficiency. Different gene mutations cause different levels of enzyme deficiency, with classes assigned to various degrees of deficiency and disease manifestation. Acute hemolysis is caused by exposure to an oxidative stressor such as infection, some foods (fava beans), drugs or various chemicals. The variant that causes chronic hemolysis is uncommon because it is related to sporadic gene mutation rather than the more common inherited gene mutation (Frank, 2005). About 160 mutations have been reported, most of which are single-base substitutions leading to amino acid replacements (Minucci et. al., 2009). Mutations are classified into four types, according to their clinical effects. Several variants, such as the the Mediterranean variant, reach the polymorphism (Wajcman et. al., 2004). The Mediterranean variant of G6PD deficiency is due to the C563CT point mutation, leading to replacement of Ser with Phe at position 188, resulting in acute haemolysis triggered by oxidants (Ingrosso et. al., 2002). Individuals with such mutations seem to have enjoyed a selective advantage because of resistance to falciparum malaria. Different mutations, each characteristic of certain populations are found.The most common African mutation G6PD is 202A376G. G6PD Mediterranean (563T) is found in Southern Europe, the Middle East and in the Indian subcontinent (Beulter, 1996).

2.2.11 Point mutation in 6-phosphogluconate dehydrogenase

The 6-phosphogluconate dehydrogenase (6PGDH) is the third enzyme of the oxidative branch of the pentose phosphate pathway. This pathway has two major functions: the production of ribulose 5-phosphate which is required for nucleotide synthesis, and the generation of NADPH which provides the major reducing power essential to protect the cell against oxidative stress and a variety of reductive biosynthetic reactions, particularly lipid production. Thus, 6PGDH plays a critical role in protecting cells from oxidative stress (He et al., 2007). Few cases of erytrocytes 6PGD deficiency in humans have been described. The episodic hemolytic events with jaundice in patients with 6PGD deficiency may be the result of a defective erythrocytes ability to counteract conditions of marked oxidative stress as happens at birth and following traumatic events. The presence of 6PGD deficiency could be mistaken for a partial G6PD deficiency if the assay of G6PD activity was performed without correcting for 6PGD activity (Vives Corrons et al., 1996; Caprari et al., 2001).

2.3 Point mutation in glutathione synthetase

Glutathione (GSH) is the most abundant intracellular thiol in living aerobic cells. GSH is present in millimolar concentrations in most mammalian cells and it is involved in several fundamental biological functions, including free radical scavenging, detoxification of xenobiotics and carcinogens, redox reactions, biosynthesis of DNA, proteins and leukotrienes, as well as neurotransmission/neuromodulation. It has been assigned several critical functions: protection of cells against oxidative damage; involvement in amino acid transport; participation in the detoxification of foreign compounds; maintenance of protein sulfhydryl groups in a reduced state; and as a cofactor for a number of enzymes. GSH is found in low levels in diseases in which increasing evidence implicate oxidative stress in the development of the disease, for example retinopathy of prematurity, necrotizing enterocolitis, bronchopulmonary dysplasia, patent ductus arteriosus and asthma. GSH is metabolised via the gamma-glutamyl cycle, which is catalyzed by six enzymes (Polekhina at al., 1999; Njålsson et al., 2005; Norgren et al., 2007). GSH is synthesized from glutamate, cysteine and glycine. The final step in its synthesis is catalysed by the enzyme glutathione synthetase (GS) The human GS enzyme is a homodimer with 52 kDa of subunits containing 474 amino acid residues, encoded by a single-copy gene located on chromosome 20q11.2 (Webb et al., 1995; Njålsson et al., 2005).

GS deficiency is a rare autosomal recessive disorder. Since the human genome contains only one GS gene, the various clinical forms of GS deficiency reflect different mutations or epigenetic modifications in the GS gene. Thus GSH acts as a feedback inhibitor of the initial step in its biosynthesis, in patients with hereditary deficiency of GS the lack of GSH leads to the formation of increased amounts of g-glutamylcysteine which is converted into 5-oxoproline by g-glutamyl cyclotransferase and excreted in massive amounts. Shi et al. identified seven mutations at the GS locus on six alleles: one splice site mutation, two deletions and four missense mutations and in patients with 5-Oxoprolinuria (pyroglutamic aciduria) resulting in GS deficiency and homozygous missense mutation in an individual affected by a milder-form of the GS deficiency, which is apparently restricted to erythrocytes and only associated with haemolytic anaemia (Shi, et al., 1996). Japanese patients with chronic nonspherocytic hemolytic anemia were found to have decreased GS activity and the others were moderately deficient in GCS. Hemolytic anemia was their only manifestation, and neither 5-oxoprolinemia nor 5-oxoprolinuria, which are usually associated with to generalized type of glutathione synthetase deficiency, was noted in patients. (Hirono et al., 1996). Dahl N. at al. described thirteen different point mutations. In vitro analysis of naturally occurring missense mutations showed that mutations could affect the stability, catalytic capacity and substrate affinities of the enzyme. Four mutant cDNAs were investigated with the mutations resulting in Leu188→Pro, Tyr270→Cys, Tyr270→His and Arg283→Cys, respectively. Each of the four mutations resulted in a considerable decrease of enzymatic activity to levels corresponding to 1 to 12% of the wild-type control value, confirming that these mutations were pathogenic. Clinically affected patients present with severe metabolic acidosis, 5-oxoprolinuria, increased rate of hemolysis, hemolytic anemia, neonatal jaundice and defective function of the central nervous system. A milder form of GS deficiency apparently restricted to erythrocytes, is associated with decreased erythrocyte GSH levels and hemolytic disease, which is usually well compensated. Complete loss of function of both GS alleles is probably lethal. Missense mutations will account for the phenotype in the majority of patients with severe GS deficiency (Dahl et al., 1997). A 141-bp deletion corresponding to the entire exon 4, whilst the corresponding genomic DNA showed a G491→A homozygous splice site mutation, and a C847→T (Arg283→ Cys) mutation in exon 9 are described in patients with GS deficiency and Fanconi nephropathy (Al-Jishi et al., 1999). A homozygous state for 656 A→G, a 808 T→C mutation of GS gene in patients with chronic haemolysis and markedly reduced erythrocytes was found in Spain (Corrons, et al., 2001). Patients with GS deficiency can be divided into three groups. Mildly affected patients have mutations affecting the stability of the enzyme, causing a compensated haemolytic anaemia; moderately affected patients have, in addition, metabolic acidosis; and severely affected patients also develop neurological defects and show increased susceptibility to bacterial infections. Moderately and severely affected patients have mutations that compromise the catalytic properties of the enzyme. 5-Oxoprolinuria appears in all three groups, but is more pronounced in the two latter groups (Njålsson .et al., 2005). 5-Oxoproline is able to promote both lipid and protein oxidation, to impair brain antioxidant defenses and to enhance hydrogen peroxide content, thus promoting oxidative stress, and is a mechanism that may be involved in the neuropathology of GS deficiency (Pederzolli et al., 2010). Approximately 25% of patients with hereditary GS deficiency die during childhood. Even though the correlation between phenotype and genotype in these patients is complex, an indication of the phenotype can be based on the type of mutation involved (Njålsson et al., 2005). Severe GS deficiency is associated with progressive retinal dystrophy of the rod-cone type, affecting the central retina with advanced macular edema in adulthood. The retinal degenerative changes in GS deficiency may be the result of the increased oxidative stress accumulated generally in the retina and also apparent in the macular area, and an insufficient level of the free radical scavenger GSH. Patients with GS deficiency may represent a model of the retinal response to oxidative stress in humans (Burstedt et al., 2009). Recently 30 different mutations in the GSS gene have been identified (Njålsson et al., 2005). The severe form of GS deficiency usually present in the neonatal period, is characterized by acute metabolic acidosis, hemolytic anemia and progressive encephalopathy (Iyori et al., 1996; Yapicioğlu et al., 2004). Diagnosis of GS deficiency is made by clinical presentation and detection of elevated concentrations of 5-oxoproline in urine and low GS activity in erythrocytes or cultured skin fibroblasts. Diagnosis can be confirmed by mutational analysis. The most important determinants for outcome and survival in patients with GS deficiency are early diagnosis and early initiation of treatment. Presently, GS deficiency is not included in newborn screening programmes in Europe. As outcome depends significantly on early start of treatment, routine inclusion of this disorder in newborn screening panels should be considered. Treatment consists of the correction of acidosis, blood transfusion, and supplementation with antioxidants (Simon et al., 2009). Patients with GS deficiency are given vitamins C and E to boost their antioxidant levels, and bicarbonate to correct metabolic acidosis (Jain et al.,1994; Ristoff et al., 2001; Njålsson et al., 2005).

2.4 Point mutation in glutathione reductase

Glutathione reductase (GR) is a key enzyme required for the conversion of oxidized glutathione (GSSG) to reduced glutathione (GSH) concomitantly oxidizing reduced nicotinamide adenine dinucleotide phosphate (NADPH). GR is a homodimeric flavoprotein with a subunit Mr of 52.4 kDa. Its 2 identical redox active sites are formed by residues from both subunits, implying that monomeric GR is not active. Human GR is encoded by a single gene, located on chromosome 8p21.1 and consisting of 13 exons. GR consists of apoglutathione reductase (apoGR) and flavin adenine dinucleotide (FAD) as a prosthetic group (Kamerbeek et al., 2007).

Acquired FAD deficiency due to low amounts of riboflavin (vitamin B2) in the diet (or failure to convert it sufficiently to FAD) may result in inactive apoGR. In that case GR activity can be restored by riboflavin administration. Due to inherited mutations, the GR protein can be absent or exhibit low catalytic activity. Whereas inherited glutathione reductase deficiency is rare, FAD deficiency is common in malnourished populations. The clinical symptoms of GR deficiency include reduced lifespan of erythrocytes, cataract, and favism (hemolytic crises after eating fava beans). A 2246-bp deletion in DNA, which results in unstable and inactive GR and a premature stop codon on one allele and a substitution of glycine 330, a highly conserved residue in the superfamily of NAD(P)H-dependent disulfide reductases, into alanine on the other allele were described in the GR gene in patients with clinical GR deficiency (Kamerbeek et al., 2007). GR deficiency may alter the clinical manifestation of an unstable hemoglobinopathy (Mojzikova at al., 2010) and may be the cause of neonatal hyperbilirubinemia (Casado et al., 1995). GR deficiency state can be asymptomatic as the residual enzyme activity might be sufficient to maintain the reduced glutathione level to prevent oxidative stress (Nakashima et al., 1978). A study on 1691 individuals from Saudi Arabia to determine the overall frequency of GR deficiency has been conducted. The overall frequency of genetic GR deficiency was 24.5% and 20.3% in males and females respectively. In addition, 17.8% of males and 22.4% of females suffered from GR deficiency due to riboflavin deficiency. This could be easily corrected by dietary supplementation with riboflavin. No cases of severe GR deficiency were identified (el-Hazmi et al., 1989; Warsy et al., 1999).

2.5 Point mutation in glutathione peroxidase

Glutathione peroxidase (GPx) is the general name of an enzyme family with peroxidase activity whose main biological role is to protect the organism from oxidative damage. There are eight well-characterized mammalian selenoproteins, including thioredoxin reductase and four isozymes of glutathione peroxidase. GPx1 is a homotetrameric selenoprotein and one of a family of peroxidases that reductively inactivate peroxides using glutathione as a source of reducing equivalents. GPx1 is found in the cytoplasm and mitochondria of all cell types, whose preferred substrate is hydrogen peroxide (Dimastrogiovanni et al., 2010).

GPx1 has been implicated in the development and prevention of many common and complex diseases, including cancer and cardiovascular disease (Lubos at al., 2011). The T allele of the GPx1 rs1050450 (C→ T) gene variant is associated with reduced enzyme activity. Significant association between the T allele and peripheral neuropathy in subjects with diabetes is observed (Tang et al., 2010). Takapoo at al. using a murine model of GPx1 deficiency (Gpx1(+/-)) found elevated hydrogen peroxide levels and increased secretion of the pro-inflammatory immunomodulator cyclophilin A (CyPA) in both arterial segments and cultured smooth muscle cells as compared to wild type. Reduction in vascular cell GPx1 activity and the associated increase in oxidative stress cause CyPA-mediated paracrine activation of smooth muscle cells. These findings identify a mechanism by which an imbalance in antioxidant capacity may contribute to vascular disease (Takapoo et al., 2011). Mice with a disrupted GPx1 gene (*Gpx1* 0/0) developed myocarditis after coxsackievirus B3 infection, whereas infected wild-type mice (*Gpx1* +/+) were resistant. Thus, GPx1 provides protection against viral-induced damage in vivo due to mutations in the viral genome of a benign virus (Beck et al., 1998). The deficiency of GPx1 promotes atherogenesis (Lubos et al., 2011). Severe acute hemoglobinemia and hemoglobinuria were described as a result a hereditary heterozygous GPx deficiency in Japan (Gondo et al., 1992). Patients with reduced GPx activity are at a high risk of developing carbamazepine-induced hemolytic crisis and/or aplastic crisis (Yamamoto et al., 2007).

2.6 Point mutation in peroxiredoxin

Peroxiredoxin (Prx) is a scavenger of hydrogen peroxide and alkyl hydroperoxides in living organisms. Six distinct mammalian Prx isozymes, types 1 to 6, have been detected in a wide range of tissues, and these have been shown to have strong antioxidant activities in vitro. In addition to their antioxidant activity, Prxs have been implicated in a number of cellular functions (Lee et al., 2003). Prx2 is an antioxidant enzyme that uses cysteine residues to decompose peroxides. Prx2 is the third most abundant protein in erythrocytes, and competes effectively with catalase and glutathione peroxidase to scavenge low levels of hydrogen peroxide, including that derived from hemoglobin autoxidation (Low, et al., 2008). Mice lacking Prdx1 are viable and fertile but have a shortened lifespan owing to the development of severe haemolytic anaemia and several malignant cancers, both of which are also observed at increased frequency in heterozygotes. The haemolytic anaemia is characterized by an increase in erythrocyte reactive oxygen species, leading to protein oxidation, haemoglobin instability, Heinz body formation and decreased erythrocyte lifespan (Neumann et al., 2003). Point mutations in gene Prx2 in humans are not described.

2.7 Point mutation in superoxide dismutase 1

Superoxide dismutase 1 (SOD1) is a primarily cytosolic enzyme of the cellular oxidative defense and acts as a protein homodimer with each monomer containing one complexed copper and zinc ion. Point mutations scattered throughout the sequence of Cu,Zn superoxide dismutase 1 (SOD1) cause a subset of amyotrophic lateral sclerosis (ALS) cases. ALS is a progressive neurodegenerative disorder affecting motor neurons (Ip et al.,

2011). The 140 Cu,Zn SOD1 gene mutations associated with ALS is described (Giannini et al., 2010). Variable penetrance and predominant lower motor neuron involvement are common characteristics in patients bearing mutations in exon 3 of the SOD1 gene (del Grande et al., 2011). Some mutations are associated with a long survival time, while others are linked to a very rapid progression (Syriani et al., 2009). With mild mechanical trauma which causes no major tissue damage, the G93A-SOD1 gene mutation alters the balance between pro-apoptotic and pro-survival molecular signals in the spinal cord tissue, leading to a premature activation of molecular pathways implicated in the natural development of ALS (Jokic et al., 2010). Mitochondria have shown to be an early target in ALS pathogenesis and contribute to the disease progression. Morphological and functional defects in mitochondria were found in both human patients and ALS mice overexpressing mutant SOD1. Axonal transport of mitochondria along microtubules is disrupted in ALS (Shi et al., 2010). Abnormal neuronal connectivity in primary motor cortex resulting from the G93A-SOD1 mutation might extend to adjacent regions and promote development of cognitive/dementia alterations frequently associated with ALS (Spalloni et al. 2011). Mutant SOD1 can alter cell cycle in a cellular model of ALS. Modifications in cell cycle progression could be due to an increased interaction between mutant G93A SOD1 and Bcl-2 through the cyclin regulator p27 (Cova et al., 2010). The D90A mutation has been identified in recessive, dominant, and apparently sporadic cases. A→C exchange at position 272 in the SOD1 gene is detected. This mutation results in an amino acid substitution of alanine for aspartate at position 90 (D90A). D90A in heterozygous state may cause predominant upper motor neuron phenotype with very slow progression (Luigetti et al., 2009). Oxidative stress markers have been found in nervous and peripheral tissues of familial and sporadic ALS patients (Cova et al., 2010). Lipid peroxidation in the erythrocytes of ALS patients was significantly increased with respect to controls (Babu et al., 2008). Recently described chronic, but moderate regenerative, haemolytic anaemia of aged SOD1-knockout mice is associated with erythrocytes modifications and sensitivity to both intra- and extra-vascular haemolysis (Starzyński et al., 2009). Deficiency of the SOD1 gene causes anemia and autoimmune responses against erythrocytes. Severity of anemia and levels of intracellular reactive oxygen species are positively correlated. Oxidation-mediated autoantibody production may be a more general mechanism for autoimmune hemolytic anemia and related autoimmune diseases. Shift in glucose metabolism to the pentose phosphate pathway and decrease in the energy charge potential of erythrocytes, increase in reactive oxygen species due to SOD1 deficiency accelerate erythrocytes destruction by affecting carbon metabolism and increasing oxidative modification of lipids and proteins. The resulting oxidation products are antigenic and, consequently, trigger autoantibody production, leading to autoimmune responses (Iuchi et al., 2007, 2009, 2010).

2.8 Point mutation in catalase

Catalase is an important anti-oxidant enzyme and physiologically maintains tissue and cellular redox homeostasis, thus plays a central role in defense against oxidative stress, it is the main regulator of hydrogen peroxide metabolism. Catalase is a tetramer of four polypeptide chains, each over 500 amino acids, it contains four porhyrin heme (iron) groups that allow the enzyme to react with hydrogen peroxide (Uchida et al., 2011).

Catalase deficiency in blood is known as acatalasemia. Deficiency of catalase may cause high concentrations of hydrogen peroxide and increase the risk of the development of pathologies for which oxidative stress is a contributing factor. Hydrogen peroxide at high concentrations is a toxic agent, while at low concentrations it appears to modulate some physiological processes such as signaling in cell proliferation, apoptosis, carbohydrate metabolism, and platelet activation. Benign catalase gene mutations in 5' noncoding region and intron 1 have no effect on catalase activity and are not associated with a disease. Decreases in catalase activity in patients with tumors is more likely to be due to decreased enzyme synthesis rather than to catalase mutations. Acatalasemia, the inherited deficiency of catalase has been detected in 11 countries (Góth et al., 2004). The molecular defects in the catalase gene, levels of m-RNA and properties of the residual catalase studied by scientists are reviewed in human (Japanese, Swiss and Hungarian) and non-human (mouse and beagle dog) acatalasemia. Japanese acatalasemia-I, the G to A transition at the fifth position of intron 4 of the catalase gene, limits the correct splicing of the mRNA, resulting in trace quantities of catalase with normal properties. The bicistronic microRNA miR-144/451 can influence gene expression by altering the activity of a key transcriptional program factor, impacting anti-oxidant-encoding genes like catalase (Yu et al., 2010). Hungarian acatalasemia type C showed a splicing mutation. In the Japanese acatalasemia II and the type A and B of Hungarian acatalasemia, deletion or insertion of nucleotides was observed in the coding regions, and a frame shift altered downstream amino acid sequences and formed truncated proteins. In the Hungarian acatalasemia D, substitution of an exon nucleotide was found. In mouse and beagle dog acatalasemia, substitution of nucleotides in the coding regions was also observed. Studies of residual catalase in Swiss mouse and beagle dog acatalasemia showed that aberrant catalase protein degrades more quickly than normal catalase in cells (Ogata et al., 2008). Japanese-type acatalasemia (Takarara disease) is characterized by the almost total loss of catalase activity in erythrocytes and is often associated with ulcerating oral lesions (Hirono et al, 1995). Polymerization of hemoglobin and aggregation of the acatalasemic erythrocytes observed upon the addition of hydrogen peroxide can be the mechanism for the onset of Takarara disease (Masuoka et al., 2006). Catalase deficiency in Hungary has been reported to be associated with increased frequency of diabetes mellitus (Vitai et al, 2005). That is human acatalasemia may be a risk factor for the development of diabetes mellitus. Catalase plays a crucial role in the defense against oxidative-stress-mediated pancreatic beta cell death (Kikumoto et al., 2009). Exon 2 and neighboring introns of the catalase gene may be minor hot spots for type 2 diabetes mellitus susceptibility mutations (Vitai et al., 2005). The catalase gene was selected as a candidate gene because of the reduction of catalase enzyme activity and concomitant accumulation of excess hydrogen peroxide observed in the entire epidermis of vitiligo patients. One of three catalase genetic markers studied was found to be informative for genotypic analysis of Caucasian vitiligo patients and control subjects. Both case/control and family-based genetic association studies of the T/C single nucleotide polymorphism (SNP) in exon 9 of the catalase gene, which is detectable with the restriction endonuclease BstX I, suggest possible association between the catalase gene and vitiligo susceptibility. The observations that T/C heterozygotes are more frequent among vitiligo patients than controls and that the C allele is transmitted more frequently to patients than controls suggest that linked mutations in or near the catalase gene might contribute to a quantitative deficiency of catalase activity in the epidermis and the accumulation of excess hydrogen peroxide (Casp et al., 2002). The increased plasma homocysteine and inherited catalase deficiency together could promote oxidative stress via hydrogen peroxide. The patients with inherited catalase deficiency are more sensitive to oxidative stress of hydrogen peroxide than the normocatalasemic family members (Góth et al., 2003). The normal activity of glutathione peroxidase could prevent the lysis of the erythrocytes in acatalasemic patients. In the presence of extremely high levels of hydrogen peroxide acute hemolysis may not be excluded; therefore, follow-up of these patients is required (Góth et al., 1995). Patients with low (inherited and acquired) catalase activities who are treated with infusion of uric acid oxidase because they are at risk of tumour lysis syndrome may experience very high concentrations of hydrogen peroxide. They may suffer from methemoglobinaemia and haemolytic anaemia which may be attributed either to deficiency of glucose-6-phosphate dehydrogenase or to other unknown circumstances. Data have not been reported from catalase deficient patients who were treated with uric acid oxidase. It may be hypothesized that their decreased blood catalase could lead to an increased concentration of hydrogen peroxide which may cause haemolysis and formation of methemoglobin. Blood catalase activity should be measured for patients at risk of tumour lysis syndrome prior to uric acid oxidase treatment. (Góth et al., 2007). Acatalasic erythrocytes metabolized glucose through the hexosemonophosphate shunt at three times the normal rate and increased this rate many times when exposed to levels of peroxide-generating drugs that had negligible effect on normal erythrocytes. When erythrocytes lacked both their hexosemonophosphate shunt and catalase, oxidative damage was greater than with either deficiency alone (Harry Jacobt et al., 1965). Under acatalasemic conditions, it was suggested that NAD(P)H is an important factor to prevent oxidative degradation of hemoglobin (Masuoka et al., 2003).

2.9 Point mutation in adenylate kinase and pyrimidine 5'-nucleotidase

Erythrocytes adenylate kinase (AK) deficiency is a rare hereditary erythroenzymopathy associated with moderate to severe nonspherocytic hemolytic anemia and, in some cases, with mental retardation and psychomotor impairment. To date, diagnosis of AK deficiency depends on demonstration of low enzyme activity in erythrocytes and detection of mutations in AK1 gene. Five variants of AK1 isoenzyme-bearing mutations (118G→A, 190G→A, 382C→T, 418-420del, and 491A→G) are found in AK-deficient patients with chronic hemolytic anemia (Abrusci et al., 2007). Pyrimidine 5' -nucleotidase (P5'N-1) deficiency is one of the frequent enzyme abnormalities causing hereditary nonspherocytic hemolytic anemia. The disease is transmitted as an autosomal recessive trait. The degree of hemolysis is generally mild-to moderate. The structural human gene for P5'N-1 is now available and fifteen different mutations have been identified so far. Some patients exhibit high residual P5'N-1 activity, suggesting that P5'N-1 deficiency is compensate by other nucleotidases and/or alternative pathways in nucleotide metabolism. No specific therapy for P5'N-1 deficiency is now available (Kondo, 1990; Chiarelli et al., 2006).

3. Conclusion

The optimum metabolism of erythrocytes depends on activity of glucose transporter type 1, glycolysis enzymes, glutathione synthetase, glutathione reductase, glutathione peroxidase, peroxiredoxin 2, superoxide dismutase 1, catalase and nucleotide metabolism. To date, all of the enzyme-deficient variants which have been investigated were caused by point mutations. Most mutations are located in the coding sequences of genes.

Expression of mutant glucose transporter 1 (GLUT1) resulted in a significant decrease in transport activity. Impaired glucose transport across brain tissue barriers results in epilepsy, mental retardation and motor disorders. Recently, mutations in GLUT1 gene have been identified as a cause in some patients with autosomal dominant paroxysmal exercise-induced dyskinesias, which in certain cases was accompanied by hemolytic anemia with echinocytosis. The causative mutations for some forms of hereditary stomatocytosis have been found to result from mutations in SLC2A1, encoding GLUT1. Stomatocytosis is associated with a cold-induced cation leak, hemolytic anemia and hepatosplenomegaly but also with cataracts, seizures, mental retardation and movement disorder.

Erythrocytes glucose metabolism only depends on hexokinase 1 (HK1) activity. HK1 deficiency is a very rare disease with a clinical phenotype of hemolysis. Glucose-6-phosphate isomerase (GPI) deficiency is one of the most common cause of congenital nonspherocytic hemolytic anemia. Patients with inherited GPI deficiency present with nonspherocytic anemia of variable severity, and with neuromuscular dysfunction. Homozygous GPI deficiency in human is responsible for chronic nonspherocytic hemolytic anemia. GPI deficiency can become clinically relevant consequence to the administration of drugs. GPI deficiency can lead to the impairment of the system that removes free radicals generated by amoxicillin, thereby resulting in oxidation of hemoglobin and destabilization of erythrocytes membranes, with acute hemolysis and severe hemoglobinuria. Phosphofructokinase (PFK) deficiency was the first recognized disorder that directly affects glycolysis. Several mutations in PFKM cause type VII glycogen storage disease (GSDVII), which is a rare disease described by Tarui (Tarui's disease). GSDVII is characterized by the coexistence of muscle disease and hemolytic process. PFK deficiency include isolated hemolytic anemia, compensated hemolysis or asymptomatic state. Portal and mesenteric vein thrombosis in patient with a known case of PFK deficiency has been described.

Aldolase A deficiency has been reported as a rare, autosomal recessive disorder. Clinical manifestations of aldolase A deficiency included transfusion-dependent anemia, increasing muscle weakness and rhabdomyolysis. Hemolytic crisis in patients with aldolase A deficiency can be provoked by fever, upper respiratory infections.

Recent evidence suggests that glyceraldehyde-3-phosphate dehydrogenase (GAPDH) is a multifunctional protein displaying diverse activities distinct from its conventional metabolic role. GAPDH has been referred to as a "housekeeping" protein and based on the view that GAPDH gene expression remains constant. Evidence of an impairment of GAPDH glycolytic function in Alzheimer's and Huntington's disease subcellular fractions despite unchanged gene expression is reported.

Phosphoglycerate kinase (PGK) deficiency is generally associated with chronic hemolytic anemia, although it can be accompanied by either mental retardation or muscular disease.

In human, phosphoglycerate mutase (PGAM) is present in three isozymes. The homodimer BB is present in erythrocytes. Only one PGAM BB deficiency has been reported. In a patient with clinical diagnosis of Hereditary Spherocytosis and partial deficiency (50%) of erythrocytes PGAM activity, a homozygous point mutation have recently been reported.

Erytrocytes enolase deficiency is rare, and its pathogenesis, inheritance and clinical manifestation have not been firmly established. Enolase deficiency causes chronic nonspecific hemolytic anemia. Chronic hemolytic anemia associated with erythrocyte enolase deficiency exacerbated by ingestion of nitrofurantoin has been described.

Pyruvate kinase (PK) deficiency is one of the most frequent red cell enzymatic defect responsible for hereditary nonspherocytic hemolytic anemia. According to the most recent database, more than 180 mutations have been reported on the PK-LR gene. Erythrocytes PK plays an important role as an antioxidant during erythroid differentiation. Glycolytic inhibition by erythrocytes PK gene mutation augmented oxidative stress, leading to activation of hypoxia-inducible factor-1 as well as downstream proapoptotic gene expression.

Glucose 6-phosphate dehydrogenase (G6PD) deficiency, the most common enzyme deficiency worldwide, causes a spectrum of diseases including neonatal hyperbilirubinemia, acute hemolysis, and chronic hemolysis. Persons with this condition also may be asymptomatic. Approximately 400 million people are affected worldwide ahd about 160 mutations have been reported. Acute hemolysis is caused by exposure to an oxidative stressor such as infection, some foods (fava beans), drugs or various chemicals.

Few cases of erytrocytes 6-phosphogluconate dehydrogenase (6PGD) deficiency in human have been described. The episodic hemolytic events with jaundice in patients with 6PGD deficiency may be the result of a defective erythrocytes ability to counteract conditions of marked oxidative stress as happens at birth and following traumatic events.

Glutathione synthetase (GS) deficiency is a rare autosomal recessive disorder. Clinically affected patients present with severe metabolic acidosis, 5-oxoprolinuria, increased rate of hemolysis, hemolytic anemia, neonatal jaundice and defective function of the central nervous system. A milder form of GS deficiency apparently restricted to erythrocytes, is associated with decreased erythrocyte GSH levels and hemolytic disease, which is usually well compensated. Complete loss of function of both GS alleles is probably lethal.

The clinical symptoms of glutathione reductase (GR) deficiency include reduced lifespan of erythrocytes, cataract, and favism (hemolytic crises after eating fava beans). GR deficiency may alter the clinical manifestation of an unstable hemoglobinopathy and may be the cause of neonatal hyperbilirubinemia. GR deficiency state can be asymptomatic as the residual enzyme activity might be sufficient to maintain the reduced glutathione level to prevent oxidative stress. Whereas inherited glutathione reductase deficiency is rare, acquired GR deficiency due to low amounts of riboflavin in the diet is common in malnourished populations.

Severe acute hemoglobinemia and hemoglobinuria has been described as a result a hereditary heterozygous glutathione peroxidase (GPx) deficiency in Japan. Patients with reduced GPx activity are at a high risk of developing carbamazepine-induced hemolytic crisis and/or aplastic crisis. Point mutations in gene peroxiredoxin 2 in human are not described.

Deficiency of the SOD1 gene causes anemia and autoimmune responses against erythrocytes. Severity of anemia and levels of intracellular reactive oxygen species are positively correlated. Oxidation-mediated autoantibody production may be a more general mechanism for autoimmune hemolytic anemia and related autoimmune diseases. Shift in glucose metabolism to the pentose phosphate pathway and decrease in the energy charge potential of erythrocytes, increase in reactive oxygen species due to SOD1 deficiency accelerates erythrocytes destruction by affecting carbon metabolism and increase oxidative modification of lipids and proteins. The resulting oxidation products are antigenic and, consequently, trigger autoantibody production, leading to autoimmune responses.

Acatalasemia, the inherited deficiency of catalase has been detected in 11 countries. Japanese-type acatalasemia (Takarara disease) is characterized by the almost total loss of catalase activity in erythrocytes and is often associated with ulcerating oral lesions. Polymerization of hemoglobin and aggregation of the acatalasemic erythrocytes observed upon the addition hydrogen peroxide can be the mechanism for the onset of Takarara disease. The patients with inherited catalase deficiency are more sensitive to oxidative stress to hydrogen peroxide. In the presence of extremely high levels of hydrogen peroxide acute hemolysis may not be excluded. Patients with low inherited catalase activities who are treated with infusion of uric acid oxidase because they are at risk of tumour lysis syndrome may experience very high concentrations of hydrogen peroxide. Inherited adenylate kinase deficiency and pyrimidine 5'-nucleotidase deficiency causes hemolytic anemia.

Under physiological conditions, changes in the activity of proteins and enzymes of erythrocytes owing to point mutations may not be appreciable, however under certain conditions for example, the neonatal period, activation of oxidative stress such as during nfection, a hypoxemia-ischemia, an acidosis, reception of some medicament, influence of toxins, point mutations in proteins and enzymes of erythrocytes can lead to premature destruction of erytrocytes, development of intravascular hemolysis and hemolytic anemia. Hence, erytrhrocyte enzyme deficiency should be considered in patients with hemolytic anaemia. Extended molecular analysis is useful for studying how several interacting gene mutations contribute to the clinical variability of erytrocytes enzymes deficiency.

4. References

Abrusci P., Chiarelli L.R., Galizzi A., Fermo E., Bianchi P., Zanella A. & Valentini G. (2007) Erythrocyte adenylate kinase deficiency: characterization of recombinant mutant forms and relationship with nonspherocytic hemolytic anemia. *Exp Hematol.* Aug;35(8):1182-9.

Aisaki K., Aizawa S., Fujii H., Kanno J. & Kanno H. (2007) Glycolytic inhibition by mutation of pyruvate kinase gene increases oxidative stress and causes apoptosis of a pyruvate kinase deficient cell line. *Exp Hematol.* Aug;35(8):1190-200.

Al-Jishi E., Meyer B.F., Rashed M.S., Al-Essa M., Al-Hamed M.H., Sakati N., Sanjad S., Ozand P.T. & Kambouris M. (1999) Clinical, biochemical, and molecular characterization of patients with glutathione synthetase deficiency. *Clin Genet.* Jun;55(6):444-9.

Alfinito F., Ferraro F., Rocco S., De Vendittis E., Piccirillo G., Sementa A., Colombo M.B., Zanella A. & Rotoli B. (1994) Glucose phosphate isomerase (GPI) "Morcone": a new variant from Italy.*Eur J Haematol.* May;52(5):263-6.

Al-Hassnan Z.N., Al Budhaim M., Al-Owain M., Lach B., Al-Dhalaan H. (2007) Muscle phosphofructokinase deficiency with neonatal seizures and nonprogressive course. *J Child Neurol.* Jan;22(1):106-8.

Babu G.N., Kumar A., Chandra R., Puri S.K., Singh R.L., Kalita J. & Misra U.K. (2008) Oxidant-antioxidant imbalance in the erythrocytes of sporadic amyotrophic lateral sclerosis patients correlates with the progression of disease. *Neurochem Int.* May;52(6):1284-9.

Beck M.A., Esworthy R.S., Ho Y.S. & Chu FF. (1998) Glutathione peroxidase protects mice from viral-induced myocarditis. *FASEB J.* Sep;12(12):1143-9.

Beulter E. (1996) G6PD: population genetics and clinical manifestations. *Blood Rev* Mar;10 (1):45-52.

Beutler E. & Gelbart T. (2000) Estimating the prevalence of pyruvate kinase deficiency from the gene frequency in the general white population. *Blood.* Jun 1;95(11):3585-8.

Bianchi M., Crinelli R., Serafini G., Giammarini C. & Magnani M. (1997) Molecular bases of hexokinase deficiency. *Biochim Biophys Acta.* May 24;1360(3):211-21.

Bianchi M. & Magnani M. (1995) Hexokinase mutations that produce nonspherocytic hemolytic anemia. *Blood Cells Mol Dis.* 21(1):2-8.

Bonnefond A., Vaxillaire M., Labrune Y., Lecoeur C., Chèvre J.C., Bouatia-Naji N., Cauchi S., Balkau B., Marre M., Tichet J., Riveline J.P., Hadjadj S., Gallois Y., Czernichow S., Hercberg S., Kaakinen M., Wiesner S., Charpentier G., Lévy-Marchal C., Elliott P., Jarvelin M.R., Horber F., Dina C., Pedersen O., Sladek R., Meyre D. & Froguel P. (2009) Genetic variant in HK1 is associated with a proanemic state and A1C but not other glycemic control-related traits. *Diabetes.* Nov;58(11):2687-97.

Boulard-Heitzmann P., Boulard M., Tallineau C., Boivin P., Tanzer J., Bois M. & Barriere M. (1984) Decreased red cell enolase activity in a 40-year-old woman with compensated haemolysis. *Scand J Haematol.* Nov;33(5):401-4.

Burstedt M.S., Ristoff E., Larsson A. & Wachtmeister L. (2009) Rod-cone dystrophy with maculopathy in genetic glutathione synthetase deficiency: a morphologic and electrophysiologic study. *Ophthalmology.* Feb;116(2):324-31

Caprari P., Caforio M.P., Cianciulli P., Maffi D., Pasquino M.T., Tarzia A., Amadori S. & Salvati A.M.(2001) 6-Phosphogluconate dehydrogenase deficiency in an Italian family. *Ann Hematol.* Jan;80(1):41-4).

Carruthers A., DeZutter J., Ganguly A. & Devaskar S.U. (2009) Will the original glucose transporter isoform please stand up! *Am J Physiol Endocrinol Metab.* Oct;297(4):E836-48.

Casado A., Casado C., López-Fernández E. & de la Torre R. (1995) Enzyme deficiencies in neonates with jaundice. *Panminerva Med.* Dec;37(4):175-7.

Casp C.B., She J.X. & McCormack W.T. (2002) Genetic association of the catalase gene (CAT) with vitiligo susceptibility.*Pigment Cell Res.* Feb;15(1):62-6.

Chiarelli L.R., Fermo E., Zanella A. & Valentini G. (2006) Hereditary erythrocyte pyrimidine 5'-nucleotidase deficiency: a biochemical, genetic and clinical overview. *Hematology.* Feb;11(1):67-72.

Cohen-Solal M., Valentin C., Plassa F., Guillemin G., Danze F., Jaisson F. & Rosa R. (1994) Identification of new mutations in two phosphoglycerate kinase (PGK) variants expressing different clinical syndromes: PGK Créteil and PGK Amiens. *Blood.* Aug 1;84(3):898-903.

Colell A., Green D.R. & Ricci J.E. (2009) Novel roles for GAPDH in cell death and carcinogenesis. *Cell Death Differ.* Dec;16(12):1573-81.

Corrons J.L., Alvarez R., Pujades A., Zarza R., Oliva E., Lasheras G., Callis M., Ribes A., Gelbart T. & Beutler E. (2001) Hereditary non-spherocytic haemolytic anaemia due to red blood cell glutathione synthetase deficiency in four unrelated patients from Spain: clinical and molecular studies.*Br J Haematol.* Feb;112(2):475-82.

Cova E., Bongioanni P., Cereda C., Metelli M.R., Salvaneschi L., Bernuzzi S., Guareschi S., Rossi B. & Ceroni M. (2010) Time course of oxidant markers and antioxidant defenses in subgroups of amyotrophic lateral sclerosis patients. *Neurochem Int.* Apr;56(5):687-93.

Cova E., Ghiroldi A., Guareschi S., Mazzini G., Gagliardi S., Davin A., Bianchi M., Ceroni M. & Cereda C. (2010) G93A SOD1 alters cell cycle in a cellular model of Amyotrophic Lateral Sclerosis. *Cell Signal.* Oct;22(10):1477-84

Dahl N., Pigg M., Ristoff E., Gali R., Carlsson B., Mannervik B., Larsson A. & Board P. (1997) Missense mutations in the human glutathione synthetase gene result in severe metabolic acidosis, 5-oxoprolinuria, hemolytic anemia and neurological dysfunction. *Hum Mol Genet.* Jul;6(7):1147-52.

de Atauri P., Repiso A., Oliva B., Vives-Corrons J.L., Climent F. & Carreras J. (2005) Characterization of the first described mutation of human red blood cell phosphoglycerate mutase. *Biochim Biophys Acta.* Jun 10;1740(3):403-10.

de Vooght K.M., van Solinge W.W., van Wesel A.C., Kersting S. & van Wijk R. (2009) First mutation in the red blood cell-specific promoter of hexokinase combined with a novel missense mutation causes hexokinase deficiency and mild chronic hemolysis. *Haematologica.* Sep;94(9):1203-10.

del Grande A., Luigetti M., Conte A., Mancuso I., Lattante S., Marangi G., Stipa G., Zollino M. & Sabatelli M. (2011) A novel L67P SOD1 mutation in an Italian ALS patient. *Amyotroph Lateral Scler.* Mar;12(2):150-2.

Dimastrogiovanni D., Anselmi M., Miele A.E., Boumis G., Petersson L., Angelucci F., Nola A.D., Brunori M. & Bellelli A. (2010) Combining crystallography and molecular dynamics: the case of Schistosoma mansoni phospholipid glutathione peroxidase. *Proteins.* Feb 1;78(2):259-70.

el-Hazmi M.A. & Warsy A.S. (1989) Glutathione reductase in the south-western province of Saudi Arabia--genetic variation vs. acquired deficiency *Haematologia (Budap).* 22(1):37-42.

Esposito G., Vitagliano L., Costanzo P., Borrelli L., Barone R., Pavone L., Izzo .P, Zagari A. & Salvatore F. (2004) Human aldolase A natural mutants: relationship between flexibility of the C-terminal region and enzyme function. *Biochem J.* May 15;380(Pt 1):51-6.

Esposito G., Vitagliano L., Costanzo P., Borrelli L., Barone R., Pavone L., Izzo P., Zagari A. & Salvatore F. (2004) Human aldolase A natural mutants: relationship between flexibility of the C-terminal region and enzyme function. *Biochem J.* May 15;380(Pt 1):51-6.

Etiemble J, Simeon J, Buc HA, Picat C, Boulard M, Boivin P. A liver-type mutation in a case of pronounced erythrocyte phosphofructokinase deficiency without clinical expression. *Biochim Biophys Acta.* 1983 Sep 13;759(3):236-42.

Flanagan J.M., Rhodes M., Wilson M. & Beutler E. (2006) The identification of a recurrent phosphoglycerate kinase mutation associated with chronic haemolytic anaemia and neurological dysfunction in a family from USA. *Br J Haematol.* Jul;134(2):233-7.

Flatt J.F., Guizouarn H., Burton N.M., Borgese F., Tomlinson R.J., Forsyth R.J., Baldwin S.A., Levinson B.E., Quittet P., Aguilar-Martinez P., Delaunay J., Stewart G.W., & Bruce L.J. (2011) Stomatin-deficient cryohydrocytosis results from mutations in SLC2A1: a novel form of GLUT1 deficiency syndrome. *Blood.* Jul. 26 Available from: <http://bloodjournal.hematologylibrary.org/content/early/2011/07/26/blood-2010-12-326645.full.pdf+html>

Fogelfeld L., Sarova-Pinchas I., Meytes D., Barash V., Brok-Simoni F. & Feigl D. (1990) Phosphofructokinase deficiency (Tarui disease) associated with hepatic glucuronyltransferase deficiency (Gilbert's syndrome): a case and family study. *Isr J Med Sci.*Jun;26(6):328-33.

Frank J.E. (2005) Diagnosis and management of G6PD deficiency. *Am Fam Physician*. Oct 1;72(7):1277-82.

Fujii H., Kanno H., Hirono A., Shiomura T. & Miwa S. (1992) A single amino acid substitution (157 Gly----Val) in a phosphoglycerate kinase variant (PGK Shizuoka) associated with chronic hemolysis and myoglobinuria. *Blood*. Mar 15;79(6):1582-5.

García M., Pujol A., Ruzo A., Riu E., Ruberte J., Arbós A., Serafín A., Albella B., Felíu J.E. & Bosch F. (2009) Phosphofructo-1-kinase deficiency leads to a severe cardiac and hematological disorder in addition to skeletal muscle glycogenosis. *PLoS Genet*. Aug;5(8):e1000615.

Giannini F., Battistini S., Mancuso M., Greco G., Ricci C., Volpi N., Del Corona A., Piazza S. & Siciliano G. (2010) D90A-SOD1 mutation in ALS: The first report of heterozygous Italian patients and unusual findings. *Amyotroph Lateral Scler*. 2010;11(1-2):216-9.

Gondo H., Ideguchi H., Hayashi S. & Shibuya T. (1992) Acute hemolysis in glutathione peroxidase deficiency. *Int J Hematol*. Jun;55(3):215-8.

Góth L. & Bigler N.W. (2007) Catalase deficiency may complicate urate oxidase (rasburicase) therapy.*Free Radic Res*. Sep;41(9):953-5.

Góth L., Rass P. & Páy A. (2004) Catalase enzyme mutations and their association with diseases.*Mol Diagn*. 8(3):141-9.

Góth L. & Vitai M. (1999) Hungarian hereditary acatalasemia and hypocatalasemia are not associated with chronic hemolysis. *Clin Chim Acta*. Jan 16;233(1-2):75-9.

Góth L. & Vitai M. (2003) The effects of hydrogen peroxide promoted by homocysteine and inherited catalase deficiency on human hypocatalasemic patients. *Free Radic Biol Med*. Oct 15;35(8):882-8.

Guis M.S., Karadsheh N. & Mentzer W.C. (1987) Phosphoglycerate kinase San Francisco: a new variant associated with hemolytic anemia but not with neuromuscular manifestations. *Am J Hematol*. Jun;25(2):175-82.

Haller J.F., Krawczyk S.A., Gostilovitch L., Corkey B.E. & Zoeller R.A. (2011) Glucose-6-phosphate isomerase deficiency results in mTOR activation, failed translocation of lipin 1α to the nucleus and hypersensitivity to glucose: Implications for the inherited glycolytic disease. *Biochim Biophys Acta*. Jul 22; Available from: <http://www.sciencedirect.com/science/article/pii/S0925443911001608 >.

Haller J.F., Smith C., Liu D., Zheng H., Tornheim K., Han G.S., Carman G.M. & Zoeller R.A. (2010) Isolation of novel animal cell lines defective in glycerolipid biosynthesis reveals mutations in glucose-6-phosphate isomerase. *J Biol Chem*. 2010 Jan 8;285(2):866-77.

Haller J.F., Smith C., Liu D., Zheng H., Tornheim K., Han G.S., Carman G.M., Zoeller R.A. Lin H.Y., Kao Y.H., Chen S.T. & Meng M. (2009) Effects of inherited mutations on catalytic activity and structural stability of human glucose-6-phosphate isomerase expressed in Escherichia coli. *Biochim Biophys Acta*. Feb;1794(2):315-23.

Harry S. Jacobt, Sidney H. Ingbar, James H. Jandl & Susan C. (1965) Bell Oxidative Hemolysis and Erythrocyte Metabolism in Hereditary Acatalasia *Journal of Clinical Investigation* (44)7:1187-99.

He W., Wang Y., Liu W. & Zhou C.Z. (2007) Crystal structure of Saccharomyces cerevisiae 6-phosphogluconate dehydrogenase Gnd1.*BMC Struct Biol* Jun 14; Vol. 7, pp. 38-47.

Hirono A., Iyori H., Sekine I., Ueyama J., Chiba H., Kanno H., Fujii H. & Miwa S. (1996) Three cases of hereditary nonspherocytic hemolytic anemia associated with red blood cell glutathione deficiency. *Blood*. 1996 Mar 1;87(5):2071-4.

Hirono A., Sasaya-Hamada F., Kanno H., Fujii H., Yoshida T. & Miwa S. (1995) A novel human catalase mutation (358 T-->del) causing Japanese-type acatalasemia. *Blood Cells Mol Dis*. 21(3):232-4.

Hjelm M., Wadam B. & Yoshida A. (1980) A phosphoglycerate kinase variant, PGK Uppsala, associated with hemolytic anemia. *J Lab Clin Med*. Dec;96(6):1015-21.

Huang I.Y., Fujii H. & Yoshida A. (1980) Structure and function of normal and variant human phosphoglycerate kinase. *Hemoglobin*. 4(5-6):601-9.

Huppke P., Wünsch D., Pekrun A., Kind R., Winkler H., Schröter W. & Lakomek M. (1997) Glucose phosphate isomerase deficiency: biochemical and molecular genetic studies on the enzyme variants of two patients with severe haemolytic anaemia.*Eur J Pediatr*. Aug;156(8):605-9.

Ingrosso D., Cimmino A., D'Angelo S., Alfinito F., Zappia V. & Galletti P. (2002) Protein methylation as a marker of aspartate damage in glucose-6-phosphate dehydrogenase-deficient erythrocytes: role of oxidative stress. *Eur J Biochem*. Apr;269(8):2032-9.

Ip P., Mulligan V.K. & Chakrabartty A. (2011) ALS-causing SOD1 mutations promote production of copper-deficient misfolded species. *J Mol Biol*. Jun 24;409(5):839-52.

Iuchi Y., Kibe N., Tsunoda S., Suzuki S., Mikami T., Okada F., Uchida K. & Fujii J. (2010) Implication of oxidative stress as a cause of autoimmune hemolytic anemia in NZB mice. *Free Radic Biol Med*. Apr 1;48(7):935-44.

Iuchi Y., Okada F., Onuma K., Onoda T., Asao H., Kobayashi M. & Fujii J. (2007) Elevated oxidative stress in erythrocytes due to a SOD1 deficiency causes anaemia and triggers autoantibody production. *Biochem J*. Mar 1;402(2):219-27.

Iuchi Y., Okada F., Takamiya R., Kibe N., Tsunoda S., Nakajima O., Toyoda K., Nagae R., Suematsu M., Soga T., Uchida K. & Fujii J. (2009) Rescue of anaemia and autoimmune responses in SOD1-deficient mice by transgenic expression of human SOD1 in erythrocytes. *Biochem J*. Aug 13;422(2):313-20.

Iyori H., Hirono A., Kobayashi N., Ishitoya N., Akatsuka J., Kanno H., Fujii H. & Miwa S. (1996) Glutathione synthetase deficiency. *Rinsho Ketsueki*. Apr;37(4):329-34.

Jain A., Buist N.R., Kennaway N.G., Powell B.R., Auld P.A. & Mårtensson J. (1994) Effect of ascorbate or N-acetylcysteine treatment in a patient with hereditary glutathione synthetase deficiency. *J Pediatr*. Feb;124(2):229-33.

Jokic N., Yip P.K., Michael-Titus A., Priestley J.V. & Malaspina A. (2010) The human G93A-SOD1 mutation in a pre-symptomatic rat model of amyotrophic lateral sclerosis increases the vulnerability to a mild spinal cord compression. *BMC Genomics*. Nov 15;11:633.

Kamerbeek N.M., van Zwieten R., de Boer M., Morren G., Vuil H., Bannink N., Lincke C., Dolman K.M., Becker K., Schirmer R.H., Gromer S. & Roos D. (2007) Molecular basis of glutathione reductase deficiency in human blood cells. *Blood*. Apr 15;109(8):3560-6.

Kanno H., Fujii H., Hirono A., Ishida Y., Ohga S., Fukumoto Y., Matsuzawa K., Ogawa S. & Miwa S.(1996) Molecular analysis of glucose phosphate isomerase deficiency associated with hereditary hemolytic anemia. *Blood*. Sep 15;88(6):2321-5.

Kanno H. (2000) Hexokinase: gene structure and mutations. *Baillieres Best Pract Res Clin Haematol*. Mar;13(1):83-8.

Kedar P., Hamada T., Warang P., Nadkarni A., Shimizu K., Fujji H., Ghosh K., Kanno H. & Colah R. (2009) Spectrum of novel mutations in the human PKLR gene in pyruvate kinase-deficient Indian patients with heterogeneous clinical phenotypes. *Clin Genet*. Feb;75(2):157-62.

Kikumoto Y., Sugiyama H., Inoue T., Morinaga H., Takiue K., Kitagawa M., Fukuoka N., Saeki M., Maeshima Y., Wang D.H., Ogino K., Masuoka N. & Makino H. (2010) Sensitization to alloxan-induced diabetes and pancreatic cell apoptosis in acatalasemic mice. *Biochim Biophys Acta.* Feb;1802(2):240-6.

Kiriyama T., Wakamatsu M., Furuta M., Kato H. & Ono K. (1993) Anesthesia for a patient with red cell aldolase deficiency. *Masui.* May;42(5):750-2.

Kishi H., Mukai T., Hirono A., Fujii H., Miwa S. & Hori K. (1987) Human aldolase A deficiency associated with a hemolytic anemia: thermolabile aldolase due to a single base mutation. *Proc Natl Acad Sci U S A.* Dec;84(23):8623-7.

Klepper J., Willemsen M., Verrips A., Guertsen E., Herrmann R., Kutzick C., Flörcken A. & Voit T. (2001) Autosomal dominant transmission of GLUT1 deficiency. *Hum Mol Genet.* Jan 1;10(1):63-8.

Kondo T. (1990) Impaired glutathione metabolism in hemolytic anemia. *Rinsho Byori.* Apr;38(4):355-9.

Kreuder J., Borkhardt A., Repp R., Pekrun A., Göttsche B., Gottschalk U., Reichmann H., Schachenmayr W., Schlegel K. & Lampert F. (1996) Brief report: inherited metabolic myopathy and hemolysis due to a mutation in aldolase A. *N Engl J Med.* Apr 25;334(17):1100-4.

Krietsch W.K., Eber S.W., Haas B., Ruppelt W. & Kuntz G.W. (1980) Characterization of a phosphoglycerate kinase deficiency variants not associated with hemolytic anemia. *Am J Hum Genet.* May;32(3):364-73.

Kugler W., Breme K., Laspe P., Muirhead H., Davies C., Winkler H., Schröter W. & Lakomek M. (1998) Molecular basis of neurological dysfunction coupled with haemolytic anaemia in human glucose-6-phosphate isomerase (GPI) deficiency. *Hum Genet.* Oct;103(4):450-4.

Kugler W. & Lakomek M. (2000) Glucose-6-phosphate isomerase deficiency. *Baillieres Best Pract Res Clin Haematol.* 2000 Mar;13(1):89-101.

Lachant N.A., Jennings M.A. & Tanaka K.R. (1986) Partial erythrocyte enolase deficiency: a hereditary disorder with variable clinical expression. *Blood* 1986; 65: 55A.

Lee T.H., Kim S.U., Yu S.L., Kim S.H., Park D.S., Moon HB, Dho SH, Kwon KS, Kwon HJ, Han YH, Jeong S, Kang SW, Shin HS, Lee KK, Rhee SG &Yu D Y. (2003) Peroxiredoxin II is essential for sustaining life span of erythrocytes in mice. *Blood.* 2003 Jun 15;101(12):5033-8.

Low F.M., Hampton M.B. & Winterbourn CC. (2008) Peroxiredoxin 2 and peroxide metabolism in the erythrocyte. *Antioxid Redox Signal.* Sep;10(9):1621-30.

Lubos E., Kelly N.J., Oldebeken S.R., Leopold J.A., Zhang Y.Y., Loscalzo J. & Handy DE. (2011) Glutathione Peroxidase-1 (GPx-1) deficiency augments pro-inflammatory cytokine-induced redox signaling and human endothelial cell activation. *J Biol Chem.* Aug 18; Available from: <http://www.jbc.org/content/early/2011/08/18/jbc.M110.205708.full.pdf+html >.

Lubos E., Loscalzo J. & Handy D.E. (2011) Glutathione peroxidase-1 in health and disease: from molecular mechanisms to therapeutic opportunities. *Antioxid Redox Signal.* Oct 1;15(7):1957-97.

Luigetti MIO, Conte AIO, Madia FIO, Marangi G., Zollino M., Mancuso I., Dileone M., Del Grande A., Di Lazzaro V., Tonali P.A. & Sabatelli M. (2009) Heterozygous SOD1 D90A mutation presenting as slowly progressive predominant upper motor neuron amyotrophic lateral sclerosis. *Neurol Sci.* Dec;30(6):517-20.

Madhoun M.F., Maple J.T. & Comp P.C. (2011) Phosphofructokinase deficiency and portal and mesenteric vein thrombosis. *Am J Med Sci.* May;341(5):417-9.

Maeda M. & Yoshida A. (1991) Molecular defect of a phosphoglycerate kinase variant (PGK-Matsue) associated with hemolytic anemia: Leu----Pro substitution caused by T/A---C/G transition in exon 3. *Blood*. Mar 15;77(6):1348-52.

Magnani M., Stocchi V., Cucchiarini L., Novelli G., Lodi S., Isa L. & Fornaini G. (1985) Hereditary nonspherocytic hemolytic anemia due to a new hexokinase variant with reduced stability. *Blood*. Sep;66(3):690-7.

Mason P. J., Bautista J. M., & Gilsanz, F. (2007) G6PD deficiency the genotype-phenotype association. *Blood Rev*. 21, 267–283.

Masuoka N., Kodama H., Abe T., Wang D.H. & Nakano T. (2003) Characterization of hydrogen peroxide removal reaction by hemoglobin in the presence of reduced pyridine nucleotides. *Biochim Biophys Acta*. Jan 20;1637(1):46-54.

Masuoka N., Sugiyama H, Ishibashi N, Wang DH, Masuoka T, Kodama H, Nakano T.(2006) Characterization of acatalasemic erythrocytes treated with low and high dose hydrogen peroxide. Hemolysis and aggregation. *J Biol Chem*. Aug 4;281(31):21728-34.

Mazzola J.L. & Sirover MA. (2001) Reduction of glyceraldehyde-3-phosphate dehydrogenase activity in Alzheimer's disease and in Huntington's disease fibroblasts. *J Neurochem*. Jan;76(2):442-9.

Merkle S. & Pretsch W. (1992) A glucosephosphate isomerase (GPI) null mutation in Mus musculus: evidence that anaerobic glycolysis is the predominant energy delivering pathway in early post-implantation embryos. *Comp Biochem Physiol B*. Mar;101(3):309-14.

Merkle S. & Pretsch W. (1993) Glucose-6-phosphate isomerase deficiency associated with nonspherocytic hemolytic anemia in the mouse: an animal model for the human disease. *Blood*. Jan 1;81(1):206-13.

Minucci A., Giardina B., Zuppi C. & Capoluongo E. (2009) Glucose-6-phosphate dehydrogenase laboratory assay: How, when, and why? *IUBMB Life*. Jan;61(1):27-34.

Miwa S., Fujii H., Tani K., Takahashi K., Takegawa S., Fujinami N., Sakurai M., Kubo M., Tanimoto Y., Kato T. & Matsumoto N. (1981) Two cases of red cell aldolase deficiency associated with hereditary hemolytic anemia in a Japanese family. *Am J Hematol*. Dec;11(4):425-37.

Mojzikova R., Dolezel P., Pavlicek J., Mlejnek P., Pospisilova D. & Divoky V. (2010) Partial glutathione reductase deficiency as a cause of diverse clinical manifestations in a family with unstable hemoglobin (Hemoglobin Haná, β63(E7) His-Asn). *Blood Cells Mol Dis*. Oct 15;45(3):219-22.

Murakami K., Kanno H., Tancabelic J. & Fujii H. (2002) Gene expression and biological significance of hexokinase in erythroid cells. *Acta Haematol*. 108(4):204-9.

Nakajima H., Raben N., Hamaguchi T. & Yamasaki T. (2002) Phosphofructokinase deficiency; past, present and future. *Curr Mol Med*. Mar;2(2):197-212.

Nakashima K., Yamauchi K., Miwa S., Fujimura K., Mizutani A. & Kuramoto A. (1978) Glutathione reductase deficiency in a kindred with hereditary spherocytosis. *Am J Hematol*. 4(2):141-50.

Neubauer B.A., Eber S.W., Lakomek M., Gahr M. & Schröter W. (1990) Combination of congenital nonspherocytic haemolytic anaemia and impairment of granulocyte function in severe glucosephosphate isomerase deficiency. A new variant enzyme designated GPI Calden. *Acta Haematol*. 83(4):206-10.

Neumann C.A., Krause D.S., Carman C.V., Das S., Dubey D.P., Abraham J.L., Bronson R.T., Fujiwara Y., Orkin S.H. & Van Etten R.A. (2003) Essential role for the peroxiredoxin Prdx1 in erythrocyte antioxidant defence and tumour suppression. *Nature*. Jul 31;424(6948):561-5.

Njålsson R. & Norgren S. (2005) Physiological and pathological aspects of GSH metabolism. *Acta Paediatr*. Feb;94(2):132-7.

Njålsson R. & Ristoff E., Carlsson K., Winkler A., Larsson A. & Norgren S. (2005) Genotype, enzyme activity, glutathione level, and clinical phenotype in patients with glutathione synthetase deficiency. *Hum Genet*. Apr;116(5):384-9

Njålsson R. (2005) Glutathione synthetase deficiency. *Cell Mol Life Sci*. Sep;62(17):1938-45.

Noel N., Flanagan J.M., Ramirez Bajo M.J., Kalko S.G., Mañú Mdel M., Garcia Fuster J.L., Perez de la Ossa P., Carreras J., Beutler E. & Vives Corrons JL. (2006) Two new phosphoglycerate kinase mutations associated with chronic haemolytic anaemia and neurological dysfunction in two patients from Spain. *Br J Haematol*. Feb;132(4):523-9.

Ogata M., Wang D.H. & Ogino K. (2008) Mammalian acatalasemia: the perspectives of bioinformatics and genetic toxicology. *Acta Med Okayama*. Dec;62(6):345-61.

Padua R.A., Bulfield G. & Peters J. (1978) Biochemical genetics of a new glucosephosphate isomerase allele (Gpi-1c) from wild mice. *Biochem Genet*. 1978 Feb;16(1-2):127-43.

Pederzolli C.D., Mescka C.P., Zandoná B.R., de Moura Coelho D., Sgaravatti A.M., Sgarbi M.B., de Souza Wyse A.T., Duval Wannmacher C.M., Wajner M., Vargas C.R. & Dutra-Filho C.S. (2010) Acute administration of 5-oxoproline induces oxidative damage to lipids and proteins and impairs antioxidant defenses in cerebral cortex and cerebellum of young rats. *Metab Brain Dis*. Jun;25(2):145-54.

Perseu L., Giagu N., Satta S., Sollaino M.C., Congiu R. & Galanello R. (2010) Red cell pyruvate kinase deficiency in Southern Sardinia. *Blood Cells Mol Dis*. Dec 15;45(4):280-3.

Pissard S., Max-Audit I., Skopinski L., Vasson A., Vivien P., Bimet C., Goossens M., Galacteros F. (2006) Wajcman H. Pyruvate kinase deficiency in France: a 3-year study reveals 27 new mutations. *Br J Haematol*. Jun;133(6):683-9.

Polekhina G., Board P.G., Gali R.R., Rossjohn J. & Parker M.W. Molecular basis of glutathione synthetase deficiency and a rare gene permutation event. *EMBO J*. 1999 Jun 15;18(12):3204-13.

Pretsch W & Merkle S. (1990) Glucose phosphate isomerase enzyme-activity mutants in Mus musculus: genetical and biochemical characterization. *Biochem Genet*. Feb;28(1-2):97-110.

Raben N., Exelbert R., Spiegel R., Sherman J.B., Nakajima H., Plotz P. & Heinisch J. (1995) Functional expression of human mutant phosphofructokinase in yeast: genetic defects in French Canadian and Swiss patients with phosphofructokinase deficiency. *Am J Hum Genet*. Jan;56(1):131-41.

Ramírez-Bajo M.J., Repiso A., la Ossa P.P, Bañón-Maneus E., de Atauri P., Climent F., Corrons J.L., Cascante M. & Carreras J. (2011) Enzymatic andmetabolic characterization of the phosphoglycerate kinase deficiency associated with chronic hemolytic anemia caused by the PGK-Barcelona mutation. *Blood Cells Mol Dis*. Mar 15;46(3):206-11.

Repiso A, Oliva B, Vives Corrons JL, Carreras J, Climent F. Glucose phosphate isomerase deficiency: enzymatic and familial characterization of Arg346His mutation. *Biochim Biophys Acta*. 2005 Jun 10;1740(3):467-71

Repiso A., Oliva B., Vives-Corrons J.L., Beutler E., Carreras J. & Climent F. (2006) Red cell glucose phosphate isomerase (GPI): a molecular study of three novel mutations associated with hereditary nonspherocytic hemolytic anemia. *Hum Mutat*. Nov;27(11):1159.

Repiso A., Ramirez Bajo M.J., Corrons J.L., Carreras J. & Climent F. (2005) Phosphoglycerate mutase BB isoenzyme deficiency in a patient with non-spherocytic anemia: familial and metabolic studies. *Haematologica*. Feb;90(2):257-9.

Rijksen G., Akkerman J.W., van den Wall Bake A.W., Hofstede D.P. & Staal G.E. (1983) Generalized hexokinase deficiency in the blood cells of a patient with nonspherocytic hemolytic anemia. *Blood*. Jan;61(1):12-8.

Ristoff E. & Larsson A. (2007) Inborn errors in the metabolism of glutathione. *Orphanet J Rare Dis*. Mar 30;2:16.

Ristoff E., Mayatepek E. & Larsson A. (2001) Long-term clinical outcome in patients with glutathione synthetase deficiency. *J Pediatr*. Jul;139(1):79-84.

Ronquist G., Rudolphi O., Engström I. & Waldenström A. (2001) Familial phosphofructokinase deficiency is associated with a disturbed calcium homeostasis in erythrocytes. *J Intern Med*. Jan;249(1):85-95.

Rossi F., Ruggiero S., Gallo M., Simeone G., Matarese S.M. & Nobili B. (2010) Amoxicillin-induced hemolytic anemia in a child with glucose 6-phosphate isomerase deficiency. *Ann Pharmacother*. Jul-Aug;44(7-8):1327-9.

Schneider S.A., Paisan-Ruiz C., Garcia-Gorostiaga I., Quinn N.P., Weber Y.G., Lerche H., Hardy J. & Bhatia K.P. (2009) GLUT1 gene mutations cause sporadic paroxysmal exercise-induced dyskinesias. *Mov Disord*. Aug 15;24(11):1684-8.

Shalev O., Leibowitz G. & Brok-Simoni F. (1994) Glucose phosphate isomerase deficiency with congenital nonspherocytic hemolytic anemia. *Harefuah*. Jun 15;126(12):699-702, 764, 763.

Shi P., Wei Y., Zhang J., Gal J. & Zhu H. (2010) Mitochondrial dysfunction is a converging point of multiple pathological pathways in amyotrophic lateral sclerosis. *J Alzheimers Dis*. 20 Suppl 2:S311-24.

Shi Z.Z., Habib G.M., Rhead W.J., Gahl W.A., He X., Sazer S. & Lieberman M.W. (1996) Mutations in the glutathione synthetase gene cause 5-oxoprolinuria. *Nat Genet*. Nov;14(3):361-5.

Simon E., Vogel M., Fingerhut R., Ristoff E., Mayatepek E. & Spiekerkötter U. (2009) Diagnosis of glutathione synthetase deficiency in newborn screening. *J Inherit Metab Dis*. 2009 Sep 2. Available from: <http://www.ncbi.nlm.nih.gov/pubmed/19728142 >.

Sirover M.A. (2005) New nuclear functions of the glycolytic protein, glyceraldehyde-3-phosphate dehydrogenase, in mammalian cells. *J Cell Biochem*. May 1;95(1):45-52.

Sirover M.A. (2011) On the functional diversity of glyceraldehyde-3-phosphate dehydrogenase: biochemical mechanisms and regulatory control. *Biochim Biophys Acta*. Aug;1810(8):741-51.

Sirover M.A. (1997) Role of the glycolytic protein, glyceraldehyde-3-phosphate dehydrogenase, in normal cell function and in cell pathology. *J Cell Biochem*. Aug 1;66(2):133-40.

Skibild E., Dahlgaard K., Rajpurohit Y., Smith B.F. & Giger U. (2001) Haemolytic anaemia and exercise intolerance due to phosphofructokinase deficiency in related springer spaniels. *J Small Anim Pract*. Jun;42(6):298-300.

Sodiende, O. (1992) Glucose-6-phosphate dehydrogenase deficiency. *Ballieres Clin. Haematol*. 5, 367–382.

Spalloni A., Origlia N., Sgobio C., Trabalza A., Nutini M., Berretta N., Bernardi G., Domenici L., Ammassari-Teule M. & Longone P. (2011) Postsynaptic alteration of NR2A subunit and defective autophosphorylation of alphaCaMKII at threonine-286 contribute to abnormal plasticity and morphology of upper motor neurons in presymptomatic SOD1G93A mice, a murine model for amyotrophic lateral sclerosis. *Cereb Cortex*. Apr;21(4):796-805.

Starzyński R.R., Canonne-Hergaux F., Willemetz A., Gralak M.A., Woliński J., Styś A., Olszak J. & Lipiński P. (2009) Haemolytic anaemia and alterations in hepatic iron metabolism in aged mice lacking Cu,Zn-superoxide dismutase. *Biochem J*. May 27;420(3):383-90.

Stefanini M. (1972) Chronic hemolytic anemia associated with erythrocyte enolase deficiency exacerbated by ingestion of nitrofurantoin. *Am J Clin Pathol*. Oct;58(4):408-14.

Syriani E., Morales M. & Gamez J. (2009)The p.E22G mutation in the Cu/Zn superoxide-dismutase gene predicts a long survival time: clinical and genetic characterization of a seven-generation ALS1 Spanish pedigree. *J Neurol Sci*. Oct 15;285(1-2):46-53.

Takapoo M., Chamseddine A.H., Bhalla R.C. & Miller F.J. (2011) Glutathione peroxidase-deficient smooth muscle cells cause paracrine activation of normal smooth muscle cells via cyclophilin A. *Vascul Pharmacol*. Jul 12. Available from: <http://www.ncbi.nlm.nih.gov/pubmed/21782974 >.

Tang T.S., Prior S.L., Li K.W., Ireland H.A., Bain S.C., Hurel S.J., Cooper J.A., Humphries S.E. & Stephens J.W. (2010) Association between the rs1050450 glutathione peroxidase-1 (C > T) gene variant and peripheral neuropathy in two independent samples of subjects with diabetes mellitus. *Nutr Metab Cardiovasc Dis*. 2010 Dec 23. Available from: <http://www.ncbi.nlm.nih.gov/pubmed/21185702 >.

Tatton W.G., Chalmers-Redman R.M., Elstner M., Leesch W., Jagodzinski F.B., Stupak D.P., Sugrue M.M. &, Tatton N.A. (2000) Glyceraldehyde-3-phosphate dehydrogenase in neurodegeneration and apoptosis signaling. *J Neural Transm Suppl*. (60):77-100.

Uchida H.A., Sugiyama H., Takiue K., Kikumoto Y., Inoue T. & Makino H. (2011) Development of Angiotensin II-induced Abdominal Aortic Aneurysms Is Independent of Catalase in Mice. *J Cardiovasc Pharmacol*. Aug 31. Available from:< http://www.ncbi.nlm.nih.gov/pubmed/21885993 >.

Valentin C., Birgens H., Craescu C.T., Brødum-Nielsen K. & Cohen-Solal M. (1998) A phosphoglycerate kinase mutant (PGK Herlev; D285V) in a Danish patient with isolated chronic hemolytic anemia: mechanism of mutation and structure-function relationships. *Hum Mutat*. 12(4):280-7.

van Wijk R., Rijksen G., Huizinga E.G., Nieuwenhuis H.K., & van Solinge W.W. (2003) HK Utrecht: missense mutation in the active site of human hexokinase associated with hexokinase deficiency and severe nonspherocytic hemolytic anemia. *Blood*. Jan 1;101(1):345-7.

Vitai M., Fátrai S., Rass P., Csordás M. & Tarnai I. Simple (2005) PCR heteroduplex, SSCP mutation screening methods for the detection of novel catalase mutations in Hungarian patients with type 2 diabetes mellitus.*Clin Chem Lab Med*. 43(12):1346-50.

Vives Corrons J.L., Colomer D., Pujades A., Rovira A., Aymerich M., Merino A. & Aguilar i Bascompte J.L. (1996) Congenital 6-phosphogluconate dehydrogenase (6PGD) deficiency associated with chronic hemolytic anemia in a Spanish family. *Am J Hematol*. Dec;53(4):221-7.

Vora S., Davidson M., Seaman C., Miranda A.F., Noble N.A., Tanaka K.R., Frenkel E.P. & Dimauro S. (1983) Heterogeneity of the molecular lesions in inherited phosphofructokinase deficiency. *J Clin Invest*. Dec;72(6):1995-2006.

Vora S., DiMauro S., Spear D., Harker D., & Danon M.J. (1987) Characterization of the enzymatic defect in late-onset muscle phosphofructokinase deficiency. New subtype of glycogen storage disease type VII. *J Clin Invest*. Nov;80(5):1479-85.

Vora S., Giger U., Turchen S., & Harvey J.W. (1985) Characterization of the enzymatic lesion in inherited phosphofructokinase deficiency in the dog: an animal analogue of human glycogen storage disease type VII. *Proc Natl Acad Sci U S A.* Dec;82(23):8109-13.

Wajcman H. & Galactéros F. (2004) Glucose 6-phosphate dehydrogenase deficiency: a protection against malaria and a risk for hemolytic accidents. *C R Biol.* Aug;327(8):711-20.

Warsy A.S. & el-Hazmi M.A. (1999) Glutathione reductase deficiency in Saudi Arabia. *East Mediterr Health J.* Nov;5(6):1208-12.

Webb G.C., Vaska V.L., Gali R.R., Ford J.H. & Board PG. (1995) The gene encoding human glutathione synthetase (GSS) maps to the long arm of chromosome 20 at band 11.2. *Genomics.* Dec 10;30(3):617-9.

Weber Y.G., Storch A., Wuttke T.V., Brockmann K., Kempfle J., Maljevic S., Margari L., Kamm C., Schneider S.A., Huber S.M., Pekrun A., Roebling R., Seebohm G., Koka S., Lang C., Kraft E., Blazevic D., Salvo-Vargas A., Fauler M., Mottaghy F.M., Münchau A., Edwards M.J., Presicci A., Margari F., Gasser T., Lang F., Bhatia K.P., Lehmann-Horn F. & Lerche H. (2008) GLUT1 mutations are a cause of paroxysmal exertion-induced dyskinesias and induce hemolytic anemia by a cation leak.*J Clin Invest.* Jun;118(6):2157-68.

West J.D., Flockhart J.H., Peters J. & Ball S.T. (1990) Death of mouse embryos that lack a functional gene for glucose phosphate isomerase. *Genet Res.* Oct-Dec;56(2-3):223-36.

Yamamoto M., Suzuki N., Hatakeyama N., Kubo N., Tachi N., Kanno H., Fujii H. & Tsutsumi H. (2007) Carbamazepine-induced hemolytic and aplastic crises associated with reduced glutathione peroxidase activity of erythrocytes. *Int J Hematol.* Nov;86(4):325-8.

Yao D.C., Tolan D.R., Murray M.F., Harris D.J., Darras B.T., Geva A. & Neufeld E.J. (2004) Hemolytic anemia and severe rhabdomyolysis caused by compound heterozygous mutations of the gene for erythrocyte/muscle isozyme of aldolase, ALDOA(Arg303X/Cys338Tyr). *Blood.* 2004 Mar 15;103(6):2401-3.

Yapicioğlu H., Satar M,. Tutak E., Narli N. &Topaloğlu A.K. (2009) A newborn infant with generalized glutathione synthetase deficiency. *Turk J Pediatr.* 2004 Jan-Mar;46(1):72-5.

Yu D., dos Santos C.O., Zhao G., Jiang J., Amigo J.D., Khandros E., Dore L.C., Yao Y., D'Souza J., Zhang Z., Ghaffari S., Choi J., Friend S., Tong W., Orange J.S., Paw B.H. & Weiss M.J. (2010) miR-451 protects against erythroid oxidant stress by repressing 14-3-3zeta. *Genes Dev.* Aug 1;24(15):1620-33.

Zanella A., Fermo E., Bianchi P. & Valentini G. (2005) Red cell pyruvate kinase deficiency: molecular and clinical aspects. *Br J Haematol.* Jul;130(1):11-25.

Zhao S., Choy B. & Kornblatt M. J. (2008) Effects of the G376E and G157D mutations on the stability of yeast enolase - a model for human muscle enolase deficiency*FEBS Journal* .275: 97–106.

12

Point Mutations in Ferroportin Disease: Genotype/Phenotype Correlation

Riad Akoum
University Medical Center – Rizk Hospital,
Lebanese American University, Beirut,
Lebanon

1. Introduction

The identification of gene mutations involved in the pathogenesis of hereditary hemochromatosis (HH) provided a better understanding of primary iron overload syndrome (Feder, 1996). HH is a genetic disorder characterized by increased dietary iron absorption despite an excess in iron stores. The result is a progressive increase in total body iron with abnormal iron deposition in the liver and the endocrine glands. Transferrin saturation and serum ferritin level are the most reliable tests for the detection of individuals with HH. Mutations in HLA-linked HFE gene result in the classical type 1 HH inherited in an autosomal recessive pattern. One major mutation, the C282Y is responsible for 85 to 90% of the cases with an estimated prevalence of 1 in 200 in Northern Europe. However, the bioclinical penetrance is incomplete and only a few suffer from overt disease. The second most common mutation is H63D and accounts for 3 to 5% of cases. Its relationship with HH is less obvious. Compound heterozygous H63D/C282Y genotype represents less than 1% and simple heterozygous genotype is not associated with biochemical abnormalities. Less common mutations in the transferrin receptor 2 (TfR2), hemojuvelin (HJV) and Hepcidin (HAMP) genes, also in the homozygous state, result in the type 2 and type 3 HH (Pietrangelo, 1999, 2007, 2010).

The non-HFE-related form caused by Ferroportin 1 (SLC40A1) gene mutation is associated with an autosomal dominant pattern of inheritance. This type 4 HH also known as ferroportin disease is emerging as the second most common inherited iron metabolic disorder. Serum ferritin levels in these patients are elevated early in the course of the disease, whereas the transferrin saturation is not elevated until later in life. The accumulation of excess iron is seen predominantly in Kupffer cells rather than in hepatocytes and there is a marginal anemia with low tolerance to phlebotomy (Pietrangelo, 1999).

Most SLC40A1 mutations occur in exon 5 and affect valine in position 162 and asparagine in position 144. Recently, two different phenotypes of ferroportin disease have been described. The M phenotype or "type 4A" characterized by iron accumulation in macrophages and due to a loss-of-function mutation leading to non-functional iron transport mutant (e.g. V162del) and the H phenotype, also called "type 4B" characterized by iron accumulation in hepatocytes and due to gain-of-function mutation leading to hepcidin-induced degradation resistance (e.g. N144H). Some mutations (e.g. Q248H) results only in genetic polymorphism without clinical manifestations (Mayr, 2010; Barton, 2003; De Domenico, 2006).

Controversial data reported before the era of molecular testing, suggested that patients with beta-thalassemia trait may develop iron overload (Edwards, 1981). However, most of these data, did not exclude the possible role of other endogenous factors including ferroportin disease (FD). Beta-thalassemia trait, when coinherited with a single H63D allele has rarely been associated with iron overload however; its co-inheritance with SLC40A1 mutation has not yet been studied.

Here we report a classical phenotype of ferroportin disease due to V162del in a Lebanese family with heterozygosity for H63D and beta-thalassemia trait. We also discuss the clinical expression of FD in the presence of genetic cofactors.

2. Family description and search strategy

The proband was a 54 years old male who presented in 1998 with fatigue and anemia. Clinical examination revealed skin pallor, splenomegaly and painful hepatomegaly. Relevant medical history included a blood transfusion 18 years earlier after a car accident and type 2 diabetes mellitus. There was no alcohol abuse or viral hepatitis. The serum ferritin concentration was 1011 ng/ml (Normal range < 400 ng/ml) and the transferrin saturation was 45%. The hemoglobin level was 10.1 g/dl (Normal: 11.5 - 17 g/dl), and the peripheral blood film showed hypochromia and aniso-poikylocytosis with target cells. The hemoglobin electrophoresis revealed a beta-thalassemia minor. The ceruloplasmin level was 474 mg/l (Normal: 155-592 mg/l) and the alpha-foetoprotein concentration was 21.37 IU/ml (Normal <5.80 IU/ml). The MRI study showed a splenomegaly, a portal vein thrombosis and a dysmorphic liver with hypertrophy of segment I. The liver biopsy revealed a fatty infiltration of the liver with iron deposits in hepatocytes and Kupffer cells and moderate portal fibrosis. Sections of liver tissue were stained with periodic acid–Schiff, Masson trichrome, Sweet's reticulin, hematoxiline/eosin and Perls Prussian blue (Figures 2 -6).

The proband's mother and one of his brothers died before the age of 50 from chronic liver disease. Their serum ferritin levels were higher than 1000 ng/ml (Figure 1). His oldest brother died from beta-thalassemia major. His 26 and 22 years old sons were healthy and presented elevated serum ferritin levels - 643 ng/ml and 744 ng/ml - with normal transferrin saturations. No liver biopsy was performed on them. His third son, 19 years old, had normal hemoglobin pattern and serum ferritin level.

The DNA from peripheral blood samples was tested with a reverse transcriptase-based assay, the Haemochromatosis StripAssay A® (Vienna Lab, Labordiagnostika, GmbH, Vienna, Austria), according to the manufacturer's instructions. This assay can detect twelve mutations in the HFE gene: V53M, V59M, H63D, H63H, S65C, Q127H, P160delC, E168Q, E168X, W169X, C282Y and Q283P, four mutations in the TfR2 gene: E60X, M172K, Y250X and AVAQ594-597del, and two mutations in the SCL40A1gene: N144H and V162del.

A systematic review of the literature was undertaken using search in Medline from 1981 for beta-thalassemia and hemochromatosis and from 2001 to 2011 for SLC40A1 novel mutations and new phenotypes.

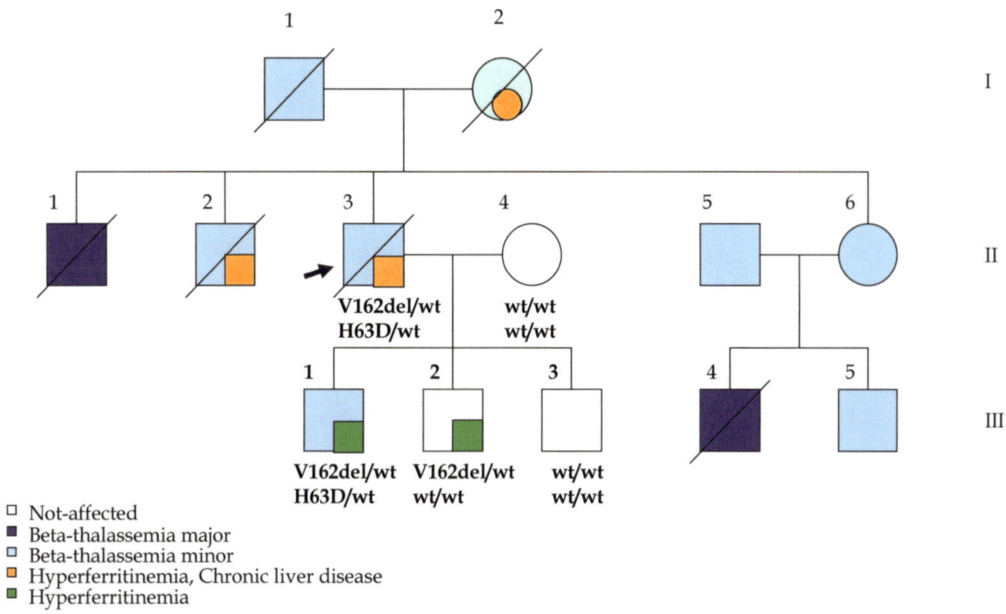

Fig. 1. Pedigree of a Lebanese family with beta-thalassemia and primary iron overload. Individuals II 3, II 4, III 1, III 2, III 3 were tested for SLC40A1 and HFE gene mutations.

2.1 Discussion and systemic review

2.1.1 Analysis of the pedigree

As shown in figure 1, the proband, his mother and one of his older brothers affected by beta-thalassemia minor died from chronic liver disease related to primary iron overload syndrome. The genetic testing showed that he was carrier of one copy of V162del mutation in SLC40A1 gene and one copy of H63D mutation in HFE gene. The two sons who carry the V162del mutation presented high serum ferritin levels with low transferrin saturation. One of them carries a single copy of H63D and beta-thalassemia trait but still remains asymptomatic. Most probably the primary iron overload syndrome transmitted in an autosomal dominant manner within this family is caused by the ferroportin disease due to V162del mutation. This mutation has a high penetrance and segregates with the clinical phenotype. The phenotypic expression is characterized by a high serum ferritin level, normal transferrin saturation; age related massive hepatocellular and macrophage iron accumulation leading to liver fibrosis. Coincidental association with H63D in two affected members and with beta-thalassemia trait in four affected members was noticed.

The role of these genetic co-factors in the aggressiveness of ferroportin disease remains to be elucidated.

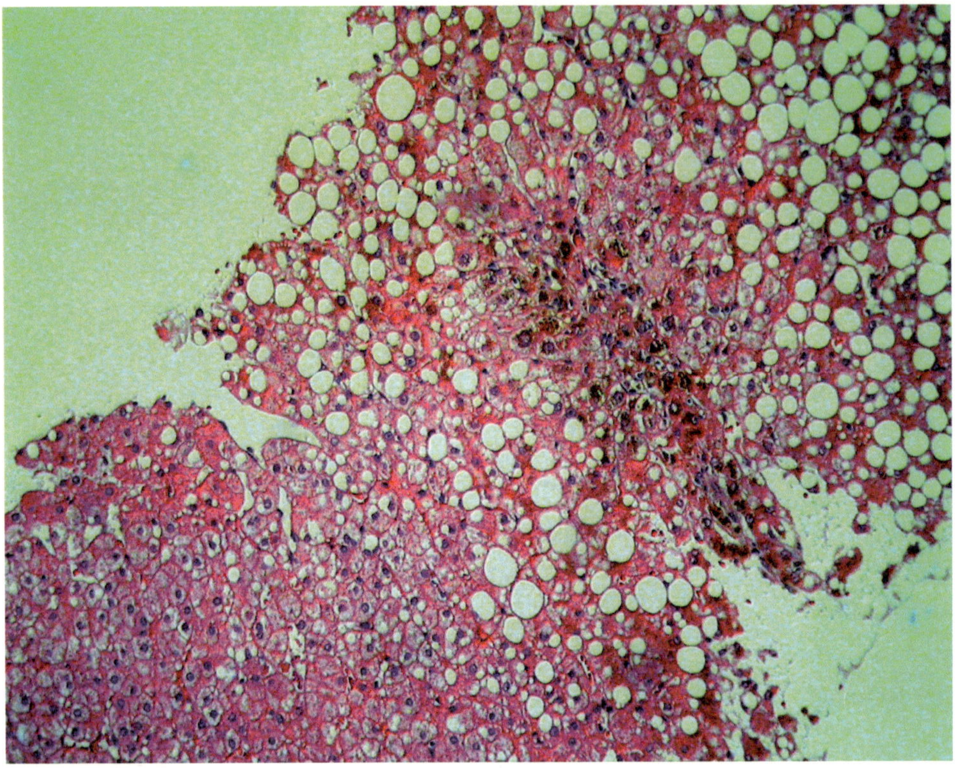

Fig. 2. Hematoxiline and Eosin stain x40. Liver siderosis and steatosis.

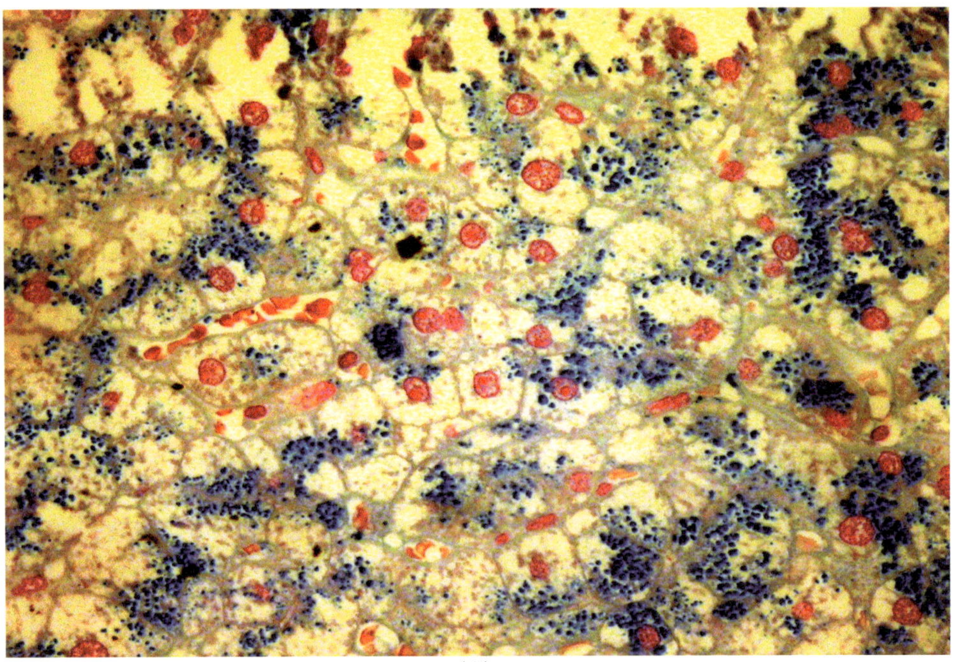

(A)

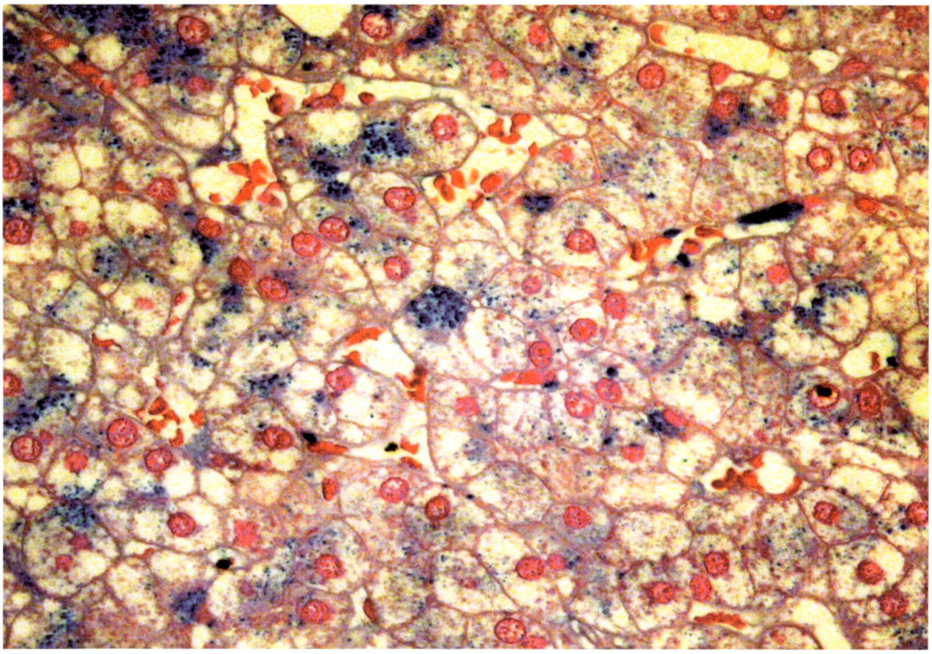

(B)

Fig. 3. Perls Prussian blue stain x400 (A and B). Grade 3 siderosis. Iron accumulation in Kupffer cells and hepatocytes

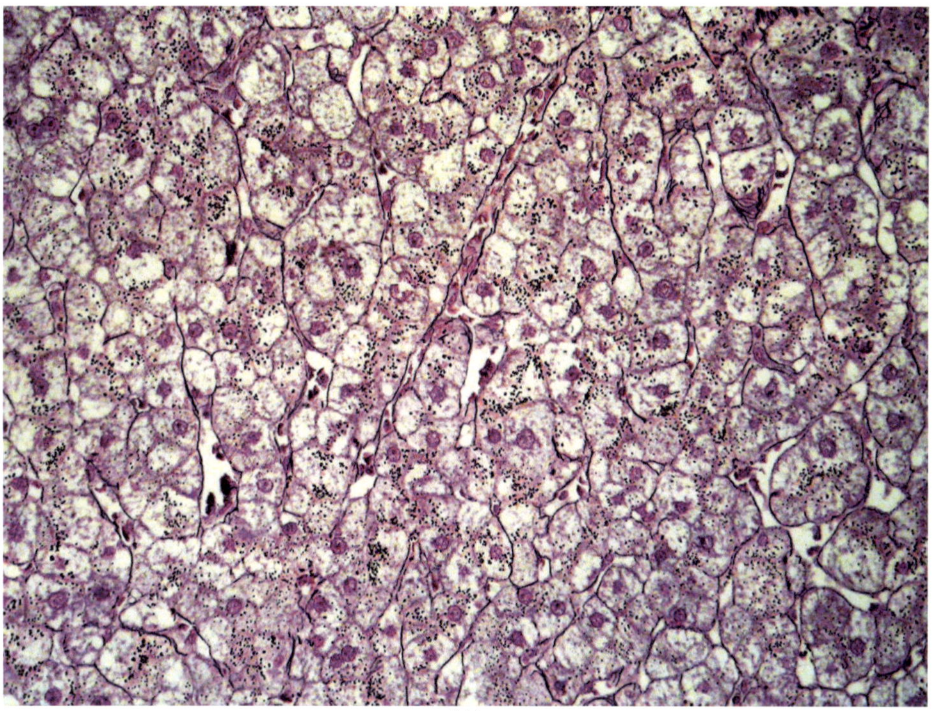

(A)

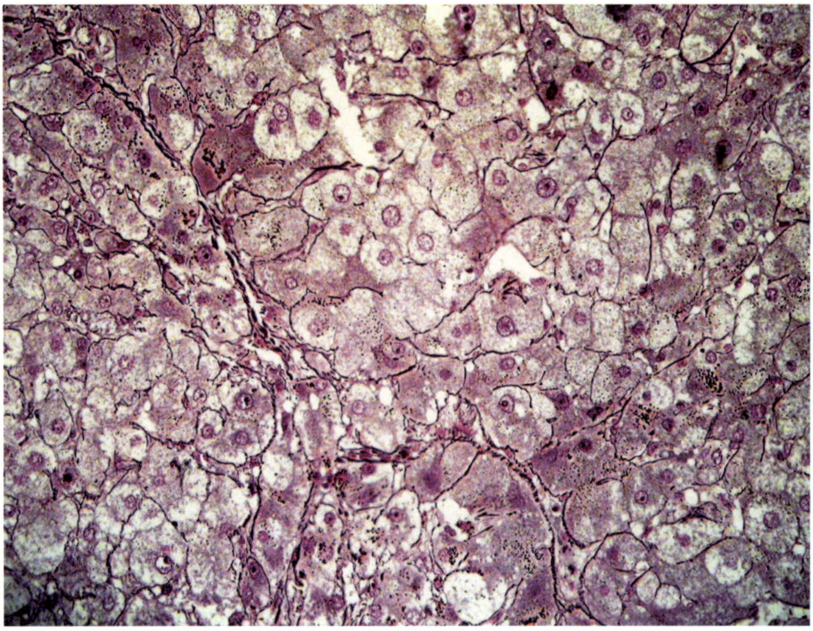

(B)

Fig. 4. Gordon Sweet's reticulin stain x100: Thick trabecula (A), and x200: Disoriented reticulin strings around the thickened trabecula (B)

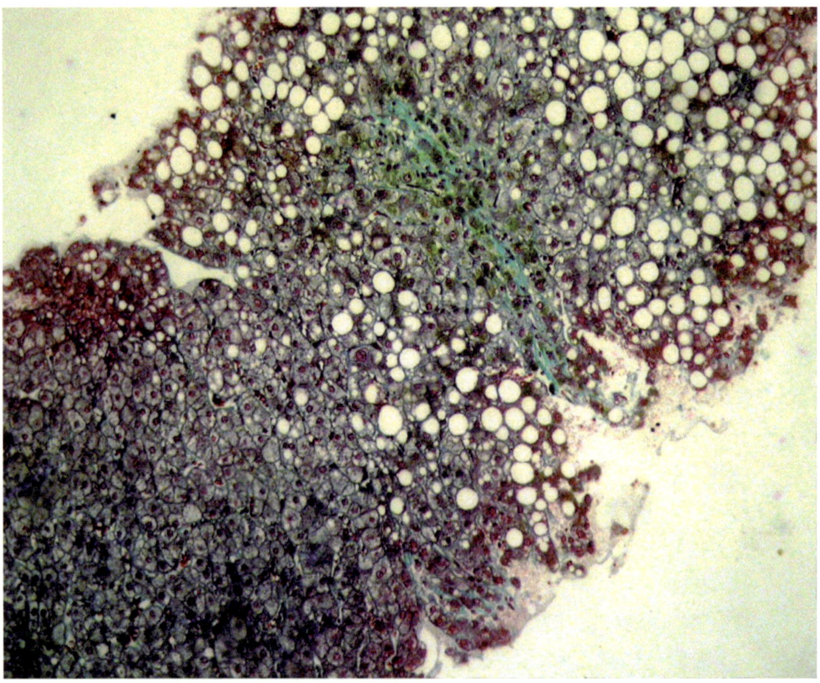

Fig. 5. Masson trichrome stain x40: Steatosis with minimal collagenous fibrosis within the stroma.

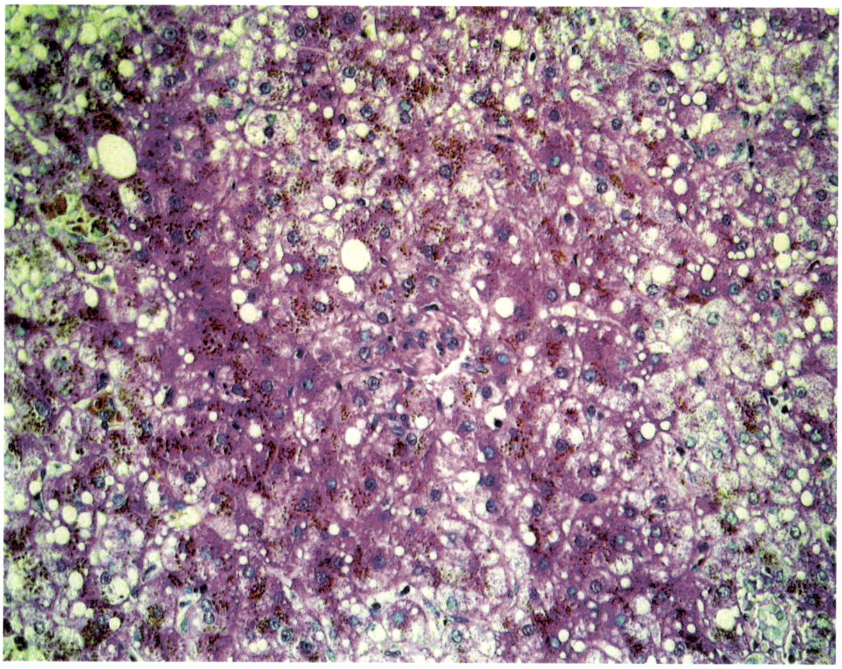

Fig. 6. Periodic-Acid Schiff stain x100. Common glycogen storage foci.

2.1.2 Genetic background and iron homeostasis

It is well known that different mutations in the same gene can result in different phenotypes and mutations in different genes can be expressed as the same phenotype. As for penetrance, carriers inherit their genotype in an autosomal dominant or recessive manner, yet they may not develop the diseased-phenotype because the altered inherited genes are incompletely penetrant. Modifier genes may affect the expression of some alleles which may increase or decrease the penetrance of a germline mutation. Furthermore, sporadic cases or phenocopies within the same pedigree have phenotype similar to affected mutation carriers. Reliable genetic testing may determine the hereditary nature of the disease and careful pedigree analysis, especially when multiple genetic conditions are co-inherited in members within the same family may help to sort out what genotype is causing what phenotype..

Iron homeostasis is balanced by the iron store. Hemoglobin level reflects the functional iron status, transferin saturation percentage reflects the iron in transport status and the serum ferritin level parallels the concentration of iron storage within the body regardless of the cell type in which it is stored. Two proteins regulate the outflow of iron through cells, Hepcidin and Ferroportin. Ferroportin is the only known mammalian iron exporter, expressed in macrophages and the basolateral membrane of enterocytes and hepatocytes. It serves as a channel through which iron is transported across the cell membrane into plasma. Up-regulation of ferroportin function enables increased iron absorption from the intestine and increased iron export to plasma from macrophages. Hepcidin mediates down-regulation of ferroportin action. Imbalances cause primary iron overload states and anemias. There is currently no available routine test to detect these two proteins in clinical practice.

Transferrin iron represents the normal form of circulating iron. Non-transferrin bound iron (NTBI) has been identified in the plasma of patients in whom transferrin saturation is significantly elevated. NTBI represents a potentially toxic form and is avidly taken-up by parenchymal cells especially hepatocytes (Brissot,2011).

2.1.3 Genetic hemochromatosis

Hereditary hemochromatosis (HH) is a primary iron overload (PIO) syndrome characterized by increased dietary iron absorption despite an excess in iron stores resulting in high transferrin saturation, high serum ferritin level and iron accumulation in liver parenchyma. It is one of the most common inherited diseases worldwide.

2.1.3.1 Hereditary hemochromatosis type 1, HFE-related

Hemochromatosis or High Fe gene (HFE) encodes for a membrane protein that is similar to MHC class I-type proteins. Following the identification of HFE gene mutations in 1996, three major mutations have been recognized to be responsible for HH in homozygous state, C282Y, H63D and S65C. The C282Y mutation has been found in more than 90% of northern European patients and in more than 80% of American patients of European origin. However, only 50-65% of Southern European patients are homozygous for this mutation (Pietrangelo, 2007, 2010). No conclusive evidence of abnormal gene expression in the heterozygous state has been found. Penetrance of HH is incomplete, usually age related and may be affected by other conditions such as hemoglobinopathies and congenital dyserythropoietic anemia. Little information about epigenetic factors influencing the penetrance is known. The precise function of the HFE protein is not fully clear.

2.1.3.2 Hereditary hemochromatosis type 4, Ferroportin disease

The availability of molecular tools has allowed investigators to identify novel mutations, non-HFE related, causing different clinical forms of hemochromatosis. The autosomal dominant form of HH was first reported in 1990, in a large family from the Solomon Islands (Eason, 1990). Serum iron indices from the family members resemble a classical HH but liver biopsies showed a pattern of iron staining in both hepatocytes and Kupffer cells with a certain degree of fibrosis and cirrhosis. In 1999, a typical pedigree was described and linked two years later to a point mutation (A77D) in ferroportin 1 gene also called FPN1, IREG1, MTP1 and SLC40A1 (Pietrangelo,1999; Montosi, 2001). At the same time a large Dutch family was identified in the Netherlands (Njajou, 2001), presenting another point mutation in the same gene (N144H). Mutations in SLC40A1 gene have then been reported from many countries throughout the world (Table 1), some of them are genetic polymorphism with slightly elevated serum ferritin levels. The most frequently reported mutations involve asparagine and valine residues in position 144 and 162. Various controversial data have been reported on the structure-function relationships of the various SLC40A1 mutants. However, phenotypic manifestations of this autosomal dominant HH named ferroportin disease (FD) are heterogeneous even between family members sharing the same SLC40A1 mutation.

Unlike HFE-related HH, FD is a genetically heterogenous iron overload syndrome with more than 40 SLC40A1 mutations reported. Most mutations have been associated with the classical form of FD characterized by hyperferritinemia, normal to low transferrin saturation and Kupffer cell iron storage. Other mutations have been associated with the non-classical form of the FD with increased transferrin saturation and hepatocellular iron storage in addition to high ferritin level and Kupffer cell iron storage. Few mutations have been reported as ferroportin gene polymorphism.

A loss-of-function mutation leads to hepcidin-independent down-regulation of ferroportin resulting in intracellular retention of the iron export pump. A gain-of-function mutation renders ferroportin resistant to inactivation by hepcidin. Functional studies have associated the classical phenotype of FD, also called M phenotype or type 4 A with the cellular iron export deficiency due to non-functional mutant and non-classical phenotype, also called H phenotype or type 4 B with the increased absorption of dietary iron due to a hyperactive mutant (De Domenico, 2006; Mayr, 2010).

2.1.4 Clinical expression of ferroportin disease and genetic cofactors

Ferroportin disease has a mild clinical expression in the absence of cofactors. Le Lan et al (Le Lan, 2011) in studying 70 affected subjects from 33 families with 19 different mutation in SLC40A1 gene showed that non-genetic co-factors such as obesity and excessive alcohol consumption are responsible for cirrhosis, fibrosis and malignant transformation cases which rather are sporadic cases in families with FD. The identification of a genetic variant in SLC40A1 is not sufficient to confirm the diagnosis of FD in patients with hyperferritinemia. Other genetically co-inherited conditions in the same individual may contribute to the development of PIO. In presenting this pedigree we mainly aimed to discuss the coexistence of multiple genetic factors that contribute to the primary iron overload condition particularly in Mediterranean areas where the β-thalassemia trait is prevalent in almost all populations and where FD seems to be present and underestimated. Although, when molecularly diagnosed FD could not by itself explain an aggressive phenotype, a comprehensive analysis of all co-inherited conditions and acquired factors seems to be relevant.

β-thalassemia minor is an asymptomatic common condition in Lebanon and the Mediterranean coast characterized by a mildly ineffective erythropoiesis that induces compensatory excess in iron absorption usually without iron overload. Moreover, β-thalassemia major and intermedia result in iron overload only through repetitive blood transfusions. Heterozygotes for HFE hemochromatosis are also asymptomatic but have been associated with mildly increased iron absorption (Zimmerman, 2008).

Whereas C282Y shows a distribution similar to HH type 1, H63D mutation is common in areas where the disease is not prevalent and its allelic frequency has great variability worldwide. It has been reported that β-thalassemia trait might increase the severity of hemochromatosis in subjects with C282Y and H63D homozygous but not heterozygous state (Piperno, 2000; Melis, 2002; Estevao, 2011).

Melis et al (Melis, 2002) demonstrated in 2002 that the H63D mutation in the homozygous state resulted in higher levels of serum ferritin and presumably iron overload in patients with β-thalassemia trait. There was no effect on ferritin levels in those with wild type/H63D or wild type/wild type genotypes. In contrast, Martins et al (Martins, 2004) showed in 2004 that the β-thalassemia trait, already related with the potential development of iron overload, tended to be aggravated with the coinheritance of H63D mutation, even when present in the heterozygous state. In a recent Brazilian analysis of 138 beta-thalassemic patients, Estevao et al found that the high levels of serum ferritin observed in beta-thalassemia heterozygotes do not depend on the inherited mutation in the beta-globin gene, and the association of beta-thalassemia heterozygous with the H63D/wild type state does not modify the iron profile in these individuals (Estevao, 2011; Oliveira, 2006). Garewal et al showed that H63D mutation which is prevalent in north Indians did not affect the iron indices in beta-thalassemia trait carriers (Garewal, 2003).

The role of SLC40A1 mutation on iron overload in beta-thalassemia carriers and inversely the role of beta-thalassemia minor on the phenotypic expression of ferroportin gene mutation have not yet been studied. Barton et al evaluated genotype and phenotype characteristics of unselected African American index patients with primary iron overload who reside in central Alabama and concluded that primary iron overload is not the result of the mutation of a single gene HFE, C282Y or ferroportin 744 G-->T (Q248H), but that common forms of heritable anemia appear to account for increased iron absorption or retention in some patients (Barton, 2003).

Arada et al in studying polymorphisms of the HFE gene and iron indices in 815 healthy Spanish subjects not affected by beta-thalassemia showed that the C282Y heterozygote, the H63D heterozygote and homozygote and the H63D/S65C compound heterozygote genotypes were associated with increased transferrin saturation relative to the wild type genotype. The latter compound genotype had the higher phenotypic expression (Arada, 2010). The SLC40A1/H63D compound heterozygosity has not yet been studied however; it may contribute to the aggravation of the iron overload picture. Table 1 shows the reported cases with this condition and the associated phenotypes. Four out of five reported cases with H63D mutation represented the mild classical form of FD while only one case report described an aggressive non-classical form with 100% transferrin saturation rate.

FD is a mild form of iron overload with heterogenous clinical presentation. It has been reported in a large cohort of patients that sex; environmental and/or acquired cofactors have prominent roles in determining the variability of the phenotypic expression. The role of co-inheritance of conditions that may interfere with the iron metabolism remains to be elucidated. In the present Lebanese pedigree, the V162del mutation is most probably the cause of the iron overload syndrome. The β-thalassemia and the H63D heterozygous state may have contributed to the aggressive phenotype in the proband.

In a systemic review of the literature and a meta-analysis of clinical, biochemical, pathological and molecular findings of FD, Mayr et al found that the biochemical penetrance of FD was 86%. Eighty probands out of 176 reported families were classified as having the classical phenotype and 53 probands the non-classical phenotype. The mean age at presentation for the non-classical form was higher. Cirrhosis was reported in only 4 patients of whom two had N144H, one C326S and one I180T mutation. Liver fibrosis was related to age but neither to hepatic iron concentration nor serum ferritin. Of the 31 different SLC40A1 mutations, six were unequivocally associated with the classical form and five with the non-classical form. Variable phenotypes were reported for nine mutations. The remaining probands were incompletely assessed. The authors concluded that because not all mutations were unambiguously correlated with the classical or non-classical phenotype in all reported patients with a particular mutation, the genotype to phenotype correlation suggests that FD has a multifactorial cause (Mayr, 2010). To determine whether bio-informatic tools SIFT (Sorting Intolerant From Tolerant) (Ng, 2003) and PolyPhen (Polymorphism phenotyping)

Author/year	Age sex	Family origin	Mutation (Protein)p.	Mutation (DNA) c.	Main symptoms	Ferritin (ng/ml)	TS	Coexisting conditions	Liver changes	Fe in liver cells
Montosi/2001	59 m	Italy	A77D	230C>A	Asymptomatic	5750	75%	None	Cirrhosis	REC
Njajou/2001	80 f	Netherlands	N144H	430A>C	Arthralgia, diabetes	>2000	88%	-	Fibrosis	REC ± HC
Wallace/2001	56 m	Australia	V162del	484-486del3	Hepatomegaly, pancytopenia	>12000	-	None	Portal fibrosis	Both
Devalia/2002	38 f	UK	V162del	484-486del3	Fatigue	>2000	40%	None	No fibrosis	Both
Cazzola/2002	-	Italy	V162del	484-486del3	-	High	<50%	None	No fibrosis	REC
Roetto/2002	26 f	Italy	V162del	484-486del3	Anemia	>1000	<20%	None	No fibrosis	REC ± HC
	58 f	Italy	V162del	484-486del3	Asymptomatic	>5000	<40%	None	No fibrosis	REC ±HC
	30 m	UK	V162del	484-486del3	Asymptomatic	>1000	<30%	None	No fibrosis	REC ±HC
Hetet/2003	61 m	France	D157G	774A>G	Asymptomatic	4069	44%	H63D/WT	-	-
	63 m	France	E182H	850G>T	Cataract	3018	16%	-	-	
	49 f	France	G323V	1272G>T	Cataract	>1700	N	-	-	
Jouanelle/2003		France (Asian)	G490D	1468G>A	-	>2000	<40%	None	-	REC ± HC
Gordeuk/2003	-	USA (African)	Q248H	744G>T	Mild anemia	>500	N	None	-	REC
Beutler/2003	-	USA (African)	Q248H	744G>T	-	High	N	-	-	REC
Rivard/2003	24 m	Canada (French)	Y64N	190T>C	Fatigue ,tremor,diarhhea	647	77%	None	Steatosis	Both
Arden/2003	48 m	Solomon Islands	N144T	431A>C	Cardiac murmur hepatomegaly	2937	80%	None	Fibrosis	Both
Wallace/2004	32 f	Australia	N144D	430A>G	Cirrhosis	High	N	Sarcoidosis	Cirrhosis	Both
Zoller/2005	68 f	Austria	V162del	484-486del3	Cholecystectomy (iron in lymph node)	5265	37%	None	-	REC
Sham/2005	young	USA	C326S	977G>C	Hepatomegaly	High	>50%	-	-	HC
Morris/2005	young	Canada	N185D	553A>G	-	High	High	-	-	-
Koyama/2005	43 m	Japan	R489S	1467A>C	Asymptomatic	822	25%	None	No fibrosis	REC ± HC
Subramaniam/2005	45 m	Australia	A77D	230C>A	Lethargy	3500	29%	None	No fibrosis	REC
Wallace/2005	36 f	Sri Lanka	V162del	484-486del3	Asymptomatic	3145	29%	None	No fibrosis	Both
Cremonesi/2006	34 m	Italy (Italian)	D181V	846A>T	Fatigue	1400	40%	None	No fibrosis	Both
	Young	Italy (Italian)	G80V	239G>T	Asymptomatic	1311	33%	None	No fibrosis	-
	Young	Italy (Chinese)	G267D	1104G>A	Asymptomatic	1153	32%	None	No fibrosis	-
Liu/2005 &	43 f	Japan	A117G	-	Chronic hepatitis	9660	92%	Chr. Hep	No fibrosis	Both
Hayashi/2006	43 m	Japan	R489S	1467A>C	Asymptomatic	822	25%	None	No fibrosis	REC
	79 m	Japan	R489S	1467A>C	Asymptomatic	2283	62%	None	No fibrosis	REC
Bach/2006	-	Spain	R88T	236G>C	-	High	N	-	-	-
	-	Spain	I180T	539T>C	-	High	N	-	-	-
Lee/2007	m	USA (Scottish)	G468S	1402G>A	-	>1000	-	H63D/WT	-	REC
Wallace/2007	72 m	New Zeeland	S338R	1014T>G	Liver function changes	1990	90%	None	Steatosis	Both
Girelli/2008	59 f	Italy	I152F	758A>T	Liver funct. Changes	1771	23%	H63D/WT,	Fibrosis	HC
	64 m	Italy	L233P	1012T>C	Diabetes	9000	75%	VHC	Fibrosis	REC +HC
Sussman/2008	47 m	USA (African)	R561G	1681A>G	Cirrhosis	2960	100%	VHC, XLSA	Fibrosis	HC
Speletas/2008	25 f	Greece	V162del	484-486del3	Mild anemia	>1000	<40%	None	-	REC
	58 f	Greece	R178G	532C>A	-	>1000	<40%	None	-	REC
Rosmorduc/2008	48 m	France	N144H	431A>G	Asymptomatic	2195	100%	None	Mild Fibrosis	HC
Pelucchi/2008	-	Italy	D157N	469G>A	-	High	N	-	-	-
	-	Italy	V72F	214G>T	-	High	N	-	-	-
Mougiou/2008	34 m	Greece	G80S	239G>?	Asymptomatic	1800	32%	None	-	REC
Lok/2009	38 m	Thailand	C326Y	977G>A	Abnormal liver function tests	4326	99%	None	-	-
Letocart/2009	35 m	Italy	Y501C	1502A>G	Asthenia, arthralgia	642	94%	None	-	-
Saja/2010	58 m	UK	D157G	470A>C	Asymptomatic	4123	32	None	Steatosis	REC
Griffith/2010	57 f	UK	R489K	1466G>A	Asymptomatic	685	39	H63D/WT	No fibrosis	REC
Mayr/2011	54 m	UK	W158C	474G>T	None	3015	21%	Ulc. Colitis	No fibrosis	REC
	41 m	UK	H507R	1520A>G	Lethargy	3097	100%	H63D/WT	Steatosis	HC
Del-Castillo-Rueda/2011	45 m	Spain	K240E	718A>G	Asymptomatic	422	71%	Chondro-sarcoma	-	-

Table 1. Reported phenotypes for various SLC40A1 gene mutations (Probands' characteristics and iron indices) HC: Hepatocytes, REC: Reticulo endothelial cells (Kupffer cells), TS: Transferin saturation, Fe in liver cells: Liver cells where iron was predominantly accumulated, XLSA: X-linked sideroblastic anemia, VHC: Viral hepatitis C, -: Data not available.

can discriminate between disease causing SLC40A1 mutation and polymorphism Mayr et al have assessed them as alternatives to predict the effect of SLC40A1 mutation on protein function and found that PolyPhen has 99% sensitivity and 67% specificity in identifying disease-causing gene variants by scoring newly-identified mutations in patients with primary iron overload as "possibly" or "probably" damaging (Mayr, 2010).

3. Conclusion

Point mutations in ferroportin gene SLC40A1 result in highly penetrant ferroportin disease genetically and phenotypically heterogeneous with mild clinical expression in the absence of cofactors. Functional analysis have identified two phenotypes, classical with normal transferrin saturation and non-classical with high transferrin saturation but locus heterogeneity still exist for each form. Variability in phenotypic expression may be related to co-inherited genetic modifiers or environmental factors.

4. References

Aranda N, Viteri FE, Montserrat C, Arija V. (2010) Effects of C282Y, H63D, and S65C HFE gene mutations, diet, and life-style factors on iron status in a general Mediterranean population from Tarragona, Spain. Ann Hematol. 2010 Aug;89(8):767-73. Epub 2010 Jan 28. ISSN: 09395555

Arden KE, Wallace DF, Dixon JL et al. (2003). A novel mutation in ferroportin 1 is associated with haemochromatosis in a Salomon Islands patient. Gut; 2003; 52: 1215-1217. (ISSN) 1468-3288

Bach V, Remacha A, Altes A et al. (2006) Autosomal dominant hereditary hemochromatosis associated with two novel Ferroportin 1 mutation in Spain. Blood Cells Mol Dis. 2006; 36(1): 41-45. ISSN (printed): 1079-9796. ISSN (electronic): 1096-0961.

Barton JC, Acton RT, Rivers CA, Bertoli LF, Gelbart T, West C, Beutler E. (2003). Genotypic and phenotypic heterogeneity of African Americans with primary iron overload. Blood Cells Mol Dis. 2003 Nov-Dec;31(3):310-9. ISSN (printed): 1079-9796. ISSN (electronic): 1096-0961

Beutler E, Hoffbrand AV, Cook JD. (2003). Iron deficiency and overload. Hematology Am Soc Hematol Educ Program. 2003:40-61. (Print ISSN) 1520-4391; (Online ISSN) 1520-4383.

Brissot P, Ropert M, Le Lan C, Loreal O. (2011). Non-transferrin bound iron: A key role in iron overloads and iron toxicity. Biochim Biophys Acta. 2011 Aug 9. ISSN: 0006-3002

Cazzola M, Cremonesi L, Papaioannou M et al. (2002). Genetic hyperferritinaemia and reticuloendothelial iron overload associated with a three base pair deletion in the coding region of the ferroportin gene (SLC11A3). Br J Haematol; 2002; 119(2): 539-546. ISSN: 1365-2141.

Cremonesi L, Forni GL, Soriani N et al. (2005). Genetic and clinical heterogeneity of ferroportin disease. Br J Haematol. 2005; 131(5): 663-670. ISSN: 1365-2141.

De Domenico I, McVey Ward D, Nemeth E et al. (2006). Molecular and clinical correlates in iron overload associated with mutations in ferroportin. Haematologica. 2006 Aug; 91(8):1092-1095. ISSN: 0390-6078 (Print) 1592-872 (online).

Del-Castillo-Rueda A, Moreno-Carralero MI, Alvarez-Sala-Walther LA, Cuadrado-Grande N, Enríquez-de-Salamanca R, Méndez M, Morán-Jiménez MJ (2011). Two novel mutations in the SLC40A1 and HFE genes implicated in iron overload in a Spanish man. Eur J Haematol. 2011 Mar;86(3):260-4. Print ISSN: 0902-4441. Online ISSN: 1600-0609.

Devalia V, Carter K, Walker AP et al. (2002). Autosomal dominant reticuloendothelial iron overload associetedwith a 3-base pair deletion in the ferropotin 1 gene (SLC11A3). Blood. 2002 Jul 15;100(2):695-7. print ISSN 0006-4971, online ISSN: 1528-0020.

Eason RJ, Adams PC, Aston CE, Searle J. (1990). Familial iron overload with possible autosomal dominant inheritance. Aust N Z J Med. 1990 Jun; 20(3):226-230. ISSN: 0004-8291.

Edwards CQ, Skolnick MH, Kushner JP. (1981). Coincidental nontransfusional iron overload and thalassemia minor: association with HLA-linked hemochromatosis. Blood. 1981 Oct; 58(4):844-848. print ISSN: 0006-4971, online ISSN: 1528-0020.

Estevão IF, Peitl Junior P, Bonini-Domingos CR. (2011). Serum ferritin and transferrin saturation levels in β^0 and $\beta(+)$ thalassemia patients. Genet Mol Res. 2011 Apr 12;10(2):632-9. ISSN: 1676-5680.

Feder JN, Gnirke A, Thomas W, Tsuchihashi Z, Ruddy DA, Basava A, Dormishian F, Domingo R Jr, Ellis MC, Fullan A, Hinton LM, Jones NL, Kimmel BE, Kronmal GS, Lauer P, Lee VK, Loeb DB, Mapa FA, McClelland E, Meyer NC, Mintier GA, Moeller N, Moore T, Morikang E, Prass CE, Quintana L, Starnes SM, Schatzman RC, Brunke KJ, Drayna DT, Risch NJ, Bacon BR, Wolff RK. (1996). A novel MHC class I-like gene is mutated in patients with hereditary haemochromatosis. Nat Genet. 1996 Aug;13(4):399-408. ISSN: 1061-4036 e ISSN: 1546-171.

Garewal G, Das R, Ahluwalia J, Marwaha RK. (2005). Prevalence of the H63D mutation of the HFE in north India: its presence does not cause iron overload in beta thalassemiatrait. Eur J Haematol. 2005 Apr;74(4):333-6. ISSN:0902 -4441 (Print) ; 1600-0609 (Electronic).

Girelli D, De Domenico I, Bozzini C et al. (2008). Clinical, pathological and molecular correlates in ferroportin disease. A study of two novel mutations. J Hepatol. 2008; 49(4):664-671. ISSN: 0168-8278.

Griffiths WJ, Mayr R, McFarlane I, Hermann M, Halsall DJ, Zoller H, Cox TM. (2010). Clinical presentation and molecular pathophysiology of autosomal dominant hemochromatosis caused by a novel ferroportin mutation. Hepatology. 2010 Mar;51(3):788-95. ISSN: 1527-3350.

Hayashi H, Wakusawa S, Motonishi S et al. (2006). Genetic background of primary iron overload syndromes in Japan. Intern Med. 2006; 45(20):1107-1111. ISSN: 1365-2796.

Hetet G, Devaux I, Soufir N et al. (2003). Molecular analyses of patients with hyperferritinemia and serum iron values reveal both L ferritin IRE and 3 new ferroportin (SLC11A3) mutations. Blood, 2003; 102(6); 1904-1910. Print ISSN 0006-4971, online ISSN 1528-0020.

Jouanelle AM, Douabin-Giquel V, Halimi C et al. (2003). Novel mutation in ferrportin 1 gene is associated with autosomal dominant iron overload. J Hepatol; 2003; 39(2): 286-289. ISSN: 0168-8278.

Kowdley KV. (2004). Iron, hemochromatosis, and hepatocellular carcinoma. Gastroenterology; 2004; 127(5): S79-86. ISSN: 0016-5085.

Koyama C, Wakusawa S, Hayashi H et al. (2005). A Japanese Family with Ferroportin Disease Caused by a Novel Mutation of SLC40A1 Gene: Hyperferritinemia Associated with a Relatively Low Transferrin Saturation of Iron. Internal Medicine; 2005; 44(9); 990-993. ISSN: 1365-2796.

Le Lan C, Mosser A, Ropert M, Detivaud L, Loustaud-Ratti V, Vital-Durand D, Roget L, Bardou-Jacquet E, Turlin B, David V, Loréal O, Deugnier Y, Brissot P, Jouanolle AM. (2011). Sex and acquired cofactors determine phenotypes of ferroportin disease. Gastroenterology. 2011 Apr;140(4):1199-1207.e1-2. ISSN: 0016-5085.

Lee PL, Gelbart T, West C et al. (2007). SLC40A1 c.140G-->A results in aberrant splicing, ferroportin truncation after glycin 330, and an autosomal dominant hemochromatosis phenotype. Acta Haematol. 2007; 118(4):237-224. ISSN: 0001-5792 (Print) ; 1421-9662 (Electronic).

Létocart E, Le Gac G, Majore S, Ka C, Radio FC, Gourlaouen I, De Bernardo C, Férec C, Grammatico P. (2009). A novel missense mutation in SLC40A1 results in resistance to hepcidin and confirms the existence of two ferroportin-associated iron overload diseases. Br J Haematol. 2009 Nov;147(3):379-85. ISSN: 0007- 1048 (Print) ; 1365-2141 (Electronic).

Liu W, Shimomura S, Imanishi H et al. (2005). Hemochromatosis with mutation of the ferroportin 1 (IREG1) gene. Intern Med. 2005 Apr; 44(4):285-289. ISSN: 1365-2796.

Lok CY, Merryweather-Clarke AT, Viprakasit V et al. (2009). Iron overload in the Asian community. Blood. 2009; 114:20-25. Print ISSN 0006-4971, online ISSN 1528-0020.

Martins R, Picanço I, Fonseca A et al. (2004). The role of HFE mutations on iron metabolism in beta-thalassemia carriers. J Hum Genet. 2004; 49(12):651-655. ISSN: 1018-4813, eISSN: 1476-5438.

Mayr R, Janecke AR, Schranz M, Griffiths WJ, Vogel W, Pietrangelo A, Zoller H. (2010). Ferroportin disease: a systematic meta-analysis of clinical and molecular findings. J Hepatol. 2010 Nov;53(5):941-9. ISSN: 0168-8278.

Mayr R, Griffiths WJ, Hermann M, McFarlane I, Halsall DJ, Finkenstedt A, Douds A, Davies SE, Janecke AR, Vogel W, Cox TM, Zoller H. (2011). Identification of mutations in SLC40A1 that affect ferroportin function and phenotype of human ferroportin iron overload. Gastroenterology. 2011 Jun;140(7):2056-63. ISSN: 0016-5085.

Melis MA, Cau M, Deidda F et al. (2002). H63D mutation in the HFE gene increases iron overload in beta-thalassemia carriers. Haematologica. 2002;87:242-245. ISSN: 0390-6078 (Print) 1592-8721 (Electronic).

Montosi G, Donovan A, Totaro A et al. (2001). Autosomal dominant hemochromatosis is associated with a mutation in ferroportin (SLC11A3) gene. J Clin Invest. 2001; 108(4): 619-623. ISSN: 0021-9738.

Morris TJ, Litvinova MM, Ralston D et al. (2005). A novel ferroportin mutation in a Canadian family with autosomal dominant hemochromatosis. Blood Cells Mol Dis. 2005 Nov-Dec; 35(3):309-314. ISSN (printed): 1079-9796. ISSN (electronic): 1096-0961.

Mougiou A, Pietrangelo A, Caleffi A et al. (2008). G80S-linked ferroportin disease: the first clinical description in a Greek family. Blood Cells Mol Dis. 2008 Jul-Aug; 41(1):138-139. ISSN (printed): 1079-9796. ISSN (electronic): 1096-0961.

Ng PC, Henikoff S. (2003). SIFT: Predicting amino acid changes that affect protein function. Nucleic Acids Res. 2003 Jul 1;31(13):3812-4. Online ISSN 1362-4962 - Print ISSN 0305-1048.

Njajou OT, Vaessen N, Joosse M et al. (2001). A mutation in SLC11A3 is associated with autosomal dominant hemochromatosis. Nat Genet. 2001; 28: 213-214. ISSN: 1061-4036, eISSN: 1546- 1718.

Oliveira TM, Souza FP, Jardim AC, Cordeiro JA, Pinho JR, Sitnik R, Estevão IF, Bonini-Domingos CR, Rahal P. (2006). HFE gene mutations in Brazilian thalassemic patients. Braz J Med Biol Res. 2006 Dec;39(12):1575-80. ISSN: 0100-879X.

Pietrangelo A, Montosi G, Totaro A et al. (1999). Hereditary hemochromatosis in adults without pathogenic mutations in the hemochromatosis gene. NEJM; 1999; 341(10): 725-732. Electronic ISSN 1533-4406 Print ISSN 0028-4793.

Pietrangelo A. (2007). Hemochromatosis: An endocrine liver disease. Hepatology. 2007; 46:1291-1301. Online ISSN: 1527-3350.

Pietrangelo A. (2010). Hereditary hemochromatosis: pathogenesis, diagnosis, and treatment. Gastroenterology. 2010 Aug;139(2):393-408. ISSN: 0016-5085.

Piperno A, Mariani R, Arosio C et al. (2000). Haemochromatosis in patients with beta-thalassaemia trait. Br J Haematol. 2000 Dec; 111(3):908-914. ISSN: 1365-2141.

Rivard SR, Lanzara C, Grimard D et al. (2003). Autosomal dominant reticuloendothelial iron overload (HFE type 4) due to a new missense mutation in the ferroportin 1 gene (SLC11A3) in a large French-Canadian family. Haematologica; 2003; 88(7): 824-826. ISSN: 0390-6078 (Print) 1592-8721 (Electronic).

Roettto A, Merryweather-Clarke AT, Daraio F et al. (2002). A valine deletion of ferroportin1: A common mutation in hemochromatosis type 4. Blood. 2002; 100(2): 733-734. Print ISSN 0006-4971, online ISSN 1528-0020.

Ropero P, Briceño O, López-Alonso G et al. (2007). [The H63D mutation in the HFE gene is related to the risk of hepatocellular carcinoma]. Rev Esp Enferm Dig. 2007 Jul; 99(7):376-81. ISSN: 1130-0108.

Rosmorduc O, Wendum D, Arrivé L et al. (2008). Phenotypic expression of ferroportin disease in a family with the N144H mutation. Gastroenterol Clin Biol. 2008 Mar; 32(3):321-327. ISSN:0399- 8320.

Saja K, Bignell P, Robson K, Provan D. (2010). A novel missense mutation c.470 A>C (p.D157A) in the SLC40A1 gene as a cause of ferroportin disease in a family with hyperferritinaemia. Br J Haematol. 2010 Jun;149(6):914-6. Online ISSN: 1365-2141.

Sham RL, Phatac PD, West C et al. (2005). Autosomal dominant hereditary hemochromatosis associated with a novel ferroportin mutation and unique clinical features. Blood Cells Mol Dis. 2005; 34(2): 157-161. ISSN (printed): 1079-9796. ISSN (electronic): 1096-0961.

Speletas M, Kioumi A, Loules G et al. (2008). Analysis of SLC40A1 gene at the mRNA level reveals rapidly the causative mutations in patients with hereditary hemochromatosis type IV. Blood Cells Mol Dis. 2008; 40(3):353-359. ISSN (printed): 1079-9796. ISSN (electronic): 1096-0961.

Subramariam VN, Wallace DF, Dixon JL et al. (2005). Ferroportin disease due to the A77D mutation in Australia. Gut; 2005 Jul; 54(7):1048-1049. ISSN 0017-5749.

Sussman NL, Lee PL, Dries AM et al. (2008). Multi-organ iron overload in an African-American man with ALAS2 R452S and SLC40A1 R561G. Acta Hematol. 2008;120(3):168-173. ISSN (printed): 0001-5792. ISSN (electronic): 1421-9662.

Wallace DF, Browett P, Wong P et al. (2005). Identification of ferroportin disease in the Indian subcontinent. Gut 2005 Apr; 54(4):567-568. ISSN 0017-5749.

Wallace DF, Clark RM, Harley HAJ et al. (2004). Autosomal dominant iron overload due to a novel mutation of ferroportin1 associated with parenchymal iron loading and cirrhosis. J Hepatol 2004; 40; 710-713. ISSN: 0168-8278.

Wallace DF, Dixon JL, Ramm GA et al. (2007). A novel mutation in ferroportin implicated in iron overload. J Hepatol. 2007 May;46(5):921-926. ISSN: 0168-8278.

Wallace DF, Pedersen P, Dixon JL et al. (2001). Novel mutation in ferroportin 1 is associated with autosomal dominant hemochromatosis. Blood; 2001; 100(2): 692-694. Print ISSN 0006-4971, online ISSN 1528-0020.

Zimmermann MB, Fucharoen S, Winichagoon P, Sirankapracha P, Zeder C, Gowachirapant S, Judprasong K, Tanno T, Miller JL, Hurrell RF. (2008). Iron metabolism in heterozygotes for hemoglobin E (HbE), alpha-thalassemia 1, or beta-thalassemia and in compound heterozygotes for HbE/beta-thalassemia. Am J Clin Nutr. 2008 Oct;88(4):1026-31. Print ISSN: 0002-9165; Online ISSN: 1938- 3207.

Zoller H, McFarlane I, Theurl I et al. (2005). Primary iron overload with inappropriate hepcidin expression in V162del ferroportin disease. Hepatology; 2005; 42(2): 466-472. Online ISSN: 1527-3350.

13

p53: Point Mutations, SNPs and Cancer

Ming Fang, Iva Simeonova and Franck Toledo
Institut Curie, Centre de Recherche, Paris, France

1. Introduction

p53 was discovered in 1979 in SV40-transformed cells as a cellular protein that forms a complex with the large T antigen (DeLeo et al., 1979; Kress et al., 1979; Lane and Crawford, 1979; Linzer and Levine, 1979). It was originally identified as an oncoprotein, but was shown to be a tumor suppressor ten years later by both *in vitro* experiments and human tumor sample studies (Baker et al., 1989; Finlay et al., 1989; Hinds et al., 1989; Nigro et al., 1989).

Since then, an impressive body of work has been performed to decipher the functions and regulation of p53. The crucial role of p53 in tumor suppression is demonstrated by the fact that the *TP53* gene is mutated in 50-70% of human sporadic cancers (Levine, 1997), and that genes encoding the p53 regulators Mouse Double Minute 2 (Mdm2) and Mdm4 (also known as MdmX) are often mutated in the other tumors (Toledo and Wahl, 2006). Furthermore, germline *TP53* mutations account for the Li-Fraumeni syndrome, a familial cancer predisposition syndrome characterized by a high tumor penetrance and early tumor onset (Malkin et al., 1990).

More than 27 000 somatic mutations and close to 600 germline mutations of *TP53* were reported (according to the *TP53* mutation database (Petitjean et al., 2007) of the International Agency for Research on Cancer (IARC) ; release R15, November 2010). In this review, we summarize what *TP53* point mutations may reveal about p53 function and cancer development, and further address the prognostic and predictive values of *TP53* point mutations or SNPs in the p53 pathway.

2. Effects of point mutations in p53: Data from tumors and mouse models

In response to diverse oncogenic stresses, the transcription factor p53 promotes transient or permanent cell cycle arrest (the latter also known as senescence), or apoptosis, hence preventing cells with a damaged genome to proliferate (Vogelstein et al., 2000). In addition, p53 regulates various processes that may contribute to its tumor suppressive functions, including glycolysis, autophagy, cell mobility, microRNA processing, ageing and suntanning (Aylon and Oren, 2010; Cui et al., 2007; Vousden and Ryan, 2009).

Due to its detrimental activities to cell proliferation, p53 needs to be tightly regulated. Mdm2 and Mdm4 are the main p53 inhibitors (Wade et al., 2010), and their essential role is demonstrated by the p53-dependent lethality of Mdm2-deficient and Mdm4-deficient mouse embryos, which die from apoptosis or proliferation arrest, respectively. Mdm2 is a E3 ubiquitin ligase that can lead to the degradation of p53 by the proteasome (Brooks and Gu, 2006), whereas Mdm4 inhibits the activity of p53 mainly by occluding the p53 transactivation domain (Marine et al., 2006). But the regulation of p53 is much more complex, as more than 160 proteins interact with p53 to regulate its activity and stability (Toledo and Wahl, 2006).

The transcription factor p53 is a 393-amino acids protein composed of 5 domains : a N-terminal transactivation domain (TAD), a proline-rich domain (PRD), a core DNA binding domain (DBD), a tetramerization domain (4D) and a C-terminal regulatory domain (CTD) (Fig. 1A). Single-base substitutions in the *TP53* coding sequence, leading to missense mutations, nonsense mutations or frameshifts, are the principal mode of p53 alteration in human cancers (Olivier et al., 2010).

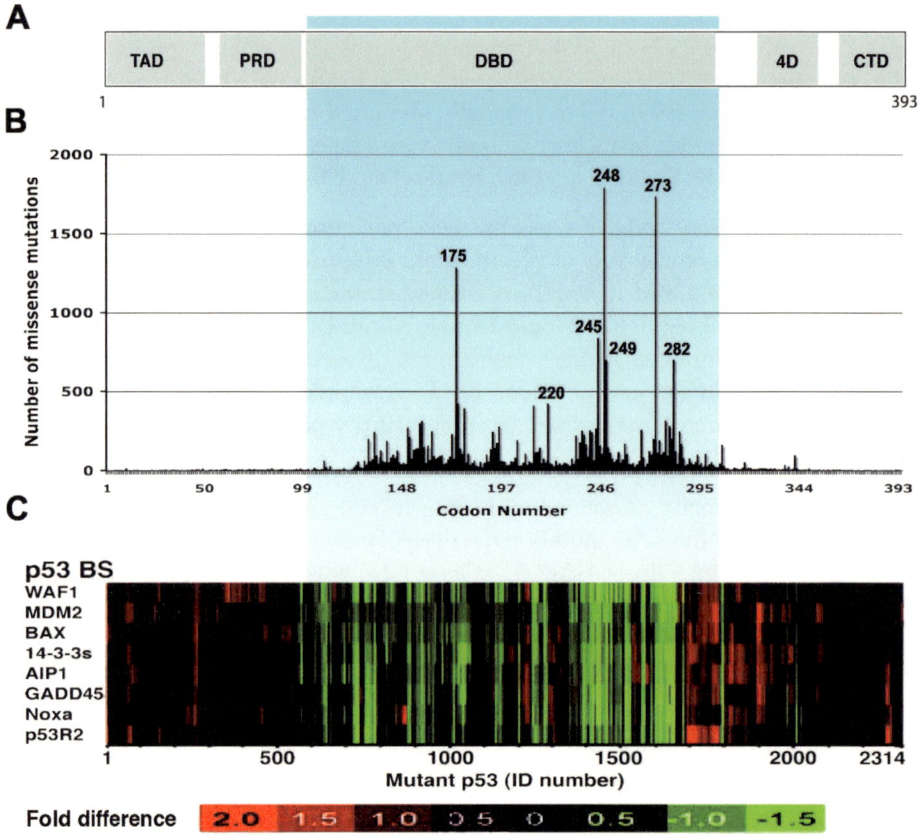

Fig. 1. *TP53* missense mutations are clustered in the DNA binding domain. (**A**) Schematic representation of the 5 domains of p53. (**B**) The number of missense somatic mutations in human cancers for each codon, according to the *IARC TP53* mutation database R15, was plotted against the p53 map. Data are from 20256 tumor missense mutations. The 7 most frequently mutated residues are indicated. (**C**) The transactivation activity of 2314 missense mutants tested in yeast and plotted against the p53 codon map. The capacity of mutants to transactivate 8 target genes (p21/WAF1, Mdm2, Bax, 14-3-3σ, AIP1, GADD45, Noxa and p53R2) relative to that of wild-type p53 is presented. (Modified from Toledo and Wahl, 2006).

2.1 *TP53* mutations in human cancers cluster in the DNA-binding domain

The functional importance of the p53 DNA-binding domain (DBD) is demonstrated by the fact that more than 70% of *TP53* mutations are missense mutations affecting residues within this domain (Fig. 1B), and leading to a decreased capacity in target gene transactivation (Fig. 1C).

Crystallographic studies showed that the p53 DBD consists of a central β-sandwich that serves as a scaffold for the DNA binding surface, composed of 2 structural motifs. The first loop-sheet-helix motif including loop L1 binds to the DNA major groove. The other half of the DNA binding surface contains two large loops L2 and L3, which interact with the DNA minor groove and can be stabilized by a zinc ion (Fig. 2). Compared to its paralogs p63 and p73, the p53 DBD has evolved to be more dynamic and unstable, with a melting temperature around 44-45°C (Joerger et al., 2006; Joerger and Fersht, 2008). Among the 7 residues most frequently mutated in human cancers, 6 are located at or close to the DNA binding surface (Fig. 2). Depending on their nature, these hotspot mutants can be classified as « contact » or « structural » mutants (Cho et al., 1994).

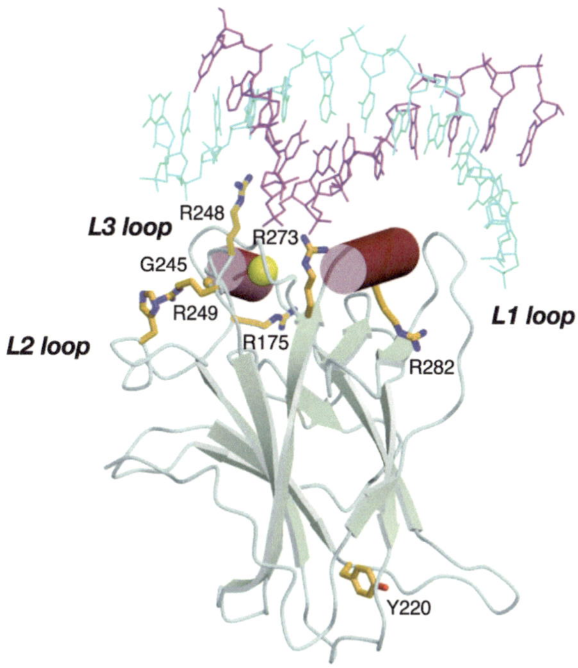

Fig. 2. Structure of the p53 DNA binding domain bound to DNA. The two strands of bound consensus DNA are shown in blue and magenta. The bound Zinc ion is shown as a golden sphere, and the 7 residues that are frequently mutated in human cancers are highlighted in orange (Modified from Joerger et al., 2006).

2.1.1 Contact mutants

Contact mutants affect the residues that interact directly with the DNA helix : residues R248 and R273 (Fig. 2). Crystallographic studies showed that R248 interacts with the minor groove of target DNA, whereas R273 contacts with the phosphate backbone at the center of a p53 binding half-site (a p53 response element is composed of 2 binding half-sites separated by 0-13 base pairs, each half site corresponding to the consensus sequence 5'-RRRCWWGYYY-3', with R = G/A ; W = A/T and Y = C/T). This group of mutants encompasses hotspot mutations R248Q, R248W, R273H and R273C. Two of these were thoroughly studied in mouse models, in which each mutation was targeted at the p53 locus by using homologous recombination in embryonic stem cells.

The mouse model $p53^{R270H}$ (equivalent to human $p53^{R273H}$) revealed the dual property of the mutant protein (Olive et al., 2004). The $p53^{R270H}$ protein could exert dominant negative effects on the wild-type protein by hetero-oligomerization. Compared to their $p53^{+/-}$ counterparts, $p53^{R270H/+}$ mouse embryonic fibroblasts (MEFs) exhibited a faster cycling rate, and $p53^{R270H/+}$ thymocytes exhibited a decreased apoptotic response to γ-irradiation. Furthermore, $p53^{R270H/+}$ mice showed an increased incidence of spontaneous B-cell lymphomas and carcinomas with frequent metastases, a tumor spectrum distinct from that observed in $p53^{+/-}$ mice. In addition, mutant $p53^{R270H}$ exhibited gain-of-function phenotypes, as evidenced by the observation of a much higher incidence of various tumor types in $p53^{R270H/-}$ mice, including high-grade carcinomas with epithelial origin and hemangiosarcomas, which are rarely found in $p53^{-/-}$ mice. The authors attributed this gain-of-function effects to the inhibition of p63 and p73 functions by the mutant p53 protein.

In another study, the two most common p53 cancer mutations, R248W and R273H, were evaluated in mice after their independent targeting at the humanized *p53* knock-in ($p53^{hupki}$) allele. This humanized allele encodes a human/mouse chimeric protein containing human p53 residues 33-332 flanked by murine N-terminal and C-terminal p53 sequences (Song et al., 2007). Both mutants had lost p53-dependent cell-cycle arrest and apoptotic responses, and each showed a more complex tumor spectrum than $p53^{-/-}$ mice, suggesting a gain-of-function. Indeed, by interacting with the Mre11 nuclease and preventing the binding of the Mre11-Rad50-NBS1 complex to DNA double-strand breaks, the mutant proteins were found to disrupt a critical DNA-damage response pathway, and thus to promote genetic instability.

2.1.2 Structural mutants

The mutations of residues that are not in direct contact with DNA but function to stabilize the DNA binding structure are referred to as structural mutants. In contrast to contact mutants, structural mutants affect the overall architecture of the DNA-binding surface and change the conformation of the protein (Cho et al., 1994). Human cancer hotspot mutations R175H, Y220C, G245S, R249S and R282W belong to this category.

The residue R175 is the third most frequently mutated p53 codon in human cancers (Fig. 1B). Two different mutations affecting this residue were analyzed *in vivo*. Mouse models expressing a $p53^{R172H}$ protein (corresponding to $p53^{R175H}$ in humans) were found to be extremely tumor-prone. $p53^{R172H}$ led to the loss of both cell cycle control and apoptosis. In addition, a dominant-negative function of the mutant protein over wild-type p53 and the acquisition of an oncogenic function through p63 and p73 inactivation were reported (Lang et al., 2004; Olive et al., 2004). Another mouse model affecting the same residue is $p53^{R172P}$. This mutant was found unable to induce apoptosis, although it retained partial cell cycle control. Compared to $p53^{-/-}$ mice, $p53^{R172P/R172P}$ mice exhibited a delayed tumor onset ; this indicated that apoptosis is not the only p53-dependent cellular response essential for tumour suppression, and that the maintenance of chromosomal stability is also important (Liu et al., 2004). More recently, further analyses of this mutant, in combination with a deficiency in Mdm2, revealed the importance of p53 and reactive oxygen species (ROS) in the regulation of pools of hematopoietic stem cells (Abbas et al., 2010).

The mutation R249S is often found in human hepatocellular carcinomas associated with exposure to aflatoxin (as detailed below). A targeted mutation leading to the expression of a murine $p53^{R246S}$ (equivalent to human $p53^{R249S}$) has, so far, only been described in embryonic stem cells (Lee and Sabapathy, 2008): this revealed a dominant negative effect of the mutant protein. Transgenic $p53^{R246S}$ mice, described earlier, suggested that this mutant might act as a promoting agent for aflatoxin-induced hepatocarcinogenesis (Ghebranious and Sell, 1998).

The properties of this group of mutant proteins were also proposed to result from their increased propensity to aggregate. The mutants R175H, R249S and R282W could coaggregate, in the cytoplasm, with wild-type p53, p63 or p73, causing deficient induction of target genes (Xu et al., 2011).

Finally, p53 was recently found to facilitate the maturation of a subset of primary miRNAs, by forming a complex with Drosha and p68. p53 point mutations in the DNA binding domain, such as R175H and R273H, were shown to disrupt the interaction between Drosha and p68 and lead to attenuated miRNA processing, suggesting another oncogenic property acquired by these p53 mutants (Suzuki et al., 2009).

2.2 Mutations in other domains of p53

In vitro and transfection studies suggested that post-translational modifications in the transactivation domain (TAD), proline-rich domain (PRD) and C-terminal domain (CTD) are important for p53 activity. Although mutations affecting these domains are extremely rare in human cancers, mouse models carrying such mutations have provided insight into p53 regulation.

2.2.1 Mutations in the Transactivation Domain (TAD)

The N-terminal p53 TAD, containing the major site of interaction with Mdm2, was initially defined as encompassing the first 40 residues of the protein. Phosphorylation of serines in the TAD were thought to be crucial for p53 activation and stabilization, by preventing Mdm2 binding and promoting p300 binding, but when mutations of such residues were targeted at the murine locus and evaluated *in vivo*, unexpected phenotypes were observed. Mutations S18A or S23A (corresponding to human S15A and S20A respectively) independently led to no or mild alterations in p53 stability, transactivation, cell cycle control and apoptosis (Chao et al., 2003; Sluss et al., 2004; Wu et al., 2002). However $p53^{S18A,S23A}$ mice, carrying mutations of the two residues, were deficent in inducing apoptosis and developped various types of late onset tumors (Chao et al., 2006). Furthermore, transfection studies led to propose that human p53 mutations of leucine 22 and tryptophan 23 into glutamine and serine (L22Q and W23S) would disrupt Mdm2 interaction and prevent the recruitement of transcription co-activators, leading to a stabilized p53 protein with reduced transactivation capacity (Lin et al., 1994). This hypothesis was confirmed in a mouse model expressing the equivalent mutant protein $p53^{L25Q,W26S}$ (referred to as $p53^{25,26}$ below) : $p53^{25,26}$

protein was very stable due to the lack of Mdm2 binding, and its ability to transactivate target genes in response to acute DNA damage was impaired. Its increased stability and residual activity led to early embryonic lethality (Johnson et al., 2005).

The work of Zhu et al. led to propose the existence of a secondary TAD domain (TAD2), adjacent to the first TAD, roughly corresponding to residues 43 to 63 (Zhu et al., 1998). The role of the two transactivation domains was further studied in a recent work, which compared the $p53^{25,26}$ mouse model to the mouse $p53^{53,54}$, with 2 mutations in the TAD2 (L53Q and W54S), and to the quadruple mutant $p53^{25,26,53,54}$ (Brady et al., 2011) (Figure 3). The similarity of $p53^{53,54}$ MEFs, but not $p53^{25,26}$ nor $p53^{25,26,53,54}$ MEFs, to wild-type cells in target gene induction after acute genotoxic stress suggested that the p53 DNA damage response relies on an intact TAD1. However, in a model of *KrasG12D*-induced lung tumorigenesis, $p53^{25,26}$ could suppress tumor formation as efficiently as wild-type p53, whereas the quadruple mutant acted as a p53 null protein. Thus, an intact TAD1 is required to achieve an acute genotoxic response, but TAD1 and TAD2 can function redundantly to supress tumors. This may explain why mutations in the TAD are rare in human cancers.

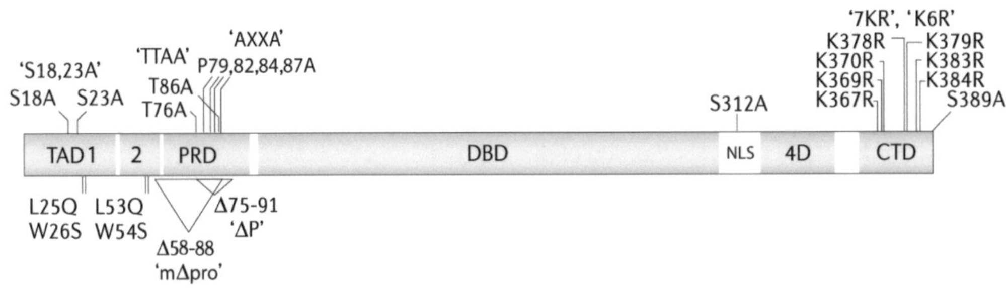

Fig. 3. Schematic representation of the murine p53 protein and the targeted mutations (outside of the DNA binding domain) that were generated. TAD (1 & 2): transactivation domain ; PRD : proline-rich domain ; DBD : DNA binding domain ; NLS : nuclear localization signal ; 4D : tetramerization domain ; CTD : C-terminal domain (Modified from Toledo and Wahl, 2006).

2.2.2 Mutations in the Proline-Rich Domain (PRD)

Human p53 lacking residues 62-91 in the PRD was found to be more sentitive to Mdm2-mediated degradation, and this was proposed to result from the loss of an essential prolyl isomerase PIN1 binding site within the PRD (Berger et al., 2005; Berger et al., 2001; Dumaz et al., 2001). The PRD might also ensure optimal p53-p300 interactions through PXXP motifs (Dornan et al., 2003). Consistent with *in vitro* findings, mouse model $p53^{\Delta P}$, lacking the amino acids 75-91 with all PXXP motifs and putative PIN1 sites deleted, displayed reduced protein stability and transactivation capacity (Toledo et al., 2006). However, $p53^{\Delta P}$ was deficient in cell-cycle control but retained a partial pro-apoptotic capacity, in striking contrast to what transfection studies had suggested. This surprising phenotype was confirmed by the observation that $p53^{\Delta P}$ rescues Mdm4-null but not Mdm2-null embryos. Another mouse model of the PRD, $p53^{m\Delta pro}$, expressing a p53 lacking residues 58-88, was reported later (Slatter et al., 2010). $p53^{m\Delta pro}$ retained a capacity to control the cell cycle in bone marrow cells, but it was not analyzed in MEFs like the $p53^{\Delta P}$ mutant, and attempts to rescue Mdm2-null or Mdm4-null embryos were not performed in a $p53^{m\Delta pro}$ context. Thus, further analyses are needed to evaluate the similarities or differences between the $p53^{\Delta P}$ and $p53^{m\Delta pro}$ mutants.

Mouse mutants with more subtle mutations in the PRD were also reported (Toledo et al., 2007). $p53^{TTAA}$, with threonines 76 and 86 mutated into alanines, removed only the putative PIN1 binding sites in the PRD. These mutations partially affected p53 stabilization upon DNA damage, but the mutant protein remained as active as wild-type p53, suggesting that PIN1 binding sites in the PRD participate in p53 stability control, but exert little effects on p53 function. In the mutant $p53^{AXXA}$, prolines 79, 82, 84 and 87 were mutated into alanines, to remove both PXXP motifs of the murine p53 PRD. The stability and activity of this mutant did not differ significantly from that of WT p53, suggesting either that the PRD has mainly a structural role, or that PXXXXP motifs present in the $p53^{AXXA}$ protein are sufficient to ensure protein-protein interactions.

2.2.3 Mutations in the C-terminal region of the protein

Several kinases may phosphorylate serines 315 and 392 in human p53. Unlike other serines or threonines in p53 that are phosphorylated by stress-related kinases, serine 315 is predominantly phosphorylated by cell cycle-related kinases. Furthermore, whether this phosphorylation regulates p53 functions positively or negatively appeared controversial after *in vitro* studies (Fogal et al., 2005; Qu et al., 2004; Zacchi et al., 2002; Zheng et al., 2002). Two mouse models expressing $p53^{S312A}$ (equivalent to a S315A mutation in human p53) were recently reported (Lee et al., 2010; Slee et al., 2010). This mutation did not affect the survival of mice under normal physiological conditions and appeared to have only mild effects on stress-responses in fibroblasts. However, the irradiation of $p53^{S312A/S312A}$ mice revealed their predisposition to develop thymic lymphomas and liver tumors, and a decreased p53 response was demonstrated in liver tumors (Slee et al., 2010). As for serine 392, *in vitro* studies revealed its phosphorylation in response to UV irradiation, correlated with p53 activation (Kapoor and Lozano, 1998; Lu et al., 1998). Mice with an equivalent mutation (S389A) were resistant to spontaneous tumors with a normal p53 stability, but presented a slightly reduced apoptotic response after UV irradiation, and a slightly higher UV-induced skin tumor occurrence (Bruins et al., 2004).

Human p53 contains 6 lysine residues in its C-terminal domain, subjected to various post-translational modifications including acetylations and ubiquitinations, long thought to be crucial for the regulation of p53 protein activity and stability (Nakamura et al., 2000; Rodriguez et al., 2000). However, mouse models expressing a p53 with 6 or 7 C-terminal lysines mutated into arginines (referred to as $p53^{K6R}$ or $p53^{7KR}$, respectively) appeared rather similar to wild-type mice, suggesting that these residues only participate in the fine-tuning of p53 responses (Feng et al., 2005; Krummel et al., 2005). More recently, $p53^{7KR}$ mice were found to be hypersensitive to γ-irradiation, due to defects in hematopoiesis (Wang et al., 2011).

2.2.4 Mutations in non-coding regions

Cancer related-mutations in intronic sequences were not studied as extensively as those in exons. Mutations in non-coding regions may affect splicing sites, potentially resulting in truncated protein products or reduced protein levels (Holmila et al., 2003). For example, an

A-to-G transition in intron 10 that eliminates a splicing acceptor site and causes a frameshift was recently reported in a pediatric adenocortical tumor (Pinto et al., 2011). *In silico* analyses suggested that the resulting mutant protein may be misfolded or may aggregate, accounting for a loss in tumor suppressor capacity.

3. p53 mutations and the etiology of human cancers

The distribution of *TP53* missense mutations in human cancers correlates with their functional impact, as the most frequent mutations severely impair sequence-specific DNA binding and transactivation. Importantly, the frequencies and types of mutations in *TP53* reflect both the selective growth advantage they confer to mutated cells, and the mutability of a particular codon to endogenous metabolites or exogenous carcinogens. Spontaneous deamination and environmental carcinogens are considered to be the main sources of mutagenesis.

3.1 Spontaneous C to T transversion

CpG dinucleotides in *TP53* are highly methylated in normal tissues, and the 5'-methylated cytosine undergoes spontaneous deamination at a higher rate than an unmethylated base, leading to a cytosine to thymidine transition. 33% of *TP53* DBD mutations occur at methylated CpG sites, affecting 5 major hotspot mutations (codons 175, 245, 248, 273 and 282), and this is considered as a main source of internal cancers (Gonzalgo and Jones, 1997).

3.2 Mutations induced by exogenous carcinogens

3.2.1 Aflatoxin & p53R249S mutations

The incidence of hepatocellular carcinoma (HCC) correlates well with the occurrence of two principal etiologic factors : hepatitis B or C infections and exposure to aflatoxins in the diet, causing a G to T transversion at codon 249 (R249S) (Aguilar et al., 1993). In high incidence areas for HCC, the molds *Aspergillus flavis* and *Aspergillus parasiticum* contaminate maize and peanuts producing aflatoxins that, once metabolized by the liver, may generate DNA adducts at several guanines in *TP53*, leading to G to T transversions. In fact, the aflatoxin adducts occur at a few codons, and the high frequency of R249S (AGG ➔ AGT) mutation results from its clonal selection during hepatocellular carcinogenesis.

3.2.2 Smoking & lung cancer

p53 mutations are common in lung cancers, with a frequency of 75% in smokers, showing a strong correlation between smoking and p53 mutations. Human lung cancers from smokers display a distinct *TP53* mutation pattern with a predominant G to T/A transversion, whereas C to T transitions are enriched in other cancer types. These smoking-induced transversions, caused by the benzo(a)pyrene metabolites in the tobacco smoke, are often observed in methylated CpG sequences at codons 157, 158, 245, 248 and 273 (Le Calvez et al., 2005). Intriguingly, the majority of G to T transversions occur on the nontranscribed strand, suggesting that the benzo(a)pyrene adducts on that strand are less efficiently removed. Thus, the distribution of *TP53* mutations in lung cancers results from the combined effects of site preference for adduct formation, differential DNA strand repair efficiencies, and clonal selection of the mutations that most affect p53 function.

3.2.3 UV & skin carcinomas

The major cause of nonmelanoma skin cancers is sunlight. In basal and squamous cell skin carcinomas, a high frequency of C to T transitions in *TP53* is observed, including tandem CC to TT transitions, considered to be the mutagen fingerprint of ultra-violet (UV) irradiation. The tandem CC to TT transitions would result from UV-induced pyrimidine dimers that escape nucleotide excision repair (NER). Consistent with this, skin tumors from *Xeroderma pigmentosum* patients, deficient in NER, exhibit a high frequency of CC to TT transitions in tumor suppressor genes such as *TP53* and *PTCH1* (Bodak et al., 1999). Importantly, the mutagen fingerprint of UV on the *TP53* gene suggests that farmers, fishermen and forestry workers are predisposed to basal cell skin carcinomas because of their occupational exposure to sunlight (Weihrauch et al., 2002).

4. Effects of Single Nucleotide Polymorphisms (SNPs) in the p53 pathway

By definition, a single nucleotide polymorphisms (SNP) affects at least 1% of a population. Numerous SNPs are present at the *TP53* locus and in genes involved in the p53 network. They may increase cancer risk and affect response to therapeutic regimens.

4.1 SNPs in *TP53* and *TP73*

4.1.1 Codon 72 Pro/Arg

The most studied SNP in *TP53* is the Proline/Arginine variation at codon 72 (referred to as p53-72Pro or p53-72Arg, respectively). This SNP is due to a change in the DNA sequence encoding the proline-rich domain of p53 (CCC or CGC). Experiments in human cell lines have suggested that the variant p53-72Arg is more efficient in inducing apoptosis, whereas p53-72Pro would be more efficent in transactivating p21 and inducing cell cycle arrest (Dumont et al., 2003; Pim and Banks, 2004; Salvioli et al., 2005; Sullivan et al., 2004). Studies of the association of these polymorphic variants with cancer risk have been controversial however (Whibley et al., 2009). Several models of 'humanized' mice designed to reproduce the p53-72Pro/Arg polymorphism were recently reported (Azzam et al., 2011; Frank et al., 2011; Zhu et al., 2010). These models revealed tissue-specific effects of the codon 72-polymorphism, which may explain the controversial findings in human studies.

4.1.2 Codon 47 Pro/Ser

The SNP p53-47 Proline or Serine (referred to as p53-47Pro or p53-47Ser hereafter), resulting from a C to T substitution at position 1 of codon 47, has been reported in populations of African origin (Felley-Bosco et al., 1993). The variant p53-47Ser, which was described to decrease the induction of some pro-apopotic genes by reducing the phosphorylation level at the adjacent serine 46 residue (Li et al., 2005), deserves further investigation.

4.1.3 Codon 217 Val/Met and codon 360 Gly/Ala

The SNP p53-217 Valine/Methionine is the only polymorphism found in the p53 DBD, which could be expected to affect p53 activity. Its function has only been tested in yeast and the p53-217Met variant showed an increased transactivation capacity (Kato et al., 2003). The SNP p53-360 Glycine/Alanine is located in the linker region adjacent to the p53 4D, and a yeast assay indicated that induction of some p53 target genes are slightly decreased with the p53-360Ala variant (Kato et al., 2003). Further studies of these SNPs in a mammalian system are required to address their role in human cancers.

Importantly, additionnal SNPs that appear specific to Chinese populations were recently reported, but their impact on cancer risk remains to be evaluated in large cohorts (Phang et al., 2011). SNPs that could influence cancer risk need to be precisely evaluated in other p53 family members as well. At present, one SNP likely relevant for cancer research has been found in *TP73*. Table 1 summarizes the identified SNPs in members of the p53 family.

Gene	Function	SNP	Molecular description	Clinical association
TP53	Tumor suppressor, transcription factor ; induces cell cycle arrest and apoptosis in response to stress	72Arg/Pro 47Pro/Ser 217Val/Met 360Gly/Ala	See text	
TP73	Transactivates p53 target genes, some isoforms inhibit p53 functions	G4C14/ A4T14	Two linked intronic SNPs, upstream of the translation starting site in position 4 and 14	A4T14 allele : increased risk of squamous cell carcinoma of the head and neck, gastric, colorectal and endometrial cancers ; G4C14 allele : increased risk of lung cancer in Chinese population

Table 1. Cancer-related SNPs in the p53 family. Data collected from (Chen et al., 2008; De Feo et al., 2009; Hu et al., 2005; Kaghad et al., 1997; Niwa et al., 2005; Pfeifer et al., 2005).

4.2 SNPs in the p53 pathway

Genes encoding p53 regulators, and p53 target genes also exhibit single nucleotide polymorphisms, which may affect p53 responses and synergize with SNPs or mutations in *TP53* to alter cancer risk and clinical outcome. The current informations on SNPs in p53 regulators and p53 target genes are summarized in Tables 2 and 3 respectively.

5. Future perspectives : The importance of p53 isoforms

Recent studies have shown that *TP53* has a complex gene structure, much like the genes encoding its family members p63 and p73. Human *TP53* encodes 12 isoforms due to the presence of multiple promoters, translation initiation sites and alternative sites of splicing (Bourdon et al., 2005; Marcel et al., 2010a). These isoforms are expressed in normal tissues in a tissue-specific manner, and at least some of them appear to participate in the regulation of full length-p53 (FL-p53) and to play a role in tumor progression (Bourdon, 2007).

The 12 human p53 protein isoforms are illustrated in Figure 4. Δ40p53, an isoform lacking the first transactivation domain (TAD1), can be obtained by alternative splicing of intron 2 or by the use of alternative translation initiation (Courtois et al., 2002; Ghosh et al., 2004; Ray et al., 2006). Under endoplasmic reticulum (ER) stress, Δ40p53 expression is increased,

Gene	Function	SNP	Molecular description	Clinical association
Mdm2	Regulates p53 stability	SNP309	T/G in intron 1. G creates a Sp1 binding site, increasing Mdm2 expression	G : increased risk for early onset tumors, particularly in young females
Mdm4	Regulates p53 activity	SNP34091	A/C in the 3'UTR region. Mdm4-C allele is a target of hsa-miR-191 but not Mdm4-A	C : later onset of ovarian carcinomas and increased response to chemotherapy
ATM	Phosphorylates and activates p53 upon DNA damage	1853 Asp/Asn	Asp or Asn at codon 1853. Asn leads to decreased activation of p53	Asn : increased colorectal cancer risk and reduced melanoma risk
NQO1	Stabilizes p53 upon oxidative stress	187 Pro/Ser	Pro or Ser at codon 187. Ser leads to loss of activity	Ser : increased cancer risk

Table 2. Cancer-related SNPs in regulators of p53. Summarized data for SNPs in Mdm2 (Bond et al., 2004; Bond and Levine, 2007; Post et al., 2010), Mdm4 (Wynendaele et al., 2010), ATM (Barrett et al., 2011; Jones et al., 2005; Maillet et al., 1999; Thorstenson et al., 2001), NQO1 (Asher and Shaul, 2005; Jamieson et al., 2007; Ross and Siegel, 2004).

Gene	Function	SNP	Molecular description	Clinical association
CDKN1A (p21)	Regulator of G1-S cell cycle progression	31 Ser/Arg	Ser or Arg at codon 31	Ser : increased esophageal, breast cancer risk ; Arg : increased type-C chronic lymphocytic leukemia
CDKN1B (p27)	Regulates cell cycle	-79C/T	C/T in 5'UTR, 79 nt upstream of the translation start site	T : increased prostate, breast, thyroid cancer risk
BAX	pro-apoptotic	-125 G/A	G/A in the promoter, 125 nt before transcription start site	A : increased risk for head and neck carcinomas and chronic lymphocytic leukemia
CASP8	pro-apoptotic	302 Asp/His	Asp or His at codon 302	His : reduced breast cancer incidence

Table 3. Cancer-related SNPs in p53 target genes. Summarized data for SNPs in p21 (Ebner et al., 2010; Johnson et al., 2009; Yang et al., 2010), p27 (Chang et al., 2004; Driver et al., 2008; Landa et al., 2010; Ma et al., 2006), Bax (Chen et al., 2007; Lahiri et al., 2007), Caspase 8 (Cox et al., 2007; MacPherson et al., 2004; Palanca Suela et al., 2009).

leading to G2 arrest (Bourougaa et al., 2010). Transgenic mice overexpressing Δ40p53 exhibit an increased cellular senescence, a slower growth rate, memory loss, neurodegeneration and accelerated ageing (Maier et al., 2004; Pehar et al., 2010).

Δ133p53 and Δ160p53 isoforms are expressed from an evolutionary conserved promoter located in intron 4 (Bourdon et al., 2005). Studies in human cells and zebrafish indicated that this internal promoter is transactivated by FL-p53 (Aoubala et al., 2011; Chen et al., 2009; Marcel et al., 2010b). Human Δ133p53 and zebrafish Δ113p53, isoforms lacking the TAD and part of the DBD, have an anti-apoptotic role (Bourdon et al., 2005; Chen et al., 2009). In addition, overexpression of Δ133p53 was found to extend cellular replicative lifespan by inhibiting p21 and miR-34 (Fujita et al., 2009). Δ133p53 is absent in normal mammary tissues, but present in breast cancers, and its overexpression is correlated with the progression of colon cancer from adenomas to carcinomas. The Δ160p53 isoform results from an alternative translation intiation site, within the same mRNA transcript that encodes Δ133p53 (Marcel et al., 2010a). The function of this isoform, identified very recently, is presently unknown.

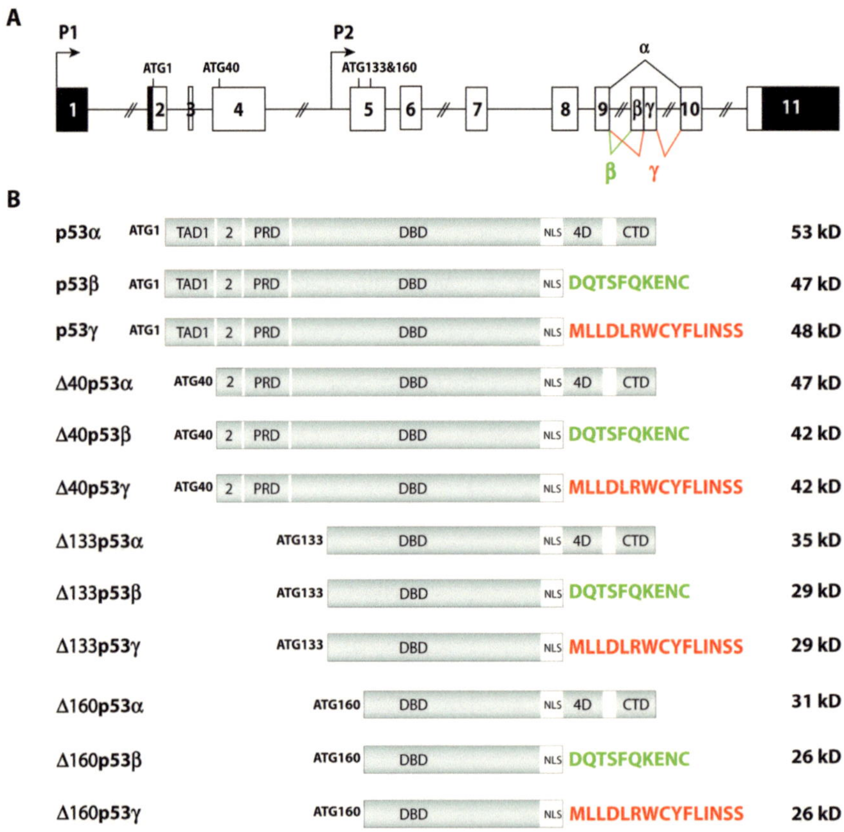

Fig. 4. *TP53* encodes 12 putative isoforms. (**A**) *TP53* gene structure with 2 promoters (P1 and P2), 4 translation initiation sites (ATG1, ATG40, ATG133 and ATG160) and 3 C-terminal alternative splicing sites (α, β and γ). (**B**) 12 protein isoforms of human p53 with their name and molecular weight listed on the left and right, respectively. The functional domains and the specific C-terminal sequences for the β and γ variants are indicated.

The use of alternative splicing sites in intron 9 results in the production of 2 isoforms with distinct C-terminal domains : p53β and p53γ (Bourdon et al., 2005). These 2 isoforms lack the oligomerization domain, but are proposed to work independently of FL-p53 by transactivating p53 target genes in a promoter-specific manner, or together with FL-p53 to modulate its target gene expression. Luciferase assays indicated that p53β could increase p53-dependent expression of *p21*, consistent with the observation that p53β cooperates with FL-p53 to accelerate replicative senescence of human fibroblasts (Fujita et al., 2009). p53γ may enhance p53 transcriptional activity on the *BAX* promoter (Bourdon et al., 2005). In a study of 127 randomly selected primary breast tumors, the expression of the p53β and p53γ were found to associate with oestrogen receptor (ER) expression and mutation of *TP53* gene, respectively (Bourdon et al., 2011). Patients expressing only mutant p53 had a poor prognosis, as expected. Interestingly however, patients with mutations in *TP53* expressing p53γ had low cancer recurrence and an overall survival as good as that of patients with wild-type p53. These results suggest that the expression status of p53 isoforms should be precisely determined in human cancers, to evaluate their relevance in cancer therapy and prognosis. Consequently, it becomes important to determine the impact of each point mutation in *TP53* on the synthesis of p53 isoforms.

6. Acknowledgements

M.F. and I.S. were supported by predoctoral fellowships from the Cancéropôle Ile de France, the Ministère de l'Enseignement Supérieur et de la Recherche and the Ligue Nationale Contre le Cancer. F.T's lab received support from the Fondation de France, the Institut National du Cancer, the Association pour la Recherche sur le Cancer, the Ligue Nationale contre le Cancer (Comité d'Ile de France) and the Emergence-UPMC program from the Université Pierre et Marie Curie.

7. References

Abbas, H.A., Maccio, D.R., Coskun, S., Jackson, J.G., Hazen, A.L., Sills, T.M., You, M.J., Hirschi, K.K., and Lozano, G. (2010). Mdm2 is required for survival of hematopoietic stem cells/progenitors via dampening of ROS-induced p53 activity. Cell Stem Cell *7*, 606-617.

Aguilar, F., Hussain, S.P., and Cerutti, P. (1993). Aflatoxin B1 induces the transversion of G-->T in codon 249 of the p53 tumor suppressor gene in human hepatocytes. Proc Natl Acad Sci U S A *90*, 8586-8590.

Aoubala, M., Murray-Zmijewski, F., Khoury, M.P., Fernandes, K., Perrier, S., Bernard, H., Prats, A.C., Lane, D.P., and Bourdon, J.C. (2011). p53 directly transactivates Delta133p53alpha, regulating cell fate outcome in response to DNA damage. Cell Death Differ *18*, 248-258.

Asher, G., and Shaul, Y. (2005). p53 proteasomal degradation: poly-ubiquitination is not the whole story. Cell Cycle *4*, 1015-1018.

Aylon, Y., and Oren, M. (2010). New plays in the p53 theater. Curr Opin Genet Dev *21*, 86-92.

Azzam, G.A., Frank, A.K., Hollstein, M., and Murphy, M.E. (2011). Tissue-specific apoptotic effects of the p53 codon 72 polymorphism in a mouse model. Cell Cycle *10*, 1352-1355.

Baker, S.J., Fearon, E.R., Nigro, J.M., Hamilton, S.R., Preisinger, A.C., Jessup, J.M., vanTuinen, P., Ledbetter, D.H., Barker, D.F., Nakamura, Y., *et al.* (1989). Chromosome 17 deletions and p53 gene mutations in colorectal carcinomas. Science *244*, 217-221.

Barrett, J.H., Iles, M.M., Harland, M., Taylor, J.C., Aitken, J.F., Andresen, P.A., Akslen, L.A., Armstrong, B.K., Avril, M.F., Azizi, E., *et al.* (2011). Genome-wide association study identifies three new melanoma susceptibility loci. Nat Genet.

Berger, M., Stahl, N., Del Sal, G., and Haupt, Y. (2005). Mutations in proline 82 of p53 impair its activation by Pin1 and Chk2 in response to DNA damage. Mol Cell Biol *25*, 5380-5388.

Berger, M., Vogt Sionov, R., Levine, A.J., and Haupt, Y. (2001). A role for the polyproline domain of p53 in its regulation by Mdm2. J Biol Chem *276*, 3785-3790.

Bodak, N., Queille, S., Avril, M.F., Bouadjar, B., Drougard, C., Sarasin, A., and Daya-Grosjean, L. (1999). High levels of patched gene mutations in basal-cell carcinomas from patients with xeroderma pigmentosum. Proc Natl Acad Sci U S A *96*, 5117-5122.

Bond, G.L., Hu, W., Bond, E.E., Robins, H., Lutzker, S.G., Arva, N.C., Bargonetti, J., Bartel, F., Taubert, H., Wuerl, P., *et al.* (2004). A single nucleotide polymorphism in the MDM2 promoter attenuates the p53 tumor suppressor pathway and accelerates tumor formation in humans. Cell *119*, 591-602.

Bond, G.L., and Levine, A.J. (2007). A single nucleotide polymorphism in the p53 pathway interacts with gender, environmental stresses and tumor genetics to influence cancer in humans. Oncogene *26*, 1317-1323.

Bourdon, J.C. (2007). p53 and its isoforms in cancer. Br J Cancer *97*, 277-282.

Bourdon, J.C., Fernandes, K., Murray-Zmijewski, F., Liu, G., Diot, A., Xirodimas, D.P., Saville, M.K., and Lane, D.P. (2005). p53 isoforms can regulate p53 transcriptional activity. Genes Dev *19*, 2122-2137.

Bourdon, J.C., Khoury, M.P., Diot, A., Baker, L., Fernandes, K., Aoubala, M., Quinlan, P., Purdie, C.A., Jordan, L.B., Prats, A.C., *et al.* (2011). p53 mutant breast cancer patients expressing p53gamma have as good a prognosis as wild-type p53 breast cancer patients. Breast Cancer Res *13*, R7.

Bourougaa, K., Naski, N., Boularan, C., Mlynarczyk, C., Candeias, M.M., Marullo, S., and Fahraeus, R. (2010). Endoplasmic reticulum stress induces G2 cell-cycle arrest via mRNA translation of the p53 isoform p53/47. Mol Cell *38*, 78-88.

Brady, C.A., Jiang, D., Mello, S.S., Johnson, T.M., Jarvis, L.A., Kozak, M.M., Kenzelmann Broz, D., Basak, S., Park, E.J., McLaughlin, M.E., *et al.* (2011). Distinct p53 transcriptional programs dictate acute DNA-damage responses and tumor suppression. Cell *145*, 571-583.

Brooks, C.L., and Gu, W. (2006). p53 ubiquitination: Mdm2 and beyond. Mol Cell *21*, 307-315.

Bruins, W., Zwart, E., Attardi, L.D., Iwakuma, T., Hoogervorst, E.M., Beems, R.B., Miranda, B., van Oostrom, C.T., van den Berg, J., van den Aardweg, G.J., *et al.* (2004).

Increased sensitivity to UV radiation in mice with a p53 point mutation at Ser389. Mol Cell Biol *24*, 8884-8894.

Chang, B.L., Zheng, S.L., Isaacs, S.D., Wiley, K.E., Turner, A., Li, G., Walsh, P.C., Meyers, D.A., Isaacs, W.B., and Xu, J. (2004). A polymorphism in the CDKN1B gene is associated with increased risk of hereditary prostate cancer. Cancer Res *64*, 1997-1999.

Chao, C., Hergenhahn, M., Kaeser, M.D., Wu, Z., Saito, S., Iggo, R., Hollstein, M., Appella, E., and Xu, Y. (2003). Cell type- and promoter-specific roles of Ser18 phosphorylation in regulating p53 responses. J Biol Chem *278*, 41028-41033.

Chao, C., Herr, D., Chun, J., and Xu, Y. (2006). Ser18 and 23 phosphorylation is required for p53-dependent apoptosis and tumor suppression. Embo J *25*, 2615-2622.

Chen, J., Ng, S.M., Chang, C., Zhang, Z., Bourdon, J.C., Lane, D.P., and Peng, J. (2009). p53 isoform delta113p53 is a p53 target gene that antagonizes p53 apoptotic activity via BclxL activation in zebrafish. Genes Dev *23*, 278-290.

Chen, K., Hu, Z., Wang, L.E., Sturgis, E.M., El-Naggar, A.K., Zhang, W., and Wei, Q. (2007). Single-nucleotide polymorphisms at the TP53-binding or responsive promoter regions of BAX and BCL2 genes and risk of squamous cell carcinoma of the head and neck. Carcinogenesis *28*, 2008-2012.

Chen, X., Sturgis, E.M., Etzel, C.J., Wei, Q., and Li, G. (2008). p73 G4C14-to-A4T14 polymorphism and risk of human papillomavirus-associated squamous cell carcinoma of the oropharynx in never smokers and never drinkers. Cancer *113*, 3307-3314.

Cho, Y., Gorina, S., Jeffrey, P.D., and Pavletich, N.P. (1994). Crystal structure of a p53 tumor suppressor-DNA complex: understanding tumorigenic mutations. Science *265*, 346-355.

Courtois, S., Verhaegh, G., North, S., Luciani, M.G., Lassus, P., Hibner, U., Oren, M., and Hainaut, P. (2002). DeltaN-p53, a natural isoform of p53 lacking the first transactivation domain, counteracts growth suppression by wild-type p53. Oncogene *21*, 6722-6728.

Cox, A., Dunning, A.M., Garcia-Closas, M., Balasubramanian, S., Reed, M.W., Pooley, K.A., Scollen, S., Baynes, C., Ponder, B.A., Chanock, S., *et al.* (2007). A common coding variant in CASP8 is associated with breast cancer risk. Nat Genet *39*, 352-358.

Cui, R., Widlund, H.R., Feige, E., Lin, J.Y., Wilensky, D.L., Igras, V.E., D'Orazio, J., Fung, C.Y., Schanbacher, C.F., Granter, S.R., and Fisher, D.E. (2007). Central role of p53 in the suntan response and pathologic hyperpigmentation. Cell *128*, 853-864.

De Feo, E., Persiani, R., La Greca, A., Amore, R., Arzani, D., Rausei, S., D'Ugo, D., Magistrelli, P., van Duijn, C.M., Ricciardi, G., and Boccia, S. (2009). A case-control study on the effect of p53 and p73 gene polymorphisms on gastric cancer risk and progression. Mutat Res *675*, 60-65.

DeLeo, A.B., Jay, G., Appella, E., Dubois, G.C., Law, L.W., and Old, L.J. (1979). Detection of a transformation-related antigen in chemically induced sarcomas and other transformed cells of the mouse. Proc Natl Acad Sci U S A *76*, 2420-2424.

Dornan, D., Shimizu, H., Burch, L., Smith, A.J., and Hupp, T.R. (2003). The proline repeat domain of p53 binds directly to the transcriptional coactivator p300 and allosterically controls DNA-dependent acetylation of p53. Mol Cell Biol *23*, 8846-8861.

Driver, K.E., Song, H., Lesueur, F., Ahmed, S., Barbosa-Morais, N.L., Tyrer, J.P., Ponder, B.A., Easton, D.F., Pharoah, P.D., and Dunning, A.M. (2008). Association of single-nucleotide polymorphisms in the cell cycle genes with breast cancer in the British population. Carcinogenesis *29*, 333-341.

Dumaz, N., Milne, D.M., Jardine, L.J., and Meek, D.W. (2001). Critical roles for the serine 20, but not the serine 15, phosphorylation site and for the polyproline domain in regulating p53 turnover. Biochem J *359*, 459-464.

Dumont, P., Leu, J.I., Della Pietra, A.C., 3rd, George, D.L., and Murphy, M. (2003). The codon 72 polymorphic variants of p53 have markedly different apoptotic potential. Nat Genet *33*, 357-365.

Ebner, F., Schremmer-Danninger, E., and Rehbock, J. (2010). The role of TP53 and p21 gene polymorphisms in breast cancer biology in a well specified and characterized German cohort. J Cancer Res Clin Oncol *136*, 1369-1375.

Felley-Bosco, E., Weston, A., Cawley, H.M., Bennett, W.P., and Harris, C.C. (1993). Functional studies of a germ-line polymorphism at codon 47 within the p53 gene. Am J Hum Genet *53*, 752-759.

Feng, L., Lin, T., Uranishi, H., Gu, W., and Xu, Y. (2005). Functional analysis of the roles of posttranslational modifications at the p53 C terminus in regulating p53 stability and activity. Mol Cell Biol *25*, 5389-5395.

Finlay, C.A., Hinds, P.W., and Levine, A.J. (1989). The p53 proto-oncogene can act as a suppressor of transformation. Cell *57*, 1083-1093.

Fogal, V., Hsieh, J.K., Royer, C., Zhong, S., and Lu, X. (2005). Cell cycle-dependent nuclear retention of p53 by E2F1 requires phosphorylation of p53 at Ser315. Embo J *24*, 2768-2782.

Frank, A.K., Leu, J.I., Zhou, Y., Devarajan, K., Nedelko, T., Klein-Szanto, A., Hollstein, M., and Murphy, M.E. (2011). The codon 72 polymorphism of p53 regulates interaction with NF-{kappa}B and transactivation of genes involved in immunity and inflammation. Mol Cell Biol *31*, 1201-1213.

Fujita, K., Mondal, A.M., Horikawa, I., Nguyen, G.H., Kumamoto, K., Sohn, J.J., Bowman, E.D., Mathe, E.A., Schetter, A.J., Pine, S.R., *et al.* (2009). p53 isoforms Delta133p53 and p53beta are endogenous regulators of replicative cellular senescence. Nat Cell Biol *11*, 1135-1142.

Ghebranious, N., and Sell, S. (1998). The mouse equivalent of the human p53ser249 mutation p53ser246 enhances aflatoxin hepatocarcinogenesis in hepatitis B surface antigen transgenic and p53 heterozygous null mice. Hepatology *27*, 967-973.

Ghosh, A., Stewart, D., and Matlashewski, G. (2004). Regulation of human p53 activity and cell localization by alternative splicing. Mol Cell Biol *24*, 7987-7997.

Gonzalgo, M.L., and Jones, P.A. (1997). Mutagenic and epigenetic effects of DNA methylation. Mutat Res *386*, 107-118.

Hinds, P., Finlay, C., and Levine, A.J. (1989). Mutation is required to activate the p53 gene for cooperation with the ras oncogene and transformation. J Virol *63*, 739-746.

Holmila, R., Fouquet, C., Cadranel, J., Zalcman, G., and Soussi, T. (2003). Splice mutations in the p53 gene: case report and review of the literature. Hum Mutat *21*, 101-102.

Hu, Z., Miao, X., Ma, H., Tan, W., Wang, X., Lu, D., Wei, Q., Lin, D., and Shen, H. (2005). Dinucleotide polymorphism of p73 gene is associated with a reduced risk of lung cancer in a Chinese population. Int J Cancer *114*, 455-460.

Jamieson, D., Wilson, K., Pridgeon, S., Margetts, J.P., Edmondson, R.J., Leung, H.Y., Knox, R., and Boddy, A.V. (2007). NAD(P)H:quinone oxidoreductase 1 and nrh:quinone oxidoreductase 2 activity and expression in bladder and ovarian cancer and lower NRH:quinone oxidoreductase 2 activity associated with an NQO2 exon 3 single-nucleotide polymorphism. Clin Cancer Res *13*, 1584-1590.

Joerger, A.C., Ang, H.C., and Fersht, A.R. (2006). Structural basis for understanding oncogenic p53 mutations and designing rescue drugs. Proc Natl Acad Sci U S A *103*, 15056-15061.

Joerger, A.C., and Fersht, A.R. (2008). Structural biology of the tumor suppressor p53. Annu Rev Biochem *77*, 557-582.

Johnson, G.G., Sherrington, P.D., Carter, A., Lin, K., Liloglou, T., Field, J.K., and Pettitt, A.R. (2009). A novel type of p53 pathway dysfunction in chronic lymphocytic leukemia resulting from two interacting single nucleotide polymorphisms within the p21 gene. Cancer Res *69*, 5210-5217.

Johnson, T.M., Hammond, E.M., Giaccia, A., and Attardi, L.D. (2005). The p53QS transactivation-deficient mutant shows stress-specific apoptotic activity and induces embryonic lethality. Nat Genet *37*, 145-152.

Jones, J.S., Gu, X., Lynch, P.M., Rodriguez-Bigas, M., Amos, C.I., and Frazier, M.L. (2005). ATM polymorphism and hereditary nonpolyposis colorectal cancer (HNPCC) age of onset (United States). Cancer Causes Control *16*, 749-753.

Kaghad, M., Bonnet, H., Yang, A., Creancier, L., Biscan, J.C., Valent, A., Minty, A., Chalon, P., Lelias, J.M., Dumont, X., *et al.* (1997). Monoallelically expressed gene related to p53 at 1p36, a region frequently deleted in neuroblastoma and other human cancers. Cell *90*, 809-819.

Kapoor, M., and Lozano, G. (1998). Functional activation of p53 via phosphorylation following DNA damage by UV but not gamma radiation. Proc Natl Acad Sci U S A *95*, 2834-2837.

Kato, S., Han, S.Y., Liu, W., Otsuka, K., Shibata, H., Kanamaru, R., and Ishioka, C. (2003). Understanding the function-structure and function-mutation relationships of p53 tumor suppressor protein by high-resolution missense mutation analysis. Proc Natl Acad Sci U S A *100*, 8424-8429.

Kress, M., May, E., Cassingena, R., and May, P. (1979). Simian virus 40-transformed cells express new species of proteins precipitable by anti-simian virus 40 tumor serum. J Virol *31*, 472-483.

Krummel, K.A., Lee, C.J., Toledo, F., and Wahl, G.M. (2005). The C-terminal lysines fine-tune P53 stress responses in a mouse model but are not required for stability control or transactivation. Proc Natl Acad Sci U S A *102*, 10188-10193.

Lahiri, O., Harris, S., Packham, G., and Howell, M. (2007). p53 pathway gene single nucleotide polymorphisms and chronic lymphocytic leukemia. Cancer Genet Cytogenet *179*, 36-44.

Landa, I., Montero-Conde, C., Malanga, D., De Gisi, S., Pita, G., Leandro-Garcia, L.J., Inglada-Perez, L., Leton, R., De Marco, C., Rodriguez-Antona, C., *et al.* (2010). Allelic variant at -79 (C>T) in CDKN1B (p27Kip1) confers an increased risk of thyroid cancer and alters mRNA levels. Endocr Relat Cancer *17*, 317-328.

Lane, D.P., and Crawford, L.V. (1979). T antigen is bound to a host protein in SV40-transformed cells. Nature *278*, 261-263.

Lang, G.A., Iwakuma, T., Suh, Y.A., Liu, G., Rao, V.A., Parant, J.M., Valentin-Vega, Y.A., Terzian, T., Caldwell, L.C., Strong, L.C., *et al.* (2004). Gain of function of a p53 hot spot mutation in a mouse model of Li-Fraumeni syndrome. Cell *119*, 861-872.

Le Calvez, F., Mukeria, A., Hunt, J.D., Kelm, O., Hung, R.J., Taniere, P., Brennan, P., Boffetta, P., Zaridze, D.G., and Hainaut, P. (2005). TP53 and KRAS mutation load and types in lung cancers in relation to tobacco smoke: distinct patterns in never, former, and current smokers. Cancer Res *65*, 5076-5083.

Lee, M.K., and Sabapathy, K. (2008). The R246S hot-spot p53 mutant exerts dominant-negative effects in embryonic stem cells in vitro and in vivo. J Cell Sci *121*, 1899-1906.

Lee, M.K., Tong, W.M., Wang, Z.Q., and Sabapathy, K. (2010). Serine 312 phosphorylation is dispensable for wild-type p53 functions in vivo. Cell Death Differ *18*, 214-221.

Levine, A.J. (1997). p53, the cellular gatekeeper for growth and division. Cell *88*, 323-331.

Li, X., Dumont, P., Della Pietra, A., Shetler, C., and Murphy, M.E. (2005). The codon 47 polymorphism in p53 is functionally significant. J Biol Chem *280*, 24245-24251.

Lin, J., Chen, J., Elenbaas, B., and Levine, A.J. (1994). Several hydrophobic amino acids in the p53 amino-terminal domain are required for transcriptional activation, binding to mdm-2 and the adenovirus 5 E1B 55-kD protein. Genes Dev *8*, 1235-1246.

Linzer, D.I., and Levine, A.J. (1979). Characterization of a 54K dalton cellular SV40 tumor antigen present in SV40-transformed cells and uninfected embryonal carcinoma cells. Cell *17*, 43-52.

Liu, G., Parant, J.M., Lang, G., Chau, P., Chavez-Reyes, A., El-Naggar, A.K., Multani, A., Chang, S., and Lozano, G. (2004). Chromosome stability, in the absence of apoptosis, is critical for suppression of tumorigenesis in Trp53 mutant mice. Nat Genet *36*, 63-68.

Lu, H., Taya, Y., Ikeda, M., and Levine, A.J. (1998). Ultraviolet radiation, but not gamma radiation or etoposide-induced DNA damage, results in the phosphorylation of the murine p53 protein at serine-389. Proc Natl Acad Sci U S A *95*, 6399-6402.

Ma, H., Jin, G., Hu, Z., Zhai, X., Chen, W., Wang, S., Wang, X., Qin, J., Gao, J., Liu, J., *et al.* (2006). Variant genotypes of CDKN1A and CDKN1B are associated with an increased risk of breast cancer in Chinese women. Int J Cancer *119*, 2173-2178.

MacPherson, G., Healey, C.S., Teare, M.D., Balasubramanian, S.P., Reed, M.W., Pharoah, P.D., Ponder, B.A., Meuth, M., Bhattacharyya, N.P., and Cox, A. (2004). Association of a common variant of the CASP8 gene with reduced risk of breast cancer. J Natl Cancer Inst *96*, 1866-1869.

Maier, B., Gluba, W., Bernier, B., Turner, T., Mohammad, K., Guise, T., Sutherland, A., Thorner, M., and Scrable, H. (2004). Modulation of mammalian life span by the short isoform of p53. Genes Dev *18*, 306-319.

Maillet, P., Vaudan, G., Chappuis, P., and Sappino, A. (1999). PCR-mediated detection of a polymorphism in the ATM gene. Mol Cell Probes *13*, 67-69.

Malkin, D., Li, F.P., Strong, L.C., Fraumeni, J.F., Jr., Nelson, C.E., Kim, D.H., Kassel, J., Gryka, M.A., Bischoff, F.Z., Tainsky, M.A., and et al. (1990). Germ line p53 mutations in a familial syndrome of breast cancer, sarcomas, and other neoplasms. Science *250*, 1233-1238.

Marcel, V., Perrier, S., Aoubala, M., Ageorges, S., Groves, M.J., Diot, A., Fernandes, K., Tauro, S., and Bourdon, J.C. (2010a). Delta160p53 is a novel N-terminal p53 isoform encoded by Delta133p53 transcript. FEBS Lett *584*, 4463-4468.

Marcel, V., Vijayakumar, V., Fernandez-Cuesta, L., Hafsi, H., Sagne, C., Hautefeuille, A., Olivier, M., and Hainaut, P. (2010b). p53 regulates the transcription of its Delta133p53 isoform through specific response elements contained within the TP53 P2 internal promoter. Oncogene *29*, 2691-2700.

Marine, J.C., Francoz, S., Maetens, M., Wahl, G., Toledo, F., and Lozano, G. (2006). Keeping p53 in check: essential and synergistic functions of Mdm2 and Mdm4. Cell Death Differ *13*, 927-934.

Nakamura, S., Roth, J.A., and Mukhopadhyay, T. (2000). Multiple lysine mutations in the C-terminal domain of p53 interfere with MDM2-dependent protein degradation and ubiquitination. Mol Cell Biol *20*, 9391-9398.

Nigro, J.M., Baker, S.J., Preisinger, A.C., Jessup, J.M., Hostetter, R., Cleary, K., Bigner, S.H., Davidson, N., Baylin, S., Devilee, P., and et al. (1989). Mutations in the p53 gene occur in diverse human tumour types. Nature *342*, 705-708.

Niwa, Y., Hirose, K., Matsuo, K., Tajima, K., Ikoma, Y., Nakanishi, T., Nawa, A., Kuzuya, K., Tamakoshi, A., and Hamajima, N. (2005). Association of p73 G4C14-to-A4T14 polymorphism at exon 2 and p53 Arg72Pro polymorphism with the risk of endometrial cancer in Japanese subjects. Cancer Lett *219*, 183-190.

Olive, K.P., Tuveson, D.A., Ruhe, Z.C., Yin, B., Willis, N.A., Bronson, R.T., Crowley, D., and Jacks, T. (2004). Mutant p53 gain of function in two mouse models of Li-Fraumeni syndrome. Cell *119*, 847-860.

Olivier, M., Hollstein, M., and Hainaut, P. (2010). TP53 mutations in human cancers: origins, consequences, and clinical use. Cold Spring Harb Perspect Biol *2*, a001008.

Palanca Suela, S., Esteban Cardenosa, E., Barragan Gonzalez, E., de Juan Jimenez, I., Chirivella Gonzalez, I., Segura Huerta, A., Guillen Ponce, C., Martinez de Duenas, E., Montalar Salcedo, J., Castel Sanchez, V., and Bolufer Gilabert, P. (2009). CASP8 D302H polymorphism delays the age of onset of breast cancer in BRCA1 and BRCA2 carriers. Breast Cancer Res Treat *119*, 87-93.

Pehar, M., O'Riordan, K.J., Burns-Cusato, M., Andrzejewski, M.E., del Alcazar, C.G., Burger, C., Scrable, H., and Puglielli, L. (2010). Altered longevity-assurance activity of p53:p44 in the mouse causes memory loss, neurodegeneration and premature death. Aging Cell *9*, 174-190.

Petitjean, A., Mathe, E., Kato, S., Ishioka, C., Tavtigian, S.V., Hainaut, P., and Olivier, M. (2007). Impact of mutant p53 functional properties on TP53 mutation patterns and tumor phenotype: lessons from recent developments in the IARC TP53 database. Hum Mutat *28*, 622-629.

Pfeifer, D., Arbman, G., and Sun, X.F. (2005). Polymorphism of the p73 gene in relation to colorectal cancer risk and survival. Carcinogenesis *26*, 103-107.

Phang, B.H., Chua, H.W., Li, H., Linn, Y.C., and Sabapathy, K. (2011). Characterization of novel and uncharacterized p53 SNPs in the Chinese population--intron 2 SNP co-segregates with the common codon 72 polymorphism. PLoS One *6*, e15320.

Pim, D., and Banks, L. (2004). p53 polymorphic variants at codon 72 exert different effects on cell cycle progression. Int J Cancer *108*, 196-199.

Pinto, E.M., Ribeiro, R.C., Kletter, G.B., Lawrence, J.P., Jenkins, J.J., Wang, J., Shurtleff, S., McGregor, L., Kriwacki, R.W., and Zambetti, G.P. (2011). Inherited germline TP53 mutation encodes a protein with an aberrant C-terminal motif in a case of pediatric adrenocortical tumor. Fam Cancer *10*, 141-146.

Post, S.M., Quintas-Cardama, A., Pant, V., Iwakuma, T., Hamir, A., Jackson, J.G., Maccio, D.R., Bond, G.L., Johnson, D.G., Levine, A.J., and Lozano, G. (2010). A high-frequency regulatory polymorphism in the p53 pathway accelerates tumor development. Cancer Cell *18*, 220-230.

Qu, L., Huang, S., Baltzis, D., Rivas-Estilla, A.M., Pluquet, O., Hatzoglou, M., Koumenis, C., Taya, Y., Yoshimura, A., and Koromilas, A.E. (2004). Endoplasmic reticulum stress induces p53 cytoplasmic localization and prevents p53-dependent apoptosis by a pathway involving glycogen synthase kinase-3beta. Genes Dev *18*, 261-277.

Ray, P.S., Grover, R., and Das, S. (2006). Two internal ribosome entry sites mediate the translation of p53 isoforms. EMBO Rep *7*, 404-410.

Rodriguez, M.S., Desterro, J.M., Lain, S., Lane, D.P., and Hay, R.T. (2000). Multiple C-terminal lysine residues target p53 for ubiquitin-proteasome-mediated degradation. Mol Cell Biol *20*, 8458-8467.

Ross, D., and Siegel, D. (2004). NAD(P)H:quinone oxidoreductase 1 (NQO1, DT-diaphorase), functions and pharmacogenetics. Methods Enzymol *382*, 115-144.

Salvioli, S., Bonafe, M., Barbi, C., Storci, G., Trapassi, C., Tocco, F., Gravina, S., Rossi, M., Tiberi, L., Mondello, C., *et al.* (2005). p53 codon 72 alleles influence the response to anticancer drugs in cells from aged people by regulating the cell cycle inhibitor p21WAF1. Cell Cycle *4*, 1264-1271.

Slatter, T.L., Ganesan, P., Holzhauer, C., Mehta, R., Rubio, C., Williams, G., Wilson, M., Royds, J.A., Baird, M.A., and Braithwaite, A.W. (2010). p53-mediated apoptosis prevents the accumulation of progenitor B cells and B-cell tumors. Cell Death Differ *17*, 540-550.

Slee, E.A., Benassi, B., Goldin, R., Zhong, S., Ratnayaka, I., Blandino, G., and Lu, X. (2010). Phosphorylation of Ser312 contributes to tumor suppression by p53 in vivo. Proc Natl Acad Sci U S A *107*, 19479-19484.

Sluss, H.K., Armata, H., Gallant, J., and Jones, S.N. (2004). Phosphorylation of serine 18 regulates distinct p53 functions in mice. Mol Cell Biol *24*, 976-984.

Song, H., Hollstein, M., and Xu, Y. (2007). p53 gain-of-function cancer mutants induce genetic instability by inactivating ATM. Nat Cell Biol *9*, 573-580.

Sullivan, A., Syed, N., Gasco, M., Bergamaschi, D., Trigiante, G., Attard, M., Hiller, L., Farrell, P.J., Smith, P., Lu, X., and Crook, T. (2004). Polymorphism in wild-type p53 modulates response to chemotherapy in vitro and in vivo. Oncogene *23*, 3328-3337.

Suzuki, H.I., Yamagata, K., Sugimoto, K., Iwamoto, T., Kato, S., and Miyazono, K. (2009). Modulation of microRNA processing by p53. Nature *460*, 529-533.

Thorstenson, Y.R., Shen, P., Tusher, V.G., Wayne, T.L., Davis, R.W., Chu, G., and Oefner, P.J. (2001). Global analysis of ATM polymorphism reveals significant functional constraint. Am J Hum Genet *69*, 396-412.

Toledo, F., Krummel, K.A., Lee, C.J., Liu, C.W., Rodewald, L.W., Tang, M., and Wahl, G.M. (2006). A mouse p53 mutant lacking the proline-rich domain rescues Mdm4 deficiency and provides insight into the Mdm2-Mdm4-p53 regulatory network. Cancer Cell *9*, 273-285.

Toledo, F., Lee, C.J., Krummel, K.A., Rodewald, L.W., Liu, C.W., and Wahl, G.M. (2007). Mouse mutants reveal that putative protein interaction sites in the p53 proline-rich domain are dispensable for tumor suppression. Mol Cell Biol *27*, 1425-1432.

Toledo, F., and Wahl, G.M. (2006). Regulating the p53 pathway: in vitro hypotheses, in vivo veritas. Nat Rev Cancer *6*, 909-923.

Vogelstein, B., Lane, D., and Levine, A.J. (2000). Surfing the p53 network. Nature *408*, 307-310.

Vousden, K.H., and Ryan, K.M. (2009). p53 and metabolism. Nat Rev Cancer *9*, 691-700.

Wade, M., Wang, Y.V., and Wahl, G.M. (2010). The p53 orchestra: Mdm2 and Mdmx set the tone. Trends Cell Biol *20*, 299-309.

Wang, Y.V., Leblanc, M., Fox, N., Mao, J.H., Tinkum, K.L., Krummel, K., Engle, D., Piwnica-Worms, D., Piwnica-Worms, H., Balmain, A., *et al.* (2011). Fine-tuning p53 activity through C-terminal modification significantly contributes to HSC homeostasis and mouse radiosensitivity. Genes Dev *25*, 1426-1438.

Weihrauch, M., Bader, M., Lehnert, G., Wittekind, C., Tannapfel, A., and Wrbitzky, R. (2002). Carcinogen-specific mutation pattern in the p53 tumour suppressor gene in UV radiation-induced basal cell carcinoma. Int Arch Occup Environ Health *75*, 272-276.

Whibley, C., Pharoah, P.D., and Hollstein, M. (2009). p53 polymorphisms: cancer implications. Nat Rev Cancer *9*, 95-107.

Wu, Z., Earle, J., Saito, S., Anderson, C.W., Appella, E., and Xu, Y. (2002). Mutation of mouse p53 Ser23 and the response to DNA damage. Mol Cell Biol *22*, 2441-2449.

Wynendaele, J., Bohnke, A., Leucci, E., Nielsen, S.J., Lambertz, I., Hammer, S., Sbrzesny, N., Kubitza, D., Wolf, A., Gradhand, E., *et al.* (2010). An illegitimate microRNA target site within the 3' UTR of MDM4 affects ovarian cancer progression and chemosensitivity. Cancer Res *70*, 9641-9649.

Xu, J., Reumers, J., Couceiro, J.R., De Smet, F., Gallardo, R., Rudyak, S., Cornelis, A., Rozenski, J., Zwolinska, A., Marine, J.C., *et al.* (2011). Gain of function of mutant p53 by coaggregation with multiple tumor suppressors. Nat Chem Biol *7*, 285-295.

Yang, W., Qi, Q., Zhang, H., Xu, W., Chen, Z., Wang, L., Wang, Y., Dong, X., Jiao, H., and Huo, Z. (2010). p21 Waf1/Cip1 polymorphisms and risk of esophageal cancer. Ann Surg Oncol *17*, 1453-1458.

Zacchi, P., Gostissa, M., Uchida, T., Salvagno, C., Avolio, F., Volinia, S., Ronai, Z., Blandino, G., Schneider, C., and Del Sal, G. (2002). The prolyl isomerase Pin1 reveals a mechanism to control p53 functions after genotoxic insults. Nature *419*, 853-857.

Zheng, H., You, H., Zhou, X.Z., Murray, S.A., Uchida, T., Wulf, G., Gu, L., Tang, X., Lu, K.P., and Xiao, Z.X. (2002). The prolyl isomerase Pin1 is a regulator of p53 in genotoxic response. Nature *419*, 849-853.

Zhu, F., Dolle, M.E., Berton, T.R., Kuiper, R.V., Capps, C., Espejo, A., McArthur, M.J., Bedford, M.T., van Steeg, H., de Vries, A., and Johnson, D.G. (2010). Mouse models for the p53 R72P polymorphism mimic human phenotypes. Cancer Res *70*, 5851-5859.

Zhu, J., Zhou, W., Jiang, J., and Chen, X. (1998). Identification of a novel p53 functional domain that is necessary for mediating apoptosis. J Biol Chem *273*, 13030-13036.

14

Transgenerational Effects of Maternal Nicotine Exposure During Gestation and Lactation on the Respiratory System

G. S. Maritz
Department of Medical Biosciences,
University of the Western Cape, Bellville,
South Africa

1. Introduction

Both genetic and environmental factors affect an individual's risk for chronic obstructive lung disease [1]. Air pollution continues to be a major public health concern in industrialized cities throughout the world. Recent population and epidemiological studies that have associated ozone and particulate exposures with morbidity and mortality outcomes underscore the important detrimental effects of these pollutants on the lung. Inter-individual variation in human responses to air pollutants suggests that some subpopulations are at increased risk to the detrimental effects of pollutant exposure, and it has become clear that genetic background is an important susceptibility factor. Environmental exposures to inhaled pollutants and genetic factors associated with disease risk likely interact in a complex fashion that varies from one population to another [2]. Investigations have suggested an influence of age on genetic susceptibility to lung cancer and other diseases, which indicate that an interaction between age and genetic background may be important in air pollution disease pathogenesis [3]. Tobacco smoke is an important contributor to the factors in the environment that impact on the health of individuals, including the fetus in the womb.

Although cigarette smoking during pregnancy is associated with adverse fetal, obstetrical, and developmental outcomes, 15–20% of all women smoke throughout the duration of pregnancy [4, 5], despite intentions to refrain from smoking during that period [6]. Approximately 75% of pregnant smokers report the desire to quit smoking [7], but only 20–30% successfully abstains from smoking during pregnancy and half of these women relapse within 6 months of parturition [8]. In some countries nicotine replacement therapy is used as a strategy to assist smokers, including pregnant mothers, to quit the habit. However, several studies showed that maternal intake of nicotine have deleterious effects on the offspring.

2. Fetal onset of adult disease

In 1990 Barker [9] noted that "The womb may be more important than the home". Up to recently the old model of adult degenerative diseases, such as emphysema, was based on the model that link the interaction between genes and an adverse environment in adult life.

The new model that is currently being developed, based on environment-gene interaction, will include programming by the environment during fetal and neonatal life. There are critical periods during which the developing organs are very plastic such as when rapid cell proliferation occurs during growth, during which it is most sensitive to environmental stressors [10]. This is because during normal development precisely timed regulation of gene transcription is essential. Only genes that are: 1) specific to a particular cell type, such as epithelial cells, and 2) to a specific developmental phase, are transcriptionally active while others are silenced. The ability to modulate gene transcription results in plasticity during lung development [11]. It is therefore conceivable that interference with this process during a phase of high plasticity will result in various metabolic, structural and functional disorders in the offspring, or reduce the capacity of the offspring to protect itself against environmental insults [10]. The type of disorder is likely to be dependent not only on the type of insult but also the timing of the insult.

Apart from the various obstetrical and developmental complications in the adult and offspring, a wide variety of *in utero* insults, such as smoking and nicotine, are associated with an increased incidence of metabolic disorders in the offspring and in subsequent generations. Holloway et al [12] showed that fetal and neonatal exposure to nicotine results in endocrine and metabolic changes in the offspring that are consistent with those observed in type 2 diabetes and high blood pressure. Regular smoking increased the risk for asthma among adolescents, especially for non-allergic adolescents and those exposed to maternal smoking during the *in utero* period. It has also been shown that maternal and grand maternal smoking during pregnancy may increase the risk of childhood asthma [13]. Smoking during pregnancy changes the *in utero* environment within which the fetus develops and in this way induce changes to the program that control lung development, maintenance and aging in the offspring in such a way that these changes are transferred to the next generation. It is clear that certain conditions in the womb can lead to genetic or epigenetic marks that can persist for many generations [14].

It has indeed been shown that maternal and grand-maternal smoking during pregnancy is linked to an increased risk of childhood asthma which suggests that it is persistent heritable effect [13]. Alterations to the epigenome [15] and transcriptome [16] are mechanisms whereby prenatal exposure to smoke induce the development of diseases like asthma and emphysema later in life (Fig.1).

Although tobacco smoke contains numerous chemicals, many of the deleterious effects of smoking on the fetus and newborn arise are attributable to nicotine [17]. Nicotine replacement therapy (NRT) has been developed as a pharmacotherapy for smoking cessation and is considered to be a safer alternative for women to smoking during pregnancy. The safety of NRT use during pregnancy has been evaluated in a limited number of short-term human trials, but there is currently no information on the long-term effects of nicotine exposure of humans during *in utero* life. However, animal studies suggest that nicotine alone may be a key chemical responsible for many of the long-term effects associated with maternal cigarette smoking on the offspring, such as impaired fertility, type 2 diabetes, obesity, hypertension, neurobehavioral defects, and respiratory dysfunction [18]. It is therefore conceivable that exposure to nicotine during fetal and early neonatal development may contribute to the development of these diseases later in the life of the individual. This is conceivable since nicotine does induce epigenetic changes as well as direct DNA damage [12].

3. Nicotine uptake and metabolism during pregnancy

Nicotine is arguably the major physiologically active component of tobacco smoke and is rapidly absorbed from the respiratory tract of smokers. The lung appears to serve as a reservoir for nicotine, which slows its entry into the arterial circulation [19]. This implies that the inhaled nicotine is gradually absorbed into the arterial circulation. It may require 30 - 60 seconds or longer for the nicotine to be absorbed. Once in the maternal circulation, nicotine readily crosses the placenta and enters the fetal circulation [20]. Once it entered the amniotic fluid it is absorbed via the skin of the fetus [21]. Nicotine enters breast milk, and can reach concentrations that are approximately 2-3 times that in maternal plasma due to the partitioning of nicotine into the high-lipid-containing [22], more acidic milk [23, 24].

Although nicotine readily crosses the placenta there, is no evidence that it is metabolized by the placenta. It is therefore likely that the blood concentrations of nicotine reached in the fetus are similar to those in the mother; however, there is no direct evidence supporting the notion. Peak nicotine levels in the pregnant mother's blood occur 15-30 minutes after it is administered [25]. Most of the nicotine that enters the fetus returns to the maternal circulation for elimination, although some enters the amniotic fluid via the fetal urine. Consequently nicotine and cotinine accumulate in the amniotic fluid of the pregnant smoker because the nicotine eliminated by the fetus is added to the nicotine coming from the blood vessels of the amniochorionic membrane [24]. The fetus is therefore likely to be exposed to nicotine even after concentrations in maternal blood have decreased. This means that the fetus is exposed to nicotine during phases of development that are characterized by high plasticity.

The clearance of nicotine and cotinine, the major product of nicotine metabolism, is increased in pregnant women [26]. This can be ascribed to an increase in liver blood flow and an increased enzymatic breakdown of nicotine and cotinine in the mother. Since the enzymatic protection mechanisms of the fetus are not well developed [27, 28], the metabolism of nicotine in the fetal liver is slow and a longer half-life of nicotine in the fetus can be expected. This is confirmed by the higher concentrations of nicotine in fetal tissue compared to maternal blood levels [29]. Consequently the cells of the developing lung and other organs are exposed to higher concentrations of nicotine for longer periods of time and thus to the adverse effects of nicotine on cell integrity. This is important as nicotine is genotoxic [30] and induces the release of oxidants [31]. Since rapidly dividing cells are more vulnerable to the effects of foreign substances such as nicotine [32], it is conceivable that nicotine exposure during gestation and early postnatal life via maternal milk may interfere with growth and development. This can be achieved in two ways: by having a direct effect on cells and/or by reducing the nutrient supply to the fetus during gestation and lactation. It has been shown that long-term nicotine exposure results in a predisposition for genetic instability [22, 33, 34]. This may result in changes in the genetic "program" that controls lung development, maintenance of lung structure and aging of lung tissue, which may render the lungs more prone to disease. Since nicotine is associated with DNA methylation [35], it is possible that it may change the program that is maintaining homeostasis in the developing lung in the long term and in this way contribute to the adult onset of diseases. In addition, a product of nicotine metabolism is nitrosamine 4-(methylnitrosamino)-1-(3-pyridyl)-1-butanone (NNK) which induces DNA damage which is associated with an increase in mutational events [36]. It is therefore possible that nicotine affects cell growth and proliferation as well as cell aging and death directly or via its metabolic end products. It may also act via other pathways such as oxidants.

4. Nicotine and oxidant/antioxidant status

It has been shown that maternal smoking is associated with increased levels of oxidative stress markers in the mother and offspring [37, 38]. There is also convincing *in vivo* and *in vitro* evidence suggesting that exposure to nicotine results in oxidative stress in fetal, neonatal and adult tissues [38, 39]. Reactive oxygen species (ROS) target mitochondria, and mitochondrial DNA has been shown to be more sensitive to the deleterious effects of ROS than nuclear DNA [40].

In addition to inducing overproduction of oxidants, nicotine exposure results in a decrease in the activity of SOD and catalase. It also results in a decrease in the levels of low molecular weight antioxidants such as vitamins C and E [41]. Along with the decrease in the antioxidant capacity of the body, concentrations of malondialdehyde (MDA) are increased, indicating oxidant damage to the cells [42, 43]. The increase in ROS levels, together with a decrease in the activities of enzymes with antioxidant function, results in an imbalance in the oxidant/antioxidant capacity. This imbalance is maintained long after nicotine withdrawal [43] and becomes worse with age [44]. Therefore, nicotine not only acts while it is in the system, but also act indirectly in later life, that is after its removal from the organs, through the disruption of the oxidant/antioxidant capacity of the individual later in life.

It is conceivable that the increased levels of nicotine-induced ROS in the fetus and suckling neonate, as a consequence of maternal smoking or NRT, will result in not only mitochondrial DNA damage but also methylation of nuclear DNA or direct DNA damage through point mutation. It is therefore likely that nicotine and ROS will result in a change in the capacity of the mitochondria to deliver energy and to participate in homeostatic mechanisms and in changing the "program" that controls growth, tissue maintenance, aging and cellular metabolism.

The above implies that the adverse effects of maternal smoking and/or nicotine intake lasts for a life-time in the offspring. Consequently the cells and DNA are continuously exposed to an unfavourable internal environment. This may induce changes in the epigenome and thus control of DNA, as well as changes in the DNA as such. This will increase the susceptibility of the offspring to develop diseases later in life.

5. Mechanisms of action of nicotine

It has been shown that long-term nicotine exposure results in a predisposition for the induction of genetic instability [32,34,45]. Gene amplification is a hallmark of gene instability. Gene instability requires two critical elements, namely an inappropriate cell cycle progression, and DNA damage. Long-term nicotine exposure, through the activation of Ras pathways and up regulation of cyclin D1, disrupts the G1 arrest. It also augments the production of ROS which may lead to DNA damage. This implies that exposure to nicotine via tobacco smoke or via NRT will make the lungs more prone to the development of cancer and other respiratory diseases, such as asthma and emphysema [46].

Various studies suggest that exposures during the intra-uterine period can increase the risk for developing diseases later in life [47]. Maternal smoking during pregnancy is associated with lower pulmonary function and increased asthmatic symptoms in childhood [13]. Studies which show that maternal as well as grand-maternal smoking during pregnancy is also associated with an increased risk of asthma in childhood. This suggests a persistent heritable effect [48]. An alterations to the epigenome is one way whereby exposure to foreign material affects disease risk later in life [49].

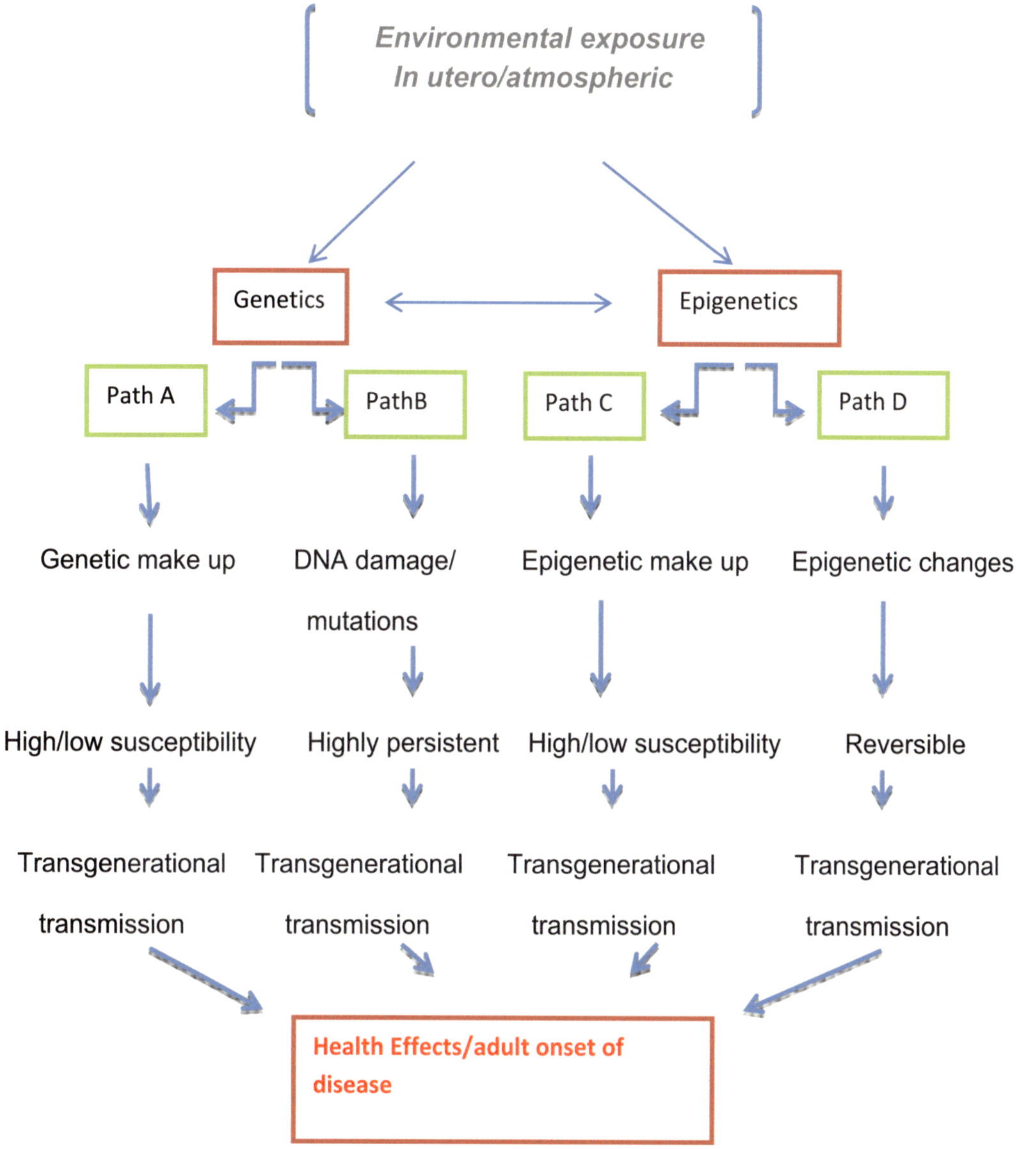

Fig. 1. The gene- vs the epigene-environment interplay. A model of possible genetic and epigenetic paths linking environmental exposures to health outcomes (Adjusted from: Bolatti and Baccarelli, 2010). [52]

Studies by Jorgenson and his co-workers [50] showed that exposure of cells to cigarette smoke containing nicotine leads to formation of double-strand DNA breaks in A549 cells in culture. It is therefore plausible that nicotine can have the same effect on type II pneumocytes in lung tissue *in vivo*. Chronic obstructive pulmonary disease (COPD), including chronic bronchitis and emphysema, is commonly thought of as an adult onset lung disease most often seen in aging people with a tobacco smoking history [51]. On the other hand, only 20% of cigarette smokers develop full-blown emphysema. COPD may also be seen in non-smokers. The question is whether the latter group is not more susceptible to COPD due to changes in the program that controls lung aging and maintenance as well as its ability to protect itself against the onslaughts of the environment Therefore, genetic susceptibility is rapidly gaining ground in recent COPD research.

Apart from genetic alterations, genetic changes such as DNA polymorphism may have no or a very small immediate impact on developing organs such as the lungs with an apparent normal phenotype during the early developmental phases of the child. Although no clear differences are seen in the new phenotype, it may have reduced compensatory capacity

resulting in a poor response to injury imposed by other stress factors, including in the environment. This environment can be *in utero* or external. The latter implies that the lifestyle of the parents may actually increase the susceptibility of the offspring to COPD.

Changes to the epigenome is one of the mechanisms whereby exposures during gestation may affect disease later in life. DNA methylation is perhaps the most known type of epigenetic mark. In mammals there are at least two very important developmental periods namely, in germ cells and in pre-implantation embryos. During these periods of development the methylation patterns are reprogrammed genome wide and consequently results in the generation of cells with a broad developmental potential [53]. This period involves demethylation and remethylation in cells in a tissue specific manner. A basic premise of epigenetic processes is that once it is established, these marks are maintained through rounds of mitotic cell division and stable for the life of the organism [54]. Thus, maternal smoking during pregnancy and early postnatal life may have lasting effects on DNA methylation and as a result influence expression and disease phenotypes across the life time of the individual [55] or result in adult onset of disease [56].

In regard to the adult onset of disease, the most sensitive developmental periods to environmental exposures, are the period of fetal development as well as the early postnatal period [57, 58]. The reason for this is that various developmental processes are occurring that, when changed permanently, will alter subsequent organ development and function [59]. Alternatively, active organ development during late fetal and early postnatal life also undergoes critical programming of the epigenome and transcriptome that is associated with cellular differentiation and organogenesis. It has indeed been shown recently that exposures to environmental toxicants, such as maternal smoking during gestation and lactation, can modify the epigenome to increase the susceptibility to adult onset of disease [58]. This may explain the increased risk for asthma among adolescents and those exposed to maternal smoking during the *in utero* period of development [51].

Nicotine is also associated with DNA damage [60]. It also induces ROS production [61] which induce DNA damage [62]. It is therefore plausible that the irreversible adverse effect on carbohydrate metabolism of lungs of rats that were exposed to nicotine via the placenta and mother's milk [63] is due to change in DNA or of the epigenetic control system. This is supported by the findings of Benyshek et al, [64] who showed that glucose metabolism of the ggrand-maternal offspring (F3) of female rats that were malnourished during development, is also adversely affected. It is likely that the structural changes that are getting progressively worse over time, were due to programming alterations during organ development *in utero* as well as during the early developmental periods. Adverse adjustment of carbohydrate metabolism may also impact negatively on the long-term maintenance of lung structure and function [65]. In addition the metabolic changes induced by maternal exposure to nicotine during pregnancy and lactation may induce premature aging of the lungs of the offspring [66] and consequently the increased risk of respiratory disease. It is therefore likely that maternal smoking, or the use of nicotine to quit smoking during pregnancy and lactation result in epigenetic changes in the lungs of the offspring which can be transferred to following generations and result in adult onset of respiratory disease.

6. Programming and future respiratory health

It has been shown that maternal nicotine exposure during critical windows of development result in offspring with a structurally and functionally normal respiratory system at birth [67]. However, as the offspring age structural changes become apparent. These include parenchymal changes that resemble emphysema and thickening of alveolar walls. The latter is due to accumulation of connective tissue in the extracellular matrix [68]. It was also shown that different structural changes appear in different age groups suggesting a programmed process [66]. This is likely due to altered gene expression in a time-specific manner. Such alterations are irreversible [69]. The data suggests that *in utero* exposure to nicotine resulted in an increase susceptibility to disease later in life. This programming is due to changes in gene expression due to altered imprinting. These changes appear to be heritable. The end result is an individual that is sensitized to be more susceptible to diseases later in life. The environmental insult could act via: 1) an *in utero* exposure that can result in pathophysiology later in life, or 2) an *in utero* exposure combined with a neonatal exposure, or 3) adult exposure that would induce the pathophysiology. The pathophysiology can lead to: 1) disease that would not normally have occurred, or 2) increase the risk for disease that would not normally have been the case or, 3) either and early onset of disease that would have normally occurred, or 4) an exacerbation of the disease [70]. Altered lung function, exacerbation of symptoms, and acceleration of disease processes seen with smoking during pregnancy might arise from direct injury suffered by the developing fetus by altering fetal gene expression [71]. It is also possible that the pathophysiology could have a long latent period from the onset during the perinatal period to the actual disease. These effects could potentially be transgenerational [72].

In conclusion, it is clear that smoking and nicotine can affect the offspring phenotype via genetic and epigenetic adjustments with long term consequences, and is an illustration of the interplay between genetic, developmental and environmental factors. The gene-environment interactions may therefore, play an important role in the etiology of complex diseases where many of these diseases such as COPD may already be induced during *in utero* development of the offspring. It has been shown that oxidative damage occur even in ex-smokers. It is therefore plausible that the effect of nicotine and smoking during gestation and lactation may have a similar persistent effect in the lungs of the offspring. If this is so, it implies that oxidants and nicotine induce irreversible damage to the epigenome and transcriptome of the lungs of the offspring. This will adversely affect the ability of the lung of the offspring to protect itself against environmental insults. Consequently the prevalence of respiratory diseases will be higher in the offspring of grand-parents or parents who smoked or used nicotine during pregnancy and lactation.

Despite a wealth of epidemiologic and experimental evidence, there is still resistance to the concept that environmental as well as other interference with early lung development have a profound effect on the vulnerability to disease later in life. Due to a lack of knowledge by health professionals and decision makers about developmental plasticity and intergenerational effects, they are not able to introduce or implement relatively simple approaches to reduce the burden of disease in particular in the low socioeconomic groups. It is, therefore, important to support approaches that will enable health professionals to introduce those who want to quit smoking to strategies other than nicotine replacement therapy; strategies that will not interfere with programming of the offspring in such a way that they may become more prone to respiratory disease later in life

7. References

[1] Mayer AS, Newman LS. Genetic and environmental modulation of chronic obstructive pulmonary disease. Resp Physiol. 2001; 128: 3-11.

[2] Kleeberger SR. Genetic aspects of pulmonary responses to inhaled pollutants. Exp Toxicol Pathol. 2005; 57 (Suppl 1):147-153.

[3] Kleeberger SR. Genetic aspects of susceptibility to air pollution. Eur Respir J Suppl.2003;40:52s-56s..

[4] Andres RL, Day MC. Perinatal complications associated with maternal tobacco use. Seminars Neonatol. 2000; 5: 231–241.

[5] Bergmann KE, Bergmann RL, Von KR, Bohm O, Richter R, Dudenhausen JW, Wahn U. Early determinants of childhood overweight and adiposity in a birth cohort study: role of breast-feeding. Int J Obesity and Related Metab Dis. 2003; 27: 162–172.

[6] Okuyemi KS, Ahluwalia JS, Harris KJ 2000 Pharmacotherapy of smoking cessation. Archives of Family Medicine. 2000; 9:270–281.

[7] Ruggiero, L., Tsoh, J. Y., Everett, K., Fava, J. L., Guise, B. J. The transtheoretical model of smoking: comparison of pregnant and nonpregnant smokers. Addict. Behav. 2000; 25: 239–251.

[8] Ebert, L. M., and Fahy, K. Why do women continue to smoke in pregnancy? Women Birth. 2007; 20: 161–168.

[9] Barker DJ. The fetal origins of adult disease. BMJ 1990; 301: 111

[10] Symonds ME, Sebert SP, Hyatt MA, Budge H. Nutritional programming of the metabolic syndrome.Nat Rev Endocrinol. 2009; 5: 604-610.

[11] Joss-Moore LA, Albertine KH, Lane RH. Epigenetics and the developmental origins of lung disease. Mol Gen Metab. 2011; doi: 10.1016/j.ymgme.2011.07.018

[12] Holloway AC, Cuu DQ, Morrison KM, Gerstein HC, Tarnopolsky MA. Transgenerational effects of fetal and neonatal exposure to nicotine. Endocrine. 2007; 3: 254-259

[13] Li YF, Langholz B, Salam MT, Gilliland FD. Maternal and grandmaternal smoking patterns are associated with early childhood asthma. Chest. 2005 Apr;127(4):1232-41.

[14] Heijmans BT, Tobi ZEW, Lumey LH, Slagboom PE. The epigenome: archive of the prenatal environment. Epigenetics 2009; 4: 526-531.

[15] Anway MD, Skinner MK. Epigenetic Transgenerational actions of endocrine disruptors. Endocrinology 2006; 147: s43-s49

[16] Skinner MK. What is epigenetic transgenerational phenotypes? F3 or F2. Reprod Toxicol. 2008; 25: 2-6.

[17] Petre MA, Petrik J, Ellis R, Inman MD, Holloway AC, Labiris NR. Fetal and neonatal exposure to nicotine disrupts postnatal lung development in rats: Role of VEGF and its receptors. Int J Toxicol. 2011; 30: 244-252.

[18] Bruin JF, Hertzel, Gerstein C, Holloway AC. Long-Term Consequences of Fetal and Neonatal Nicotine Exposure: A Critical Review. Toxicoll Sci. 2010; 116, 364–374.

[19] Brewer, B.G.; Roberts, A.M.; Rowell, P.P. Short-term distribution of nicotine in the rat lung. Drug Alcohol. Depend. 2004, 75, 193-198.

[20] Matta, S.G.; Balfour, D.J.; Benowitz, N.L.; Boyd, R.T.; Buccafusco, J.J.; Caggiula, A.R.; Craig, C.R.; Collins, A.C.; Damaj, M.I.; Donny, E.C.; Gardiner, P.S.; Grady, S.R.; Heberlein, U.; Leonard, S.S.; Levin, E.D.; Lukas, R.J.; Markou, A.; Marks, M.J.; McCallum, S.E.; Parameswaran, N.; Perkins, K.A.; Picciotto, M.R.; Quik, M.; Rose, J.E.; Rothenfluh, A.; Schafer, W.R.; Stolerman, I.P.; Tyndale, R.F.; Wehner, J.M.; Zirger, J.M. Guidelines on nicotine dose selection for in vivo research. Psychopharmacology (Berl) 2007, 190, 269-319.

[21] Onuki, M.; Yokoyama, K.; Kimura, K.; Sato, H.; Nordin, R.B.; Naing, L.; Morita, Y.; Sakai, T.; Kobayashi, Y.; Araki, S., Assessment of urinary cotinine as a marker of nicotine absorption from tobacco leaves: a study on tobacco farmers in Malaysia. J. Occup. Health 2003, 45, 140-145.

[22] Sastry, B.V.; Chance, M.B.; Hemontolor, M.E.; Goddijn-Wessel, T.A. Formation and retention of cotinine during placental transfer of nicotine in human placental cotyledon. Pharmacology 1998, 57, 104-116.

[23] Dahlstrom, A.; Lundell, B.; Curvall, M.; Thapper, L. Nicotine and cotinine concentrations in the nursing mother and her infant. Acta Paediatr. Scand. 1990, 79, 142-147.

[24] Luck, W.; Nau, H.; Hansen, R.; Steldinger, R. Extent of nicotine and cotinine transfer to the human fetus, placenta and amniotic fluid of smoking mothers. Dev. Pharmacol. Ther. 1985, 8, 384-395.

[25] Suzuki, K.; Horiguchi, T.; Comas-Urrutia, A.C.; Mueller-Heubach, E.; Morishima, H.O.; Adamsons, K. Placental transfer and distribution of nicotine in the pregnant rhesus monkey. Am. J. Obstet. Gynecol. 1974, 119, 253-262.

[26] Dempsey, D.A.; Benowitz, N.L. Risks and benefits of nicotine to aid smoking cessation in pregnancy. Drug Saf. 2001, 24, 277-322.

[27] Frank, L.; Sosenko, I.R. Prenatal development of lung antioxidant enzymes in four species. J. Pediatr. 1987, 110, 106-110.

[28] Hayashibe, H.; Asayama, K.; Dobashi, K.; Kato, K. Prenatal development of antioxidant enzymes in rat lung, kidney, and heart: marked increase in immunoreactive

superoxide dismutases, glutathione peroxidase, and catalase in the kidney. Pediatr. Res. 1990, 27, 472-475.

[29] Lambers, D.S.; Clark, K.E. The maternal and fetal physiologic effects of nicotine. Semin. Perinatol. 1996, 20, 115-126.

[30] Kleinsasser, N.H.; Sassen, A.W.; Semmler, M.P.; Harreus, U.A.; Licht, A.K.; Richter, E. The tobacco alkaloid nicotine demonstrates genotoxicity in human tonsillar tissue and lymphocytes. Toxicol. Sci. 2005, 86, 309-317.

[31] Bruin, J.E.; Petre, M.A.; Raha, S.; Morrison, K.M.; Gerstein, H.C.; Holloway, A.C. Fetal and neonatal nicotine exposure in Wistar rats causes progressive pancreatic mitochondrial damage and beta cell dysfunction. PLoS One 2008, 3, e3371.

[32] Rehan, V.K.; Wang, Y.; Sugano, S.; Santos, J.; Patel, S.; Sakurai, R.; Boros, L.G.; Lee, W.P.; Torday, J.S. In utero nicotine exposure alters fetal rat lung alveolar type II cell proliferation, differentiation, and metabolism. Am. J. Physiol. Lung Cell Mol. Physiol. 2007, 292, L323-L333.

[33] Guo, J.; Chu, M.; Abbeyquaye, T.; Chen, C.Y. Persistent nicotine treatment potentiates amplification of the dihydrofolate reductase gene in rat lung epithelial cells as a consequence of Ras activation. J. Biol. Chem. 2005, 280, 30422-30431.

[34] Hartwell, L.H.; Kastan, M.B. Cell cycle control and cancer. Science 1994, 266, 1821-1828.

[35] Soma T, Kaganoi J, Kawabe A, Kondo K, Imamura M, Shimada Y. Nicotine induces the fragile histidine triad methylation in human esophageal squamous epithelial cells. Int. J. Cancer. 2006; 119, 1023–1027.

[36] Cloutier J-F, Drouin R, Weinfeld M, O'Connor TR, Castonguay A. Characterization and Mapping of DNA Damage Induced by Reactive Metabolites of 4-(methylnitrosamino)-1-(3-pyridyl)-1-butanone (NNK) at Nucleotide Resolution in Human Genomic DNA. J. Mol. Biol. 2001; 313: 539-557

[37] Noakes, P.S.; Thomas, R.; Lane, C.; Mori, T.A.; Barden, A.E.; Devadason, S.G.; Prescott, S.L. Association of maternal smoking with increased infant oxidative stress at 3 months of age. Thorax 2007, 62, 714-717.

[38] Orhon, F.S.; Ulukol, B.; Kahya, D.; Cengiz, B.; Baskan, S.; Tezcan, S. The influence of maternal smoking on maternal and newborn oxidant and antioxidant status. Eur. J. Pediatr. 2009, 168, 975-981

[39] Husain K, Scott BR, Reddy SK, Somani SM. Chronic ethanol and nicotine interaction on rat tissue antioxidant defense systems. Alcohol 2001; 25: 89-97.

[40] Droge, W., Free radicals in the physiological control of cell function. Physiol. Rev. 2002, 82,

[41] Zaken, V.; Kohen, R.; Ornoy, A. Vitamins C and E improve rat embryonic antioxidant defense mechanism in diabetic culture medium. Teratology 2001, 64, 33-44.

[42] Halima, B.A.; Sarra, K.; Kais, R.; Salwa, E.; Najoua, G. Indicators of oxidative stress in weanling and pubertal rats following exposure to nicotine via milk. Hum. Exp. Toxicol. 2010, 29, 489-496.

[43] Ozokutan, B.H.; Ozkan, K.U.; Sari, I.; Inanc, F.; Guldur, M.E.; Kilinc, M. Effects of maternal nicotine exposure during lactation on breast-fed rat pups. Biol. Neonate 2005, 88, 113-117.

[44] Bruin, J.E.; Petre, M.A.; Raha, S.; Morrison, K.M.; Gerstein, H.C.; Holloway, A.C. Fetal and neonatal nicotine exposure in Wistar rats causes progressive pancreatic mitochondrial damage and beta cell dysfunction. *PLoS One* 2008, *3*, e3371.

[45] Guo J, Chu M, Abbeyquaye T, Chen CY. Persistent nicotine treatmant potentiates amplification of the dihydrofolate reductase gene in rat lung epithelial cells as a consequence of Ras activation and antioxidant status. J Biol Chem 2005; 280: 30422-30431.

[46] Chu M, Guo J, Chen CY. Long-term Exposure to Nicotine, via Ras Pathway, Induces Cyclin D1 to Stimulate G1 Cell Cycle Transition. J Biol Chem. 2005; 280: 6369–6379.

[47] Holloway, A.C.; Cuu, D.Q.; Morrison, K.M.; Gerstein, H.C.; Tarnopolsky, M.A. Transgenerational effects of fetal and neonatal exposure to nicotine. Endocrinol 2007, *31*, 254-259.

[48] Whitelaw NC, Whitelaw E. Transgenerational epigenetic inheritance in health and disease. Gemetics and Dev. 2008; 18: 273-279.

[49] Waterland RA, Michels KB. Epigenetic epidemiology of the developmental origins of disease. Annu Rev Nutr 2007; 27: 363-388

[50] Jorgensen ED, Zhao H, Traganos F, Albino AP, Darzynkiewicz Z. DNA damage response induced by exposure of human lung adenocarcinoma cells to smoke from tobacco- and nicotine-free cigarettes. Cell Cycle. 2010; 9. [Epub ahead of print]

[51] Gilliland FD, Islam T, Berhane K, Gauderman WJ, McConnell R, Avol E, Peters JM. Regular smoking and asthma incidence in adolescents. Am J Respit Crit Care Med. 2006; 174: 1094-1100.

[52] Bollati V, Baccarelli A. Environmental epigenetics. Heredity 2010; 105: 105-112.

[53] Reik W, Dean W, Walter J. Epigenetic reprogramming in mammalian development. Science 2001; 293: 1089-1093.

[54] Jirtle RL, Skinner MK. Environmental epigenetics and disease susceptibility. Nat Rev Genet 2007; 8: 253-262.

[55] Morgan HD, Santos F, Green K, Dean W, Reik W. epigenetic reprogramming in mammalas. Hum Mol Genet. 2005; 14: R47-R58.

[56] Breton CV, Byun H-M, Wenetn M, Pan F, Yang A, Gilliland D. Prenatal tobacco smoke exposure affects global and gene-specific DNA methylation. Am J Respir Crit Care Med. 2009; 180: 462-467.

[57] Heindel JJ. Role of Exposure to Environmental Chemicals in the Developmental Basis of Reproductive Disease and Dysfunction. Semin Reprod Med 2006; 24: 168-177.

[58] Bateson P. Developmental plasticity and evolutionary biology. J Nutr. 2007: 137;1060-1062.

[59] Ginzkey C, Kampfinger K, Friehs G, Köhler C, Hagen R, Richter E, Kleinsasser NH. Nicotine induces DNA damage in human salivary glands. Toxicol Lett. 2009;184: 1-4.

[60] Kajekar R. Environmental factors and developmental outcomes in the lung. Pharmacol. Ther. 2007; 114; 129-145.

[61] Zhao Z, Reece EA. Nicotine-induced embryonic malformations mediated by apoptosis from increasing intracellular calcium and oxidative stress. Birth Defects Res B Dev Reprod Toxicol. 2005; 74: 383-391.

[62] Wiseman H, Halliwell B. Damage to DNA by reactive oxygen and nitrogen species: role in inflammatory disease and progression to cancer. Biochem J 1996; 313: 17-29.

[63] Maritz, G. Pre- and postnatal carbohydrate metabolism of rat lung tissue. The effect of maternal nicotine exposure. Arch. Toxicol. 1986, 59, 89-93.

[64] Benyshek DC, Johnston CS, Martin JF. Glucose metabolism is altered in the adequately-nourished grand-offspring (F3 generation) of rats malnourished during gestation and perinatal life. Diabetologia 2006; 49: 1117-1119.

[65] Maritz GS, Windvogel S. Is maternal copper supplementation during alveolarisation protecting the developing rat lung against the adverse effects of maternal nicotine exposure? A morphometric study. Exp Lung Res 2003; 29: 243-260.

[66] Maritz GS, Mutemwa M, Kayigire AX. Tomato juice protects the lungs of the offspring of female rats exposed to nicotine during gestation and actationh. Ped Pulmonol. 2011; DOI: 10.1002/ppul.21462

[67] Maritz GS, Windvogel S. Does maternal nicotine exposure during different phases of lung development influence the progam that regulates the maintenance of lung integrity in the offspring? A comparative morphologic and morphometric study. Trends Comp Biochem Physiol. 2005; 11: 69-75.

[68] Sekhon HS, Proskocil BJ, Clark JA, Spindel ER. Prenatal nicotine exposure increases connective tissue expression in foetal monkey pulmonary vessels. Eur Respir J. 2004 Jun;23(6):906-15.

[69] Gluckman PD, Hanson MA, Buklijas T, Low FM, Beedle AS. Epigenetic mechanisms that underpin metabolic and cardiovacular diseases. Nat. Rev Endocrinol 2009; 5: 401-408.

[70] Skinner MK, Manikkam M, Guerero-Bosagna C. Epigenetic trnsgenerational actions of environmental factors in disease etiology. Trends Endocrinol Metab. 2010; 21: 214-222.

[71] Rousse RL, Boudreaux MJ, Penn AL. In utero environmental tobacco smoke exposure alters gene expression in lungs of adult BALB/c mice. Environ Hlth Perspect. 2007; 115: 1757-1766.

[72] Asami S, Manabe H, Miyake J, Tsurudome Y, Hirano T, Yamaguchi R, Itoh H, Kasai H. Cigarette smoking induce an increase in oxidative DNA damage, 8-hydroxydeoxyguanosine, in a central site in human lung. Carcinogenesis 1997; 18: 1763-1766.

15

Synthetic Point Mutagenesis

Roman A.G. Schaeken, Joke J.F.A. van Vugt and Colin Logie
Molecular Biology Department,
Nijmegen Centre For Molecular Life Sciences,
Radboud University Nijmegen,
The Netherlands

1. Introduction

Over the last 5 decades, because of the revolution in recombinant DNA technology, site-directed mutagenesis became one of the most powerful tools in molecular life sciences. Its power lies in the ability to manipulate a specific DNA sequence in a definable and often predetermined way. Subsequently, genetic changes are correlated with a change in phenotype. Hence, this method offers the possibility to test protein functions down to the individual amino acid level and to characterize single nucleotides within regulatory RNA and DNA elements. In addition, synthetic point mutagenesis makes it possible to test whether specific mutations in a gene are benign or detrimental and thus lead to disease or not, in a model organism (Smith, 1985).

2. Point mutagenesis, a historical perspective

During the 1920's, Hermann Joseph Muller, was the first scientist to report the effects of mutagens on DNA. He demonstrated that there was a quantitative relation between the exposure to x-ray radiation and lethal mutations in *Drosophila.* He used this technique later on to create *Drosophila* mutants for his genetic research. Furthermore, he noted that x-rays could not only mutate genes in fruit flies but also have effects on the human genome (Crow, 2005).

In 1941, Charlotte Auberauch demonstrated similar results as Muller using mustard gas as a mutagen in microbes and *Drosophila.* Within her studies several biological effects of mutations were described such as mosaicism and the heritability of mutations when occurring in the gametes (Sobels, 1975).

In 1978, Hutchison *et al.* (Hutchison et al., 1978) were among the first to describe site-directed mutagenesis using synthetic oligonucleotides. They demonstrated that a chemically synthesized oligonucleotide annealed to a phage genome could produce a specific mutation when incorporated in a closed circular phage genome by *in vitro* enzymatic reactions. The basic procedure was to use a mutation-bearing oligonucleotide as a primer for DNA polymerase to synthesize a mutant single-stranded genome. A ligase was included so that the newly elongated DNA strand was ligated into the circular vector (Smith, 1985; Hutchison et al., 1971; Hutchison et al., 1978). Later on, several other techniques were described, including site-directed mutagenesis of double-strand plasmid DNA vectors and targeted random mutagenesis using chemical reagents (Botstein et al., 1985). A major downside of these site directed point mutagenesis techniques was that they were time-consuming. In particular the introduction of the mutated target sequence into the appropriate plasmid vector systems required multiple time-consuming steps. Furthermore, designed mutations were often obtained at low frequencies (Ho et al., 1989).

The development of the Polymerase Chain Reaction (PCR) technique by Mullis in 1983 provided opportunities to resolve these drawbacks. PCR uses two synthetic oligonucleotides as primers to exponentially amplify a specific DNA sequence. The primers are complementary to the ends of the amplified DNA and are oriented in opposite directions. Exponential amplification of target DNA occurs in multiple cycles of DNA duplex denaturation, primer annealing to single strand DNA and annealed primer extension by DNA polymerase. PCR is familiar as a method for the detection of a specific DNA sequence (Bartlett et al., 2003). As exemplified below, this method is also commonly applied to modify DNA sequences by design, using protocols that are collectively known as PCR-mediated site-directed mutagenesis.

3. Site-directed mutagenesis I: PCR synthesis of bacterial plasmid vectors

Site-directed mutagenesis is an important method to investigate the relationship between a given gene and its function. The technique is based on hybridization of a synthetic DNA primer containing the desired point mutation(s) with single-stranded target DNA encompassing the gene of interest. The hybridized DNA primer is extended by a DNA polymerase creating double-stranded DNA that can eventually be transformed into a host cell and cloned (Carter, 1986).

Over the years optimization has taken place, creating a rapid and simple to execute protocol to alter plasmid-borne genes with high fidelity in a specific and precise fashion *in vitro*.

One of the first methods used mutagenic primers which, after PCR, incorporate point mutations close to the PCR fragment's ends. After PCR amplification the PCR products had to be cleaved with restriction enzymes and inserted in place of the wild-type sequence in a bacterial plasmid vector. However, the above site directed point mutagenesis protocol was limited by the (non)availability of restrictions sites in the close vicinity of the DNA sequence to be mutated. Furthermore, wild-type clones were recovered at a high frequency, making it tedious to isolate the desired mutant clones (Kadowaki et al., 1989). Hemsley *et al.* (Hemsley et al., 1989) improved the protocol by using an adaptation of inverse PCR, amplifying the whole circular plasmid to incorporate mutations at any site of the plasmid without relying on restriction sites in the close vicinity. This approach was fast and simple, and only a small amount of plasmid template DNA was required. Still, after PCR, linear instead of circular mutated plasmid DNA was obtained and this was physically separated from the original plasmid and circularized by ligation before transformation in *E. coli*. Despite these improvements the frequency of transformed bacteria harboring the desired mutant plasmid was still relatively low (Hemsley et al., 1989). Furthermore, the rates of unwanted random base substitution in these PCR reactions varied according to the reaction conditions, the precise DNA sequence and the DNA polymerase that had been used. Optimization of DNA polymerase fidelity in several PCR applications reduced the error-rate and thereby increased efficiency. The 3'→5' exonuclease activity of proofreading DNA polymerases is one of the most important replication error correction mechanisms *in vivo* (Eckert et al.,

1991). Where former studies used thermostable DNA polymerases without 3'→5' exonuclease activity, nowadays thermostable DNA polymerases with proofreading activity are included to reduce the error-rate. For PCR controlled mutagenesis a balance between proofreading and mutagenesis is sought so as to allow introduction of desired point mutations into the target DNA sequence but not other mismatches. Combining two different DNA polymerases not only reduced the random error-rate but also allowed efficient amplification of considerably longer PCR fragments. This led to the invention of 'long-distance PCR' where fragments up to 40kb in length are amplified, solving some of the technical limitations ascribed to gene and plasmid size (Barnes, 1994).

Current site-directed mutagenesis of plasmid-borne DNA sequences (eg. Figure 1) use two complementary mutagenic overlapping primers that bind to the two complementary sequences at the site of the desired mutation and amplify the entire plasmid. Mutated plasmids are created through heteroduplex formation between the wild type template and the mutation-bearing primers during the first PCR cycles, normally using a mixture of DNA polymerases with and without proofreading activity, where consecutive cycles realize amplification. Where former mutagenesis protocols had trouble separating the mutated plasmid from the original template, newly marketed techniques resolved this problem. Restriction enzymes, like *Dpn*I (target sequence, 5'-G^{me}ATC-3') are specific for methylated and hemimethylated *E. coli* DNA and will degrade the original plasmid by enzymatic digestion (Figure 1) (Fisher et al., 1997; Li et al., 2002). The mutant PCR products, however, will be preserved from cleavage because they are enzymatically synthesized *in vitro* using unmethylated adenosine, contrary to the original plasmid templates produced by *E. coli* which are methylated at every GATC palyndrome. Although after amplification by PCR the mutant plasmid DNA is not a pristine closed double stranded DNA plasmid, the presence of single strand nicks is not an obstacle for transformation in bacteria, indicating that endogenous bacterial enzymes repair the PCR products (Figure 1). Overall, this technology offers the possibility to easily engineer and obtain mutated cloned plasmids in a highly efficient fashion in less than one week (Aslam 2010).

4. Site-directed mutagenesis II: Vector engineering via homologous recombination in bacteria

A second modern point mutagenesis protocol relies on homologous recombination of PCR products in bacteria and was pioneered by the Stewart laboratory at the EMBL in the late 1990s.

Homologous recombination is a class of genetic recombination in which genetic information is exchanged between two identical or nearly identical DNA molecules. In eukaryotes homologous recombination is used to repair several types of DNA damage and it plays a vital role during meiosis, creating genetic diversity in sexually reproducing populations. In bacteria, the main function of homologous recombination is to rescue DNA replication forks that collapsed due to template strand DNA damage. Bacteriophages also code for homologous recombination enzymes, indicating that they employ homologous recombination to maintain themselves at some yet undetermined point of their life cycle. Furthermore, bacterial homologous recombination also occurs during conjugation when plasmid and/or chromosomal DNA is transferred between bacterial cells in a process called horizontal gene transfer.

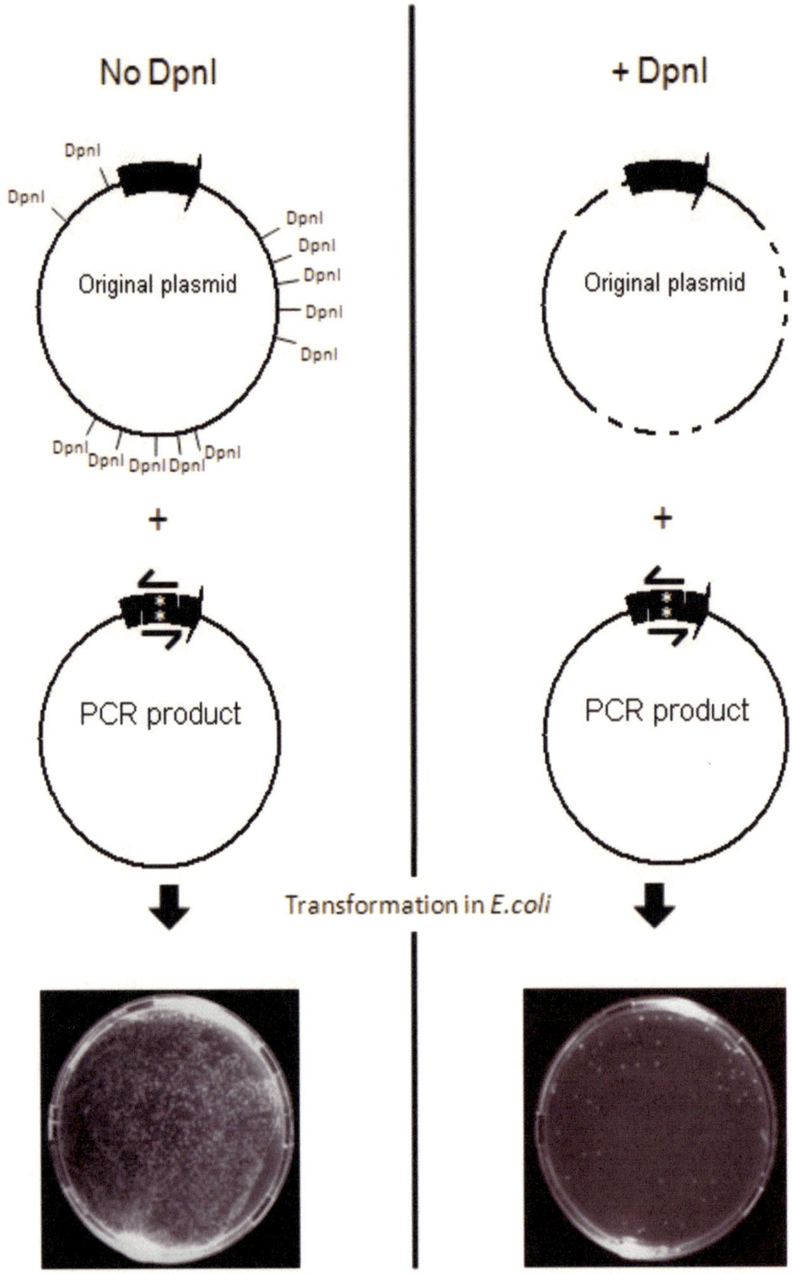

Fig. 1. Bacterial plasmid vector mutagenesis by PCR. A purified bacterial plasmid with the sequence to be mutated is amplified by two complementary PCR primers (black arrows) bearing the desired point mutation (indicated by a white star). The *Dpn*I methylated-DNA-specific restriction enzyme is then used to destroy the original bacterial DNA vector, leaving only the mutant PCR version of the plasmid intact (right hand side). Destruction of the original template greatly reduces the number of *E. coli* clones, most of which now harbour the desired mutant plasmid.

Recombinogenic engineering, also known as 'recombineering' exploits homologous recombination to modify a DNA molecule inside bacteria in a precise and specific manner (Figure 2). Modification of a DNA molecule is accomplished by generating a synthetic targeting DNA construct (e.g. by PCR amplification) containing two regions that are homologous to regions flanking the target site. The targeting construct is introduced into an appropriate bacterial host cell that already bears the locus to be modified. Homologous recombination factors first resect the double strand DNA ends of the targeting construct into 3′ single strand DNAs that align the construct with the double strand target locus and then insert it there via DNA polymerization at the invading 3′ end, followed by resolution of the resulting Holliday junctions. This is the case for simple modifications, such as inserting or deleting a DNA sequence. In many cases a second recombination step is performed to remove the selectable and counter selectable gene (Figure 2). One major advantage of this technique is that the sequences of homology regions can be selected freely, so long as they are unique, which makes it possible to specifically alter DNA sequences in bacteria at almost any position. The second advantage of two step recombineering is that it is possible to design strategies whereby the resultant mutant DNA bears no sequence alterations other than the desired mutation (Muyrers et al., 2000a; 2001).

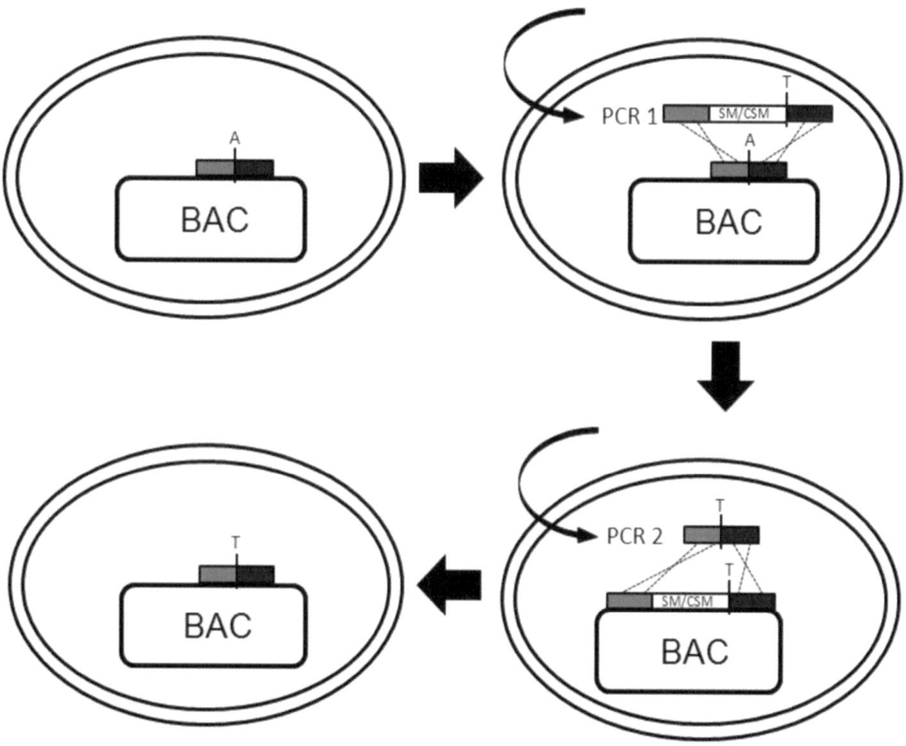

Fig. 2. Bacterial artificial chromosome point mutagenesis Two PCR products, bearing ~ 50 bp homology arms (gray and black boxes) are used in sequence to select bacteria harbouring, firstly a chromosome with the desired point mutation together with a selectable/counter selectable gene and secondly to remove the selectable/counter selectable marker, leaving only the desired point mutation.

Bacterial artificial chromosomes (BAC) are usually more than 100 kb large, rendering their ex-vivo manipulation exceedingly difficult, mainly because these giant DNA molecules tend to fragment through exposure to shearing forces typically associated with liquid solution manipulation. Because BACs are vectors that can carry very large inserts, they do offer the opportunity to manipulate complete mammalian genes because the genomic DNA inserts include gene promoters, exons, introns and regulatory regions. BACs thus provide a milieu to modify higher eukaryote chromosomal segments. Recombineering can be applied to introduce precise changes in the nucleotide sequence of BACs in bacteria via homologous recombination factors and to then transfer the engineered DNA back into a mammal. The first part of this procedure has been named ET recombination, as it precisely engineers BACs using the homologous recombination factors RecE and RecT enzymes of the RAC prophage or the equivalent Redα and Redβ proteins of Lambda phage. RecT and Redβ are DNA strand annealing factors (Erler et al., 2009) whilst RecE and Redα are their partner 5'→3' exonucleases (Muyrers et al., 2000b). ET recombination relies on synthetic linear DNA fragments that contain at least 50 nucleotide long homology arms, which are normally generated by PCR, to mediate homologous recombination at the desired region on the target (BAC) DNA. The use of linear targeting DNA fragments increases the efficiency of gene modification significantly because double strand DNA ends are the actual substrates for the RecE and Redα exonucleases.

A two-step use of ET recombination was developed to create subtle changes in DNA in bacteria, such as point mutations. The two-step protocol is based on a fusion protein that permits selection as well as counter selection. Hence, mutagenesis is divided in a selection and a counter selection step. In the first step, PCR is applied to create a linear DNA fragment containing the (counter)selectable fusion gene, the desired point mutation and 50 nucleotide homology arms identical to the target DNA (Figure 2). Once that is successfully introduced by ET recombination, a second PCR fragment containing the original sequence of the BAC region and the desired point mutation is introduced into competent bacteria. This second PCR product enables a homologous recombination event that precisely deletes the counterselectable marker. The bacteria with the desired mutation are then selected by killing all the bacteria that still harbor the counterselectable gene. This two-step ET recombination can be applied to introduce single nucleotide substitutions as well as kilobase-sized insertions or deletions at any position in a desired locus encompassed by a BAC. Site-directed mutagenesis can also be performed on the actual bacterial chromosome, on BACs as exemplified here, or on any other double stranded DNA that is stably propagated in bacteria (Muyrers et al., 2001).

5. Conclusion

Over the years site-directed mutagenesis became an important tool to specifically mutate DNA molecules by design. Multiple studies contributed to the development of several techniques that can incorporate different kinds of mutations in rapid, simple and efficient ways. PCR fragment-mediated mutagenesis is one of these techniques. It permits efficient point mutagenesis of genes borne on plasmid vectors. On the other hand, combining PCR with recombineering in bacteria results in methodologies that can be applied to modify megabase-sized DNA fragments borne on artificial bacterial chromosomes, relying on the high fidelity associated with in vivo DNA replication. Subsequent transfer of such modified

BAC DNA into mice makes it possible to study the consequences of subtle chromosomal alterations, down to single nucleotide changes, within the native chromosomal environment. Application of these techniques on a large scale is leading to a better fundamental understanding of biology and disease aetiology (Skarnes et al., 2011) as well as providing opportunities to improve on what nature has offered to date.

6. References

Aslam A, and Logie C (2010). Histone H3 Serine 57 and Lysine 56 Interplay in Transcription Elongation and Recovery from S-Phase Stress. *PLoS ONE* 5: e10851. doi:10.1371/journal.pone.0010851

Barnes WM (1994). PCR amplification of up to 35-kb DNA with high fidelity and high yield from lambda bacteriophage templates. *Proc Natl Acad Sci U S A* 91: 2216-2220.

Bartlett JM, and Stirling D (2003). A short history of the polymerase chain reaction. *Methods Mol Biol* 226: 3-6.

Botstein D, and Shortle D (1985). Strategies and applications of in vitro mutagenesis. *Science* 229: 1193-1201.

Carter P (1986). Site-directed mutagenesis. *The Biochemical journal* 237: 1-7.

Crow JF (2005). Timeline: Hermann Joseph Muller, evolutionist. *Nat Rev Genet* 6: 941-945.

Eckert KA, and Kunkel TA (1991). DNA polymerase fidelity and the polymerase chain reaction. *PCR methods and applications* 1: 17-24.

Erler A, Wegmann S, Elie-Caille C, Bradshaw CR, Maresca M, Seidel R, Habermann B, Muller DJ, and Stewart AF (2009). Conformational adaptability of Redbeta during DNA annealing and implications for its structural relationship with Rad52. *J Mol Biol* 391: 586-598.

Fisher CL, and Pei GK (1997). Modification of a PCR-based site-directed mutagenesis method. *BioTechniques* 23: 570-571, 574.

Hemsley A, Arnheim N, Toney MD, Cortopassi G, and Galas DJ (1989). A simple method for site-directed mutagenesis using the polymerase chain reaction. *Nucleic Acids Res* 17: 6545-6551.

Ho SN, Hunt HD, Horton RM, Pullen JK, and Pease LR (1989). Site-directed mutagenesis by overlap extension using the polymerase chain reaction. *Gene* 77: 51-59.

Hutchison CA, 3rd, and Edgell MH (1971). Genetic assay for small fragments of bacteriophage phi X174 deoxyribonucleic acid. *J Virol* 8: 181-189.

Hutchison CA, 3rd, Phillips S, Edgell MH, Gillam S, Jahnke P, and Smith M (1978). Mutagenesis at a specific position in a DNA sequence. *J Biol Chem* 253: 6551-6560.

Kadowaki H, Kadowaki T, Wondisford FE, and Taylor SI (1989). Use of polymerase chain reaction catalyzed by Taq DNA polymerase for site-specific mutagenesis. *Gene* 76: 161-166.

Li F, and Mullins JI (2002). Site-directed mutagenesis facilitated by DpnI selection on hemimethylated DNA. *Methods Mol Biol* 182: 19-27.

Muyrers JP, Zhang Y, Benes V, Testa G, Ansorge W, and Stewart AF (2000a). Point mutation of bacterial artificial chromosomes by ET recombination. *EMBO Rep* 1: 239-243.

Muyrers JP, Zhang Y, Buchholz F, and Stewart AF (2000b). RecE/RecT and Redalpha/Redbeta initiate double-stranded break repair by specifically interacting with their respective partners. *Genes Dev* 14: 1971-1982.

Muyrers JP, Zhang Y, and Stewart AF (2001). Techniques: Recombinogenic engineering--new options for cloning and manipulating DNA. *Trends Biochem Sci* 26: 325-331.

Skarnes WC, Rosen B, West AP, Koutsourakis M, Bushell W, Iyer V, Mujica AO, Thomas M, Harrow J, Cox T, *et al.* (2011). A conditional knockout resource for the genome-wide study of mouse gene function. *Nature* 474: 337-342.

Smith M (1985). In vitro mutagenesis. *Annu Rev Genet* 19: 423-462.

Sobels FH (1975). Charlotte Auerbach and chemical mutagenesis. *Mutat Res* 29: 171-180.